Onco-critical Care

Vinod Kumar • Nishkarsh Gupta
Seema Mishra
Editors

Onco-critical Care

An Evidence-based Approach

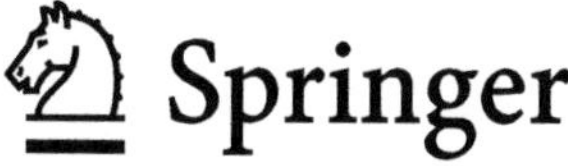

Editors
Vinod Kumar
Department of Onco-Anesthesia
and Palliative Medicine
Dr. B.R.A. Institute Rotary Cancer Hospital
All India Institute of Medical Sciences
New Delhi, India

Nishkarsh Gupta
Department of Onco-Anesthesia
and Palliative Medicine
Dr. B.R.A. Institute Rotary Cancer Hospital
All India Institute of Medical Sciences
New Delhi, Delhi, India

Seema Mishra
Department of Onco-Anesthesia
and Palliative Medicine
Dr. B.R.A. Institute Rotary Cancer Hospital
All India Institute of Medical Sciences
New Delhi, India

ISBN 978-981-16-9931-3 ISBN 978-981-16-9929-0 (eBook)
https://doi.org/10.1007/978-981-16-9929-0

This Springer imprint is published by the registered company Springer Nature Singapore Pte Ltd.
The registered company address is: 152 Beach Road, #21-01/04 Gateway East, Singapore 189721, Singapore

Foreword

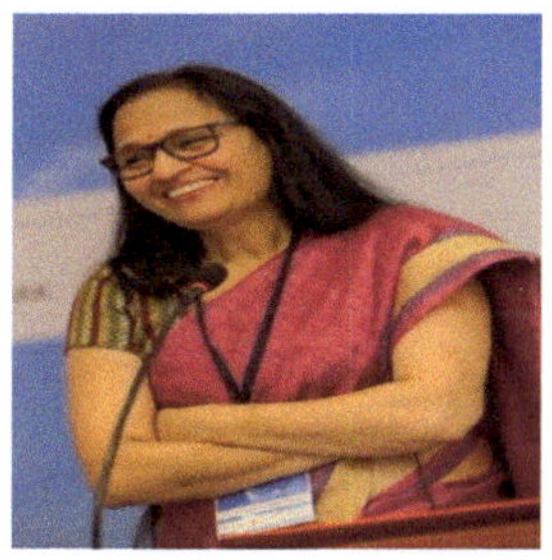

Cancer is not new to humanity, and its evidence has been described in the Chinese and Arabic medical writings. Taking a look at the present times, it is clear that the cancer epidemic is engulfing the world including India. The natural course of the disease has changed over the last decade. With the increase in the number of patients presenting with malignancy, and associated vast clinical and financial implications, early detection and prompt management is required to reduce morbidity and mortality. Also, the need for critical care healthcare services is expanding. We need dedicated professionals with skill, knowledge, and expertise in managing cancer patients not only in the outpatient department and operation theatre but also in ICUs. There are many factors which work against timely response from critical care specialists. Firstly, there is a huge gap between demand and supply of critical care specialists especially those trained to handle oncological cases. Secondly, the technology and huge cost involved in taking care of onco-critical cases puts an extra burden on healthcare set-ups. And perhaps the most important factor is that onco-critical care does not exist as subspeciality in our country to date. Most critical care organizations have not acknowledged this lack of access, do not have an oncologic section and allocate minimal space for lectures in their curriculum about the specific problems only seen in these populations. There is an urgent need to develop a robust and organized response along with evidence-based approach to manage onco-critical patients. This textbook edited by Dr Vinod Kumar, Dr Nishkarsh Gupta and Dr Seema Mishra elucidates all the important theoretical and practical aspects pertaining to research and management of patients in oncological set-up who need critical care support in a concise and precise manner. From an Indian perspective, this textbook is first of its class. It would be of great help to all the residents and clinical practitioners who are involved in the management of cancer patients. I would like to extend my best wishes and congratulate Dr Vinod Kumar and all the authors to come up with this idea and bringing out a much-needed evidence-based textbook highlighting all the aspects regarding onco-critical care.

Sushma Bhatnagar
Department of Onco-Anesthesia and Palliative Medicine
Dr. B.R.A. Institute Rotary Cancer Hospital
All India Institute of Medical Sciences, New Delhi, New Delhi, India

Preface

Critical care in cancer patients is complex and different from routine care for non-malignant patients. These patients are immunocompromised, malnourished and have specific concerns due to cancer-related complications, treatment-related toxicities, and severe infections. The intensivist must understand about pathophysiology, diagnosis, and management of common cancer-related issues. The optimal management of cancer patients requires expertise in oncology, critical care, and palliative medicine. There is a dearth of books explaining about critical care needs of cancer patients comprehensively. So, we felt the need for a book that is comprehensive and provides insight into the care of cancer patients in the intensive care unit.

This book contains 43 chapters. Each chapter has been prepared by experts in the field of critical care. It contains chapters on basic intensive care starting with the organization and design of the Oncocritical care unit followed by staffing and admission and discharge criteria. As these patients are immunocompromised and prone to infections, we had included chapters on infection control practices, antibiotic stewardship programmes, and sepsis management. This is followed by chapters on fluid and electrolyte management and blood transfusion. A sizeable number of patients are transferred to ICU for the management of complications due to chemotherapy and radiotherapy. Some of the oncosurgical procedures like CRS-HIPEC, head and neck surgery, thoracic surgery, and major abdominal surgeries necessitate intensive care for optimal management in the postoperative period as these surgeries involve extensive surgical resection with major fluid shift and intraoperative inotropes and vasopressor.

Few oncology patients with extensive disease may reach the spectrum of best supportive care when definitive treatment is not feasible. So, we had included chapters on palliative care which will help in decision making regarding initiation of palliation and end-of-life care. Overall, we had tried to cover diverse topics which confront intensivists in oncology ICU. This book will provide an evidence-based approach to postgraduate students and practitioners to understand about critical care needs of patients suffering from malignancies. It will help them develop critical thinking and encourage discussion toward improving the overall care of the patients and their families. This book will fulfil the needs of the postgraduate MD anaesthesia, DM Oncoanaesthesia, fellows in critical care, fellows in Onco-anaesthesiology, fellows in Onco-critical care, MSc (nursing) in critical care students to provide systemic care to the patients.

New Delhi, India Vinod Kumar

Contents

About the Editors

Vinod Kumar is additional professor in the Department of Onco-Anaesthesia & Palliative Medicine at Dr BRA IRCH, All India Institute of Medical Sciences (AIIMS), New Delhi, India. He received his training in anaesthesia from PGIMER, Chandigarh, India. Dr Kumar has a teaching experience of 12 years and guides MD (palliative medicine) and DM (onco-anaesthesiology) residents for research. He has many publications in peer-reviewed national and international journals to his credit and has edited a book. Dr Kumar is a reviewer for various national and international journals. He is a member of national anaesthesia, airway, and palliative care societies. He is an invited faculty for various national and international conferences.

Nishkarsh Gupta is working as additional professor in the Department of Onco-Anaesthesia & Palliative Medicine at Dr BRA IRCH, All India Institute of Medical Sciences (AIIMS), New Delhi, India. He has done graduation and post-graduation in anaesthesiology from Maulana Azad Medical College (MAMC), New Delhi. Thereafter, he completed DNB (anaesthesiology), postgraduate diploma in hospital administration and fellowship in palliative medicine. Dr Gupta has a teaching experience of 15 years and guides MD (palliative medicine) and DM (onco-anaesthesiology) residents for research. He has 150 publications to his credit in various international and national journals. He has also edited 2 books and contributed 15 book chapters. Dr Gupta is actively involved in research and working on 4 AIIMS-funded projects. He is on the editorial board and serves as reviewer of many journals.

Seema Mishra is working as professor in the Department of Onco-Anaesthesia & Palliative Medicine at Dr BRA IRCH, All India Institute of Medical Sciences (AIIMS), New Delhi, India. She has a teaching experience of 23 years. She is currently acting as chief and co-guide of 24 students of DM (onco-anaesthesiology) and 15 students of MD (palliative medicine) for thesis research. Dr Mishra has more than 150 publications in peer-reviewed national and international journals to her credit. She is a reviewer for various national and international journals. She is actively involved in various research projects at AIIMS, New Delhi. Dr Mishra is an invited faculty for various national and international conferences. She is a member of national and international societies of anaesthesia, pain and palliative care. She is working as executive member of Indian Association of Palliative Care. She is a member of advisory board of the *Indian Journal of Palliative Care*. She has also been working as a national faculty member of Indian Institute of Palliative Care affiliated certificate course in palliative care since 2009. She was also involved in development of various policies at AIIMS (pain policy and end-of-life care policy).

1 Design and Organization of Oncology ICU

Renu, Vinod Kumar, and Nishkarsh Gupta

1.1 Introduction

The incidence of cancer is rising and overall survival of cancer patients is improving due to advancement in chemotherapeutic regimens and surgical options [1]. So, more patients will require intensive care in future due to cancer related complications, treatment toxicities and severe infection. Designing an ICU for oncology patient is significant as these patients are malnourished, immunosuppressed and tend to require prolonged hospitalization compared to general population [2]. An ICU (intensive care unit) is a complex and highly specialized division of a hospital for the purpose of treatment of seriously ill people. It is meticulously designed, located, built and furnished. It is a division with a dedicated nursing, medical and ancillary staff who are tuned to the requirement of the specialty. It has its own policies, protocols, and standard operative procedures to take care of critically ill patients [3].

1.2 ICU Design

1.2.1 Location

ICU should be located above ground floor. It should be adjacent to operation theatre and emergency department. Pharmacy, pathology, radiology suite, sterile supplies,

Renu (✉)
School of Planning & Architecture, New Delhi, India

V. Kumar
Department of Onco-Anesthesia and Palliative Medicine, Dr. B.R.A. Institute Rotary Cancer Hospital, All India Institute of Medical Sciences, New Delhi, India

N. Gupta
Department of Onco-Anesthesia and Palliative Medicine, Dr. B.R.A. Institute Rotary Cancer Hospital, All India Institute of Medical Sciences, New Delhi, Delhi, India

V. Kumar et al. (eds.), *Onco-critical Care*,
https://doi.org/10.1007/978-981-16-9929-0_1

infection control and blood bank should be in the same building. Corridors, elevators, and ramps should be large enough to allow for bed/trolley mobility. The ICU should have a single entry/exit point that is manned [4, 5].

1.3 ICU Design and Bed Space

Beds may be arranged in U or L shape with nursing counter in the centre.

In the patient care area, 150–200 square feet for every bed is recommended. The ICU ought to have 100–150% additional space to accommodate stockpiling, nursing station, patient/specialists/staff area, and attendant's quarters, showing region, relative's region, and bathrooms. There should be a buffer space between the area for patient attendants and the area for medical professionals [6].

1.4 Single-Occupancy Cubicles/Rooms

The patient care area should be between 200 and 250 square feet. Depending on demands and bedside treatments such as ECMO, RRT, and so on, it may be beneficial to create one or two larger rooms or sections. It is advised that 10% (one to two) of the isolation rooms be used to treat immunocompromised and/or infected patients. There should be 20% more space in these rooms. Two rooms/cubicles/beds may be separated by a partition for the privacy of patients. Standard curtains are commonly used in ICUs to soften the aesthetics of the environment; however, they may become dirty or misplaced, impairing privacy.

An indestructible permanent or removable partition made of aluminum, wood, or fiber can be used to divide two rooms. Permanent partitions, on the other hand, may limit the ability to temporarily increase floor area if required. Electronic windows may be offered while designing. The glass or fiber of these windows is transparent when the switch is off and opaque when the switch is on. Installation of such window is expensive although cost may decrease in future. Transparent windows help in elevating the mood of the patient and help him in orientation with time [7].

1.5 Requirement of ICU Beds in Hospital as per Norms

Number of intensive care beds required in a tertiary care facility can range from 5 to 25% of absolute medical clinic beds, depending on the facility's specialty. ICUs with less than six beds are inefficient, and they may not provide enough clinical training or exposure to the ICU's skilled HR. It is difficult to operate an ICU with a bed strength of more than 12, and severe issues in management and result may occur. If more than 12 beds are needed, a second ICU may be built. As a result, overall bed strength in the ICU is advised to be between 8 and 12 [8].

1.6 Panels at the Head-End and at the Pendant

How to plan bedside design is one of the most crucial decisions. The two most prevalent methods are head-end wall panels or free-standing/hanging systems (power columns), which are typically suspended from the ceiling. Each one can be permanent or mobile and adjustable. It can occur on patient's right or left side. Flexibility is typically a good thing. Panels on head wall systems do not allow patients to move freely due to dangling wires and tubes.

Though hanging pendants appear to be more scientific, but head-end panels are used in the majority of ICUs in India. Pendants, rather than head-end panels, may be scrutinized by new ICU planners. Power columns that are adaptable can rotate or move from side to side. Power column mounts are frequently adjustable as well. Ceiling-mounted, movable, rotatory devices can help clear the debris from the floor and free up a lot of space. However, if the weight of the power column cannot be structurally supported, then this may not be feasible. It is recommended that the monitoring equipment be situated at eye level. Doctors and nurses may suffer from persistent head tilting, which can cause cervical neck pain and problems.

In the ICU, getting to the top of the bed in an emergency and weaving through different tangled wires is a common problem. At the same time, the patient should not feel hemmed in or surrounded by apparatus, nor should he or she be frightened unnecessarily. So, bed should be kept at least 2 feet away from the head wall. For that, a wooden plank which is 2 feet wide and 6 inches thick should be placed between wall and head end of the bed.

It will keep the bed away from the wall and provide a space for caregivers to stand in the event of an emergency without causing too many problems. A fixed ring of lines connected together can be used to route lines.

1.7 Isolation Rooms

Ten percent of the beds (1 or 2) may be utilized as isolation rooms for patients with febrile neutropenia, GVHD, and other post-stem cell transplant problems. Each patient should be given an alarm bell with both sound and light indications, and he should be trained how to use it when necessary. These isolation rooms usually have an anteroom or airlock lobby which acts as a barrier against potential loss of pressurization, controls entry and exit of air and provides a control area for transfer of supplies without contaminating the patient care area. An anteroom can be shared between.

1.8 Negative Pressure Isolation Room

There is requirement for patients infected/suspected with organisms transmitted through airborne droplets of <5 μm in diameter. In these rooms, windows are kept closed. Outside of the room, the air pressure is higher than within the room. In this way, potentially contaminated air or other potentially dangerous particles will not migrate outside into uncontaminated areas when the door is opened. Pressure differential of 2.5 Pa is kept between the two. An externally directed airflow into the room comes from neighboring areas, such as corridors and anterooms, in a clean to filthy direction. Room air should be vented to the outside, but if filtered with a HEPA filter, it can be recirculated [9]. A minimum of 12 air changes are required per hour and one must maintain a minimum 0.01-inch water column (WC). An airflow difference of 150–200 cubic feet per minute 9CFM) should be there to maintain pressure difference in a well-sealed room. They should be located at the entry of the entry of the ICU so that these patients do not have to pass through the other patient areas. A negative pressure room should have a hand wash basin preferably with hands free operation, ensuite shower and toilet, self-closing door, supply air ducts independent of the rest of the building.

1.9 Positive Pressure Isolation Room

They are needed to prevent contagious disease away from immunocompromised patients like those with cancer and/or transplants. These rooms should contain more supply air than exhaust air. These room require at least 12 air changes per minute and must have a difference of 0.01 inch WC positive pressure differential to ensure protection form airborne contamination. In relation to the corridor, there is a positive air flow i.e., flow of air from the room to the adjacent outside space. HEPA filter must be used if air is recirculated.

1.10 ICU Heating, Ventilation, and Air Conditioning System

Air conditioning is necessary to regulate temperature, humidity, and air flow in the intensive care unit. Temperature should be maintained with a focus on the patients' and ICU personnel's comfort. A temperature range of 16–25 °C is found to be suitable [10].

1.11 Utilities

In order to satisfy the needs of the patients and critical care team in both regular and emergency scenarios, oxygen, water, electrical power, compressed air, environmental control systems, vacuum, and lighting system must all ensure compliance with regulatory and accreditation agencies. A utility column is the best source of oxygen, electrical power, vacuum (freestanding, ceiling mounted, or floor mounted),, and compressed air which should also house temperature and lighting controls. Utility columns, when placed correctly, allow simple access to the patient's head and, if necessary, emergency airway care. It is possible to provide utility services on the head wall if utility columns aren't feasible.

1.12 Electrical Services

The ICU should have its own power backup that starts immediately in the event of a power loss. This electricity should be enough to keep the ICU equipment running and maintain the temperature despite the fact that most of the vital ICU equipment have battery backup. Stabilization of the voltage is also required. In the ICU, an UPS (uninterrupted power supply) system is preferred.

At least 50% of electrical outlets with proper labelling are connected to a continuous power source (UPS). An ICU's electrical panel, which should be located in the utility room, should contain a circuit breaker for each receptacle or cluster.

If the ICU does not have an UPS (uninterrupted power supply), there should be at least four UPS points on each panel, as well as a suitable number of lights and computers [11].

1.13 Lighting

Typical nursing duties, such as charting, can be carried out using general overhead illumination plus ambient light, while encouraging a comforting atmosphere for patients. No more than 30 foot-candles (fc) of total brightness should be used [12].

Lighting controls should be placed on variable-control dimmers situated directly outside the room. This allows for night-time illumination adjustments from outside the room, minimizing sleep interruption during patient surveillance. For long periods of time, night lighting should not exceed 6.5 fc, and for short periods of time, it should not exceed 19 fc.

1.14 ICU Noise Level

The International Noise Council advises that noise levels in ICUs be kept to a minimum of 45 decibels during day, 40 decibels in the evening, and 20 decibels at night [13].

1.15 Furniture and Furnishing

The countertops and furnishings should be durable enough to survive a lot of usage, as well as easy to clean and maintain. Metal to metal fasteners should be used for connections.

The fabric should be sturdy, colorfast, static-resistant, and flame if feasible, and countertops should be solid, nonporous, and stain-resistant. Patient's surrounding can be made comfortable by allowing him to keep few modest personal objects.

1.16 Coverings for the Floor, Walls, and Ceiling

Floors should be easy to maintain, non-slippery, durable, and sound absorbing while also increasing the aesthetic feel of the place. Carts and beds should be able to roll over it without difficulty.

1.17 Walls

Walls should be durable, easy to clean and maintained. It should be flame and mildew resistant. To minimise abuse and noise while simultaneously facilitating patient mobility and ambulation, door stoppers and handrails should be properly placed.

1.18 Ceiling

Ceiling is the most visualized surface by the patient. It is important that the ceiling be stain-resistant and break-proof in order to prevent eye strain from bright spotlights or fluorescent lighting [14].

1.19 Water Supply

There should be provision for clean water as hand washing, storage tanks, water filtration, and drinking water is required in the ICU [15].

1.20 Waste Disposal

An alcohol-based antimicrobial rapid hand wash solution should be accessible on every bed, so that the caregiver (doctor, nurse, relative or paramedic) can wash their hands before they touch the patient. For fear of spreading foul odors and infections, no material/dirty linen/soiled linen should be permitted to linger in the ICU for lengthy periods of time and should be disposed of as soon as feasible. Linen that has become soiled should be replaced on a regular basis and at predetermined intervals.

1.21 Central Nursing Station

Central nursing station is the soul of ICU. At this place, all of the resident physicians, nurses, and other support workers gather to discuss information and maintain track of records. All computers and digital information systems, as well as stationery, registers, and other documents, are housed here. Patients must be seen from this area regardless of whether the nurse is seated or standing, hence taller chairs are typically necessary. The central monitoring system is desirable in the oncology ICU as it connects a series of patient monitors together and back to a central monitor.

1.22 Storage

It's crucial to select what should be kept by the bedside, at the nursing station and in the nursing store. Supplies which are required often and urgently should be easily available and easy to locate. While keeping a big inventory can be costly and waste precious time. Making supplies more accessible may improve their utilization. Some overly careful or astute employees may seek to hide or hoard them. Designs that are both cost-effective and efficient are required. Ideas from nursing staff and ICU technicians should be pooled while designing space for storage.

Supplies should be categorized by activity and their usage such as chest trays, central lines, skin care trays, catheterization trays, and intracranial pressure tray, etc. They can be named or color-coded.

JCAHO now mandates secure storage when pharmaceuticals are maintained at the bedside; these stores can contain disposables, medicines, injections, records, and tabs etc. Using trolleys for supplies at the bedside loaded for different subgroups of patients, including as medical, surgical, cardiac patients, and trauma, who all have different demands, can help save space in the room. Staff nurses may have received special training to provide such care and tasks.

1.23 Communications

The patient cubicles, staff station, conference rooms, staff lounge and staff-overnight stay rooms should all have a voice intercommunication system. The plan may additionally contain supply spaces and a visitors' lounge/waiting room. Connections to important departments including the blood bank, radiology, pharmacy, and clinical laboratories should be created whenever possible. There should be a way to communicate internally and externally in the event of a system failure which is in addition to conventional telephones available in each ICU.

1.24 Wash Basins and Scrubs

Near the staff station and patient bed areas, handbasins and clinical hand-washing facilities are required. It is recommended that there be one clinical hand-washing station for every two patient beds, and one for every patient's room or cubicle.

1.25 Support Areas for Staff

Doctors duty rooms (male and female), nurses lounge, medication counters, changing rooms, meeting room for discussion of medical professionals and family meeting, toilets, janitor room, pantry, equipment room (mobile X-ray, USG) and utility rooms for dirty and clean utility should be provided.

1.26 Waiting Area

A separate waiting area for patient's family member is must with seating arrangement. Lockers, prayer area, food, beverages, drinking water, and rest rooms should be provided. There should be a separate interview room and a separate waiting area for anxious relatives, as well as overnight rooms for relations, should be provided.

Provision for renal replacement therapy (RRT) should be there as some of the cancer patients may need during their care. For this one RRT (HD/CRRT) bed with RO/de-iodinated water supply outlets should be set aside for HD machines.

1.27 The ICU's Equipment

The least fundamental equipment necessary for the ICU's successful and safe operation is known as essential equipment. While desired equipment is that which will improve the ICU's ability to manage patients and provide high-quality care. Below are the list of equipment required in setup of ICU. This list is not all inclusive.

- ICU equipment ICU bed with mattress,
- Air mattress,
- ICU ventilator,
- non-invasive ventilation mask,
- high flow nasal cannula,
- Stretcher trolley,
- Chair for staff and relatives,
- Procedure trolley,
- emergency crash cart,
- linen cart, multiparameter monitor,
- Computer,
- intravenous stand,
- syringe pump, infusion pump, sequential compression device.

1.28 Conclusion

Care delivery costs, clinical outcomes, and organizational performance are all influenced by critical care facility architecture. For organizations participating in design and construction projects, consultants with experience will connect with customers and make important design choices based on the best available evidence.

References

1. SEER stat fact sheet: cancer of any site. Seer.cancer.gov. Accessed 2 Feb 2022.
2. Koch A, Checkley W. Do hospitals need oncological critical care units? J Thorac Dis. 2017;9(3):E304–9.

3. Rungta N, Zirpe KG, Dixit SB, Mehta Y, Chaudhry D, Govil D, et al. Indian Society of Critical Care Medicine experts committee consensus statement on ICU planning and designing, 2020. Indian J Crit Care Med. 2020;24(Suppl 1)
4. American Institute of Architects Committee on Architecture for Health and the U.S. Department of Health and Human Services—Guidelines for Construction and Equipment/Hospital and Medical Facilities. AIA Press, 1996.
5. Marshall JC, Bosco L, Adhikari NK, Connolly B, Diaz JV, Dorman T, et al. What is an intensive care unit? A report of the task force of the world Federation of Societies of intensive and critical care medicine. J Crit Care. 2017;37:270–6.
6. Chaudhury H, Mahmood A, Valente M. Advantages and disadvantages of single versus multiple occupancy rooms in acute care environments: a review and analysis of the literature. Environ Behav. 2005;37:760–86.
7. Bracco D, Dubois M-J, Bouali R, Eggimann P. Single rooms may help to prevent nosocomial bloodstream infection and cross-transmission of methicillin-resistant Staphylococcus aureus in intensive care units. Intensive Care Med. 2007;33:836–40.
8. Williams SV. How many intensive care beds are enough? Crit Care Med. 1983;11(6):412–6.
9. Lee SY, Choi SH, Park JE, et al. Crucial role of temporary airborne infection isolation rooms in an intensive care unit: containing the COVID-19 outbreak in South Korea. Crit Care. 2020;24:238.
10. Minvielle E, Dervaux B, Retbi A, Aegerter P, Boumendil A, Jars-Guincestre MC, et al. Culture, organization, and management in intensive care: construction and validation of a multidimensional questionnaire. J Crit Care. 2005;20:126–38.
11. Wunsch H, Gershengorn H, Mayer S, Claassen J. The effect of window rooms on critically ill patients with subarachnoid hemorrhage admitted to intensive care. Crit Care. 2011;15:R81.
12. Hamilton D, Thompson D. What's new in ICU design? Critical Connections, Society of Critical Care Medicine; 2005. p. 1–10.
13. Grumet GW. Pandemonium in the modern hospital (editorial). N Engl J Med. 1993;328:433–7.
14. O'Connell NH, Humphreys H. Intensive care unit design and environmental factors in the acquisition of infection. J Hosp Infect. 2000;45:255–62.
15. Andreas Valentin and Patrick Ferdinande (ESICM Working Group on Quality Improvement): Recommendations on basic requirements for intensive care units: structural and organizational aspects Intensive Care Med 2011;1(37):1575–1587.

ICU Staffing, Models, and Outcomes in Onco-Critical Care Unit

2

Saurabh Vig, Anuja Pandit, and Swati Bhan

2.1 Introduction

The 'Intensive Care Unit' (ICU) in any hospital houses critically ill patients and is specifically designed, staffed and equipped to monitor and manage the life threating illnesses and other complications which may be seen in critically sick patients [1]. Thus, an ICU is a area of the hospital which is cost intensive to maintain and operate and requires precise management to be economically viable for any hospital.

Historically, the concept of a designated area for the management of critically ill patients has developed with major historical events of the world. The World War 1 saw the development of the so called 'shock wards' for the resuscitation of soldiers in hypovolemic shock with colloids and crystalloids. This progressed to surgical wards with the onset of blood transfusion and surgeries for management of wounds sustained in the battlefield. The concept of a 'respiratory unit' with mechanical ventilatory support emerged during the polio epidemic which saw widespread use of ventilators for respiratory support [2]. Organ specific based intensive care was first described in neurosurgery as 'brain teams' looking after the perioperative care of neurosurgical patients [3].

With the progress of medicine and development of various medical and surgical branches ICUs in the present-day scenario are super specialized units where medical or surgical patients requiring intensive round the clock monitoring and management are admitted. ICU's are graded into three levels (level 1, 2 and 3) on the basis of the size and speciality of the hospital housing these units [4]. The basic guidelines on skeletal and structural formation of an ICU according to the level of care the number of beds to be housed, number of beds in a chamber, the spacing and

S. Vig (✉) · A. Pandit · S. Bhan
Onco-Anaesthesia & Palliative Medicine, National Cancer Institute, AIIMS, New Delhi, India

V. Kumar et al. (eds.), *Onco-critical Care*,
https://doi.org/10.1007/978-981-16-9929-0_2

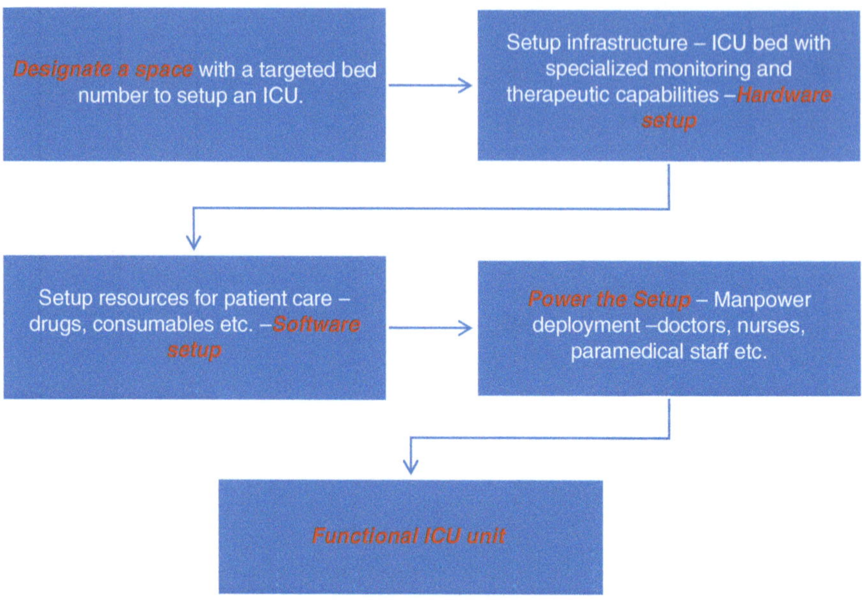

Fig. 2.1 Showing the basic steps of designing and operating a ICU

distance between the beds, the equipment's required for proper functioning of an ICU according to its level of care are well defined in litrature [4].

Majority of the ICUs in the developed as well as developing nations are designed and operated in the basic steps as outlined in Fig. 2.1.

2.1.1 Staffing Patterns in ICU—Current Concepts and Practices -

Doctors or intensivists, nursing and other para medical staff like physiotherapists, phlebotomists, cleaning staff, equipment in charge, store in charge etc. are integral to the functioning of any ICU.

Worldwide critical care society guidelines insist on a fixed nursing ratio for ICU patients [1, 4, 5], a nurse patient ratio of 1:1 for ventilated and other critically ill patients and a ratio of 1:2 or 1:3 for less sick patients. However, literature does not exactly specify the staffing pattern and numbers for doctors or intensivists for proportion of patients in any ICU. A statement released in 2013 from the Society of Critical Care Medicine states that intensivist patient ratio less favourable than 1:14 negatively impacted patient care, teaching training and staff wellbeing [6]. However, this statement has not been implemented as a standard guideline by the various critical care societies around the world. The reason behind this is that an ICU trained doctor or an 'Intensivist' is a scarce manpower resource all over the world in all types of medical systems be it a government sponsored institute or a private medical centre or hospital.

To understand the dynamic concept of staffing an intensivist in ICU and its related outcomes one first needs to understand the working modes of ICU and patient care delivery, as these models call for different types of staffing for smooth running of the ICU.

2.2 Working Modes of an ICU

ICU is an interwoven and complex organisation which deals with patients from various specialities. There are multiple stakeholders for each patient right from the primary physician, the intensivist in the ICU to the various doctors which may called for their speciality reference. The primary stakeholder may be the intensivist or the primary care physician depending on the working model of the ICU. The staffing patterns, duty hours of the ICU and the role of a trained intensivist varies according to the working model adopted by the ICU.

The various working models described for ICU's are summarized in Table 2.1.

Table 2.1 Summarizing working models for an ICU [7]

Working Model	Closed ICU	Open ICU	Semi closed ICU	Semi open ICU.
Salient features	Admission and discharge rights only with the intensivist All decisions on patient care and management are taken by the critical care team The initial physician becomes only an observer with no active role in patient management Practised predominantly in ICU'S in Europe and Australia Can easily be applied and practised in 'academic institutes	Admission and discharge—any physician with hospital admission rights can admit the patient directly to the ICU Primary care provider—management and decision making remains in the hands of the primary care provider ICU just provides a place of intensive monitoring (eg. vasopressor infusion and invasive monitoring), better nursing care etc	Hybrid model between closed and open model Admission rights—anyone can admit the patient in ICU Management—critical team is automatically consulted and comanages all patients with the primary physician	Hybrid model between closed and open model Anyone with admitting rights can admit a patient Critical team is consulted for all patients *but* all patients are not comanaged

(continued)

Table 2.1 (continued)

Working Model	Closed ICU	Open ICU	Semi closed ICU	Semi open ICU.
Advantages	Unidirectional flow of command and a single decision-making team for the patient, thus no confusion in medical decision making	Primary physician is the decision maker—thus continuity of care is maintained Less labour intensive and not dependent on critical care specialist	Aims at best of both open and closed system—i.e., continuity of care with primary physician and specialist care by the intensivist	Opinion of critical care is sought initially and then whenever require leaving the entire decision making on the primary physician
Drawbacks	Most labour intensive of all the systems	The specialized care of an intensivist trained in managing critically ill patients is missing Primary physician may not be expert in certain ICU procedures and techniques (ventilatory management, bedside procedures)	Two managing teams (primary physician and the intensivist) may lead to conflict of ideas and thoughts and may delay or negatively impact clinical decisions	Daily involvement of a critical care specialist is missing

2.3 Staffing of an ICU

After a basic understanding of the working models of ICU its is quite clear that the closed model of ICU will be the most labour intensive with respect to employing trained intensivists, the open system will be the least labour intensive with no involvement of the intensivist and the semi closed and semi open will be somewhat in between of the two, with the semi closed system requiring more staff than the semi open as intensivists comanage all cases in semi closed whereas are consulted only on need basis in semi open system.

Staffing a closed or semi closed ICU with intensivists would be economically more costly on any hospital system. From an administrative point of view the costs incurred to staff a closed or semi closed ICU should be supported by positive patient outcomes. The earliest concrete evidence in this regard was given by Pronovost and co-workers in their systematic review published in 2002 addressing the question of relation between ICU physician staffing and patient outcomes [8]. In this paper ICU physician staffing and patient related outcomes like length of stay (LOS), mortality etc. were studied from 1965 to 2001. They grouped the generated data into a '*low intensity staffing model*' where intensivist or the ICU physician is not directly involved in patient care or is only electively consulted (an open or semi open model of ICU care). The second group was '*high intensity staffing model*' where an intensivist was the primary care provider or was mandatorily involved and comanaged all patient (closed or semi closed model of ICU care). They concluded that the high intensity staffing was associated with a lower hospital mortality, lower ICU mortality and lower LOS in the ICU and thus translated into better patient outcomes.

The '*Leapfrog Group*' a consortium of purchasers and providers of health care [9], this group aims to improve healthcare system outcomes, minimize preventable errors, rate the various healthcare systems of America and aims to bring about a system of transparency in the functioning of healthcare in America. This group issues guidelines and sets standards for health care systems housing ICU for staffing and functioning of the ICU.

The Leapfrog group in their 2021 document on ICU physician staffing (IPS) [10] state that—the quality of care in an ICU is broadly determined by (a) whether "intensivists" are providing care and (b) model of care delivery in the ICU (open vs. closed ICU). The Leapfrog group defines 'Intensivist' as a board-certified physician additionally certified in the speciality of critical care medicine. A physician eligible for a subspecialty certification in critical care may be a specialist in medicine, emergency medicine, anaesthesia or paediatrics.

The Leapfrog group IPS safety standard guidelines with an aim to minimize preventable errors and enhance positive outcomes in patient care can be summarized as [10]—

1. Certified intensivists to be present on site to exclusively manage (closed model) or comanage (semi-closed model) all the patients in medical or surgical ICU for optimum outcomes.
2. The onsite intensivist to be present for a period of 8 h per day in the day time for 7 days a week for exclusive clinical care in the ICU.
3. When intensivist is not present onsite or working via telemedicine—more than 95% of calls/texts/messages from the ICU are to be returned and answered to within 5 min.
4. An onsite 'Effector' i.e., a trained medical person to carry out order given by the intensivist (when not present on site or working via telemedicine) to be present on site and physically reach any patient within 5 min to carry out orders given by the intensivist.

The recommendations have been made in line and based on the evidence generated in the sentinel paper on ICU staffing by Pronovost et al. [8].

2.4 Physician Staffing Models of an ICU

Basic 3 models are described for ICU staffing [7], these are mainly—

(a) Academic model
(b) Modified academic model
(c) Open model.

The salient features of each with its advantages, drawbacks, cost benefit analysis for the hospital are summarized in Table 2.2.

2.4.1 Outcomes with Different Staffing Models

While relatively clear that the academic model will have the maximum benefit and positive impact on patient outcomes, 24-h intensivist on floor versus day time intensivist followed by on call/ telemedicine was a matter of debate. Literature on patient outcome in the recent years has shed light on this question.

Table 2.2 Table describing various physician staffing models for ICU setup

Staffing model	Academic model	Modified academic model	Open model
Salient features.	A team of attending consultant and resident trainees 24 h on floor of the ICU Default model for closed ICU and large teaching institutes	24-h coverage by a certified intensivist not necessarily on ICU floor during this period Physician assistants (PA) and advanced practice providers (APP) on floor of the ICU 24 h a day in shifts to carry out orders of the intensivist within 5 min as per Leapfrog guidelines	Consulting intensivist only when required and do not take over or comanage patients In line with Open or semi open ICU setup May be used mainly by small Level I ICU units
Advantages	Maximum coverage and theoretically minimal chances of lapses in patient care	Better utilization of the scarcest manpower i.e., certified intensivist The concept of 'Telemedicine' can be implemented with this model	Minimal costs to the institution
Draw backs	Resource heavy and maximum costs for the system Difficult to find faculties for night shifts and resident trainees for 24-h shift duties Poor work life balance for doctors	The PA's and APP's have to be trained in common ICU procedures like lumbar puncture, ventilator management, central line placement etc. for optimal care High risk procedures like intubations, intercostal drain placement etc. may still need on site specialist backup	Not in line with the Leapfrog guidelines Poor patient outcomes and inconsistent care

In an official systematic review and metanalysis on night time intensivist staffing sone by the American Thoracic Society concluded that Night time intensivist staffing did not have any superior outcome in mortality and length of hospital stay as compared to day time dedicated intensivist coverage [11]. Similar conclusions were echoed in a retrospective study in over 65,000 patients, night time intensivist ICU staffing had a positive impact on outcomes when applied to low intensity ICU care and had no impact on outcomes when applied on day time intensivist covered ICU setups [12].

To conclude, a high intensity (closed or semi closed) staffing model definitely improves overall outcomes as compared to low intensity staffing but the same cannot be said for night time intensivist in all types of ICU's. with advanced in medical care and communication techniques especially with the advent of telemedicine the evidence in favour of night time intensivist has declined in recent literature.

The future of telemedicine in ICU looks promising, a systematic review and metanalysis on impact of telemedicine on patient outcomes collected data from 13 eligible studies from 35 ICU's and included 41,000 patients. This study concluded that tele ICU coverage was associated with lower ICU mortality and LOS but did not translate into lower in hospital mortality or shortened LOS [13]. In the same year a prospective stepped clinical practice study by Craig M Lily and co-workers on 6290 patients in 7 ICU's showed that implementation of a tele ICU was associated with reduced in hospital mortality and reduced hospital LOS [14]. The key feature in this study which led to its success was that the tele ICU consult providers had full independence in patient care and could order any necessary interventions just as an in-house intensivist.

Thus, the ideal staffing system of an ICU would be a closed type of ICU with high intensity 24-h in-house intensivist. However, keeping in mind the limited available certified intensivists in any medical system and literature clearly showing day time high intensity staffing to be equally effective the most practical system in any ICU setup be it a teaching hospital or a private setup would be a closed or semi-closed type of ICU with high intensity day time staffing with a physician patient ratio of not more than 1:14 and well-trained PA's or APP's for night time cover. Telemedicine can be practised in a robust manner with all decisions and responsibilities resting on the shoulders of intensivist in charge and a well trained on ground medical staff.

2.5 Burnout Among Intensivists

An ICU is a highly stressful workplace with a high-pressure environment. Such work conditions put the workforce both physicians and paramedical staff under extreme stress and make them prone for burnout [15].

Various factors which put the ICU physicians under extreme stress and at risk of burnout are [15–17]—

- Long working hours and shift timings.
- Regular night shifts with no time for family.

Admission and Discharge in the Critical Care in Oncology Setting

3

A. R. Karthik and Vinod Kumar

3.1 Introduction

Cancer patients require admission to the Intensive Care Unit (ICU) for various indications. Not all cancer patients requiring ICU admission benefit from the same. Some patients with reversible pathologies and increased life expectancy benefit more from intensive care than others. Patients with irreversible organ damage and reduced life expectancy occupy the ICU bed depriving needy patients of the required level of care. Hence inclusion of admission criteria is required for optimal utilization of the available ICU beds in the Oncology setting [1]. Similar to admission to ICU, appropriate discharge timing is essential to prevent ICU related complications in prolonged admission and to utilize the bed for the next deserving patient.Discharge of patients from the ICU includes conditions when the patient has improved so that there is no further need of ICU care or when the patient has deteriorated or remained status quo and further intensive care management would prove futile. Hence evidence-based discharge criteria would further support optimal utilization of ICU beds.

3.2 Common Indications for ICU Admissions in the Cancer Patient

Prognosis in cancer patients has recently improved dramatically due to early diagnosis, advanced surgical procedures, newer chemotherapeutic agents and immunotherapy agents, targeted radiotherapy and improved supportive care measures. Thus, those conditions which were once considered non-responsive to treatment have

A. R. Karthik
Onco-anesthesia & Palliative Medicine, Dr BR Ambedkar IRCH AIIMS, New Delhi, India

V. Kumar (✉)
Department of Onco-Anesthesia and Palliative Medicine, Dr. B.R.A. Institute Rotary Cancer Hospital, All India Institute of Medical Sciences, New Delhi, India

V. Kumar et al. (eds.), *Onco-critical Care*,
https://doi.org/10.1007/978-981-16-9929-0_3

become amenable to treatment or control [2]. The most common indications for ICU admissions in a cancer patient are presented below.

- A postoperative patient who has undergone a major resection/reconstructive procedure or patients with multiple comorbidities undergoing oncological procedures will require intensive care management in the immediate postoperative period. Most of these admissions would be planned.
- A patient may be emergently admitted to the ICU because of unanticipated surgical or anaesthetic complications in the perioperative period.
- Oncological emergencies like superior vena cava (SVC) syndrome, hypercalcemia of malignancy, acute haemorrhage, blast crisis, leucostasis, cardiac tamponade will need to be managed in the ICU.
- About one-fifth of patients with hematopoietic stem cell transplants (HSCT) need to be taken care in isolation rooms of the ICU to support recovery from transplant and treat complications associated with it [3].
- Oncology patients who have suffered a complication due to chemotherapy such as febrile neutropenia, sepsis and septic shock, tumour lysis syndrome, pneumonia and respiratory insufficiency will require intensive care.
- Patients with airway related malignancies with impending airway obstruction would initially be stabilized in the Emergency Department (ED) and later be shifted to the ICU.

The above list is not exhaustive and is given just to highlight the diversity in the admission indications.

3.3 Oncology ICU Vs a General ICU

The presence of a malignancy per se would tend to weigh down in the probability of getting an ICU bed in a multispeciality setup owing to the enormous number of non-malignant patients requiring intensive care. However, in an oncology setting, the mere presence of a malignancy is ruled out as a factor for denial of ICU admission. Oncology ICUs have evolved into multidisciplinary units with inputs from various clinical and paraclinical specialities rather than being a closed unit managed by an intensivist. The admission criteria must be individualized to each unit depending on various parameters discussed below. A blanket protocol would not be appropriate for every unit due to the interplay of various factors in the effective utilization of ICU beds.

3.4 Admission Criteria

The following parameters can be taken as a guide to formulate decisions regarding acceptance or denial of ICU admissions.

1. Presence and severity of comorbidities
2. Type and stage of the malignancy

3. Reversibility of the current condition
4. Performance and physical status of the patient before the current event
5. Availability of the resources and expertise to manage the condition
6. Objective ICU admission scores
7. Benefit vs futility of providing critical care

1. Presence and severity of comorbidities

   Patients with life-limiting and end stage organ dysfunction unrelated to cancer with limited life expectancy would score down on the admission criteria even if the underlying malignancy is amenable to treatment. However, the decision based on this parameter needs to be taken on an individual case-to-case basis.
2. Type and stage of malignancy

   The nature of malignancy and stage gives a hint at the overall prognosis after hospitalization. Oncology treatment has advanced a lot recently and advanced malignancies which were not amenable to treatment earlier or where treatment caused unacceptable side effects, have become treatable now with acceptable side effect profile. Hence consultation with an oncologist is becoming essential in prognostication of cancer patients requiring critical care.
3. Reversibility of current condition

   Where the indication of ICU admission is a reversible complication of oncology therapy or a reversible pathology due to the underlying malignancy, ICU admission is warranted because denying admission would prevent further oncology treatment or would negatively impact the quality of life. A retrospective study of 175 ICU admissions in breast cancer patients concluded that the in-hospital mortality was more related to the acute complications inciting the event rather than the overall cancer characteristics [4].
4. Performance and physical status of the patient before the current event

   The Eastern Cooperative Group (ECOG) scale of performance status (Table 3.1) is a useful tool in evaluating the overall severity of the cancer. A higher ECOG status even before the current inciting event denotes reduced usefulness of intensive care in improving the quality of life of the patient [6]. However, if the higher ECOG status is due to some reversible pathology, all attempts at intensive management should be given at the first go.

Table 3.1 ECOG performance status [5]

Grade	ECOG Performance Status
0	Fully active, able to carry on all pre-disease performance without restriction
1	Restricted in physically strenuous activity but ambulatory and able to carry out work of a light or sedentary nature, e.g., light house work, office work
2	Ambulatory and capable of all selfcare but unable to carry out any work activities; up and about more than 50% of waking hours
3	Capable of only limited selfcare; confined to bed or chair more than 50% of waking hours
4	Completely disabled; cannot carry on any selfcare; totally confined to bed or chair
5	Dead

5. Availability of the resources and expertise to manage the condition
   All medical and surgical conditions are not amenable to treatment in all medical centres. Centres should appreciate their limitations as to availability of resources and expertise and should transfer patients to a centre with the required resources after initial stabilization. Continuation of care during transport should be ensured.
6. Objective ICU admission scores
   Various scoring systems have been formulated to predict morbidity and mortality during ICU admissions. These include the multiple versions (I, II, III) of Acute Physiology and Chronic Health Evaluation (APACHE) scores, the Simplified Acute Physiology Score—II (SAPS II). Oncology specific prediction models such as the Intensive Care Mortality Model (ICMM) incorporated oncology therapy related organ dysfunction into the APACHE scoring. The Sequential Organ Failure Assessment (SOFA) score when assessed on a daily basis has been shown to particularly useful in patients with sepsis, shock and hematologic malignancy [7]. However, no score is perfect and the reliability and predictability of the scores varies with patients and conditions. Yet these scores are objective criteria and serve to avoid personal bias in decision making. So, these scores should be considered in triaging but not to be solely relied upon.
7. Benefit vs. futility of providing critical care
   If intensive care management produces increased disability and reduced quality of life the decision to continue such care should be solely made by the patient and caretakers after careful consideration of the pros and cons of continuing treatment even though such treatment offers increased quantity of life.

However, the final decision of accepting or denying admission to ICU should be taken on an individual case-to-case basis considering all the factors discussed above.

3.5 Course of ICU Stay and Discharge Criteria

Unlike multispecialty ICUs, the aim of management in the Oncology ICU would be many a time to not treat the primary disease but to tide over a complication or crisis. Based upon the admission criteria, the aim of ICU stay will vary [8].

1. **Full Code ICU Management**
   If the disease and the inciting event is largely curable, the aim of ICU stay would be curative. All available curative measures would be initiated, and the patient would receive all treatment modalities as any other ICU patient. The probable indications include reversible disease pathology, patients in remission, iatrogenic complications and availability of potential curative treatment options. A consensus statement from Germany and Austria suggests that a full code ICU management protocol should be provided to all critically ill malignancy patients whose long-term prognosis is in line with the prognosis of the underlying malignancy [6].Patients must be periodically reviewed on whether full code management is to be continued [9].

2. **Trial of ICU Care**

   If there is no clear-cut picture as to whether the inciting condition is treatable or not, a trial of full code ICU care is warranted. In these borderline patients a full code ICU care trial is given for a few days and progress is noted. The response to treatment will further direct whether the patient would continue receiving complete ICU care protocol or would require de-escalation of treatment [10]. De-escalation of treatment would require the consensus of all the stakeholders including the patient (if communicable), caretakers, primary treating physician and ICU team. Legal and ethical issues would also have to be considered when it comes to de-escalation of treatment. There is no definite evidence as to what the duration of ICU trial should be. However a duration of 4 days for solid tumours and 10 days for haematological malignancies seems to be a valid choice [11].
3. **Palliative Care in the ICU**

   If a condition warrants ICU care and the treatment of that inciting event would improve the quality of life, then such a patient should not be denied ICU admission even if the disease process is irreversible and untreatable. Examples would be a palliative stenting of the airway to relieve airway obstruction, palliative diversion procedures for intestinal obstruction etc. These patients should not receive full code ICU management and mostly would receive non-invasive or less invasive organ support measures. Palliative care integration in the ICU reduces cost and length of stay without considerable impact on mortality [12]. In patients with advanced stage malignancies with rapidly evolving irreversible multi-organ failure, the goals of care should be reconsidered. In such cases an early integration of end-of-life-care can reduce the burden on the patients and their caregivers. This should include discussions with all stakeholders on withholding or withdrawal of life-sustaining measures, options for distress management, and dignity preserving care.

Discharge of patients from the ICU must be contemplated when the patient has improved from his/her admitting status and is physiologically stable so that further management is possible in a hospital ward. Scores such as the APACHE II at discharge seem to correlate well in identifying patients who are prone to deterioration after discharge. Such patients may be transferred to a step-down unit like a High Dependency Unit (HDU) before shifting to the ward. This transition would reduce readmissions to the ICU in this patient population. Continuation of care would be efficient if the ICU physician briefs the doctor at the receiving unit regarding the patient's history, course of ICU stay, and realistic goals of further care. Discharge at odd hours is not preferred [13]. If a patient under trial of ICU care has failed the trial, then further course of action should be decided taking the opinion of all stakeholders. It might even include a discharge to home or a hospice.

The status of patients admitted to an ICU should be reviewed continuously to identify patients who may no longer need ICU care.

This includes:

A. When a patient's physiologic status has stabilised and the need for ICU monitoring and care is no longer necessary
B. When a patient's physiological status has deteriorated and / or become irreversible and active interventions are no longer beneficial, withdrawal of therapy should be carried out in the intensive care unit. Patient should only be discharged to the ward if bed is required.

3.6 Triage

Due to the limited number of ICU beds, triaging may be necessary.

The following factors will be taken into consideration in triaging:

- Diagnosis
- Severity of illness
- Age and functional status
- Co-morbid disease
- Physiological reserve
- Prognosis
- Availability of suitable treatment
- Response to treatment to date
- Recent cardiopulmonary arrest
- Anticipated quality of life

3.7 Discharge Will Be Based on the Following Criteria

1. Stable haemodynamic parameters
2. Stable respiratory status (patient extubated with stable arterial blood gases) and airway patency
3. Oxygen requirements not more than 60%
4. Intravenous inotropic/vasopressor support and vasodilators are no longer necessary. Patients on low dose inotropic support may be discharged earlier if ICU bed is required.
5. Cardiac dysrhythmias are controlled
6. Neurologic stability with control of seizures
7. Patients who require chronic mechanical ventilation (e.g. motor neuron disease, cervical spine injuries) with any of the acute critical problems reversed or resolved
8. Patients with tracheostomies who no longer require frequent suctioning

References

1. Nasir SS, Muthiah M, Ryder K, Clark K, Niell H, Weir A. ICU deaths in patients with advanced cancer: reasonable criteria to decrease potentially inappropriate admissions and lack of benefit of advance planning discussions. Am J Hosp Palliat Med. 2017;34(2):173–9.
2. Soubani AO. Critical care prognosis and outcomes in patients with cancer. Clin Chest Med. 2017;38(2):333–53.
3. Pène F, Salluh JIF, Staudinger T. Has survival increased in cancer patients admitted to the ICU? No Intensive Care Med. 2014;40(10):1573–5.
4. Destrebecq V, Lieveke A, Berghmans T, Paesmans M, Sculier J-P, Meert A-P. Are intensive cares worthwhile for breast cancer patients: the experience of an oncological ICU. Front Med [Internet]. 2016 [cited 2021 Sep 7];3. http://journal.frontiersin.org/article/10.3389/fmed.2016.00050/full.
5. Oken M, Creech R, Tormey D, Horton J, Davis T, McFadden E, et al. Toxicity and response criteria of the eastern cooperative oncology group. Am J Clin Oncol. 1982;5(6):649–55.
6. Consensus of the German Society of Hematology and Medical Oncology (DGHO), Austrian Society of Hematology and Oncology (OeGHO), German Society for Medical Intensive Care Medicine and Emergency Medicine (DGIIN), and Austrian Society of Medical and General Intensive Care and Emergency Medicine (ÖGIAIN), Kiehl MG, Beutel G, Böll B, Buchheidt D, Forkert R, et al. Consensus statement for cancer patients requiring intensive care support. Ann Hematol. 2018 Jul;97(7):1271–82.
7. Shelton BK. Admission criteria and prognostication in patients with cancer admitted to the intensive care unit. Crit Care Clin. 2010 Jan;26(1):1–20.
8. Azoulay É, Afessa B. The intensive care support of patients with malignancy: do everything that can be done. Intensive Care Med. 2006;32(1):3–5.
9. Kostakou E, Rovina N, Kyriakopoulou M, Koulouris NG, Koutsoukou A. Critically ill cancer patient in intensive care unit: issues that arise. J Crit Care. 2014;29(5):817–22.
10. Lecuyer L, Chevret S, Thiery G, Darmon M, Schlemmer B, Azoulay É. The ICU trial: a new admission policy for cancer patients requiring mechanical ventilation*. Crit Care Med. 2007;35(3):808–14.
11. Shrime MG, Ferket BS, Scott DJ, Lee J, Barragan-Bradford D, Pollard T, et al. Time-limited trials of intensive Care for Critically ill Patients with cancer: how long is long enough? JAMA Oncol. 2016;2(1):76.
12. Kyeremanteng K, Gagnon L-P, Thavorn K, Heyland D, D'Egidio G. The impact of palliative care consultation in the ICU on length of stay: a systematic review and cost evaluation. J Intensive Care Med. 2018;33(6):346–53.
13. Nates JL, Nunnally M, Kleinpell R, Blosser S, Goldner J, Birriel B, et al. ICU admission, discharge, and Triage guidelines: a framework to enhance clinical operations, development of institutional policies, and further research. Crit Care Med. 2016;44(8):1553–602.

4 Predicting Outcomes in Onco-Critical Care

Anirban Hom Choudhuri, Priyanka Harisinghani, and Nidhi Gupta

4.1 Introduction

The dimensions of cancer treatment are diverse and distinct. From the stage of early screening to late palliation, it is beset with decisions based upon prediction. The need for prophylactic surgery, the effects of neoadjuvant therapy, the dose of radiation etc. are all major end-points based upon predictions. Therefore, for matching expectations with results in patients admitted in the intensive care unit (ICU) outcome prediction is absolutely necessary.

The causes for ICU admission after cancer are many and the type and stage of cancer influence the course of ICU stay. This is in sharp contrast to critical illness of non cancer origin where the outcome after admission is primarily determined by the severity of antecedent illness alone. For e.g. the outcome of abdominal sepsis following non cancer diseases can be predicted more reliably by using conventional scoring systems viz. APACHE, SOFA, MODS etc. but not after non cancer diseases where the scores become less reliable due to lesser specificity. So there arises the need for revalidating the scores or modifying them by reviewing the original database and using statistical tools for measuring the additional risks posed by cancer. The task is often cumbersome due to the dynamic nature of illness and variable trajectories for various cancers.

It is also well accepted that patient outcomes and cancer outcomes are distinct and that many patient outcome parameters viz. survival, quality of life etc. are of greater relevance to the physician than the pure cancer outcome parameters viz. dose, toxicity, cure, etc. The chapter focuses on evidence based prediction of the various outcomes in cancer settings from the prism of critical illness.

A. H. Choudhuri (✉) · N. Gupta
Anesthesia & Intensive Care, GIPMER, New Delhi, India

P. Harisinghani
Anesthesia & Critical Care, Safdarjung Hospital & VMMC, New Delhi, India

V. Kumar et al. (eds.), *Onco-critical Care*,
https://doi.org/10.1007/978-981-16-9929-0_4

4.2 General Principles of Outcome Prediction

Most researchers follow a data mining or machine learning method to create a prediction model to determine a particular type of clinical outcome. Some prefer a mathematical model to predict multiple clinical outcomes simultaneously. A few use hybrid models that perform continuous prediction of multiple clinical outcomes. Although these models have variable accuracy, they can perform a wide range of outcome prediction and can serve as better guide for comprehensive care than subjective assessment alone. The figure (Fig. 4.1) shows the different approaches used for these models.

4.3 Development of a Prediction Score in Critical Care

To develop a prediction score, the outcome has to be defined precisely. The mortality described in critical care is usually ICU mortality or in-hospital mortality or mortality at 28 days. Likewise, the morbidity can signify either duration of ICU stay or duration of mechanical ventilation or duration of vasopressor and inotropic support etc. The variables chosen to identify the outcomes must be standardized. Often the cohort datasets contain more variables than that can be used for analysis and in

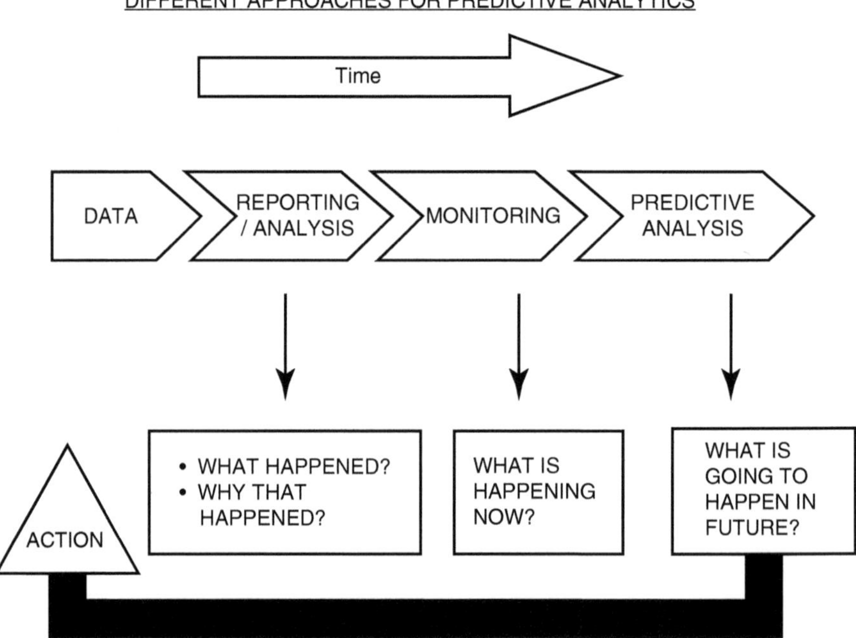

Fig. 4.1 Different approaches for predictive analytics

such cases the most sensitive and predictive variables are chosen. It is known that inclusion of more than ten variables can reduce the efficiency, feasibility and convenience of the prediction models. Some predictors which are found to be valuable in earlier models can be treated as candidate variables but not all predictors are included in the final model. The selection of predictors is guided by clinical relevance and judgement to exclude less relevant and user unfriendly variables and variables with false positive associations. The categorical and continuous variables are coded and arranged separately. A regression analysis is then performed using either a full model approach or a stepwise selection approach. Finally, the new score is evaluated for its predictive power and is validated both internally and externally in an independent dataset.

The underlying figure represents a schematic description of the steps in development of prediction score (Fig. 4.2).

4.4 Causes of ICU Admission in Cancer Patients

The common causes of ICU admission in cancer patients are in table listed (Table 4.1). Postoperative admission after elective surgery is the most common surgical cause. This group of patients has the best prognosis. Shock (cardiogenic, hypovolemic or sepsis) is the most common medical cause of admission. Patients with cardiogenic shock have the worst prognosis. Survival in sepsis is dependent on various factors but mainly depend on the initial severity and the delay in treatment initiation. It has been observed that mortality after cancer sepsis varies widely with age and is highest in the young adults. It is also associated with frequent readmissions. This gap decreases with advancing age and becomes similar at around 85 years of age. The reason for similar mortality with advancing age is ascribed to immunosenescence which results in similar kind of immune dysfunction in both cancer and non cancer patients [1].

Infections are frequent in hematological malignancies due to both neutropenia and primary immune suppression. The risks are related to the degree of neutropenia which is determined by absolute neutrophil count (ANC) and can manifest without any fever.

Respiratory failure is a common cause of admission in patients with both hematological malignancies and solid tumors. This may follow pneumonias, drug toxicities; transfusion associated acute lung injuries (TRALI) and direct pulmonary metastases.

Metabolic and electrolyte disturbances, renal failure, neurological complications and acute pulmonary embolism are other causes for admission. It is observed that both mortality and the duration of hospital stay are higher in neutropenic patients with hematological malignancies than after solid tumors [2]. The underlying table shows the differences in features and outcome between neutropenic and non-neutropenic sepsis (Table 4.2).

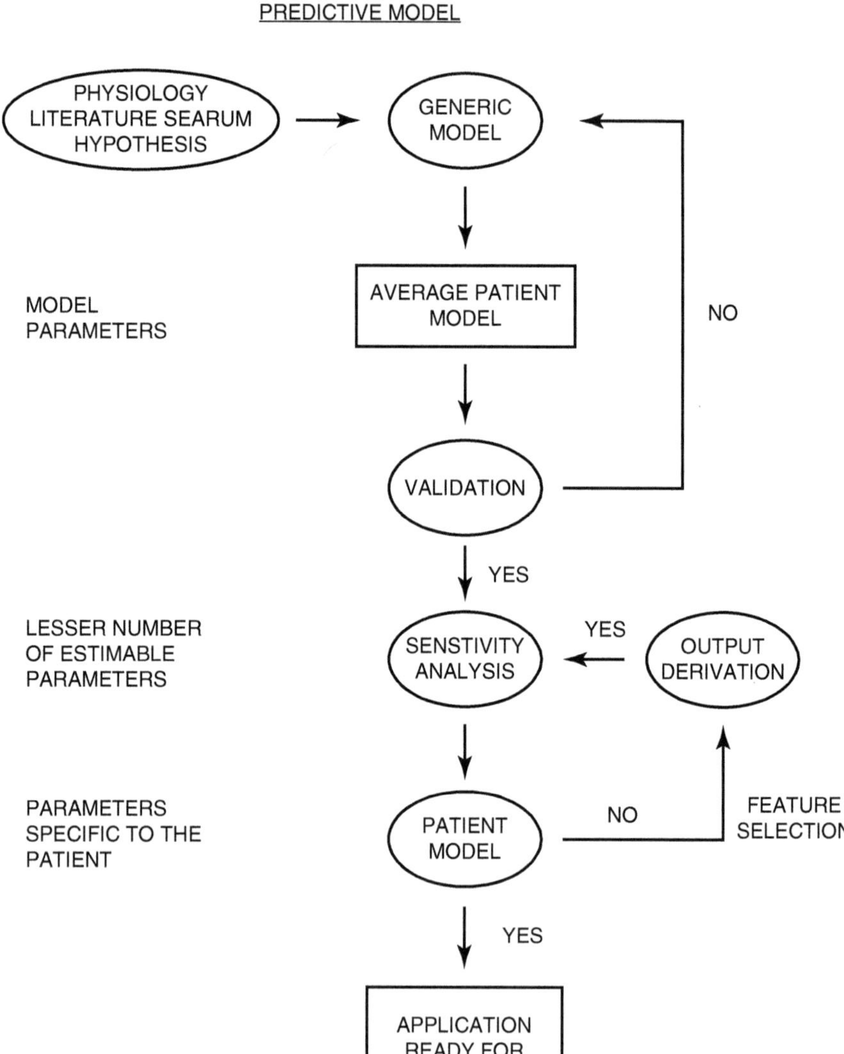

Fig. 4.2 Steps involved in the development of predictive model

4.5 Outcome Prediction in Adult Patients

The table below (Table 4.3) compares and contrasts the various severity assessment scores used in the ICU. It has been observed that general scoring systems calculated on the first day of ICU admission (APACHE, SAPS II, SOFA) provided fairly

Table 4.1 Causes of ICU admission in cancer patients

Early (between diagnosis to start of definitive therapy)	Intermediate (during intermediate therapy)	Late (after definitive therapy or in end stage disease)
• Sepsis • Metabolic & electrolyte disturbances • Neurological disorders	• Post operative • Sepsis • Tumor related complications • Treatment related complications • Heart failure • Renal failure	• Shock • Sepsis • Multiorgan failure • Palliative/End-of-life

Table 4.2 Differences in features and outcome between neutropenic and non-neutropenic sepsis

	Non- neutropenic	Neutropenic
Race	No predilection	More common in whites
Severity score	Usually lower	Usually higher
Bacteremia	Less common	More common
Shock at presentation	Uncommon	Common
Nature of malignancy	No predilection for any particular malignancy	More common in hematological malignancies
Diabetes	More common	Less common
Plasma protein	Lower IL-6, IL-8, G-CSF	Higher IL-6, IL-8, G-CSF
Risk of AKI	Lower	Higher
Mortality	Both 30 & 60 day mortality is lower	Both 30 and 60 day mortality higher

IL-6- Interleukin 6, IL-8- Interleukin 8, G-CSF- Granulocyte colony stimulating factor

accurate prediction about ICU mortality with good discrimination and acceptable calibration [3]. APACHE (most commonly APACHE II) is the preferred scoring system in most ICUs because of its easy comprehensibility, familiarity, capacity to allow comparisons between standardized mortality rates (SMR) over time and easier representation of lower standardized mortality rate (SMR), in case present. However there are some limitations too. The response of the physiological variables to treatment and resuscitation can fluctuate. In one study, APACHE II was predictive of 76.3% of non-survivors and 86.6% of survivors (overall accuracy, 81.8%); SOFA was predictive of 62.7% of non-survivors and 83.6% of survivors (accuracy, 73.8%); and SAPS II was predictive of 69.5% of non-survivors and 83.6% of survivors (accuracy, 77.0%) [3].

In another study, SOFA score had a strong prognostic accuracy for mortality in cancer with sepsis with an AUROC of 0.79 (95% of CI, 0.71–0.87). This was much above qSOFA which had an AUROC of 0.66 (95% CI, 0.56–0.75). However when lactate was added to qSOFA, its prognostic value improved to an AUROC of 0.77 (95% CI, 0.69–0.85) which was similar to SOFA [4].

SAPS II which has been found to be a good predictor of mortality after surgical resection of rectal carcinoma has also been tried in many ICUs. It has shown very

Table 4.3 A comparison of the different severity scores

Sl. No.	Characteristics	APACHE II	SAPS II	SOFA
1	Development	1985	1993	1996
2	Type	General risk prognostication score	General risk prognostication score	Organ dysfunction assessment score
3	Collection of data	First 24 h in ICU	First 24 h in ICU	First 24 h in ICU
4	Max Score	71	217	24
5	Selection of variables and their weights	Panel of experts	Multiple logistic regression analysis	Panel of experts
6	Age	Yes	Yes	No
	Surgical status	Yes	Yes	No
	Chronic health status	Yes	Yes	No
	Physiology	Yes	Yes	No
	GCS	No	No	Yes
	MAP	No	No	Yes
	Serum Creatinine	No	No	Yes
	Urine output	No	No	Yes
	$PaO_2/F iO_2$ ratio	No	No	Yes
	Mechanical ventilation	No	No	Yes
	Platelet Count	No	No	Yes
	Serum Bilirubin	No	No	Yes
7	Number of variables	17	17	7
8	Mortality prediction	YES	YES	YES

APACHE Acute Physiology and Chronic Health Evaluation, *SAPS* Simplified Acute Physiology Score, *SOFA* Sequential Organ Failure Assessment, *GCS* Glasgow Coma Scale, *MAP* Mean Arterial Pressure

good discrimination between survivors and non-survivors. Unfortunately it's used has been mostly confined to the surgical ICUs. Few studies have evaluated the performance of both APACHE II and SAPS II in the same population of critically ill cancer patients and found no major difference between the two while some have found the best variables predictive of ICU mortality to be ICM (ICU cancer mortality model) and APACHE II scores [5, 6]. Schellongowski et al. found that the ability of SAPS II to discriminate between survivors and non-survivors (AUROC, 0.82) was better than that of APACHE II (AUROC, 0.78). All scores had acceptable calibration, but the statistical significance for the Hosmer-Lemeshow goodness-of-fit tests was marginally better for SAPSII [7]. The importance of APACHE II has been further observed in determining the risk of flap failure in head and neck cancer patients undergoing microvascular surgery. The complications were less when the patients were managed in the critical care unit on the basis of their admission APACHE II score [8]. APACHE II score >10 and bilateral neck dissection ($RR = 3.57$; $p = 0.01$) has been found as risk factors for post operative complications in oral cancer and increased length of hospital stay [9].

Despite these observable differences, APACHE II and SAPS II are more often chosen for outcome prediction in critical care owing to their applicability in wide range of settings.

4.6 Outcome Prediction in Paediatric Malignancies

It has been reported that at least 1 in 3 or 4 children with cancer is admitted in the ICU at least once during their disease course. They are admitted due to cancer associated conditions viz. tumour lysis or treatment related complications viz. immunosuppression, infection etc. Mortality in the ICU is higher after haematological malignancies than solid tumours, in children with systemic infections and those presenting with organ failure [10, 11]. The Paediatric Risk of Mortality Score (PRISM) is a physiology based score developed and validated by Pollack and colleagues from the Physiologic Stability Index using 1415 patients from 9 PICUs in the United States between 1984 and 1985. The PRISM score consists of 14 physiological parameters, in comparison with 34 parameters in Physiologic Stability Index, recorded during the first 24 hours after admission to PICU [12]. Although three generations of PRISM score were subsequently developed and widely used in paediatric ICUs, their inaccuracies in oncology led to the advent of oncology PRISM (O-PRISM) consisting of the standard PRISM score in addition to other factors as graft versus host disease grade, C-reactive protein level, and macroscopic bleeding [13]. The choice of paediatric oncology ICU stay (POICU) as an outcome parameter found good correlation with both O-PRISM and PRISM III-12 scores. However inaccuracies still persist between these scores and crude mortality rates [14–16].

4.7 Conclusion

Since none of the prognostic factors are unequivocally predictive of outcome the search for predicting models is unending. Most models represent the population in which they have been developed and lack clarity about others. Therefore a periodic assessment of the predictive performance of the models is necessary for proper benchmarking. Furthermore, important ergonomic aspects viz. nurse: patient ratio & cost of ICU care needs incorporation for meticulous understanding of the merits and drawbacks.

References

1. Hensley MK, Donnelly JP, Carlton EF, Prescott HC. Epidemiology and outcomes of cancer-related versus non-cancer-related sepsis hospitalizations. Crit Care Med. 2019;47:1310–6.
2. Osmani AH, Jabbar AA, Gangwani MK, Hassan B. Outcomes of high risk patients with febrile neutropenia at a tertiary care Center. Asian Pac J Cancer Prev. 2017;18:2741–5.
3. Kopterides P, Liberopoulos P, Ilias I, Anthi A, Pragkastis D, Tsangaris I, Tsaknis G, Armaganidis A, Dimopoulou I. General prognostic scores in outcome prediction for cancer patients admitted to the intensive care unit. Am J Crit Care. 2011 Jan;20(1):56–66.

4. Chae BR, Kim YJ, Lee YS. Prognostic accuracy of the sequential organ failure assessment (SOFA) and quick SOFA for mortality in cancer patients with sepsis defined by systemic inflammatory response syndrome (SIRS). Support Care Cancer. 2020;28:653–9.
5. Sculier JP, Paesmans M, Markiewicz E, Berghmans T. Scoring systems in cancer patients admitted for an acute complication in a medical intensive care unit. Crit Care Med. 2000;28:2786–92.
6. Berghmans T, Paesmans M, Sculier JP. Is a specific oncological scoring system better at predicting the prognosis of cancer patients admitted for an acute medical complication in an intensive care unit than general gravity scores? Support Care Cancer. 2004;12:234–9.
7. Schellongowski P, Benesch M, Lang T, et al. Comparison of three severity scores for critically ill cancer patients. Intensive Care Med. 2004;30:430–6.
8. Grant CA, Dempsey GA, Lowe D, Brown JS, Vaughan ED, Rogers SN. APACHE II scoring for the prediction of immediate surgical complications in head and neck cancer patients. Plast Reconstr Surg. 2007;119:1751–8.
9. de Melo GM, Ribeiro KC, Kowalski LP, Deheinzelin D. Risk factors for postoperative complications in oral cancer and their prognostic implications. Arch Otolaryngol Head Neck Surg. 2001;127:828–33.
10. Faraci M, Bagnasco F, Giardino S, Conte M, Micalizzi C, Castagnola E, Lampugnani E, Moscatelli A, Franceschi A, Carcillo JA, Haupt R. Intensive care unit admission in children with malignant or nonmalignant disease: incidence, outcome, and prognostic factors: a single-center experience. J Pediatr Hematol Oncol. 2014;36:e403–9.
11. Diaz MA, Vicent MG, Prudencio M, Rodriguez F, Marin C, Serrano A, Sevilla J, Casado J, Madero L. Predicting factors for admission to an intensive care unit and clinical outcome in pediatric patients receiving hematopoietic stem cell transplantation. Haematologica. 2002;87:292–8.
12. Pollack MM, Ruttimann UE, Getson PR. Pediatric risk of mortality (PRISM) score. Crit Care Med. 1988;16:1110–6.
13. Schneider DT, Lemburg P, Sprock I, et al. Introduction of the oncological pediatric risk of mortality score (O-PRISM) for ICU support following stem cell transplantation in children. Bone Marrow Transplant. 2000;25:1079–86.
14. Pollack MM, Patel KM, Ruttimann UE. PRISM III: an updated Pediatric risk of mortality score. Crit Care Med. 1996;24:743–52.
15. Meyer S, Gottschling S, Biran T, et al. Assessing the risk of mortality in paediatric cancer patients admitted to the paediatric intensive care unit: a novel risk score? Eur J Pediatr. 2005;164:563–7.
16. Ehlenbach WJ, Cooke CR. Making ICU prognostication patient centered: is there a role for dynamic information? Crit Care Med. 2013;41:1136–8.

Clinical Imaging in Oncological ICU

5

Vijay Kubihal, S. H. Chandrashekhara, and G. S. Triveni

Imaging plays significant role in the management of critically ill cancer patients. It is essentially to establish diagnosis at ICU admission, and also to evaluate various catheters and tubes used in critically ill cancer patients [1, 2]. Two most commonly used modalities include portable radiography, and bedside ultrasonography (USG). In addition, computed tomography(CT), magnetic resonance imaging (MRI), and interventional radiological (IR) procedures may play a significant role in the management of special clinical scenarios [3–6].

5.1 Imaging Modalities

Commonly used imaging modalities in ICU setting include portable radiograph, bedside ultrasound (USG), computed tomography (CT), and magnetic resonance imaging (MRI) [7].

(a) Portable radiograph

Portable radiograph is the most commonly used modality in ICU patients. Bedside chest radiograph is most common radiograph performed. American college of radiology (ACR) recommendation for portable chest radiograph include (1) daily

V. Kubihal
Department of Radiodiagnosis, All India Institute of Medical Sciences New Delhi, New Delhi, India

S. H. Chandrashekhara (✉)
Department of Radiodiagnosis, IRCH, All India Institute of Medical Sciences New Delhi, New Delhi, India

G. S. Triveni
Department of Obstetrics and Gynaecology, Lady Hardinge Medical College, New Delhi, India

V. Kumar et al. (eds.), *Onco-critical Care*,
https://doi.org/10.1007/978-981-16-9929-0_5

chest radiograph in critically ill cancer patients requiring mechanical ventilation, and in ICU patients with cardiopulmonary disease; (2) immediate post procedure radiograph to access the position of central venous line, intercostal drainage tube, endotracheal tube, tracheotomy tube, and feeding tube [8]. Often, supine anteroposterior radiograph is only possible view in ICU patients, and carries few inherent limitations that include poor inspiratory effort, cardiac magnification, and difficulty in diagnosis of pleural effusion, pneumothorax, and pneumoperitoneum [7].

Abdominal radiograph is infrequently performed in critically ill cancer patients admitted to ICU. Common indications for abdominal radiograph include suspected bowel obstruction or bowel perforation [7].

(b) Bedside ultrasound (USG)

Bedside USG is a valuable tool in the management of critically ill cancer patients admitted to ICU. Advantages of USG include portability, easy availability, cheap, and lack of ionising radiation [7].

Point of care ultrasonography (POCUS) is performed by clinician at the patient's side, to answer the specific clinical question needed for immediate management of critically ill patients. Common indications for POCUS include identification and monitoring of shock, and fluid responsiveness, screening of extremities for deep vein thrombosis, chest USG to look for pneumothorax, or pleural effusion, and basic point of care cardiac evaluation. Though, POCUS by attending clinician plays very important role in the immediate management of critically cancer patients, it is not substitute for diagnostic USG by radiologist or cardiologist [7, 9, 10].

Common limitations to the use of USG in ICU settings include operator dependency, and high acoustic impedance by bowel gas, excess adipose tissue, bandages, and dressings [7].

(c) Computed tomography (CT)

CT is particularly important in specific clinical scenario, where it difficult to establish diagnosis by use of bedside radiograph or USG. It is particularly important in evaluation of pulmonary diseases, pulmonary thromboembolism, source of infection, central nervous system disorder, oncological emergencies, and post-operative complications. Although CT is excellent diagnostic modality, it's routine use in ICU patients is limited, as the patient needs to be shifted to radiology department for CT scan, which requires prior preparations, and skilled manpower. Even then, there is chance of complications during transit, or on table, and often times, the patients may be considered unsuitable to shift to the radiology department for CT scan. Also, critically ill cancer patients may commonly have impaired renal parameters, and use of intravenous iodinated contrast is contraindicated in such patients, unless haemodialysis is planned. Alternatively, non-contrast CT, USG, and non-contrast MRI can be done, depending on the clinical question that needs to be answered [7].

(d) Magnetic resonance imaging (MRI)

MRI has a very good soft tissue resolution, and is particularly very useful in evaluation of disorders of central nervous system, and hepatobiliary diseases, in the ICU setting. Limitations that prevent routine use of MRI in ICU setting include requirement to shift the patients to the MRI suite, requirement of non -ferromagnetic support, and monitoring devices, longer acquisition time, and difficulty in monitoring patients inside the MRI scanner [7].

5.2 Oncological and Non-oncological Emergencies Requiring ICU Admission in Cancer Patients

Common indications for ICU admission in cancer patients include post-operative recovery/complications, sepsis, respiratory failure, oncological emergencies, and bleeding complications [11]. Common diagnosis in cancer patients that may require admission to oncological ICU are discussed below.

5.2.1 Opportunistic Infections

Cancer patients are often prone to opportunistic infection, particularly of fungal origin, due to compromised immune system, that may result from chemotherapy, immunosuppressive therapy, or graft versus host disease [2]. Lung is the most common site of infection, and pneumonia is the common cause of death in cancer patients [12]. CT is the imaging modality of choice for evaluation of the source of sepsis, and diagnosis of lung infections [2].

Invasive pulmonary aspergillosis is common opportunistic infection, seen in ~1% to 8% of patients with solid tumour, and ~20–50% of patients with acute leukaemia. CT findings in invasive pulmonary aspergillosis include nodules or consolidation with adjacent ground glass opacity forming 'halo sign', and less commonly, central ground glass opacity with rim of consolidation forming 'reverse halo sign' (Fig. 5.1). Air crescent sign, that occurs due to necrosis with in nodule, can be seen in later stage of disease, and is considered as the sign of recovery, and good prognosis [2].

Pneumocystis jiroveci infection is another common opportunistic infection seen in immunocompromised cancer patients. CT findings of pneumocystis jiroveci pneumonia include bilateral ground glass opacity, predominantly in perihilar distribution, and lung cysts of variable size. 'Crazy paving' and consolidation may also be seen [2].

Neutropenic enterocolitis is an important opportunistic infection, particularly seen in patients with leukaemia, on cancer chemotherapy, or in patients with bone marrow transplantation. CT findings include wall thickening, and abnormal wall enhancement, particular affecting caecum, proximal ascending colon, and terminal

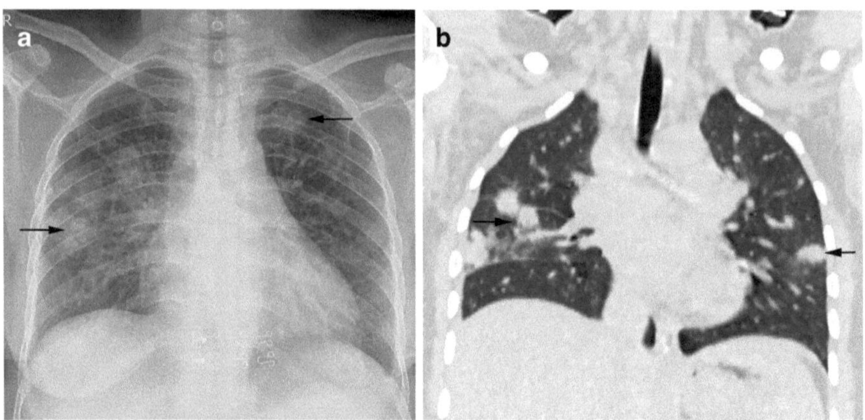

Fig. 5.1 Fungal pneumonia in a patient with AML. (**a**) Chest radiograph, PA view, and (**b**) coronal chest CT, lung window, shows multiple nodules (*black arrows*) in bilateral lungs with peripheral ground glass opacity s/o halo sign

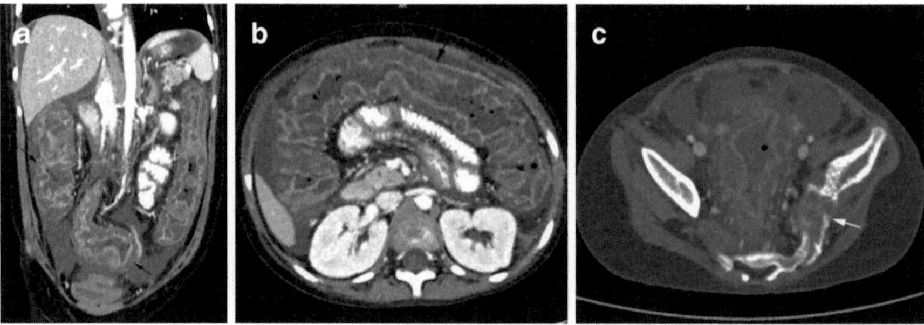

Fig. 5.2 Neutropenic enterocolitis in patient with iliac blade PNET, post chemotherapy. (**a**) Coronal contrast enhanced CT, and (**b**) axial contrast enhanced CT images show long segment bowel wall thickening and mural stratification, involving large bowel from caecum till rectum (*black arrows*). (**c**) axial bone window CT image shows expansile mass in the left iliac blade (*white arrow*). Ascites noted

ileum, along with inflammatory changes in adjacent fat (Fig. 5.2). Early diagnosis and effective treatment of this condition is required to prevent bowel wall necrosis, and perforation, and thus associated morbidity and mortality [13].

5.2.2 Intracranial Hypertension

Intracranial hypertension is serious complication that can occur in cancer patients either due to (1) extensive parenchymal metastasis, commonly from lung cancer, breast cancer, and melanoma (2) intra-tumour bleed with in hyper vascular metastasis, commonly from melanoma, renal cell carcinoma, and choriocarcinoma, (3) non communicating hydrocephalous from tumour obstructing fourth ventricle, aqueduct

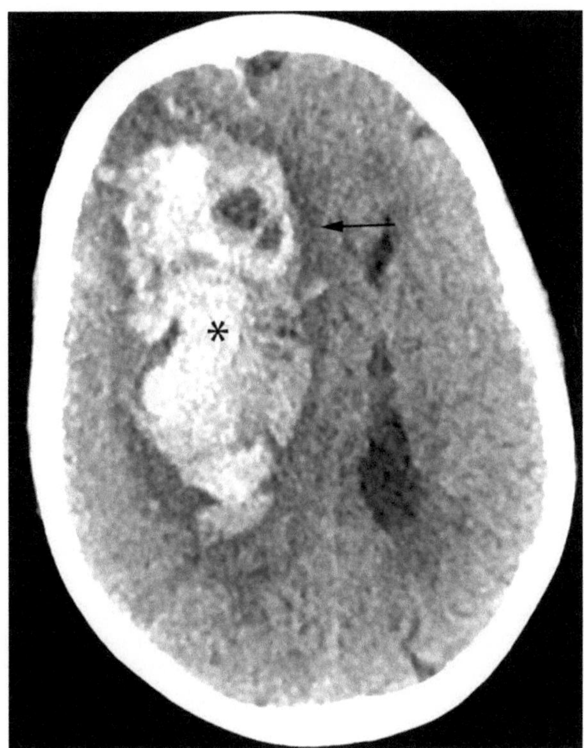

Fig. 5.3 Intracranial bleed in patient with CLL. Axial non-contrast CT image shows bleed with in right cerebral hemisphere (*black asterisk*), with significant midline shift towards the left side (*black arrow*)

of sylvius, and foramen of Monroe, (4) communicating hydrocephalous from diffuse leptomeningeal carcinomatosis [13] or (5) intracranial bleed due to cancer or cancer treatment related coagulopathy (Fig. 5.3).

CT is often the first imaging done to evaluate intracranial hypertension in critically ill cancer patients. It can demonstrate the presence of mass effect, herniation of brain parenchyma, acute intracranial haemorrhage, or hydrocephalous. MRI is the imaging modality of choice and is indicated when CT fails to establish the cause for intracranial hypertension [13].

5.2.3 Thoracic Emergencies

Common thoracic findings seen in critically ill cancer patients in oncological ICU include pleural effusion, pericardial effusion, pulmonary thromboembolism, airway obstruction, and drug induced pulmonary toxicity.

(1) Pleural effusion

Pleural effusion can be either of benign or malignant aetiology. Common benign causes include opportunistic infections, reduced oncotic pressure, and obstruction

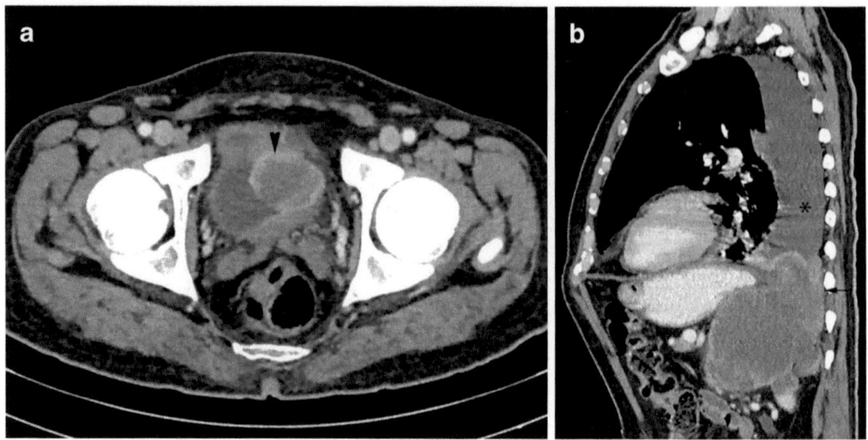

Fig. 5.4 Sub diaphragmatic deposit and pleural effusion in patient with carcinoma UB. (**a**) axial contrast enhanced CT, and (**b**) sagittal contrast enhanced CT images show enhancing UB mass (*black arrowhead*), with sub diaphragmatic deposit invading diaphragm (*black arrow*), and pleural effusion (*black asterisk*)

to lymphatic drainage from malignancy. Pleural spread of cancer, commonly of lung, breast or ovarian origin, results in malignant pleural effusion [13, 14].

Pleural effusion can often be seen on both chest radiograph and USG, while USG can also demonstrate complexity of effusion, and loculations, if present. Malignant pleural effusion can have similar appearance to simple benign pleural effusion on imaging. Malignant pleural effusion can sometimes be identified on CT by the presence of nodular or thick circumferential pleural thickening [13, 14] (Fig. 5.4)

(2) Pericardial effusion/cardiac tamponade

Pericardial effusion in cancer patients can be due to opportunistic infections, cancer chemotherapy or radiotherapy, or due to involvement by cancer itself, commonly from breast and lung cancers. Cardiac tamponade occurs when pericardial effusion is large enough to reduce venous return and thus, cardiac output [12, 14].

On chest radiograph, pericardial effusion causes globular cardiomegaly, with 'water bottle appearance' of cardiac silhouette. On USG, pericardial effusion is seen as anechoic space between heart and pericardium. Pericardial effusion is readily seen on CT (Fig. 5.5). Malignant pericardial effusion at times, can be seen as nodular pericardial thickening. On CT, presence of reflux into intravenous contrast into IVC, enlargement of IVC, hepatic veins, and SVC, and periportal portal oedema could point towards cardiac tamponade [12, 14].

(3) Pulmonary embolism (PE)

1–2.5% of cancer patients can develop PE [2]. Cancer patients are at increased risk of PE due to their hypercoagulable state, local tumour effects, cancer therapy

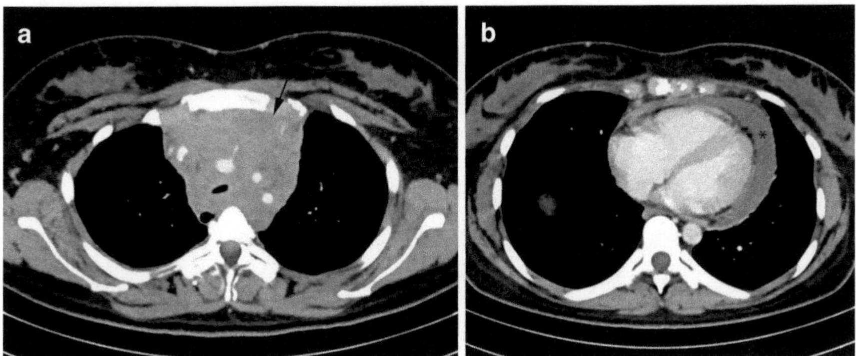

Fig. 5.5 Pericardial effusion in a patient with mediastinal lymphoma. (**a**) and (**b**) axial contrast enhanced CT images show infiltrating mediastinal mass, encasing trachea, and mediastinal vessels, and pericardial effusion

related factors, and prolonged immobilization. Patients with PE can be asymptomatic or may present with tachycardia, tachypnoea, dyspnoea, and chest pain. Cardiac failure can occur in patients with massive PE [2, 14].

Chest radiograph is insensitive technique to detect PE. However, there are certain radiographic sign that when present can sometimes help in early identification of PE. Common described signs of PE on chest radiograph include Hampton's hump seen as peripheral wedge shaped area of increased density due to lung infarction, Westermark sign seen as area of increased lucency distal to obstructed pulmonary artery, resulting from decreased pulmonary blood flow, Fleischner sign seen as enlargement of central pulmonary artery proximal to obstruction [2, 3]. USG evaluation of extremity veins can sometimes show deep venous thrombosis, which predisposes to PE [14]. PE in ICU patients is best evaluated with CT pulmonary angiogram. CT findings in acute PE include filling defect from thrombus with in pulmonary artery, having acute angles with the vessel wall, and 'polo mint' or 'tram track appearance' from contrast surrounding the acute thrombus (Fig. 5.6). Peripheral wedge shaped consolidation (pulmonary infarction) can sometimes be seen distal to obstructed pulmonary artery. In addition, features of right ventricular dysfunctions should be looked for, that include abnormal shape of interventricular septum, increased right ventricle diameter to left ventricle diameter ratio (>0.9–1.5), and contrast reflux into IVC. These when present can point towards the severe disease [2, 3].

(4) Airway obstruction

Airway obstruction can result from wither endoluminal or extraluminal pathology or both. Common endoluminal causes include bronchogenic carcinoma, primary tracheobronchial tumour (mucoepidermoid carcinoma, and adenoid cystic carcinoma), and carcinoid tumour. Extra luminal causes include compression of airway by large metastatic mediastinal lymph nodes, or from primary mediastinal

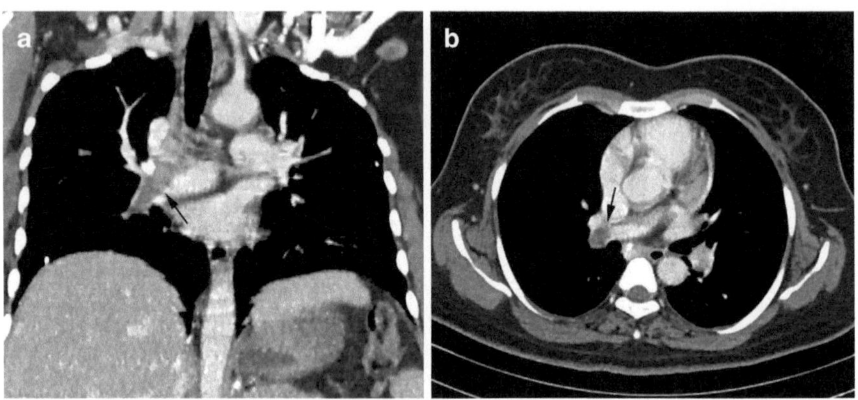

Fig. 5.6 Pulmonary thromboembolism in patient with endometrial carcinoma. (**a**) coronal, and (**b**) axial contrast enhanced CT images shows right pulmonary artery intraluminal filling defect suggestive of pulmonary thromboembolism

mass. Central airway obstruction can result in acute respiratory failure, whereas, bronchial and peripheral airway obstruction, often results in less severe symptoms from consolidation or atelectasis distal to obstruction [2, 12].

Chest radiograph can sometimes show mediastinal mass, tracheal deviation and airway narrowing. CT is the excellent imaging modality to evaluate airway obstruction, identify the cause, and to look at secondary findings in lung that such as consolidation or atelectasis distal to obstruction. Airway obstruction is best evaluated with bronchoscopy, which in addition to identifying the site of obstruction, can be used to obtain tissue sample, and stent placement, if required [2, 12].

(5) Drug related lung toxicity

10–20% of patients with cancer on anticancer therapy can develop drug related lung toxicity [2], either from direct pneumocyte injury (as seen with bleomycin) (Fig. 5.7), injury to vascular endothelium (as seen with docetaxel, and gemcitabine), or from autoimmune/hypersensitivity reaction (as seen with mTOR inhibitors, taxanes, and cyclophosphamide) [2].

Common patterns of drug related lung toxicity include diffuse alveolar damage (DAD), organising pneumonia, eosinophilic pneumonia, and diffuse pulmonary haemorrhage (DPH). Diffuse alveolar damage (DAD) often shows mid and lower zone predominance, and is characterised by diffuse or scattered ground glass opacity and interlobular septal thickening. Consolidation and pleural effusion can sometimes be seen. Organising pneumonia is often seen as patchy focal consolidation, predominantly in the peripheral or peri-bronchovascular distribution. Eosinophilic pneumonia is often characterised by homogeneous consolidation, with peripheral or upper zone predominance. Diffuse pulmonary haemorrhage (DPH) is often seen as diffuse ground glass opacity, with relative apical sparing, with or without consolidation or crazy paving pattern [2].

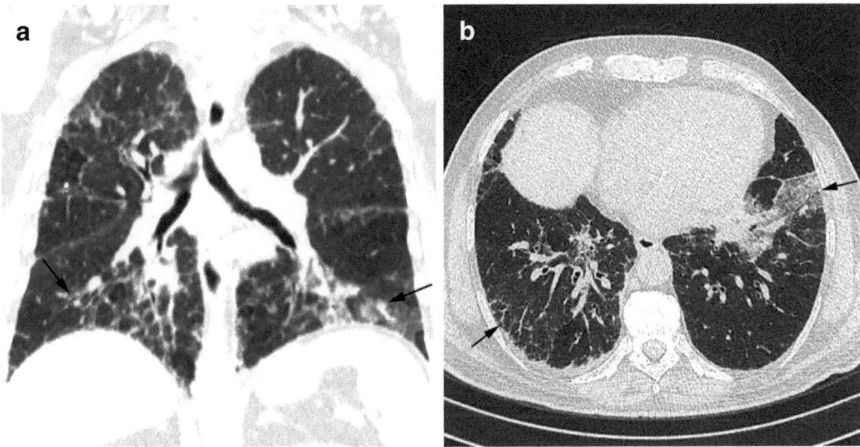

Fig. 5.7 Bleomycin toxicity in a patient with non-Hodgkin's lymphoma. (**a**) coronal, and (**b**) axial, lung window, CT images show reticulations and ground glass opacity in bilateral lungs, with basal predominance, consistent with bleomycin toxicity

5.2.4 Abdominal Emergencies

Common abdominal emergencies seen in critically ill cancer patients requiring admission to oncological ICU include intestinal obstruction, intestinal perforation, and bowel infarction.

(1) Intestinal obstruction

5–15% of cases of intestinal obstruction can be attributed to neoplastic aetiology [2]. Even in cancer patients, the two most common causes of intestinal obstruction are post-surgery adhesions, and inflammatory stricture. Malignant causes include primary bowel mass or extraluminal mass compromising bowel lumen. Also, functional bowel obstruction can be seen in cancer patients secondary to drugs (such as vinca alkaloids, and narcotics), peritonitis, and peritoneal carcinomatosis involving myenteric plexus [2, 12, 13].

In mechanical intestinal obstruction, abdominal radiograph can show gaseous distension of intestinal loops, with absent air in the intestinal loops distal to obstruction. Air fluid levels can be appreciated on lateral decubitus or erect abdominal radiograph. Functional intestinal obstruction is seen as dilatation of both small and large intestine, with no point of transition. CT is excellent modality to evaluate site, and cause of intestinal obstruction (Fig. 5.8) [2, 12, 13].

(2) Intestinal perforation

Perforation is one of the serious complication in gastrointestinal malignancy. It can be due to cancer necrosis, cancer chemotherapy or secondary to long standing intestinal obstruction [2, 12].

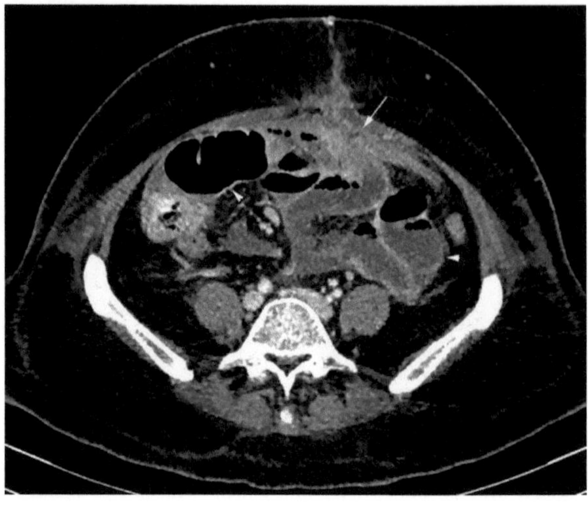

Fig. 5.8 Small bowel obstruction (*white arrow head*) in a patient with surgical site recurrence of carcinoma ovary (*white arrow*)

Often, erect chest radiograph or cross table abdominal radiograph are first investigation. It can sometimes show free peritoneal air. However, radiograph is limited in sensitivity for diagnosis of bowel perforation. CT is the investigation of choice. Direct signs seen on CT are bowel wall discontinuity, and free peritoneal air. Indirect signs of bowel perforation include abnormal wall enhancement, bowel wall thickening, and adjacent inflammatory changes or collection [2].

(3) Bowel infarction

Intestinal infarction in cancer patients can be due to mesenteric vessels thrombosis/embolism from hypercoagulable state, or direct vascular invasion by the mass. CT angiogram is the modality of choice. Mesenteric vessels, secondary bowel wall changes, and associated complications such as perforation, can be very well seen on CT [2].

5.2.5 Bleeding Complications

In cancer patients, bleeding complications can occur secondary to bleeding from highly vascular tumour, tumour breakdown and rupture, or due to associated coagulopathy. Massive haemoptysis, and severe intra-abdominal bleed, are the serious complications that can be seen in cancer patients. CT angiogram is the imaging modality of choice. It can demonstrate site, and cause of bleeding, and also allow assessment of supplying arteries, useful for planning embolization procedures, if need arises (Fig. 5.9) [13].

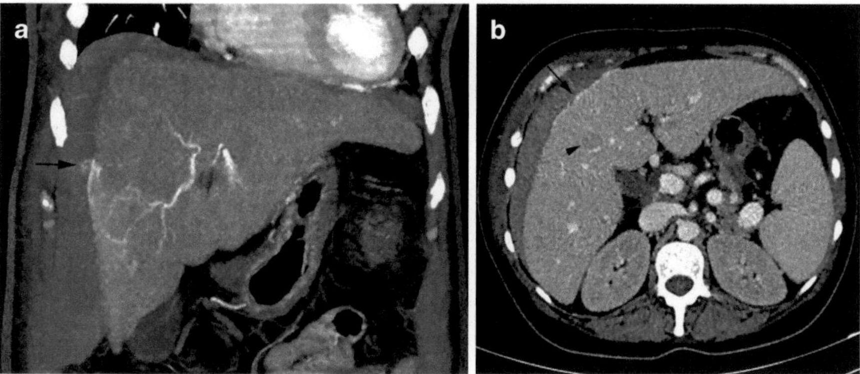

Fig. 5.9 Active biopsy site contrast extravasation in patient with multiple myeloma. (**a**) coronal maximum intensity projection, and (**b**) axial contract enhanced CT images show active extravasation (*black arrow*) from the liver surface, with adjacent hematoma. Multiple hypo enhancing liver lesions also noted

5.3 Evaluation of Catheters and Tubes Used in Critically Ill Cancer Patients

Various catheters and tubes are often used in management of cancer patients in oncological ICU. Imaging is essential to confirm their position and to detect any complications that can occur [3, 15]. Chest radiograph is most commonly used imaging modality for the purpose. Common catheters and tubes used in oncological ICU are briefly discussed below.

(1) Endotracheal (ET) tube

Normal position: ET tube should be seen with in tracheal lucency, with tip around 2–6 cms above the carina [3, 15] (Fig. 5.10).

Complications: Procedure related complication include wrong intubation into bronchus or oesophagus, tracheal perforation, and oesophageal perforation. Delayed complications include barotrauma, and tracheal stenosis [3, 15].

(2) Nasogastric (NG) tube

Normal position: NG tube is seen to course in the midline, across the diaphragm, with tip around 10 cms distal to GE (gastroesophageal) junction [3, 15].

Complications: Procedure related complications include malposition of NG tube beyond the stomach, coiled with in the mouth, or with in pleura, and oesophageal or enteric perforation. Delayed complications include aspiration, tube migration, and tube breakage [3, 15].

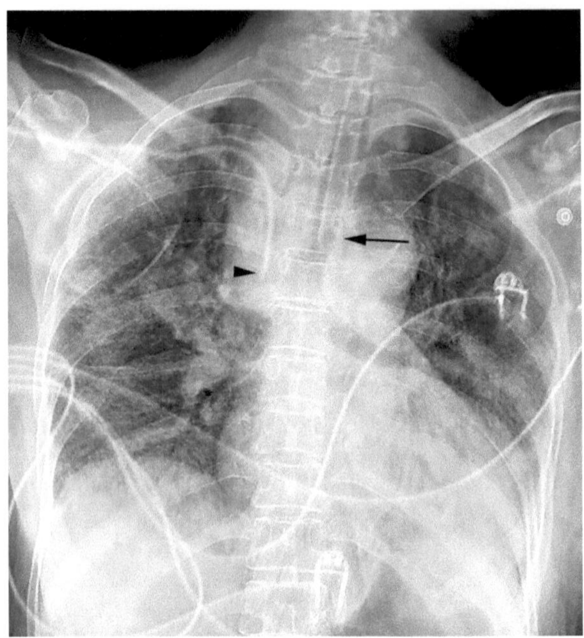

Fig. 5.10 Normal position of endotracheal tube with the tracheal lucency (*black arrow*) with tip 2 to 6cms above carina. Central is also noted with tip along the course of SVC (*black arrowhead*)

(3) Intercostal drainage (ICD) tube

Normal position: ICD tube should be seen with in pleural cavity, directed antero-superiorly in pneumothorax, and posteroinferiorly in pleural effusion [3, 15] (Fig. 5.11).

Complications: Procedure related complications include malposition of ICD tube with in lung parenchyma, mediastinum, pericardium, across the diaphragm, or with in subcutaneous tissue. Delayed complications include re-expansion pulmonary oedema [3, 15].

(4) Central venous line, or dialysis catheter

Normal position: central venous line or dialysis catheter are placed with in SVC, through internal jugular vein or subclavian vein, with tip at the cavo-atrial junction [3, 15].

Complications: Procedure related complications include incorrect placement with in the right atrium or ventricle, which can be potentially arrhythmogenic, in azygous vein, or with in extra-vascular space including pleura, mediastinum, and pericardium. Delayed complications include catheter migration, and thrombosis [3, 15].

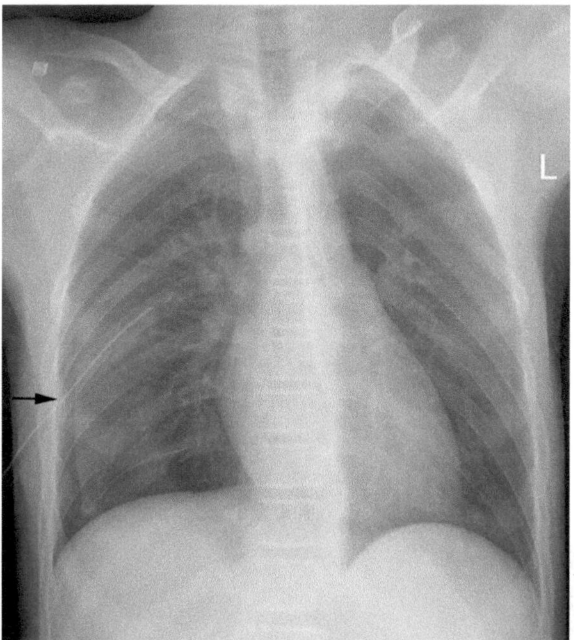

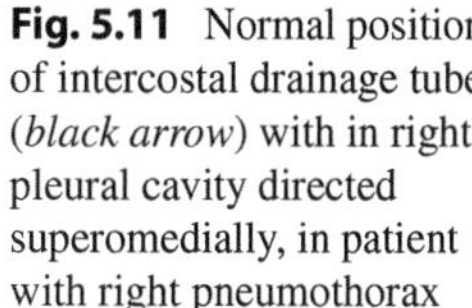
Fig. 5.11 Normal position of intercostal drainage tube (*black arrow*) with in right pleural cavity directed superomedially, in patient with right pneumothorax

5.4 Interventional Radiology (IR) in Management of Critically Ill Cancer Patients

IR procedures, either at bedside or at IR suite, can be very useful in the management of critically ill cancer patients [5, 6]. Common IR procedure performed in oncological ICU include

(1) Percutaneous drainage or aspiration of collection is recommended by society of cardiovascular and interventional radiology standards of practice committee, when there is suspicion of infected collection, or when the collection is large enough to cause significant symptoms, or when characterization of collections is necessary.
(2) Central venous line placement is the most common IR procedure in oncological ICU. It provides intermediate or long term vascular access for cancer chemotherapy, total parenteral nutrition, medications, and blood sampling. Even though, central venous line can be placed as blind procedure based on the anatomical landmarks, use of image guidance can significantly improve the success rate and reduce the complications.
(3) Embolization of bleeding artery can be done in case of severe bleeding complications of cancer.
(4) IV filter can be placed in critically ill cancer patients at risk of PE [5, 6].

5.5 Summary

Imaging plays a crucial role in everyday monitoring and management of cancer patients admitted in oncological ICU. Imaging is essential for diagnosis of oncological and non-oncological emergencies requiring admission to oncological ICU, and also to evaluate various catheters and tubes used in ICU. Portable radiograph and ultrasonography are the two commonly used imaging modalities in ICU patients, and computed tomography, and magnetic resonance imaging are often reserved for conditions that are not readily explained by radiograph or ultrasound. Interventional radiology procedures also play an important part in management of critically ill cancer patients. Thus, the multidisciplinary approach involving clinician and radiologist, is often required in the management of cancer patients admitted in oncological ICU.

References

1. Hill JR, Horner PE, Primack SL. ICU Imaging. Clin Chest Med. 2008 Mar;29(1):59–76.
2. Iacobellis F, Perillo A, Iadevito I, Tanga M, Romano L, Grassi R, et al. Imaging of oncologic emergencies. Semin Ultrasound CT MRI. 2018 Apr;39(2):151–66.
3. Lohan R. Imaging of ICU patients. In: Chawla A, editor. Thoracic imaging [Internet]. Singapore: Springer Singapore; 2019 [cited 2021 Jan 4]. p. 173–94. http://link.springer.com/10.1007/978-981-13-2544-1_7.
4. Maury E, Arrivé L, Mayo PH. Intensive care medicine in 2050: the future of medical imaging. Intensive Care Med. 2017 Aug;43(8):1135–7.
5. Nicolaou S, Talsky A, Khashoggi K, Venu V. Ultrasound-guided interventional radiology in critical care. Crit Care Med. 2007;35(Suppl):S186–97.
6. O'Neill SB, O'Connor OJ, Ryan MF, Maher MM. Interventional radiology and the care of the oncology patient. Radiol Res Pract. 2011;2011:160867.
7. Porté F, Basit R, Howlett D. Imaging in the intensive care unit. Surg Oxf. 2009;27(11):496–9.
8. Godoy MCB, Leitman BS, de Groot PM, Vlahos I, Naidich DP. Chest radiography in the ICU: part 1, evaluation of airway, enteric, and pleural tubes. Am J Roentgenol. 2012;198(3):563–71.
9. Johnson GGRJ, Kirkpatrick AW, Gillman LM. Ultrasound in the surgical ICU: uses, abuses, and pitfalls. Curr Opin Crit Care. 2019;25(6):675–87.
10. Choi WJ, Ha YR, Oh JH, Cho YS, Lee WW, Sohn YD, et al. Clinical guidance for point-of-care ultrasound in the emergency and critical care areas after implementing insurance coverage in Korea. J Korean Med Sci. 2020;35(7):e54.
11. Kostakou E, Rovina N, Kyriakopoulou M, Koulouris NG, Koutsoukou A. Critically ill cancer patient in intensive care unit: issues that arise. J Crit Care. 2014;29(5):817–22.
12. Handa A, Nozaki T, Makidono A, Okabe T, Morita Y, Fujita K, et al. Pediatric oncologic emergencies: clinical and imaging review for pediatricians. Pediatr Int. 2019;61(2):122–39.
13. Guimaraes MD, Bitencourt AG, Marchiori E, Chojniak R, Gross JL, Kundra V. Imaging acute complications in cancer patients: what should be evaluated in the emergency setting? Cancer Imaging. 2014;14(1):18.
14. Gaunt T, D'Arco F, Smets AM, McHugh K, Shelmerdine SC. Emergency imaging in paediatric oncology: a pictorial review. Insights Imaging. 2019;10(1):120.
15. Bentz MR, Primack SL. Intensive care unit imaging. Clin Chest Med. 2015;36(2):219–34.

Role of Point of Care Ultrasound in Oncocritical Care Unit

6

Ridhima Bhatia, Damarla Haritha, and Puneet Khanna

6.1 Introduction

The use of ultrasound is rapidly gaining popularity in all areas including emergency department, operation theatre and intensive care units (ICU). Not only, it is rapid, non-invasive, inexpensive but also can be easily performed bedside without exposure to radiations, thus, making it ideal to use in unstable patient.

Historically, ultrasound was used only by the radiologists. However, with the advancement in the technology and more compact nature of the equipment lead to the emergence of Point-of-care (POC) ultrasound which is defined as bed side ultrasonography performed by the clinician to understand the hemodynamic condition in real time.

According to the previous studies, use of ultrasound in the emergency department has shown to improve diagnostic accuracy and decrease time to consultation and length of stay in the emergency department. In addition, POC ultrasound has been useful in management of critical conditions including pericardial effusion, pulmonary embolism, cardiac arrest and sepsis. Furthermore, use of ultrasound for procedural guidance has proven to be cost-effective with decreased complication rates and improved patient safety.

This real time imaging aids in quick diagnosis and management of the patients in the critical care setting avoiding the potential harm of transporting the patient, thus, making POCUS standard of care in the ICU. POCUS can be divided into single-targeted ultrasound examinations (STU, one or two scanning sites) and multiple-targeted ultrasound examinations (MTU) depending on the purpose (Fig. 6.1). This

R. Bhatia
Fortis Hospital, Faridabad, India

D. Haritha · P. Khanna (✉)
All India Institute of Medical Sciences, New Delhi, India

V. Kumar et al. (eds.), *Onco-critical Care*,
https://doi.org/10.1007/978-981-16-9929-0_6

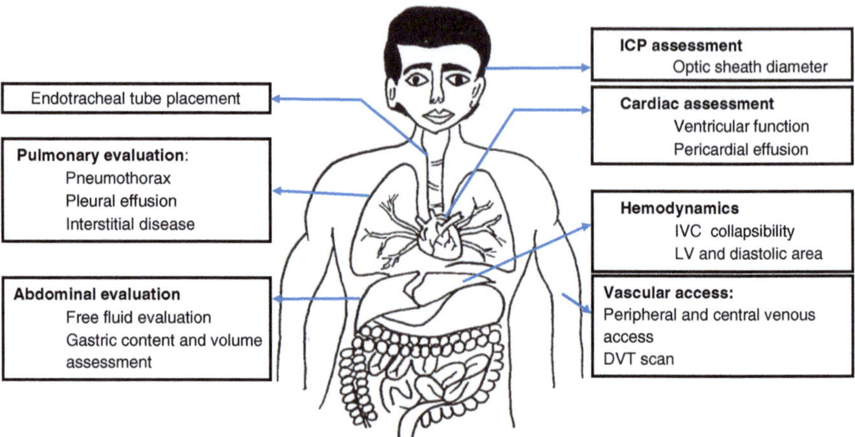

Fig. 6.1 Sites of POCUS Examination

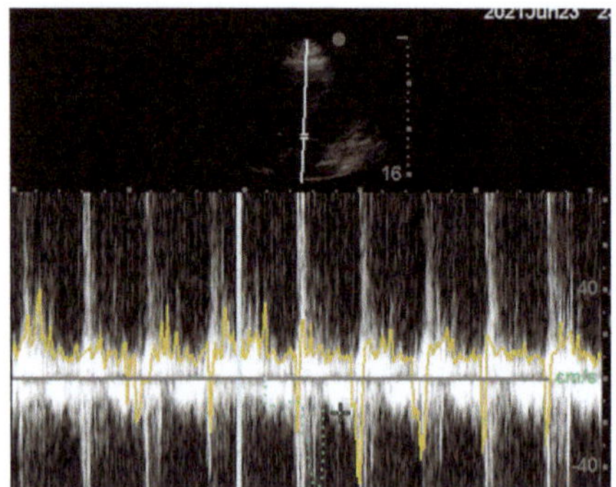

Stroke volume (SV) = Cross sectional area of LV outflow tract * Velocity time integral of LV Cardiac output = SV * Heart rate

Fig. 6.2 Velocity time integral of Left ventricle to estimate cardiac output

chapter shall briefly discuss the role of POCUS in managing critically ill oncologic patients

6.2 Single Targeted Ultrasound Examination

6.2.1 Point-of-Care Cardiac Ultrasound

The point-of-care echocardiography (POCE) is used for rapid assessment of cardiac anatomy and function in the critically ill patient. The examination includes five standard views including parasternal long axis, parasternal short axis, apical four chamber, subcostal and suprasternal notch views and can be performed in few minutes (Fig. 6.2).

POCE allows the immediate recognition of life-threatening emergencies such as pericardial effusion, cardiac tamponade and aid in the management (pericardiocentesis). Furthermore, bed side echo can be used to assess the cardiac anatomy, a global contractility and the hemodynamic status such as preload, cardiac activity and afterload. Subsequently, this forms the basis of goal directed fluid therapy. The common findings suggestive of hypovolemia include a small calibre inferior vena cava (<2 cm diameter) which collapses during inspiration and vigorous, hyperkinetic contractions obliterating the ventricles in systole.

Other uses of echocardiography include monitoring the evolution of disease, to observe the response to potentially therapeutic interventions, such as inotropic drugs, and to search for new problems that arise during the course of a critical illness.

6.2.2 Thoracic Ultrasound

Thoracic ultrasound is usually performed on patients in respiratory failure in the critical care setting. Not only it is fast, safe and cheaper, but also more informative compared with anteroposterior chest radiograph and equally effective as chest tomography. It can be used to diagnose various causes of dyspnea including pneumothorax, pleural effusion, cardiogenic and non-cardiogenic pulmonary edema, alveolar consolidation (Acute respiratory distress, pneumonia, atelectasis) or any combination.

Ever since the introduction of Bedside Lung Ultrasound in Emergency (BLUE) protocol in 2008 by intensivist Daniel Lichtenstein, several studies have proven the effectiveness of lung ultrasound in many clinical scenarios (Flowchart 6.1). POC thoracic ultrasound is nearly 100% sensitive for the diagnosis of pneumothorax and more accurate in quantifying the pleural effusion.

In his protocol Lichtenstein describes the basic lung ultrasound findings used in the ICU. *A-lines* are the horizontal repetitions of the pleural lines (Figs. 6.3 and 6.4). Presence of these along with the *lung sliding* indicates that the visceral pleural surface is moving freely with respiration against the parietal pleura, and defines a normal aeration pattern. Also, lung sliding rules out a pneumothorax with a negative predictive value of 100% at the site of the ultrasound probe. However, presence of *lung point*, that is the point where normal pleural interface contacts the boundary of the pneumothorax, is 100% specific for pneumothorax (Fig. 6.5).

The other type of lines seen are hyperechoic comet tail artifacts called *B-lines,* which appear due to edematous interlobar septa and indicate the presence of an *alveolar interstitial syndrome*. Bilateral, multiple B-lines usually stipulate pulmonary edema and whereas, unilateral indicate mostly infection. As B-lines are dynamic and disappear with the improvement of the underlying process, repeat ultrasound exams can be used to monitor a patient's response to treatment.

Next, thoracic ultrasound can be used to detect alveolar consolidations which appear similar to the liver, a pattern referred to as *hepatisation of the lung*.

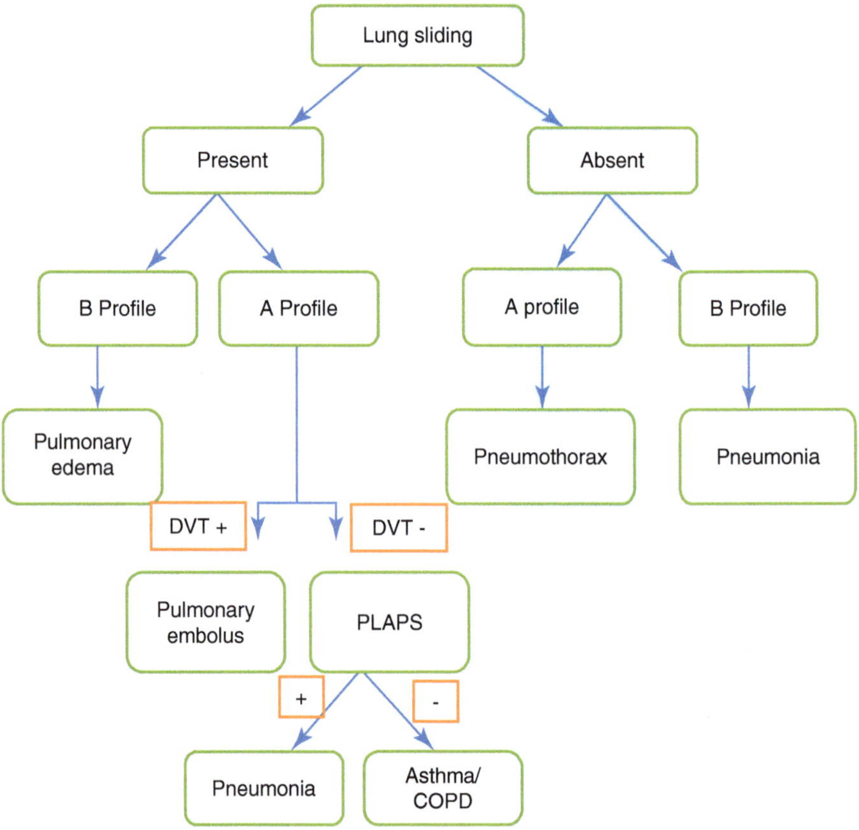

- Lung sliding
  - Present
    - B Profile → Pulmonary edema
    - A Profile
      - DVT + → Pulmonary embolus
      - DVT - → PLAPS
        - + → Pneumonia
        - - → Asthma/ COPD
  - Absent
    - A profile → Pneumothorax
    - B Profile → Pneumonia

Flowchart 6.1 BLUE Protocol

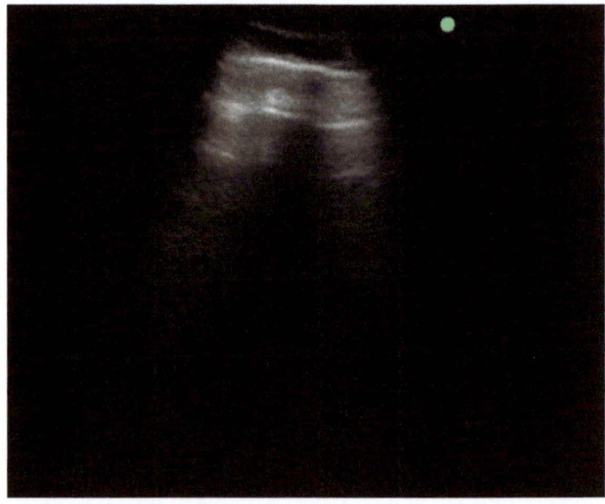

Fig. 6.3 A lines in Lung ultrasound

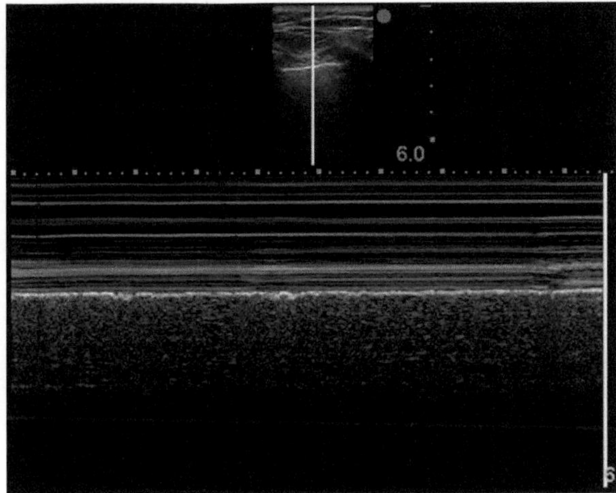

Fig. 6.4 Seashore sign—Normal pleura on M mode

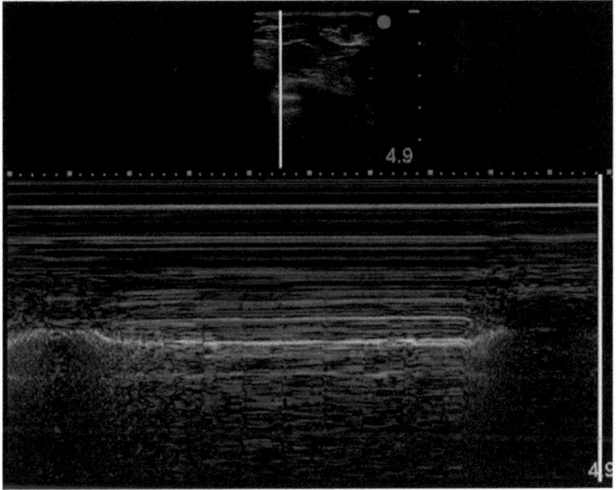

Fig. 6.5 Barcode sign in pneumothorax

Furthermore, profiles defined in the BLUE-protocol by Lichtenstein aid in rapid diagnosis of the common causes of acute respiratory failure with an accuracy >90%.

6.2.3 Evaluation of DVT and Pulmonary Embolism

Deep Vein Thrombosis (DVT) and pulmonary embolism are a frequent cause of morbidity and mortality in the ICU. The diagnosis of DVT can be rapidly made using the two-dimensional compression ultrasound without a Doppler study.

Thrombus in a vein typically appears as an intraluminal echogenic focus with non-compressible walls. However, fresh, immature thrombi may not be echogenic, and thus, the primary diagnostic criteria is a lack of vessel compressibility and not visualisation of the thrombus.

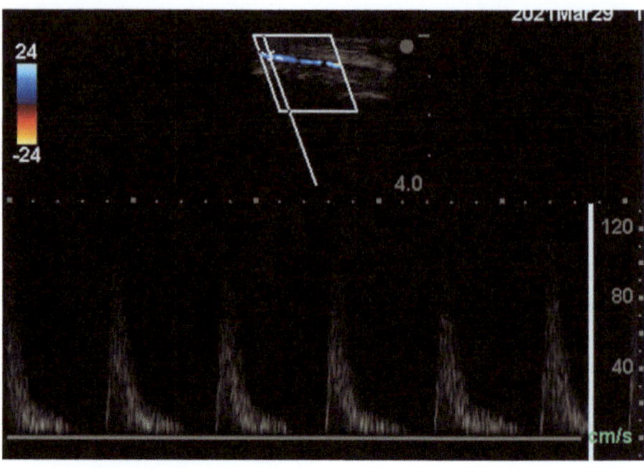

Fig. 6.6 Normal Doppler in femoral vessels

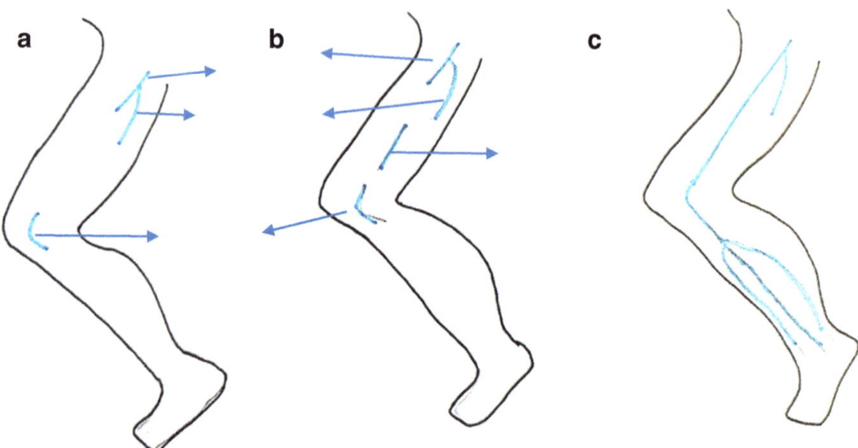

Fig. 6.7 (**a**) 2-point leg USG, (**b**) 3-point leg USG, (**c**) whole leg USG

Enlarged right ventricle, D-shaped left ventricle and the presence of DVT in a hypotensive patient suggests pulmonary embolism (Figs. 6.6 and 6.7).

6.2.4 Abdominal Ultrasound

Fluid responsiveness can be assessed using the changes in the diameter of inferior vena cava along with respiration by placing a phased array probe in the subcostal view of cardiac ultrasound (Fig. 6.8). The IVC diameter is measured at maximum and minimum and calculated using the following formula.

$$IVC\ collapsibility = IVC_{\text{max}} - IVC_{\text{min}} / IVC_{\text{max}}$$

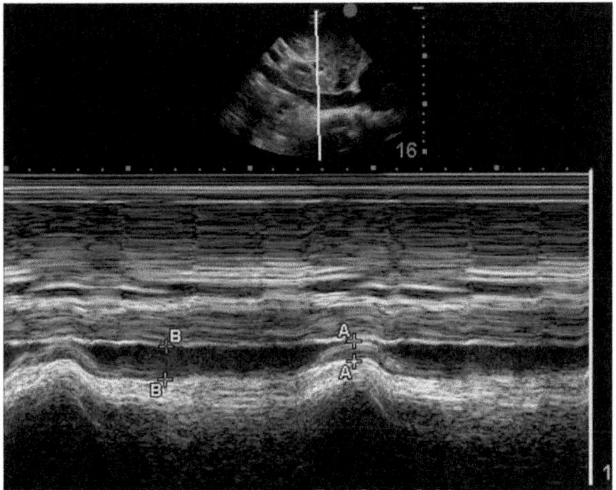

Fig. 6.8 IVC distensibility

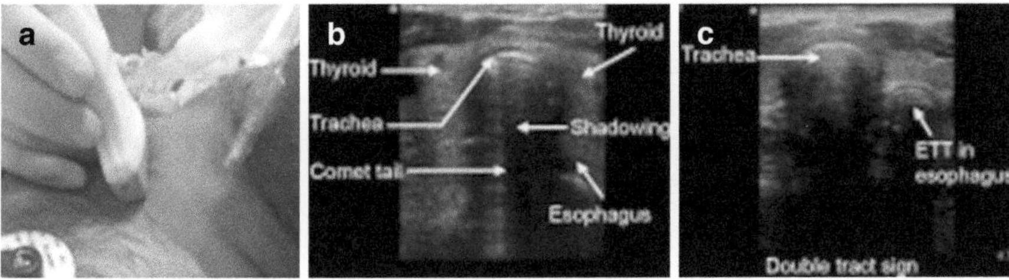

Fig. 6.9 (**a**) Transverse probe just above the suprasternal notch; (**b**) Normally trachea appears as hyperechoic curve with artifact (comet tail) and shadowing. The esophagus is usually seen more distally and on side of the screen as an oval structure with hypoechoic center and a hyperechoic wall; and (**c**) Intubation of esophagus reveals an adjacent hyperechoic curvilinear structure with comet tail artifact and shadowing, consistent with endotracheal tube in the esophagus. This has been referred to as the "double tract sign"

6.2.5 Ultrasound Guided Procedures

Application of ultrasound in the *neurological setting* includes: B-mode sonography to monitor hydrocephalus and intracranial hemorrhage, transcranial Doppler (TCD) for diagnosing brain death, and transcranial color-coded sonography to monitor cerebral autoregulation and intracranial pressure. Ultrasonography can be employed for clinical decision-making, intervention for airway management and for assessing pathology of the upper and lower airways. It can also be used to confirm the position of endotracheal tube (Fig. 6.9).

6.2.6 Soft Tissue and Musculoskeletal Ultrasound

Musculoskeletal ultrasound is a rapid, sensitive technique and better technique compared to radiograph for detecting the presence of joint effusions. Also,

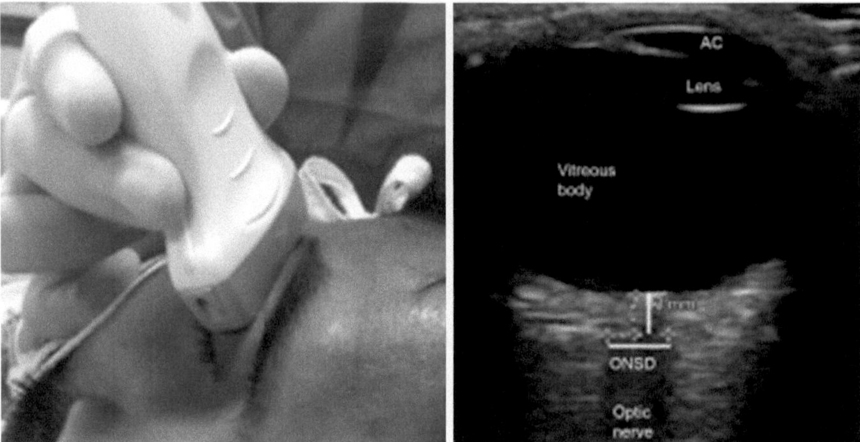

Fig. 6.10 Measuring ONSD

ultrasound can be used for arthrocentesis. Additionally, it can be used to diagnose some fractures including injuries that are difficult to diagnose using conventional radiography, such as scaphoid, sternum and occult rib and to identify radiolucent foreign materials such as glass or wood.

6.2.7 Ocular Ultrasound

The common use of ocular POCUS in the ICU is to determine optic sheath nerve diameter (ONSD) as an indicator of increased intracranial pressure. Based on the concept that the optic nerve is an extension of the central nervous system, the technique was first described by Helmke and Hansen in 1997. ONSD is determined using 7.5 MHz US probe placed on the superior and lateral aspect of the orbit and angled caudally and medially (Figure). The nerve is visualised as a hypoechoic structure just posterior to the globe (Figure). After identification of the nerve, the optic nerve sheath diameter (ONSD) is measured. A "normal" ONSD on ocular US is <5 mm for adults, <4.5 mm for children aged 1–15 years old, and <4 mm for infants. 67 Values above the stated ONSD are considered abnormal. The sensitivity and specificity of ocular US and abnormal ONSD based on multiple studies are 77–100% and 63–100%, respectively (Fig. 6.10).

6.3 Multiple Targeted Ultrasound Examination

6.3.1 POCUS in Cardiac Arrest

POCUS has become a common prognostic and diagnostic tool during cardiac resuscitation, particularly when combined with rhythm strip data. The transthoracic cardiac ultrasound should be performed within 10 s of stopping chest compressions for a pulse check and not cause delays in chest compressions. If the heart cannot be visualized within seconds after the chest compressions are stopped, POCUS should be aborted and reattempted after 5 cycles of compression. The first recommended approach is subcostal followed by parasternal and apical.

POCUS examinations of the thorax, abdomen, and inferior vena cava can be performed during chest compressions. In patients with pulseless electrical activity (PEA) in particular, it can prove to be helpful in revealing anatomic causes of PEA such as tension pneumothorax, cardiac tamponade and pulmonary embolism. For instance, presence of increased right ventricular strain, new tricuspid regurgitation, pericardial effusion or absence of lung sliding can direct towards the reversible cause of PEA, thus rapidly directing the intensivist to perform tube thoracostomy, pericardiocentesis or thrombolysis.

In addition, POCUS during cardiac arrest can be used for prognosis. Various studies have shown that the absence of any organized systolic contractions after three rounds of advanced cardiac life support medications suggests a minimal likelihood of return of spontaneous circulation. Subsequently, this intra-arrest information can help guide the resuscitation timeline and appropriate use of the resources.

6.3.2 POCUS in Shock

POCUS in the undifferentiated shock patient can help in the rapid differentiation between the major shock types: distributive (i.e., septic), cardiogenic, hypovolemic (i.e., bleeding or other volume loss), and obstructive. To standardize this assessment, there are several scan protocols which mostly involve the ultrasound imaging of the heart, the lungs, the vena cava and a focused assessment of the abdomen to look for free fluid. Table 6.1 summarizes the sonographic findings in various kinds of shock. In a study by Atkinson et al, early multisystem POC ultrasound improved diagnostic accuracy of the treating physician in the first 15 min of patient presentation by 30%. Recognising the type of shock can further help in guiding the management such as fluids, vasopressors etc.

Table 6.1 Sonographic findings in major shocks

	Distributive shock	Cardiogenic shock	Hypovolemic shock	Obstructive shock
Cardiac findings	Spectrum from hyperdynamic to decreased left ventricular function	Decreased left ventricular function	Hyperdynamic	Dilated right ventricle or pericardial effusion
Inferior Vena Cava findings	Range from collapsible to dilated	Non-collapsible	Collapsible	Non-collapsible
Lung findings	Negative	B lines present	Negative	Focal or Negative
Abdominal findings	Negative	Negative	Evaluate for hemorrhage	Negative

To conclude, Point-of-care ultrasound is evolving as a practice changing technology to care for the critically ill patient. The ability to look inside the human body in real time without the risk of radiation helps intensivists narrow the differential diagnoses, initiation of proper management, and thus improving the overall patient care.

Suggested Reading

Adhikari S, Amini R, Stolz LA, Blaivas M. Impact of point-of-care ultrasound on quality of care in clinical practice. Rep Med Imaging. 2014;7:81–93.

Balmert N, Espinosa J, Arafeh MO, Costello J, Markle S. Integration of bedside ultrasound into the ICU—a review of indications, techniques and interventions. J Emerg Crit Care Med. 2018;2:17.

Choi WJ, Ha YR, Oh JH, Cho YS, Lee WW, Sohn YD, Cho GC, Koh CY, Do HH, Jeong WJ, Ryoo SM. Clinical guidance for point-of-care ultrasound in the emergency and critical care areas after implementing insurance coverage in Korea. J Kor Med Sci. 2020;35(7)

Melgarejo S, Schaub A, Noble VE. Point of care ultrasound: an overview. American College of Cardiology. 2019.

Sobczyk D, Nycz K, Andruszkiewicz P, Weirzbicki K, Stapor M. Ultrasonic Caval indices do not significantly contribute to predicting fluid responsiveness immediately after coronary artery bypass grafting when compared to passive leg raising. Cardiovasc Ultrasound. 2016;14:23.

Zaidi G. Point-of-Care Ultrasonography in Critical Care. Curr Pulmonol Rep. 2017;3:161–3.

7 Analgesia in Oncology Critical Care

Madan Narayanan and Tim Keady

7.1 Incidence

Patients suffering from cancer often require admission to intensive care unit (ICU) either primarily due to the malignancy, to the treatment of the primary condition (surgery, chemotherapy) or complications either of the primary disease process (e.g., metastasis) or treatment (e.g., pulmonary complications, neutropenic sepsis, drug toxicity).

Pain is defined as an unpleasant sensory and emotional experience associated with actual or potential tissue damage or described in terms of such damage [1]. Though not specific to the cancer population, as high as 70% of patients report experiencing pain during their treatment in the general intensive care [2].

7.2 Causes of Pain

Pain could be present at rest or induced during interventions. The causes of pain in ICU are summarised in Table 7.1. Factors like young age, prior surgery, pre-existing anxiety or depression, number of comorbidities, length of ICU stay are predictors of higher self-reported pain intensity. Of all interventions, arterial catheter insertion, chest or wound drain removal, turning and repositioning, and tracheal suctioning are associated with the greatest increase in pain intensity [3].

M. Narayanan (✉)
Consultant in Anaesthesia & Intensive Care, Frimley Park Hospital NHS Foundation Trust, Surrey, UK

T. Keady
Clinical Fellow Anaesthesia and Intensive Care, Frimley Park Hospital NHS Foundation Trust, Surrey, UK

V. Kumar et al. (eds.), *Onco-critical Care*,
https://doi.org/10.1007/978-981-16-9929-0_7

Table 7.1 Causes of pain in ICU

Specific to intensive care	• Interventions—endotracheal intubation, tracheostomy, central/arterial lines, chest drains, dressing changes, urinary catheters, nasogastric tubes • Routine care—position changes, physiotherapy, endotracheal suctioning
Medical conditions	• Pneumonia—pleuritic chest pain • Myocardial infarction/angina • Abdominal pathology—cholecystitis, pyelonephritis, peritonitis, pancreatitis • Pre-existing arthritis
Postoperative	• Surgical incisions • Abdominal/chest drains
Neuropathic pain	• Infiltrative disease, pressure effect (e.g., lymph nodes, Pancoast tumor) • Cancer chemotherapy • Paraneoplastic syndromes • Phantom pain syndromes
Metastasis	• Bony metastatic deposits • Pathologic fractures

Table 7.2 Deleterious effects of uncontrolled pain on organ systems

System	Effect
Cardiovascular	• Sympathoadrenal stimulation—tachycardia, hypertension • Increased myocardial oxygen consumption • Myocardial ischaemia (in susceptible patients)
Respiratory	• Hyper/hypo ventilation • Atelectasis • Pulmonary complications
Neurology	• Poor sleep • Agitation/delirium
Psychology	• Transition to chronic pain • Post-traumatic stress disorder • Depression/anxiety
Metabolic	• Systemic inflammatory response • Increased catabolism • Hyperglycemia • Immunosuppression • Hypercoagulability • Impaired wound healing
Patient experience	• Increased length of hospital and ICU stay • Poor experience

7.3 Short- and Long-Term Consequences of Untreated Severe Pain

Pain is widely regarded as the fifth vital sign, and it induces a myriad of deleterious physiological changes in most organ systems (Table 7.2). The deleterious effects stem from sympathoadrenal stimulation and triggering the systemic inflammatory response. Poorly recognised and managed pain can lead to worse patient outcomes both in the short and long term.

7.4 Assessment of Pain in ICU

Less than 50% of intensive care professionals assess pain and even when it is done, the assessment is infrequent [4]. Pain assessment in mechanically ventilated patients is independently associated with a reduction in the duration of ventilator support and of duration of ICU stay [5]. Lack of training in assessment of pain is the commonly cited factor for poor pain management.

Studies evaluating the validity of vital signs for pain assessment produced inconsistent results, and in the general ICU patients, there was no observed association between vital sign changes and patient self-reported pain scores. Hence, vital signs should not be used alone to assess pain in critically ill adults [6].

Pain scoring systems for use in ICU have been adapted and used as a continuum from their perioperative use. The choice of the appropriate scale depends on the sedation levels and the ability of the patient to communicate.

The pain scales commonly used in ICU in patients:

Who are able to communicate:

(i) Visual Analogue scale (VAS): Patients mark their pain on a 100 mm horizontal line, with verbal descriptors at each end (0: no pain; 100: very severe pain). The score is obtained by measuring the distance in millimetres from the left end of the line.

(ii) Numerical Rating Scale (NRS): Patients rate pain on an 11-point scale (0: no pain; 10: severe pain).

(iii) Verbal Descriptor Scale (VDS): patients rate their pain as none, mild, moderate, severe or extreme.

Who are unable to communicate:

(i) Behavioural Pain Scale (BPS): this scale uses clinical observations of facial expression, upper limb movements, and synchrony with mechanical ventilation. BPS ranges from 3 to 12, scores >6 require pain management (Table 7.3) [4].

(ii) Critical Care Pain Observation Tool (CPOT): the scale uses a four-component clinical observation of: facial expression, body movements, muscle tension, and compliance with the ventilator for intubated patients or vocalization for extubated.

In ICU patients who are able to communicate, the NRS in the visual format is the best self-reported pain scale and the VDS should be considered in patients unable to use numerical scales. The CPOT and the BPS remain the best validated and robust scales for assessing pain in critically ill adults unable to self-report. In deeply sedated and paralyzed patients, newer approaches like heart rate variability

Table 7.3 The behavioural pain scale [4]

Clinical observation	Score
Facial expression	
• Relaxed • Partially tense • Totally tense • Grimace	1 2 3 4
Movement of upper limbs	
• Relaxed • Partially flexed • Totally flexed • Totally contracted	1 2 3 4
Mechanical ventilation	
• Tolerating movements • Coughing but tolerating most of the time • Fighting the ventilator • Impossible to control ventilation	1 2 3 4

Reproduced with kind permission from Woulters Kluwer Health

(Analgesia Nociception Index) and pupillary size (Pupillary Pain Index) are being explored, but they require validation prior to clinical implementation.

7.5 Pharmacotherapy

The choices for management of pain in ICU can be classified as systemic and locoregional techniques depending on the aetiology of the pain. A multimodal approach employing both systemic and loco-regional techniques improve the quality of analgesia whilst minimising the side effects. There is evidence to suggest an algorithm-based approach to pain management where analgesia is goal directed and titrated to effect improves outcomes [7].

The key choice of the technique depends on a detailed risk benefit analysis and keeping in mind the pharmacokinetic and pharmacodynamic differences in this cohort of patients. Specific issues which warrant alterations to the choice of drug, route of drug administration, dosage, frequency of administration and risk of side effects include—altered protein binding, acid base characteristics, reduced splanchnic blood flow due to inotropes, hepatic and renal dysfunction. Similarly, the pharmacodynamic effects may be exaggerated due to altered drug sensitivity, drug interactions, and alterations to the effect site (e.g., blood brain barrier in meningeal carcinomatous infiltration) [8].

Systemic Analgesia

A large proportion of patients remain deeply sedated in ICU with very little assessment and attention paid towards assessment and treatment of baseline or procedural pain [9]. Analgo-sedation protocols (Fig. 7.1), where pain is treated first with opioids and targeted sedation levels are associated with reduced duration of mechanical ventilation and lower use of sedatives [10]. Though systemic opioids remain the

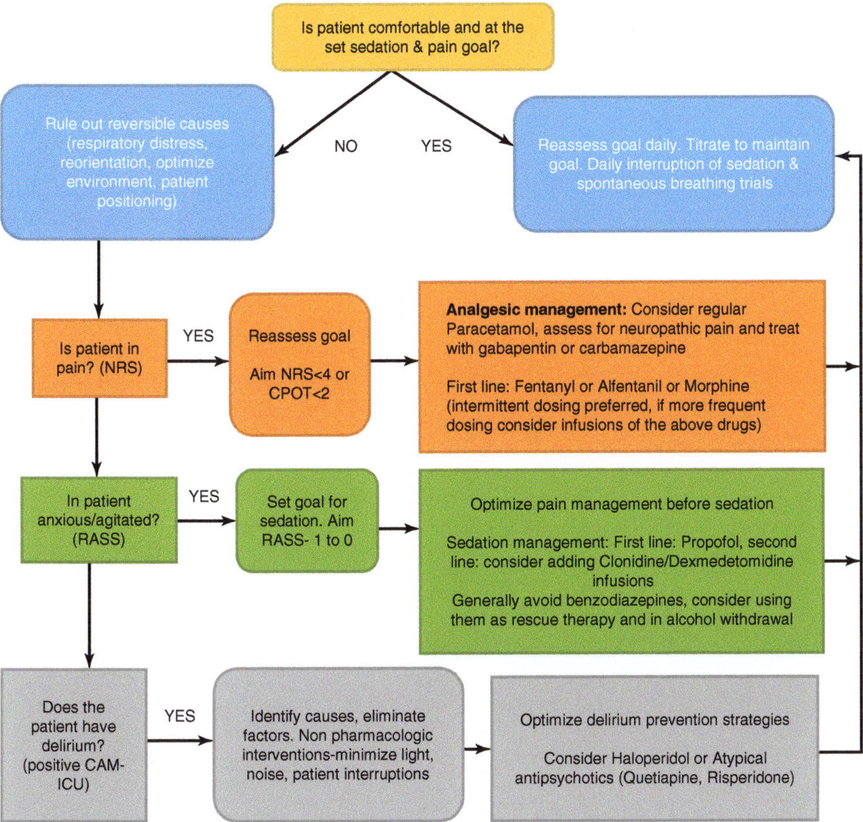

Fig. 7.1 Composite pain, agitation and delirium management guideline in mechanically ventilated adult ICU patients. *NRS* numerical rating scale, *CPOT* critical care pain observation tool, *RASS* Richmond agitation and sedation scale, *CAM-ICU* confusion assessment method for ICU. Adapted from Barr et al. [6]

mainstay of drugs used for analgesia, a multimodal approach which involves different classes of drugs, pain receptors and signalling pathways is preferred as they offer synergism in drug action with reduced side effects.

The analgesic drugs can be classified into

- Opioid analgesics—Morphine, diamorphine, fentanyl, alfentanil, oxycodone, codeine.
- Non-opioid analgesics—paracetamol, non-steroidal anti-inflammatory agents (NSAID's).
- Adjuncts—Tramadol, tricyclic antidepressants, gabapentinoids, alpha-2 agonists, ketamine & magnesium.

The dosage, routes of administration, and special considerations of the commonly used opioid analgesics and adjuvants are summarised in Table 7.4.

Table 7.4 Commonly used drugs for pain management in ICU.

Drug	Onset	Half life	Dosage	Special considerations
Fentanyl	1–2 min	2–4 h	B: 1–2 μg kg^{-1} I: 1–10 μg kg^{-1} h^{-1} PCA: 10–25 μg bolus, lock out: 5–15 min, 4 h limit 400–800 μg. Patches: 25–100 μg h^{-1}	Metabolised in the liver with no active metabolites. Accumulation in hepatic impairment. May accumulate in ESRF. Less hypotension than with morphine. Highly lipid soluble, duration of action is significantly prolonged when continuous infusions are used for prolonged periods. Transdermal patches used in palliative care.
Morphine	5–10 min	3–4 h	B: 0.1–0.2 mg kg^{-1}; I: 0.05–0.1 mg kg^{-1} h^{-1} PCA: 1–3 mg bolus, lock out: 5–15 min, 4 h limit: 30–70 mg IM/SC: 10 mg fourth hourly PO: 5–20 mg fourth hourly	Metabolised by glucouronidation, active metabolites Morphine-6-glucouronide (M6G), Morphine-3-glucouronide (M3G). Oral bioavailability poor 15–65%. M6G is more potent than morphine and accumulates in renal impairment and M3G can cause delirium. Caution in both hepatic and renal impairment. Morphine causes histamine release.
Alfentanil	1–2 min	1.6 h	B: 10–30 μg kg^{-1} I: 20–60 μg kg^{-1} h^{-1}	Less lipid soluble, quick onset and offset. Dose related, short duration respiratory depression, elderly patients particularly sensitive. Clearance prolonged in hepatic impairment (cirrhosis) but unaffected in renal impairment.
Remifentanil	1–3 min	3–10 min	B: 1 μg kg^{-1} I: 0.05–2 μg kg^{-1} min^{-1}	Hydrolysis by plasma esterases. No active metabolites. No accumulation in hepatic/renal failure. Use **IBW if body weight >130% IBW. Used more often in the neuro-intensive care for early neurology assessment.

Table 7.4 (continued)

Drug	Onset	Half life	Dosage	Special considerations
Pethidine	5–10 min	4 h	B: 0.5–1 mg kg^{-1}; I: 0.1–0.3 mg kg^{-1} h^{-1} PO: 50–150 mg fourth hourly PCA: 10–30 mg bolus, lock out: 5–15 min, 4 h limit 80–300 mg	Active metabolites—norpethidine, pethidinic acid. Antimuscarinic effects, hypotension, interactions with Mono-amino Oxidase inhibitors (MAOI). Metabolites accumulate in renal failure and can cause seizures.
Oxycodone		4–6 h	s.c. 2.5–5 mg fourth hourly PO: 5–10 mg fourth hourly	Predictable and higher oral bioavailability 60–87%, caution in hepatic and renal impairment. Used both in acute pain and in cancer/palliative pain.
Tramadol		4–6 h	i.v./i.m.: 50–100 mg iv four to sixth hourly PO: 50–100 mg four to sixth hourly	High oral bioavailability, only partial antagonism by naloxone, causes less respiratory depression. Accumulates in renal and hepatic impairment. Contraindicated with concomitant use of MAOI. Caution in patients with epilepsy.
Codeine		4–6 h	i.m.: 30–60 mg fourth hourly PO: 30–60 mg fourth hourly	50% oral bioavailability, 10% undergoes O-demethylation to morphine, less effective against severe pain. CYP 2D6 polymorphisms produce unpredictable effects. Poor metabolizers have inadequate pain relief; ultra-rapid metabolizers may have respiratory depression.
Diamorphine		3–4 h	i.v. bolus: 0.05–0.1 mg kg^{-1} i.m./s.c.: 5–10 mg fourth hourly PO: 5–10 mg fourth hourly	Metabolised to active components—monoacetyl morphine and morphine by esterases. Highly lipid soluble, less likely to cause respiratory depression when administered intrathecally. Mainly used for cancer pain and palliative care as subcutaneous infusions

(continued)

Table 7.4 (continued)

Drug	Onset	Half life	Dosage	Special considerations
Ketamine		2.5–4 h	B: 0.1–1 mg kg^{-1}; I: 0.125–0.5 mg kg^{-1} h^{-1}	Metabolite nor-ketamine is less potent and has hypnotic effect. Oral bioavailability 20%. Contraindicated in cases with ischaemic heart disease, raised intracranial pressure, significant hypertension and psychotic states.
α-2 agonists Clonidine			B: 2–5 μg kg^{-1}; I: 0.3 μg kg^{-1} h^{-1} PO: 50–150 μg	Reduced myocardial ischaemia, sedation and hypotension at higher doses
Dexmedetomidine			B: 1 μg kg^{-1}; I: 0.2–1 μg kg^{-1} h^{-1}	Not available orally.
Gabapentinoids Gabapentin		5–9 h	PO: 900–3600 mg/day in 3 divided doses	Bioavailability of gabapentin inversely related to dose.
Pregabalin		5–7 h	50–300 mg/day in 2–3 divided doses	Both gabapentinoids have no hepatic metabolism and are excreted largely unchanged in the urine. Dose adjustment in renal impairment.
Amitryptyline			PO: 10–100 mg	Useful in neuropathic pain. Caution in elderly, start at night time at low dosage. Avoid in heart blocks and QT prolongation.
Magnesium			B: 40 mg kg^{-1} I: 10 mg kg^{-1} h^{-1}	Delayed tendon reflexes in high doses/prolonged infusions. Prolongs duration of action of neuromuscular blockers.
Nefopam			PO: 30–90 mg eighth hourly	
Paracetamol			1 g PO/iv four to sixth hourly	

Above doses are guides and vary widely for individual patients. **B* Bolus (Bolus doses are titrated in aliquots for achieving pain relief), *I* infusion, *PCA* patient-controlled analgesia, *PO* per oral, ***IBW* ideal body weight, *ESRF* end stage renal failure (Adapted with kind permission from Oxford university press). Narayanan et al. [8]

Systemic opioids are the standard in pain management in ICU. But some of the side effects of opioids may prolong LOS in ICU and worsen outcome (Table 7.5). Non-opioid adjuvants have opioid sparing effects. Intravenous acetaminophen (Paracetamol) decreased pain scores, morphine consumption with significantly improved time to extubation, sedation scores and nausea rates in surgical ICU patients but was associated with an increased risk of hypotension [11]. Low dose

Table 7.5 Complications and side effects of commonly used analgesic in ICU

Drug	Systemic side effects
Opioids	Cardiovascular—Hypotension, bradycardia. Respiratory—Delayed ventilator weaning, increased length of stay, cough suppression. Gastrointestinal—Ileus, nausea/vomiting, constipation. Central nervous system—Respiratory depression, Sedation, delirium, confusion, hallucination, hyperalgesia, physical dependence, addiction, dysphoria, seizures, drug withdrawal. Others—Immunosuppression, pruritus, urinary retention, muscle rigidity, dry mouth.
NSAID's	GI bleeding, renal dysfunction, reduced platelet aggregation
Non opioid analgesics	
Ketamine	Delirium, hallucinations, nausea, vomiting.
Clonidine/ dexmedetomidine	Sedation, dizziness, hypotension, bradycardia, dry mouth.
Gabapentin/ pregabalin	Somnolence, dizziness, confusion, convulsions, fatigue, ataxia.
Nefopam	Tachycardia, glaucoma, seizure, delirium
Amitriptyline	Dry mouth, sedation, blurred vision, arrhythmias, postural hypotension.

ketamine has significant opioid sparing effects, but its use should be only be considered in ICU after a careful risk benefit analysis due to its undesirable psychomimetic side effects (delirium, hallucinations). Neuropathic agents (gabapentin, pregabalin) reduced pain intensity and opioid consumption in ICU patients with Guillain Barre Syndrome [12]; sedative, cognitive dysfunction and need for enteral route precludes their generalisability to all ICU patients without a neuropathic element to pain. NSAID's are not routinely recommended in ICU due to their high risk-benefit profile and serious side effects (gastrointestinal bleeding, acute kidney injury). There is paucity of data on the role of selective cyclooxygenase-2 (COX-2) inhibitors in critically adult ICU patients. Evidence from non-ICU studies supports the use of i.v. Lidocaine in reducing pain intensity after abdominal surgery. The benefits of i.v. lidocaine are at best modest; with significant pharmacokinetic variability and the risk of cardiac or neurotoxicity in the ICU patients, the safety concerns outweigh the benefits of its routine use.

7.6 Side Effects and Complications

Prolonged use of any drug is associated with a side effect profile which may even obscure the benefits for which it was commence, hence all drugs should be reviewed on a daily basis. The presence of cardiovascular or respiratory failure was associated with the use of sedatives and opioids [9]. The common side effect profile of the analgesics used are summarised in Table 7.5.

Regional Analgesia

Systemic analgesia is associated with significant side effects (Table 7.5), which may prolong the duration of ICU/hospital stay and lead to a poor patient experience. Though poorly studied in ICU patient population, regional anaesthesia (RA) has the potential to offer excellent pain relief while minimising the side effects. Though epidural analgesia (EA) has not been to definitively proven to reduce cancer recurrence or long-term mortality [13], thoracic epidural analgesia (TEA) facilitates early weaning from ventilatory support after lung surgery, lung transplant, and cytoreductive abdominal surgery.

Specific factors to consider in the ICU population are the altered pharmacokinetics of the local anaesthetics (LA) due to hypoalbuminaemia, renal or hepatic dysfunction which may predispose to LA toxicity and necessitate dosage adjustments [14]. The pharmacodynamics alterations may lead to increased sensitivity or exaggerated effects like hypotension in vasopressor dependant or hypovolemic patients. The environmental factors due to unfamiliarity may predispose to drug errors or wrong injections via indwelling regional anaesthesia catheters. Regional catheters can frequently dislodge during routine ICU care like position changes and physiotherapy. Recognition of side effects or complications of regional techniques may be delayed by factors such as sedation, critical care weakness, and delirium [14].

The indication & choice of technique depends on skills and a detailed risk benefit analysis specific to on an individual patient (Table 7.6).

The complications of RA techniques in ICU patients, though unquantified may possibly be higher than the perioperative setting. These complications can go unrecognised and have catastrophic consequences increasing the morbidity and length of

Table 7.6 Indications of RA

Indications of RA	Regional anaesthetic options
Surgical resections for malignancy in specific organ systems	
Thoracotomy—lung resection/ pneumonectomy	Thoracic epidural Paravertebral blocks
Laparotomy (hepatectomy, bowel resection)	Neuraxial-epidural/spinal TAP blocks: classical and Subcostal approaches Rectus sheath blocks Local infiltration analgesia
Rib fractures (metastatic deposits)/rib resection	Thoracic epidural Paravertebral blocks Interpleural block Intercostal blocks Serratus plane blocks
Limb fractures (pathological)/ limb amputations	Lower limb: spinal/epidural Plexus (Lumbar + Sacral), fascial plane blocks (fascia iliaca blocks) and peripheral nerve blocks (femoral, sciatic, popliteal) Upperlimb: brachial plexus blocks and peripheral nerve blocks

Table 7.6 (continued)

Indications of RA	Regional anaesthetic options
Non-Surgical indications due to primary or chemotherapy induced complications	
Acute pancreatitis	Thoracic epidural; coeliac plexus block
Neuralgia & complex regional pain syndromes (CRPS) Ischaemic limb	Sympatholytic blocks
Painful procedures in ICU	
Chest drains	Intercostal blocks
Central lines insertion Tracheostomy	Superficial cervical plexus block
Debridement/dressing changes	Upper and lower limb blocks as above

Adapted with kind permission from Oxford university press. Venkataraju et al. [14]

ICU stay. Infective complications include sepsis, meningitis, vertebral canal abscess due to neuraxial techniques. Bleeding complications due to haemostatic abnormalities include neuraxial or extra-neuraxial hematoma, hypovolemia, hypotension and local compressive effects. Pneumothorax or diaphragm paresis due to upper limb or trunk blocks can delay weaning from mechanical ventilation. Similarly, nerve damage, neuropraxia especially of lower limbs, significantly hampers mobilisation and rehabilitation.

Non-pharmacologic Measures

Modalities like hypnosis, massage, music therapy, relaxation techniques and cryotherapy are supported by low quality evidence and hence have conditional recommendations for their use in specific cohorts of ICU patients. They are attractive due to their low harm profile but are limited by resources.

References

1. Loeser JD, Treede RD. The Kyoto protocol of IASP basic pain terminology. Pain. 2008;137:473–7.
2. Puntillo KA. Pain experiences of intensive care unit patients. Heart Lung. 1990;19:526–33.
3. Delvin JW, Skrobik Y, Gelinas C, et al. Clinical practice guidelines for the prevention and management of pain, agitation/sedation, delirium, immobility, and sleep disruption in adult patients in the ICU. Crit Care Med. 2018;46(9):825–73.
4. Payen J, Bru O, Bosson J, et al. Assessing pain in critically ill sedated patients by using a behavioural pain scale. Crit Care Med. 2001;29:2258–63.
5. Payen JF, Bosson JL, Chanques G, Mantz J, Labarere J, Investigators DOLOREA. Pain assessment is associated with decreased duration of mechanical ventilation in the intensive care unit: a post Hoc analysis of the DOLOREA study. Anesthesiology. 2009;111(6):1308–16.
6. Barr J, Fraser GL, Puntillo K, Ely EW, Gelinas C, Dasta JF, Davidson JE, Devlin JW, Kress JP, Joffe AM, Coursin DB, Herr DL, Tung A, Robinson BR, Fontaine DK, Ramsay MA, Riker RR, Sessler CN, Pun B, Skrobik Y, Jaeschke R. Clinical practice guidelines for the management of pain, agitation, and delirium in adult patients in the intensive care unit. Crit Care Med. 2013;41:263–306.

7. Skrobik Y, Ahern S, Leblanc M, et al. Protocolized intensive care unit management of analgesia, sedation, and delirium improves analgesia and subsyndromal delirium rates. Anesth Analg. 2010;111:451–63.
8. Narayanan M, Venkataraju A, Jennings J. Analgesia in intensive care: Part-1. BJA Educ. 2016;16(2):72–8.
9. Payen JF, Chanques G, Mantz J, et al. Current practices in sedation and analgesia for mechanically ventilated critically ill patients: a prospective multicenter patient-based study. Anesthesiology. 2007;106:687–95.
10. Faust AC, Rajan P, Sheperd LA, Alvarez CA, McCorstin P, Doebele RL. Impact of an analgesia-based sedation protocol on mechanically ventilated patients in a medical intensive care unit. Anesth Analg. 2016;123(4):903–9.
11. Memis D, Inal MT, Kavalci G, et al. Intravenous paracetamol reduced the use of opioids, extubation time, and opioid-related adverse effects after major surgery in intensive care unit. J Crit Care. 2010;25:458–62.
12. Pandey CK, Bose N, Garg G, et al. Gabapentin for the treatment of pain in Guillain-Barré syndrome: a double-blinded, placebo-controlled, crossover study. Anesth Analg. 2002;95:1719–23.
13. Grandhi RK, Lee S, Abd-Elsayed A. The relationship between regional anesthesia and cancer: a metaanalysis. Ochsner J. 2017;17:345e61.
14. Venkataraju A, Narayanan M. Analgesia in intensive care: Part 2. BJA Educ. 2016;16(12):397–404.

8 Sedation and Neuromuscular Blockade in Oncology Critical Care

Tim Keady and Madan Narayanan

8.1 Sedation

8.1.1 The Need for Sedation in ICU

Sedatives are frequently administered to critically ill patients to relieve anxiety, reduce the stress of being mechanically ventilated, and prevent agitation-related harm [1]. However these medications may predispose patients to prolonged ventilation, delirium or other morbidities [2, 3].

The need for sedation should therefore be considered carefully. The ideal state of a patient in ICU is comfortable, alert and in no distress. Common causes of distress include anxiety, delirium, pain, dyspnoea and neuromuscular paralysis. The cause of distress should therefore be identified and treated before pharmacologic sedation. This is exemplified by the concept of analgosedation where pain is treated first, and thereafter sedative agents are considered. This is especially relevant in cancer patients where pain control is a high priority.

In 2018, the Society for Critical Care Medicine released the PADIS guidelines on which much of the following chapter is based. These were updated from the 2013 guidelines to include the prevention of immobility and sleep provision as key components of best practice in caring for critically ill patients.

8.1.2 Risk Factors for Delirium and Agitation

Delirium is an acute fluctuant confusional state that is common in ICU. There are modifiable and non-modifiable risk factors for its development in critically ill patients.

T. Keady · M. Narayanan (✉)
Frimley Park Hospital, Surrey, UK

V. Kumar et al. (eds.), *Onco-critical Care*,
https://doi.org/10.1007/978-981-16-9929-0_8

8.1.2.1 Modifiable Risk Factors

- Benzodiazepine use (reported by multiple high-quality studies) [1]
- Blood transfusions (in surgical and trauma patients) [1]

8.1.2.2 Non-Modifiable Risk Factors

- Episode of coma or deep sedation [4]
- Older age
- History of dementia
- Emergency surgery or trauma prior to admission
- Increasing APACHE and ASA scores

Conversely, opioid use and mechanical ventilation have been strongly shown not to alter the risk of delirium [1].

Delirium in critically ill adults is strongly associated with hospital length of stay and cognition at 3 and 6 months. However, it has been shown not to be associated with PTSD and not consistently with ICU length of stay, disposition to a place other than home, functionality or mortality [1].

Agitation in ICU is of course a safety concern and should be managed carefully by treating the cause, and with pharmacological and non-pharmacological methods. However, subsyndromal and hypoactive delirium is common, and pharmacologic management does not appear to affect clinical outcomes other than the incidence of delirium itself. Furthermore, antipsychotics are often continued unnecessarily into the patients discharge medications. Society guidelines have therefore recommended avoiding the risks of antipsychotics and other medications in these cases unless there is a safety concern [1].

8.1.3 Goals and Sedation Scores

For years sedation was considered a necessary adjunct to critical care. A combination of factors has led to a paradigm shift. This includes the emergence of advanced ventilation modes, rapidly titratable sedative agents, increased placement of tracheostomy tubes, increased recognition of ICU acquired weakness as well as economic pressures and new high-quality evidence.

Today, the most common goals are the provision of anxiolysis and rest, the reduction of distress, and the blunting of awareness where communication is not possible.

The goal of sedation may also be related to a disease process such as seizure management or raised intracranial pressure, or it may be used to reduced oxygen utilization, facilitate procedures, maintain safety or for palliation.

Thus, a clear definition for the goal of sedation remains elusive and case dependent.

A variety of validated sedation scores are in widespread use however. One of the simplest and most commonly used is the Richmond Agitation Sedation Scale

Table 8.1 Richmond agitation sedation scale (RASS)

+4	Combative
+3	Very agitated
+2	Agitated
+1	Restless
0	Alert and calm
−1	Drowsy
−2	Light sedation
−3	Moderate sedation
−4	Deep sedation
−5	Unrousable

(RASS) seen in Table 8.1. Tools like this allow sedation targets to be more objective, prescriptive and protocolised.

8.1.4 Protocolised Sedation Algorithms

There is a clear vogue today for light sedation. This is most likely due to the benefits of a reduction in time to extubation, and the rate of tracheostomy [5, 6]. More recent RCTs have demonstrated that light sedation does not appear to affect mortality however, and it has no clear effect either way on delirium, PTSD, depression or self–extubation [1].

There are several other caveats when considering the evidence for a sedation protocol. Firstly, there is no consensus on the definition of light, moderate or deep sedation or the effect of depth of sedation on patient centred outcomes. Secondly, the magnitude of the reduction in time to extubation and tracheostomy rate is small [1]. Thirdly, most studies in this area used benzodiazepines in their sedation regimens, and since this medication is no longer recommended, the validity of these studies today may be questioned.

Despite the above, a variety of methods for targeting an appropriate level of sedation are in use today. The two most often used are Daily Sedative Interruption (DSI) and Nursing-Protocolised sedation—either continuous infusion or intermittent bolus. No significant differences exist between them in achieving a safe and light level of sedation [1]. However DSI protocols may increase nursing workload compared with protocolised sedation alone [4].

8.1.5 Monitoring

After initiation of pharmacotherapy, the goal of monitoring should be to avoid excess sedation. This may be achieved using scoring systems to assess not only sedation but also delirium and pain. Commonly used scoring systems include the similarly named Sedation-Agitation Scale (SAS) scored from 1 to 7, the Richmond

Agitation Sedation Scale (RASS) scored from −5 to +4, and the Ramsay Sedation Scale (RSS) scored from 1 to 6. Commonly used delirium scales include the Confusion Assessment Method for the ICU (CAM-ICU) and the Intensive Care Delirium Screening Checklist (ICDSC). Both are simple and valid tools for detecting delirium.

More objective scores are also in use, particularly during deep sedation and/or muscle relaxation. Most research has focused on Bispectral Index (BIS) monitoring where some small studies have shown reductions in total in total sedative use, faster wakening times and less agitation, however, more research is needed in this area [1].

8.1.6 Pharmacotherapy

Pharmacotherapy is indicated when the cause of a patient's distress cannot be remedied, and non-pharmacological treatments cannot sufficiently control the situation. The most used sedatives in ICU are benzodiazepines, opioids, propofol, dexmedetomidine, ketamine and anti-psychotics.

As there is no ideal agent, selection of a therapy should be individualized to the patient and situation.

- Pain and dyspnoea are best treated with an opioid. See Chap. 7 for more detail.
- In the case of delirium, the most recent guidelines discourage the routine use of antipsychotic agents such as quetiapine and olanzapine [1]. They are often continued into the patients discharge medications and continued exposure to these agents can result in significant morbidity and financial burden. However, they are useful in managing agitation and the symptoms of delirium such as anxiety, fearfulness, hallucinations and delusions. There is also evidence from the Dahlia study for the use of dexmedetomidine for delirium in the instance where it is precluding safe extubation [7].
- For agitation due to stress or anxiety, propofol or dexmedetomidine are preferred over benzodiazepines
  - Dexmedetomidine was found to be non-inferior to propofol and midazolam for sedation in in the Prodex-Midex studies.
  - However, the more recent large multicentre RCT, the SPICE III study, which compared early dexmedetomidine infusion to usual care found only minor differences in ventilator and ICU free days [8].
  - Clonidine may be used as an analgesic adjunct or to transition away from dexmedetomidine infusions. It is not licensed for sedation and data on the safety and efficacy of clonidine infusions are lacking.
  - Propofol has the added benefit of anti-emetic properties which may be useful in cancer patients.
- Barbiturates such as thiopental are occasionally used where patients are not responding to other agents. Drawbacks to its use include profound cardiorespiratory depression, and a prolonged elimination half-life.

- Ketamine is rarely used and not licensed for infusion in ICU. Unwanted psychoactive effects such as hallucinations, confusion and delirium as well as cardiorespiratory changes limit its use. It is however, a useful analgesic adjunct.

8.1.7 Acute Withdrawal Syndrome of Long-Term Analgesia and/or Sedation in the ICU

Opioids such as fentanyl and morphine are frequently administered for long periods of time in ICU for their analgo-sedative effects. Withdrawal symptoms such as sweating, vomiting, lacrimation, hypertension, fever, and anxiety are common on discontinuation—up to 32% of patients in ICU for 1 week or more may suffer from these [9]. If the agent has been administered for a short period of time, i.e., less than 7 days, it is reasonable to discontinue over a few hours. A more gradual reduction of 10–25% per day may be required if tachyphylaxis has developed.

Benzodiazepine withdrawal causes similar symptoms to opioid withdrawal as well as increasing the risk of seizures. Management strategies may include slow weaning of the infusion and the addition of regular lorazepam.

In the case of deeply sedated patients with prolonged ICU stays, it may be necessary to completely stop sedative infusions due to medication accumulation.

There have not been any controlled trials and there is no consensus on the best strategy for avoiding withdrawal. Oral methadone has been used due to its desirable effects such as NMDA antagonism and long half-life [10]. Oral and intravenous clonidine and dexmedetomidine infusions have been used but data are limited to case reports.

8.2 Concept of Minimal Sedation

According to the American Society of Anaesthesiologists, minimal sedation (anxiolysis) is a drug-induced state during which patients respond normally to verbal commands. Although cognitive function and physical coordination may be impaired, airway reflexes, and ventilatory and cardiovascular functions are unaffected.

A recent trial of non-sedation (analgesia only) vs light sedation showed no difference in mortality, ICU or ventilator free days, or delirium [11].

8.3 Mobilization and Rehabilitation

Survivors of ICU frequently experience long-term sequelae such as ICU acquired muscle weakness (ICUAW). It can occur in 25–50% of critically ill patients. As well as mitigating ICUAW, mobilisation may be beneficial in the management of delirium and pain although there is no evidence for an effect on mortality [1].

8.4 Sleep

Poor sleep is a common source of significant distress among critically ill patients. The interplay of severe illness, medications, cerebral perfusion, delirium and sleep is complex but an evolving area of research. There is insufficient evidence to support the use of medications such as dexmedetomidine and melatonin to promote sleep. However, dexmedetomidine may improve sleep architecture and melatonin is cheap and has few side effects. Due to REM suppression and haemodynamic effects, it is suggested propofol should not be used for sleep promotion. Non-pharmacological methods such as sleep promoting protocols involving earplugs and eyeshades may have some benefit in improving sleep and reducing delirium but their effectiveness remains to be proven [1].

8.4.1 Complications and Prevention

See Table 8.2 for a summary of the complications of sedation and how they may be prevented.

8.5 Neuromuscular Paralysis

8.5.1 Role of Paralysis and Neuromuscular Blocking Agents in the ICU

Neuromuscular blocking agents have a number of clinical uses in ICU on which there is broad agreement. However, consensus is lacking in some areas such as in the management of moderate to severe respiratory failure in the setting of ARDS. This debate is especially relevant in the critically ill cancer patient where the

Table 8.2 Complications of sedation and how they may be prevented

Complications of Under-Sedation	Prevention of Complications
Agitation	Validated delirium monitoring tools
Pain	Validated sedation scales
Increased stress response	Protocolised sedation strategies
Accidental removal of medical devices	Using light or minimal sedation
Increased clinician workload	Prevention of prolonged immobility
	Facilitation of sleep
Complications of over-sedation	Avoiding benzodiazepines
Cardiorespiratory effects	Appropriate blood transfusion targets
Drug side effects and interactions	Processed EEG monitoring
Continuation of antipsychotics post ICU	Management of withdrawal symptoms
Delirium	
Prolonged ventilation	
Prolonged ICU stay	

risk of respiratory failure and mortality is high, but advanced therapies such as ECMO may not be appropriate [12].

Where sedation and analgesia strategies alone have failed, or are not appropriate, some clinical indications for neuromuscular blockade include the following: [13].

- Facilitation of lung-protective mechanical ventilation in the case of severe hypoxemia
- Prevention of shivering due to therapeutic hypothermia post cardiac arrest
- Management of the increased muscle activity of certain medical conditions, such as tetanus or neuroleptic malignant syndrome
- Elimination of unwanted movement or ventilator dyssynchrony in the setting of raised ICP, raised intra-abdominal pressure, pulmonary haemorrhage or refractory status asthmaticus
- Facilitation of procedures commonly needed for critically ill cancer patients such as intubation, bronchoscopy, endoscopy, bronchoalveolar lavage, or biopsy

Critically ill cancer patients are at high risk of ARDS [14]. This may be infective or non-infective in origin. Causes specific to cancer patients include chemotherapy-related pulmonary toxicity. The utility of neuromuscular blockade in this setting has been extensively investigated, however, uncertainty still exists. The ACURASYS study in 2010 showed mortality benefit from 48 hours of cisatracurium infusion for patients with severe ARDS [15]. On the basis of this and other trials, society guidelines suggested NMBA infusions for patients with moderate to severe ARDS [16]. The second major RCT, the ROSE study, was published in 2019 and found no benefit from NMBA infusion and deep sedation compared with light sedation [17]. Society guidelines were subsequently adjusted to recommend against the routine use of NMBA infusions where light sedation alone is tolerated [18]. NMBA use has therefore become more limited recently to the aforementioned indications.

8.5.2 Need for Sedation During Neuromuscular Blockade

NMBAs have no sedative, amnestic or analgesic properties. In small case series, patients who were paralysed without adequate sedation reported continuous feelings of fear, nervousness and discomfort [19]. However patients have also reported feelings of being cared for and remembered emotional support from staff and family [20]. Guideline recommendations are therefore that sedative and analgesic drugs should be administered prior to and during neuromuscular blockade, with the goal of achieving deep sedation [16].

Where NMBA infusions are used, processed EEG monitoring is sometimes employed to ensure sufficient sedation. Data surrounding the validity of these monitors in critically ill patients are lacking, however a positive correlation between BIS and the Sedation Agitation Scale has been noted in one small study of non-paralysed patients [21]. Given increasing knowledge and interest among intensivists in the interpretation of EEG waveforms, where clinical assessment is equivocal, processed EEG monitoring may have a role [22].

8.5.3 Choice of Neuromuscular Blocking Agents

A variety of NMBAs exist and the choice between them depends on the indication and the patients' comorbidities.

- For rapid sequence intubation, the agent most often used is the non-depolarising agent rocuronium. The depolarising agent succinylcholine is rarely used in intensive care due to the potential for hyperkalemia in this high risk population. It is also a trigger for malignant hyperthermia, can cause elevated intraocular and intracerebral pressure and has higher potential for anaphylaxis than other agents.
- Rocuronium and vecuronium are intermediate acting agents that are commonly used as bolus doses in ICU. Sugammadex is effective in reversing neuromuscular blockade due to both rocuronium and vecuronium by forming a tight complex with those compounds followed by renal excretion.
- Atracurium or cisatracurium are the preferred agents for infusions as their metabolism is unrelated to renal or hepatic function [13]. The side effect of histamine release that occurs with atracurium use is not seen with its cis-isomer, cisatracurium. They are both primarily eliminated through Hoffman degradation.
- Pancuronium is a long-acting agent with vagolytic properties that make it useful for cardiac surgery. However it should be used with caution in critically ill cancer patients due to the risk of exacerbating and prolonging muscle weakness.

8.5.4 Monitoring Depth of Paralysis

Peripheral nerve stimulation with train of four (TOF) monitoring may be a useful adjunct in the assessment of neuromuscular paralysis. It involves stimulating a nerve four times and counting the number of muscle twitches seen. A TOF count of 0/4–1/4 is a typical target for deep paralysis. While this is a useful objective measure, several factors including the characteristics of the patient, the staff and the equipment may affect its accuracy. For instance, a patient with a TOF count of 0/4 may still exhibit respiratory effort or a cough on suctioning. A small RCT which compared protocol driven neuromuscular paralysis with TOF monitoring vs clinical assessment alone showed no difference in paralysis time, recovery time or total dose administered [23]. It is therefore recommended to perform clinical assessment of the level of neuromuscular blockade and consider the incorporation of peripheral nerve stimulation where issues arise [16].

Table 8.3 Complications and methods for their prevention

Complications	Prevention
ICU acquired weakness	Avoid NMBA infusions where possible Limit the infusion duration to less than 48 h Avoid long acting agents
Corneal drying, scarring, ulceration and infection	Passive eyelid closure and artificial tears
Tachycardia, histamine release	Avoid pancuronium Consider cisatracurium in place of atracurium
Awareness under neuromuscular blockade	Ensure deep sedation and analgesia with regular clinical assessment and consider processed EEG monitoring
Venous thromboembolism	Consider passive mobilization, elastic compression stockings and pharmacological prophylaxis
Skin breakdown, slowed GI motility, diaphragmatic atrophy	Supportive care, changes in position and early mobilisation

8.5.5 Complications and Prevention

ICU acquired weakness (ICUAW) is a syndrome that may persist long after the patient has been discharged from ICU and the hospital. It likely results from several factors including critical illness neuromyopathy and disuse atrophy, but it is unclear whether neuromuscular blockade is a major contributor [13]. No difference in ICU acquired weakness was noted in either major RCT assessing the benefits of NMBA infusions—the ACURASYS and ROSE studies. Other factors which may contribute to ICUAW include corticosteroid use, prolonged bed rest and immobility, aminoglycoside use and sepsis with multi-organ failure [24].

A summary of complications and methods for their prevention can found in in Table 8.3.

References

1. Devlin JW, Skrobik Y, Gélinas C, et al. Clinical Practice Guidelines for the Prevention and Management of Pain, Agitation/Sedation, Delirium, Immobility, and Sleep Disruption in Adult Patients in the ICU. *Critical Care Medicine* [Internet] NLM (Medline); 2018 [cited 2021 Feb 13]; 46: e825–73 http://journals.lww.com/00003246-201809000-00029.
2. Hughes CG, McGrane S, Pandharipande PP. Sedation in the intensive care setting [Internet]. Clinical pharmacology: advances and applications. Dove Press; 2012 [cited 2021 Feb 16]. p. 53–63.
3. Kollef MH, Levy NT, Ahrens TS, Schaiff R, Prentice D, Sherman G. The use of continuous IV sedation is associated with prolongation of mechanical ventilation. Chest American College of Chest Physicians. 1998;114:541–8.
4. Mehta S, Burry L, Cook D, et al. Daily sedation interruption in mechanically ventilated critically ill patients cared for with a sedation protocol: A randomized controlled trial. *JAMA—Journal of the American Medical Association* [Internet] American Medical Association; 2012 [cited 2021 Feb 15]; 308: 1985–92. www.jama.com.

5. Strøm T, Martinussen T, Toft P. A protocol of no sedation for critically ill patients receiving mechanical ventilation: a randomised trial. *The Lancet* [Internet] Elsevier B.V.; 2010 [cited 2021 Mar 8]; 375: 475–80. https://pubmed.ncbi.nlm.nih.gov/20116842/.
6. Tanaka LMS, Azevedo LCP, Park M, et al. Early sedation and clinical outcomes of mechanically ventilated patients: A prospective multicenter cohort study. *Critical Care* [Internet] BioMed Central Ltd.; 2014 [cited 2021 Mar 8]; 18. https://pubmed.ncbi.nlm.nih.gov/25047960/.
7. Reade MC, Eastwood GM, Bellomo R, et al. Effect of dexmedetomidine added to standard care on ventilator-free time in patients with agitated delirium a randomized clinical trial. *JAMA—Journal of the American Medical Association* [Internet] American Medical Association; 2016 [cited 2021 Feb 15]; 315: 1460–8. https://pubmed.ncbi.nlm.nih.gov/26975647/.
8. Shehabi Y, Howe BD, Bellomo R, et al. Early sedation with dexmedetomidine in critically ill patients. New England Journal of Medicine Massachusetts Medical Society. 2019;380:2506–17.
9. Cammarano WB, Pittet JF, Weitz S, Schlobohm RM, Marks JD. Acute withdrawal syndrome related to the administration of analgesic and sedative medications in adult intensive care unit patients. *Critical Care Medicine* [Internet] Crit Care Med; 1998 [cited 2021 Feb 16]; 26: 676–84. https://pubmed.ncbi.nlm.nih.gov/9559604/.
10. Al-Qadheeb NS, Roberts RJ, Griffin R, Garpestad E, Ruthazer R, Devlin JW. Impacto de Metadona Enteral en la Habilidad Para Apartar de Opioides Infundidos Continuamente a Adultos en Estado Crítico en Ventilación Mecánica: Estudio de caso Control. *Annals of Pharmacotherapy* [Internet] Ann Pharmacother; 2012 [cited 2021 Feb 16]; **46**: 1160–6 Available from: https://pubmed.ncbi.nlm.nih.gov/22872749/
11. Olsen HT, Nedergaard HK, Strøm T, et al. Nonsedation or light sedation in critically ill, mechanically ventilated patients. New England Journal of Medicine Massachusetts Medical Society. 2020;382:1103–11.
12. Azoulay E, Schellongowski P, Darmon M, et al. The intensive care medicine research agenda on critically ill oncology and hematology patients. Intensive Care Medicine Springer Verlag. 2017:1366–82.
13. de Backer J, Hart N, Fan E. Neuromuscular Blockade in the 21st Century Management of the Critically Ill Patient [Internet]. Chest. Elsevier Inc; 2017 [cited 2021 Mar 4]. p. 697–706. https://pubmed.ncbi.nlm.nih.gov/27818334/.
14. Azoulay E, Lemiale V, Mokart D, et al. Acute respiratory distress syndrome in patients with malignancies. *Intensive Care Medicine* [Internet] Springer Verlag; 2014 [cited 2021 Mar 1]; 40: 1106–14 Available from: https://pubmed.ncbi.nlm.nih.gov/24898895/
15. Papazian L, Forel J-M, Gacouin A, et al. Neuromuscular Blockers in Early Acute Respiratory Distress Syndrome. *New England Journal of Medicine* [Internet] Massachusetts Medical Society; 2010 [cited 2021 Mar 4]; 363: 1107–16. http://www.nejm.org/doi/abs/10.1056/NEJMoa1005372.
16. Murray MJ, DeBlock H, Erstad B, et al. Clinical Practice Guidelines for Sustained Neuromuscular Blockade in the Adult Critically Ill Patient. *Critical Care Medicine* [Internet] Lippincott Williams and Wilkins; 2016 [cited 2021 Mar 1]; 44: 2079–103. http://journals.lww.com/00003246-201611000-00016.
17. Moss M, Huang DT, Brower RG. Early Neuromuscular Blockade in the Acute Respiratory Distress Syndrome. *New England Journal of Medicine* [Internet] Massachusetts Medical Society; 2019 [cited 2021 Mar 1]; **380: 19**97–2008. http://www.nejm.org/doi/10.1056/NEJMoa1901686.
18. Alhazzani W, Belley-Cote E, Møller MH, et al. Neuromuscular blockade in patients with ARDS: a rapid practice guideline. *Intensive Care Medicine* [Internet] Springer Science and Business Media Deutschland GmbH; 2020 [cited 2021 Mar 1]; 46: 1977–86. http://link.springer.com/10.1007/s00134-020-06227-8.
19. Wagner BKJ, Zavotsky KE, Sweeney JB, Palmeri BA, Hammond JS. Patient recall of therapeutic paralysis in a surgical critical care unit. Pharmacotherapy: The Journal of Human Pharmacology and Drug Therapy. 1998;18:358–63.

20. Ballard N, Robley L, Barrett D, Fraser D, Mendoza I. Patients' recollections of therapeutic paralysis in the intensive care unit. American Journal of Critical Care American Association of Critical-Care Nurses. 2006;15:86–94.
21. Arbour R, Waterhouse J, Seckel MA, Bucher L. Correlation between the Sedation-Agitation Scale and the Bispectral Index in ventilated patients in the intensive care unit. *Heart and Lung: Journal of Acute and Critical Care* [Internet] Heart Lung; 2009 [cited 2021 Mar 4]; 38: 336–45. https://pubmed.ncbi.nlm.nih.gov/19577705/.
22. Sewell L, Abbas A, Kane N. Introduction to interpretation of the EEG in intensive care Learning objectives. 2019.
23. Baumann MH, McAlpin BW, Brown K, et al. A prospective randomized comparison of train-of-four monitoring and clinical assessment during continuous ICU cisatracurium paralysis. *Chest* [Internet] American College of Chest Physicians; 2004 [cited 2021 Mar 4]; 126: 1267–73. https://pubmed.ncbi.nlm.nih.gov/15486392/.
24. Fan E, Dowdy DW, Colantuoni E, et al. Physical complications in acute lung injury survivors: A two-year longitudinal prospective study. *Critical Care Medicine* [Internet] Lippincott Williams and Wilkins; 2014 [cited 2021 Mar 6]; 42: 849–59. https://pubmed.ncbi.nlm.nih.gov/24247473/.

Blood Gas Analysis and Acid-Base Disorders

9

Nitin Rai and Dalim Kumar Baidya

Human body maintain homeostasis by many physiological processes which keep a fine tuning of pH between 7.35 to 7.45. This pH enables various essential processes like oxygen delivery to tissue, maintaining protein structure in the proper configuration and helps in carrying out various biochemical reactions smoothly. Two types of acids contribute to daily acid load—respiratory (or volatile) acids and metabolic (or fixed) acids. Respiratory acid is carbon dioxide produced by complete oxidation of carbohydrates and fatty acids [1]. Although CO_2 itself is not an acid as per Bronsted-Lowry system as it does not contain a hydrogen, instead it has a potential to create an equivalent amount of carbonic acid (H_2CO_3). Daily basal CO_2 production is 12,000 to 13,000 mmols/day. All acids other then H_2CO_3 are fixed acids as those are not eliminated by lungs. These acids are produced due to incomplete metabolism of carbohydrates (e.g. lactate), fats (e.g. acetoacetate or b-hydroxybutyrate) and protein (e.g. sulphate, phosphate) and are eliminated by kidneys. Daily production is about 70 to 100 mmoles of H^+ per day in an adult.

9.1 Buffers

Any acid base disturbance is compensated by buffers system in the body, respiratory response by alteration in arterial pCO_2 or renal response by alteration in HCO_3^- elimination [1, 2]. Buffering is a rapid physico-chemical phenomenon carried out by various buffers like-intracellular (proteins, phosphates), blood (bicarbonates,

N. Rai
Department of Critical Care Medicine, King George Medical University, Lucknow, India

D. K. Baidya (✉)
Department of Anaesthesiology, Pain Medicine and Critical Care, All India Institute of Medical Sciences, New Delhi, India

V. Kumar et al. (eds.), *Onco-critical Care*,
https://doi.org/10.1007/978-981-16-9929-0_9

haemoglobin, plasma proteins), interstitial fluids (bicarbonates protein), urine (phosphate, ammonia) and bone buffer [3]. Extracellular buffers contributes to 43% of total buffering (by bicarbonate & protein buffers) and remaining 57% is contributed by intracellular buffers [4]. Respiratory response to acid base perturbation occurs rapidly within minutes to hours by alteration in ventilation. Being able to cross cell membranes easily, respiratory response mainatains intracellular pH as well as extracellular pH. Renal response is much slower process (several days to reach maximum capacity) and involves adjustment of bicarbonate excretion by the kidney.

9.2 Respiratory Regulation of Acid Base Disorders

Respiratory regulation involves adjustment of pH due to pCO_2 changes from adaptation in ventilation. This is an inherently rapid process by virtue of CO_2 being lipid soluble and crossing cell membrane rapidly [5]. The quantification of respiratory variation can be estimated by two equations which provide the connection between alveolar ventilation, pCO_2 and pH. These are

$$\text{First, paCO}_2 \text{ is proportional to} [V_{CO2}/V_A] \tag{9.1}$$

where:

- $paCO_2$ = Arterial partial pressure of CO_2
- V_{CO2} = Carbon dioxide production by the body
- V_A = Alveolar ventilation

Second, Henderson Hasselbach Equation

$$\text{pH} = 6.1 + \log \text{HCO}_3 - \\ 0.03\,\text{pCO}_2 \tag{9.2}$$

Where:

- HCO_{3-}: in millimoles per litre
- $PaCO_2$: partial pressure of arterial CO2 in mmHg
- pK: Acid dissociation constant
- 0.03 the solubility of CO_2 in blood

9.3 Renal Regulation of Acid Base Disorders

Kidneys are responsible for excretion of the fixed acids and this is also a critical role even though the amounts involved (70–100 mmols/day). This action is mediated by 2 processes—Excretion of the fixed acids (1 mmol/kg/day) and Reabsorption of filtered bicarbonate at proximal convoluted tubules [5].

9.4 Technicalities of Blood-Gas Analysis

9.4.1 Site Selection

Common sites for arterial sampling includes radial, brachial, axillary femoral or dorsalis pedis artery. There is no evidence that any site is superior to the others. However, being more accessible and comfortable for the patients radial artery is used most often. Allen's test or modified Allen's test can be performed prior to sampling the radial artery to demonstrate collateral flow from the ulnar artery through the superficial palmar arch [6, 7].

9.4.2 Transport and Analysis

Analysis of the sample should be done immediately after sampling. In the event of any delay, arterial blood sample should be placed on ice. Delayed analysis results in increased potassium, phosphates, proteins and LDH. Ongoing metabolism during the delay results in reduced bicarbonate, decreased glucose and increased lactate [8]. Properly timed sample reduces oxygen consumption by leukocytes or platelets (i.e., leukocyte or platelet larceny), which can cause a factitiously low partial pressure of arterial oxygen (PaO_2). Delayed analysis result in falsely low PaO_2 and high $PaCO_2$ (increases at the rate of 3–10 mmHg/hour). [9].

9.4.3 Sources of Errors

Presence of air bubble in an ABG sample can significantly affect $PaCO_2$ and PaO_2 values. $PaCO_2$ and PaO_2 values move towards that of room air (PaO_2 room air is about 150 mm Hg, $PaCO_2$ room air is approximately zero) [10].

Heparin acts as another source of preanalytical error. It can decrease the pH (as heparin and extreme anionic charge and near-total dissociation at physiologic pH) and dilute the $PaCO_2$, resulting in a falsely low value. N+, K+, Cl−, Ca++, glucose, and lactate values also decrease by dilution with liquid heparin.[11] Dead space volume of a standard 5 ml syringe with 1 inch 22 guage needle is 0.2 ml, filling the syringe dead space with heparin provides sufficient volume to anticoagulate a 4 ml blood sample.

Types of syringes also affect the results. O_2 diffuses out at higher PaO_2 from plastic syringes. Glass syringes are less pervious to O_2. Though glass syringes may be preferred, differences are usually not of clinical significance. pH & pCO_2 values unaffected by types of syringes.

Solubility of CO_2 and O_2 is increased in hypothermia [12]. This principle is utilized in temperature based interpretation of blood gases values—*pH stat and alpha stat*. During pH-stat acid-base management, the patient's pH is maintained at a constant level by managing pH at the patient's temperature. pH-stat pH management is temperature-corrected. Compared to alpha-stat, pH stat (which aims for a pCO_2 of

40 and pH of 7.40 at the patient's actual temperature) leads to higher pCO_2 (respiratory acidosis), and increased cerebral blood flow. While, during alpha-stat acid-base management, the ionization state of histidine is maintained by managing a standardized pH (measured at 37C). Alpha-stat pH management is not temperature-corrected—as the patient's temperature falls, the partial pressure of CO_2 decreases (and solubility increases), thus a hypothermic patient with a pH of 7.40 and a pCO_2 of 40 (measured at 37C) will, in reality, have a lower pCO_2 (because partial pressure of CO_2 is lower), and this will manifest as a relative respiratory alkalosis coupled with decreased cerebral blood flow [13, 14].

Clotted sample, haemolysis by inappropriately small needle, haemolysis by syringe vacuum and poorly calibrated ABG analyser are another sources of error.

9.5 Various Models of Acid-Base Interpretation

Three common interpretation models for blood gas analysis are

1. Boston/Physiological approach
2. Copenhagen/Base excess approach
3. Stewart/Physicochemical approach

9.5.1 Boston/Physiological Approach

This approach was developed by Schwartz and colleagues at Tufts University in Boston. Based on Henderson Hasselbach Equation, the Boston approach adapts carbonic acid–bicarbonate buffer system. A primary change in the partial pressure of carbon dioxide (pCO_2) causes a secondary "adaptive" response in the bicarbonate concentration and vice versa and further changes in carbon dioxide or bicarbonate reflect additional changes in acid–base status. The six primary acid–base disorders has been described—two metabolic disorders (acidosis and alkalosis) and four respiratory disorders—acute respiratory acidosis and alkalosis, and chronic respiratory acidosis and alkalosis. Patients with known acid-base disturbances evaluated and using acid–base maps mathematic relationship between $PaCO_2$ and HCO_3- is established.[15].

Boston approach is the most frequently used approach for bed side ABG analysis. The details are presented later in the chapter.

Corrected anion gap is used to account for UMAs (unmeasured anions like albumin), in presence of which uncorrected anion gap may be normal [16]. It is calculated as

$$\text{Anion gap corrected}\left(\text{for albumin}\right) = \text{Calculated anion gap} \\ + 2.5\,\text{x}\left(\text{Normal albumin g / dL} - \text{Observed albumin g / dL}\right)$$

Anion gap assessment in Boston approach evaluates mixed acid-base disorders using delta ratio method. Delta ratio delta identify if the presence of high anion gap metabolic acidosis 'pure' or if there is coexistant normal anion gap metabolic acidosis (NAGMA) or metabolic alkalosis [17]. Delta ratio is

Increase in AG or AG-12/Decrease in HCO_3^- or 24-HCO_3^-

- Interpretation, 0.4—Normal AG metabolic acidosis
- 0.4–1.0—High AG+ Normal AG metabolic acidosis
- 1–2—Pure high AG metabolic acidosis
- >2—High AG metabolic acidosis + Metabolic alkalosis

The advantages of Boston approach is that it is a physiological, simplest, most rigorous and most serviceable of all the approaches. Drawbacks include-Assumption that pCO_2 & HCO_3 are independent, all buffering of metabolic acids are mediated by HCO_3^-, buffering by intracellular buffers is ignored and does ot many complex acid-base abnormalities like acute acidosis in setting of hypoalbuminemia, hyperchloremic acidosis and lactic acidosis [18].

9.5.2 Copenhagen/Base Excess Approach

The Copenhagen method involves the use of standard base excess (SBE) to distinguish between respiratory and metabolic influences on acid base balance. SBE, also known as the **base excess of extracellular fluid** (BEECF), is a calculated variable from pH, $PaCO_2$ and haematocrit. ABG machine calculates SBE for anaemic blood, with a Hb of 50 g/L using algorithms based on Van Slyke equation, to account for whole blood buffering [19]. Copenhagen approach uses three steps for acid base disorders-

- First step: To evaluate standard base excess in relation to pH and PCO_2
- Second step: To determine secondary response
- Third step: Partition of standard base excess (to consider mixed metabolic acid–base disorders)

The advantages of base excess approach are—SBE value is readily available from most blood gas machines, useful for evaluating acid–base disorders, four calculations of $PaCO_2$ and SBE to evaluate secondary response and easier to remember and perform.

9.5.3 Stewart/Physicochemical Approach

This approach was introduced by Peter Stewart in 1978 [20]. It is based on two main principles-electroneutrality (Sum of all positively charged ions = sum of all negatively charged ions in aqueous solutions) and Conservation of mass (Total concentration = Dissociated + Undissociated forms). pH or $[H^+]$ concentration in the body is determined by two variables, independent and dependent. The independent variables are $PaCO_2$ (controlled by respiratory system), strong ion difference/SID (controlled by kidney) and weak acid/Atot-include serum albumin, phosphate and globulins (controlled by liver and metabolic state). Dependent variables are [H+], [OH−], [HCO_3−].

Normal value of SID ranges between 38–44 mmol/L. (value less than 38 mmmol/L is interpreted as SID acidosis and higher than 44 mmol/L is SID alkalosis) [21].

Stewart approach identifies 6 acid base disorders-Respiratory acidosis and alkalosis, SID acidosis and alkalosis, Increased Atot acidosis and decreased Atot alkalosis.

$$\mathrm{SID_a} = \left([\mathrm{Na}+]+[\mathrm{K}+]+[\mathrm{Mg}++]+[\mathrm{Ca}++]\right)-\left([\mathrm{Cl}-]+[\mathrm{lactate}]\right)$$
$$\mathrm{SID_e} = [\mathrm{HCO_3}-]+[\mathrm{albumin}]+[\mathrm{phosphates}]$$

Where, SID_a is strong ion difference apparenrent and SID_e is strong ion difference effective. The difference between SID_a and SID_e is stong ion gap (SIG) and SIG is close to zero in normal situations. SIG Quantifies amount of unmeasured anions present in the plasma. [20, 21].

Advantages of Stewart approach are quantitative mathematical explanation of acid-base disorders, a more scientific approach which apply concepts of physical chemistry to traditional acid-base concepts and a logical framework for design of resuscitation fluids. Disadvantages are complex, complicated, and difficult to apply approach at bedside, substantially different to well-validated classical Boston approach, numerous variables creates confusion and no evidence that this approach has any influence on mortality.

9.6 What to Correct, How Much to Correct and How to Correct?

Being the most commonly used approach, physiological/Boston approach is selected here as a primary method for correction of acid base disorders.

9.7 Approach to Patient with Metabolic Derangements

Bedside approach to patient with metabolic acid base disorders involve

- Identification of presence of metabolic acidosis (pH < 7.30, serum [HCO_3^-] < 24 mEq/l)/metabolic alkalosis (pH > 7.40, serum [HCO_3^-] > 24 mEq/l)
- Respiratory compensation-adequate or inadequate
- Estimation of AG (anion gap) in the presence of metabolic acidosis
- Acknowledge presence of mixed disorders using delta ratio

9.7.1 Expected Respiratory Compensation to Metabolic Acidosis [15]

Rule 1: for Metabolic Acidosis

$$\text{Expected pCO2} = 1.5\left[\text{HCO}_3\right] + 8\left(\text{Range} : +/-2\right)$$

9.7.2 Anion Gap

Anion gap (AG) is used for evaluation of metabolic acidosis. The sum of the positive and negative ion charges in plasma are equal in vivo: [Na+] + [K+] + [Ca2+] + [Mg2+] + [H+] + unmeasured cations = [Cl−] + [HCO_3−] + [CO_3^{2-}] + [OH−] + albumin+phosphate+sulfate+lactate+unmeasured anions (e.g., inorganic anions) [22–24]. Other ions being in extremely low concentration, following formulas are used to estimate AG [25]:

$$\text{AG}\left(\text{simple}\right) = ([\text{Na} + -\left(\left[\text{Cl} -\right] + \left[\text{HCO3} -\right]\right) = 12 - 14\,\text{mEq} / \text{L}$$

$$\text{AG}\left(\text{conventional}\right) = (\left[\text{Na} =\right] + \left[\text{K} +\right] - \left(\left[\text{Cl} -\right] + \left[\text{HCO3} -\right]\right) = 14\,\text{to}\,18\,\text{mEq} / \text{L}$$

$$\text{AG}\left(\text{modern}\right) = (\left[\text{Na} =\right] + \left[\text{K} +\right] - \left(\left[\text{Cl} -\right] + \left[\text{HCO3} -\right] + \left[\text{Lactate}\right]\right) = 14\,\text{to}\,18\,\text{mEq} / \text{L}$$

Corrected anion gap is used to account for UMAs (unmeasured anions like albumin), in presence of which uncorrected anion gap may be normal.[16] It is calculated as

$$\text{Anion gap corrected}\left(\text{for albumin}\right) = \text{Calculated anion gap} + 2.5\,\text{x}\left(\text{Normal albumin g} / \text{dL} - \text{Observed albumin g} / \text{dL}\right)$$

9.8 Causes and Treatment of High Anion Gap Metabolic Acidosis

L-Lactic acidosis	Correction of underlying disorder, correction of shock, improving oxygenation, removing offending drugs, treatment of seizures, Hemodialysis may be indicated in resistant cases
Diabetic ketoacidosis	Fluids and insulin
Methanol toxicity	Oral charcoal, soda bicarbonate, fomepizole
Salicylate toxicity	Alkalinization of urine, Haemodialysis
Ethylene glycol	Ethanol or fomepizole
Propylene glycol toxicity	Stop the drug infusion
Impaired lactate clearance in liver failure	Supportive management, NAC
D-Lactic acidosis	sodium bicarbonate and antimicrobial agents

9.9 Nonanion Gap Acidosis

Bicarbonate loss is the primary pathophysiology for nonanion gap acidosis. Cl^- is raised maintaining the anion gap to normal. Gastrointestinal losses and renal etiology are the primary causes of nonanion gap acidosis and urine anion gap (UAG) is used to distinguish between them.

$$\text{UAG} = \left(\text{Urine}\left[\text{Na}+\right] + \text{Urine}\left[\text{K}+\right]\right) - \left(\text{Urine}\left[\text{Cl}-\right]\right)$$

The UAG is normally zero or slightly positive. In the setting of a nonanion gap acidosis, the appropriate renal response would be to increase ammonium excretion, as NH4Clcausing the UAG to become negative, usually ranging from −20 to −50 mEq/L. This is seen in nonrenal causes of.

nonanion gap acidosis, such as severe diarrhea. In renal derangements, like chronic kidney disease (CKD) and distal renal tubular acidosis (RTA), the UAG will remain positive or become only slightly negative.

Normal anion gap metabolic acidosis
1. Loss of bicarbonate
• Gastrointestinal conditions (diarrhea, ureteral diversions, biliary or pancreatic fistulas)
2.Renal tubular acidosis-Type 1, 2 and 4
3. Other causes: fluid resuscitation with saline, hyperalimentation (lysine, histidine, or arginine hydrochloride), administration of hydrochloride, ammonium chloride, cholestyramine, hippuric acid, sulfuric acid

9.10 Metabolic Alkalosis

The diagnosis of metabolic alkalosis is sometimes a clinical one, but it is often found incidentally of laboratory work. A higher serum bicarbonate level in association with hypokalemia is highly suggestive of metabolic alkalosis.

Rule 2: Respiratory compensation for a Metabolic Alkalosis [15]

$$\text{Expected pCO2} = 0.7\left[\text{HCO}_3\right] + 20\left(\text{Range} : +/-2\right)$$

9.11 Causes of Metabolic Alkalosis

Urine chloride concentration (U_{Cl-}) a useful tool in the diagnosis and management of metabolic alkalosis [26].

Chloride Responsive ($U_{Cl} \leq 25$ mEq/L)	Chloride Resistant (UC > 25 mEq/L)
Gastrointestinal losses-vomiting, Nasogastric suction – Post hypercapnia – Cystic fibrosis – Prior loop/thiazide diuretics use – Chloride losing diarrhoea-villous adenoma, laxative abuse **Treatment**—administration of 0.9% or 0.45% NaCl, potassium repletion	**With high B.P** – Primary/secondary hyperaldosteronism, Cushing's syndrome, recent diuretics use, renal artery stenosis, rennin secreting tumor, hydroxylase deficiencies, licorice intake **With normal B.P** – Bartter syndrome, Gitelman syndrome **Other causes** – Alkali intake or administration Milk alkali syndrome – Severe potassium depletion **Treatment**—Treat the underlying cause, potassium repletion, Acetazolamide (metabolic alkalosis associated with volume overload complicated by the need for continued attempts at diuresis), intermittent hemodialysis with the bicarbonate bath decreased to the lowest allowable value or a continuous hemofiltration modality using primarily a nonbicarbonate, noncitrate replacement fluid.

9.12 Approach to Respiratory Acid–Base Disorders [27, 28]

Bedside approach to patient with respiratory acid base disorders involve

- Identification of presence of respiratory acidosis (pH < 7.30, $PaCO_2$ > 45 mm Hg)/respiratory alkalosis (pH > 7.40, $PaCO_2$ < 45 mm Hg)
- Metabolic compensation-adequate or inadequate
- Determine if mixed acid base disorder is present
- Treat the underlying causes

9.13 Expected Metabolic Compensation to Respiratory Derangements [15]

Rule 3: Acute Respiratory Acidosis

$$\text{Expected}\left[\text{HCO}_3\right] = 24 + \left\{\left(\text{Actual pCO}_2 - 40\right)/10\right\}$$

Rule 4: Chronic Respiratory Acidosis

$$\text{Expected}\left[\text{HCO3}\right] = 24 + 4\left\{\left(\text{Actual pCO2} - 40\right)/10\right\}$$

Rule 5: Acute Respiratory Alkalosis

$$\text{Expected}\left[\text{HCO3}\right] = 24 - 2\left\{\left(40 - \text{Actual pCO2}\right)/10\right\}$$

Rule 6: Chronic Respiratory Alkalosis

$$\text{Expected}\left[\text{HCO3}\right] = 24 - 5\{\left(40 - \text{Actual pCO2}\right))/10\}\left(\text{range} : +/{-2}\right)$$

The 0.008 rule: The pH change in response to an acute respiratory acid-base disturbance

$$\text{pH} = 7.40 - \left(\left(\text{PaCO}_2 - 40\right) \text{x}\, 0.008\right))$$

The 0.003 rule: The pH change in response to a chronic respiratory acid-base disturbance

$$\text{pH} = 7.40 - \left(\left(\text{PaCO}_2 - 40\right) \text{x}\, 0.003\right))$$

9.14 Causes of Respiratory Derangements

Respiratory acidosis	Respiratory alkalosis
Decreased alveolar ventilation – Central respiratory depression e.g. by drugs or post-ictally – Neuromuscular disorders resulting in weakness – Lung or chest wall defects resulting in restriction – Airway obstruction, e.g. after a seizure – Inadequate mechanical ventilation	Respiratory control centre – Head injury, stroke – Anxiety, fear, stress, pain – Salicylates – Pregnancy – Chronic liver disease – Hypoxia
Increased inspired fraction of CO_2 – Rebreathing of CO_2-containing expired gas – Addition of CO_2 to inspired gas – Insufflation of CO_2 into body cavity (eg for laparoscopic surgery)	Pulmonary receptors – Pulmonary embolism – Pneumonia – Asthma – Pulmonary oedema
Increased metabolic CO_2 production – Malignant hyperthermia – Thyrotoxicosis – Phaeochromocytoma – Sepsis – Liver failure	
Treatment – Addressing the underlying etiology (bronchodilators for patients with asthma and chronic obstructive pulmonary disease, reversal of medication/drug effects, treatment of pulmonary edema, treatment of neuromuscular diseases, and mechanical ventilation	Treatment – Addressing the underlying etiology (Decreasing minute ventilation in mechanically ventilated patients, reassurance and anxiolytics for psychogenic hyperventilation, acetazolamide to induce a metabolic acidosis to compensate for the respiratory alkalosis caused by high altitudes)

References

1. Adrogue HE, Adrogue HJ. Acid-base physiology. Respir Care. 2001 Apr;46(4):328–41.
2. Johnston DG, Alberti KG. Acid-base balance in metabolic acidoses. Clin Endocrinol Metab. 1983 Jul;12(2):267–85.
3. Hasan A. Buffer systems. In: Handbook of blood gas/acid-base interpretation. London: Springer; 2013. https://doi.org/10.1007/978-1-4471-4315-4_4.
4. Worthley LI. Hydrogen ion metabolism. Anaesth Intensive Care. 1977 Nov;5(4):347–60. pmid:23014.
5. Hamm LL, Nakhoul N, Hering-Smith KS. Acid-base homeostasis. Clin J Am Soc Nephrol. 2015;10(12):2232–42.
6. Bartella AK, Flick N, Kamal M, Steegmann J, Kloss-Brandstätter A, Teichmann J, Hölzle F, Lethaus B. Hand perfusion in patients with physiological or pathological Allen's tests. J Reconstr Microsurg. 2019 Mar;35(3):182–8.
7. Romeu-Bordas Ó, Ballesteros-Peña S. Reliability and validity of the modified Allen test: a systematic review and metanalysis. AbrEmergencias. 2017;29(2):126–35.
8. Tanner M, Kent N, Smith B, Fletcher S, Lewer M. Stability of common biochemical analytes in serum gel tubes subjected to various storage temperatures and times pre-centrifugation. Ann Clin Biochem. 2008;45(4):375–9.
9. Hess CE, Nichols AB, Hunt WB, Suratt PM. Pseudohypoxemia secondary to leukemia and thrombocytosis. N Engl J Med. 1979;301:361.
10. Biswas CK, Ramos JM, Agroyannis B, Kerr DN. Blood gas analysis: effect of air bubbles in syringe and delay in estimation. Br Med J (Clin Res Ed). 1982;284(6320):923–7. https://doi.org/10.1136/bmj.284.6320.923.
11. Bageant RA. Variations in arterial blood gas measurements due to sampling techniques. Respir Care. 1975;20:565.
12. Ashwood ER, Kost G, Kenny M. Temperature correction of blood-gas and pH measurements. Clin Chem. 1983;29(11):1877–85.
13. Tarik Kiziltan H, Baltali M, Bilen A, Seydaoglu G, Incesoz M, Tasdelen A, Aslamaci S. Comparison of alpha-stat and pH-stat cardiopulmonary bypass in relation to jugular venous oxygen saturation and cerebral glucose-oxygen utilization. Anesth Analg. 2003;96(3): 644–50.
14. Sakamoto T, Kurosawa H, Shin'oka T, Aoki M, Isomatsu Y. The influence of pH strategy on cerebral and collateral circulation during hypothermic cardiopulmonary bypass in cyanotic patients with heart disease: results of a randomized trial and real-time monitoring. J Thorac Cardiovasc Surg. 2004;127(1):12–9.
15. Berend K, de Vries APJ, Gans ROB. Physiological approach to assessment of acid–base disturbances. N Engl J Med. 2014;371:1434–45.
16. Figge J, et al. Crit Care Med. 1998;26:1807.
17. Tsapenko MV. Modified delta gap equation for quick evaluation of mixed metabolic Acid-base disorders. Oman Med J. 2013;28(1):73–4. https://doi.org/10.5001/omj.2013.18.
18. Adrogué HJ, Gennari FJ, Galla JH, Madias NE. Assessing acid-base disorders. Kidney Int. 2009;
19. Kofstad J. Base excess. Clin Chim Acta. 2001.
20. Stewart PA. Independent and dependent variables of acidbase control. Resp Physiol. 1978;33:9–26.
21. Stewart PA. How to understand acid-base: a quantitative acid-base primer for biology and medicine. New York: Elsevier; 1981.
22. Feldman M, Soni N, Dickson B. Influence of hypoalbuminemia or hyperalbuminemia on the serum anion gap. J Lab Clin Med. 2005;146:317–20.
23. Moe OW, Fuster D. Clinical acid-base pathophysiology: disorders of plasma anion gap. Best Pract Res Clin Endocrinol Metab. 2003;17:559–74.

24. Kellum JA. Making strong ion difference the "Euro" for bedside acid-base analysis. In: Vincent JL, editor. Yearbook of intensive care and emergency medicine. Berlin: Springer; 2005. p. 675–85.
25. Emmett M, Narins RG. Medicine (Baltimore). 1977;56:38.
26. Soifer JT, Kim HT. Approach to metabolic alkalosis. Emerg Med Clin North Am. 2014;32(2):453–63.
27. Epstein SK, Singh N. Respiratory acidosis. Respir Care. 2001;46(4):366–83.
28. Foster GT, Vaziri ND, Sassoon CS. Respiratory alkalosis. Respir Care. 2001;46(4):384–91.

Oxygen Therapy in Cancer Patients

10

Uma R. Hariharan, Shweta Bhopale, Kiran Mahendru, and Rakesh Garg

10.1 Introduction

Oxygen is the breath of life. Oncology patients may need oxygen therapy at various stages of their treatment. Oxygen therapy is a medical management strategy of supplementing oxygen at higher concentrations in patients showing features suggestive of hypoxemia or hypoxia [1]. Oxygen needs to be used with great caution as a medication in indicated situations. Unscrupulous use of Oxygen in cancer patients may be deleterious rather than being useful. This chapter focuses on the various aspects of oxygen therapy in oncology patients, their indications, types of oxygen delivery devices, monitoring, side-effects, and their role in palliative care. The usefulness of hyperbaric oxygen therapy is also discussed in this chapter.

10.2 Oxygen Cascade

It describes the sequential transfer of oxygen from the atmosphere to the cellular organelles (mitochondria). It is a cascade because in each step there is a fall in PaO_2 (partial pressure of oxygen). It determines the oxygen delivery to tissues down the pressure gradients (step-wise decrease in oxygen partial pressures). Oxygen cascade is important to understand the nuances of oxygen therapy. Tissues have no storage mechanism for this vital substance and hence, depend on the continuous

U. R. Hariharan
ABVIMS & Dr Ram Manohar Lohia Hospital and PGIMER, New Delhi, India

S. Bhopale · R. Garg (✉)
Oncoanaesthesia & Palliative Medicine, AIIMS, New Delhi, New Delhi, India

K. Mahendru
Dayanand Medical College & Hospital Ludhiana, Ludhiana, Punjab, India

V. Kumar et al. (eds.), *Onco-critical Care*, https://doi.org/10.1007/978-981-16-9929-0_10

supply of oxygen in tandem with the metabolic demands. The following are the major steps in the oxygen cascade [2]:

a. Oxygen uptake from the atmosphere by the lungs
b. Oxygen carrying capacity of the blood
c. Global delivery from lungs to tissue
d. Regional distribution of oxygen
e. Diffusion from capillary to cell
f. Cellular use of oxygen

The alveolar-arterial oxygen gradient is indicative of the oxygen absorption and its delivery [3]. Normal PAO_2–PaO_2 (A-a) gradient or the alveolar to arterial oxygen difference is 1 KPa. The alveolar (A) to arterial (a) oxygen gradient is indicative of alveolo-capillary membrane functionality for adequate gas exchange. This can increase tremendously in respiratory failure patients, which can be encountered in some cancer patients, especially in terminal stages of metastatic disease. The gradient is normal in cases of alveolar hypoventilation. Alveolar hypoventilation [4] as a cause of hypoxia is reflected by a fall in alveolar and arterial PO_2 with increasing $PaCO_2$. Alveolo-capillary unit pathology widens this gradient, eg hypoxemia due to V/Q mismatch, diffusion limitation, and shunt. The three main causes [5] of arterial hypoxemia requiring oxygen therapy include *alveolar hypoventilation*; *diffusion abnormalities* and *ventilation-perfusion mismatch*. The major causes of alveolar hypoventilation in cancer patients include phrenic nerve invasion, opioid overdose, invasive chest wall tumors, or peri-operative anesthetic complications. The common causes of diffusion impairment in cancer include malignant pleural effusion, pleural thickening or fibrosis, invasive mesotheliomas, and pulmonary metastases. Causes of hypoxemia due to ventilation-perfusion (V/Q) mismatch [6] include asthma, COPD (smoking), bronchiectasis, interstitial lung disease (chemotherapy or radiotherapy-induced), and pulmonary hypertension (drug-induced). Patients with hypoxemia due to shunt respond poorly to supplemental oxygen and its major causes in cancer patients include secondary pneumonia, severe anemia (bone marrow suppression, large vascular tumors, or operative massive blood loss), pulmonary edema, and development of ARDS (acute respiratory distress syndrome) during cancer treatment.

10.3 Principles of Oxygen Therapy

The 21% of oxygen in atmospheric air is sufficient for normal human respiration. In cancer patients with various systemic diseases like COPD exacerbation, febrile neutropenias, thrombo-embolic states, metastatic disease, and chemo-or-radio-therapy-induced complications, supplemental oxygen is required to improve oxygen content and delivery to tissues. The major carrier of oxygen in the blood is hemoglobin and measured using a pulse oximeter [7]. The minor proportion is in soluble form and assessed via measurement of PaO_2 (normal values in healthy adults 80–100 mmHg).

This dissolved oxygen can be improved by supplemental oxygen, which can also reduce the work of breathing. Oxygen therapy is indicated for hypoxia and hypoxemia. Supplied oxygen without added moisture can be used as low-flow via nasal cannula or a mask, with the advantage of reduced bacterial contamination. They may lead to drying out of upper airway mucosa and thickening of secretions. A humidified oxygen can be used for high-flow oxygen (>4 L/min) with greater patient comfort as well as a greater risk of bacterial contamination [8].

10.4 Indications of Oxygen Therapy in Cancer Patients

The indications of oxygen therapy in cancer patients are numerous, the most important being hypoxemia [9]. It can be administered in institutional or domiciliary settings [10]. Indications of oxygen therapy in cancer patients can be divided into the following four categories (Table 10.1):

A. Acute indications: Medical emergencies

Cancer patients may require oxygen in acute conditions like shock, sepsis, anaphylaxis, transfusion reactions, major trauma, acute heart failure, pulmonary embolism, myocardial infarction, asthma exacerbation, acute respiratory failure, etc. Generally, these are given in ICUs or HDUs, with or without ventilatory support and monitoring.

B. Chronic indications: Chronic medical conditions

Cancer patients with severe COPD, pulmonary metastasis, restrictive lung disease, lung cancer, malignant pleural effusions, cancer cachexia, etc., may require oxygen therapy on a daily or frequent basis. It can be in the domiciliary or institutional settings.

C. Perioperative indications: Surgical and anesthetic course

Cancer patients requiring surgical procedures (diagnostic and therapeutic) require oxygen therapy during the perioperative period.

Table 10.1 Need of oxygen therapy in cancer patients

Serial No.	Indication of oxygen in oncology	Examples
1.	Acute	Medical emergencies like sepsis
2.	Chronic	Long-term conditions like COPD
3.	Peri-operative	Diagnostic & Therapeutic procedures under anesthesia
4.	Palliative	End-stage cancer for comfort

Table 10.2 Various types of oxygen delivery devices

Sr no.	Type of oxygen delivery device	Example	FiO_2/flow rate
1.	Variable Performance (Low-Flow)	Nasal cannula/prongs; Simple mask; Mask with reservoir; Partial Rebreathing & Non-rebreathing mask	21–100%/1–15 L/min
2.	Fixed Performance (High-flow)	Air-entraining Venturi mask	24–60%/4–12 L/min
3.	High flow systems	High-flow nasal cannula/High flow nasal prongs/ High flow nasal oxygen therapy (washes out 2 and creates positive nasopharyngeal pressure, used in hypoxemic respiratory failure)	Heated & Humidified 2 at 21–100% FiO_2 @ upto 60 litres/min.
4.	Other methods	Non-invasive positive pressure devices (deliver positive pressure either with the tight-fitting mask or a helmet and provides CPAP)	40–100% FiO_2 either by the ventilator or stand-alone device

D. Palliative indications: End-stage cancer

Terminally ill cancer patients may require oxygen as part of palliative therapy to provide comfort to the patient and relieve dyspnea.

10.5 Types of Oxygen Delivery Devices

The type of oxygen delivery device decides the oxygen concentration delivered [11]. (Table 10.2). The various oxygen delivery devices include low-flow or high flow systems, with or without humidity, and with or without a reservoir bag. Oxygen therapy equipment consists of the oxygen-delivery system (consisting of an oxygen source, regulator, delivery device) and oxygen cylinders (made of aluminum filled with pressurized oxygen). There are several types of oxygen cylinders [12], the common ones being D type (425 L), Jumbo D type (640 L), and E type (680 L).

Oxygen delivery devices can be grouped into the following:

1. Nasal cannula: It provides supplemental oxygen to breathing patients at the low inspired concentration (Flow rate of 1–6 L/min with FiO_2 25–45%) (Fig. 10.1).
2. Simple face masks: Used at 5–8 L/min flow and delivering oxygen concentration 28–50%. (Fig. 10.2)
3. Non-rebreather mask (reservoir mask): Deliver high concentrations of supplemental oxygen (Flow rate of 10–16 L/min with FiO_2 80–90%), useful in acute situations (Figs. 10.3 and 10.4).
4. Blow-by delivery: Especially useful for children who will not tolerate traditional face masks on the face.
5. Venturi mask or air-entrainment masks: It delivers a pre-determined oxygen concentration (color-coded mask ports with FiO_2 ranging from 24 to 60% over a

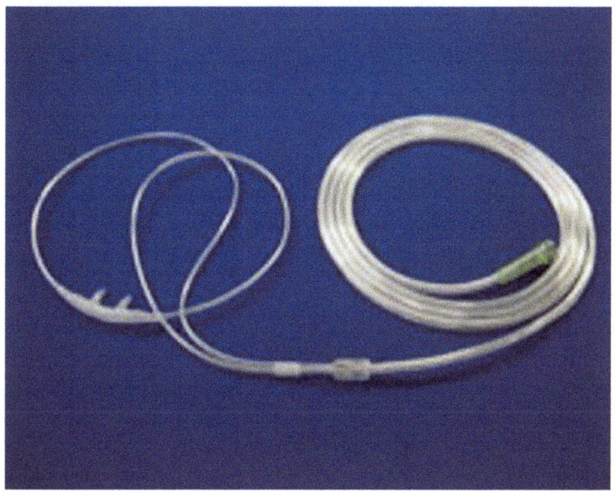

Fig. 10.1 Nasal Cannula

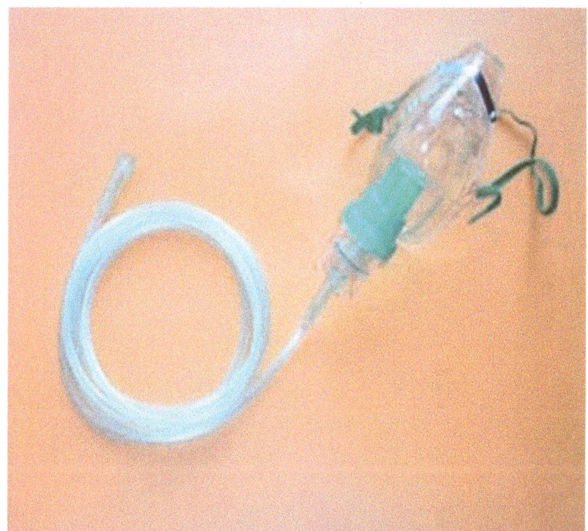

Fig. 10.2 Simple face mask

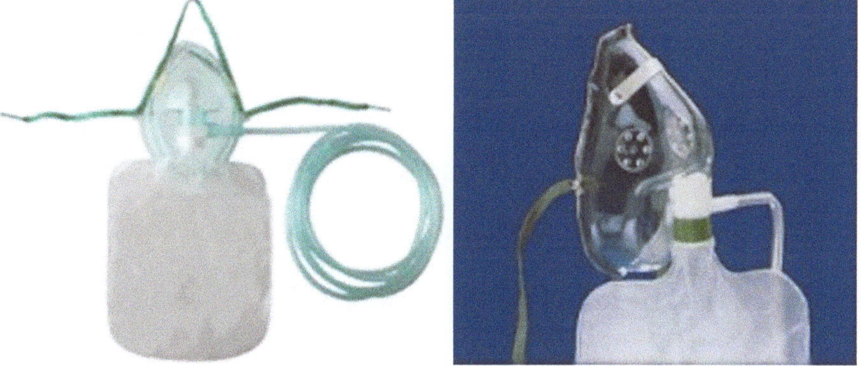

Figs. 10.3 and 10.4 Non-rebreather mask

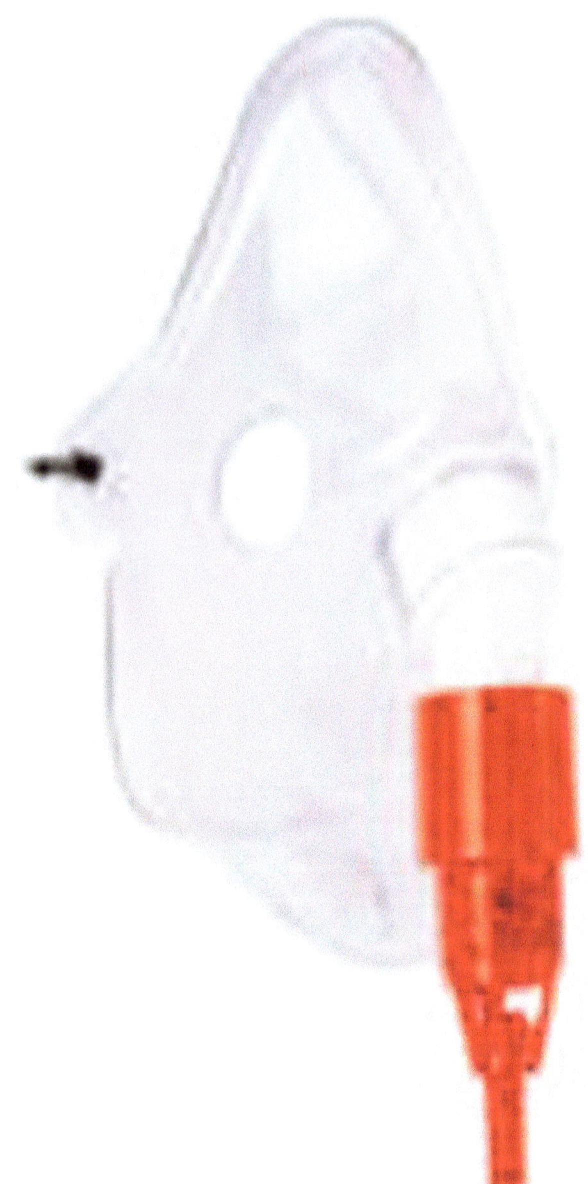

Fig. 10.5 Venturi Mask

flow rate range of 2–15 L/Min) (Fig. 10.5). It is particularly useful in COPD patients.

6. Demand oxygen delivery systems (DODS): It delivers oxygen as triggered by patient inhalation or with patient-controlled use of push-button. It conserves oxygen as compared to other steady-flow devices. They are useful in performing resuscitation as rescue breaths (100% O_2) can be delivered with the press of a button.

Fig. 10.6 T-piece

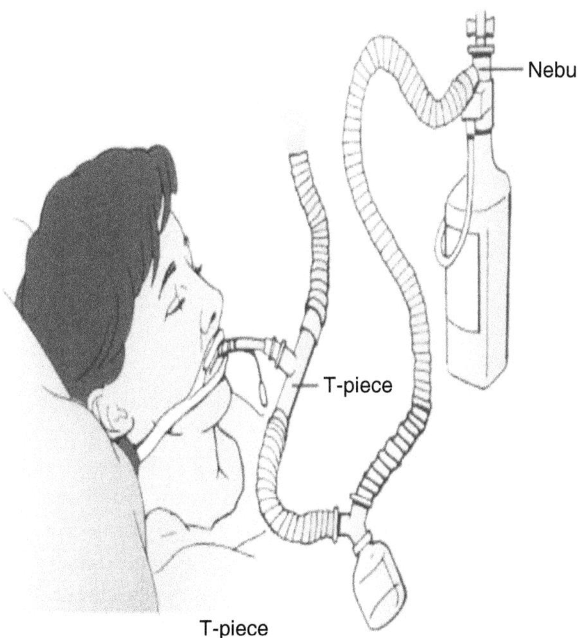

7. Humidified High flow nasal oxygen cannula: Provides 100% FiO_2 at flow rates of 60 L/min.
8. Tracheal delivery systems:

a. Tracheostomy masks—Delivers FiO_2 of 30–80% at a flow rate of 8–10 L/min via a small plastic dome that fits over tracheostomy site;
b. T-piece: It is a T-shaped tubing device that can be connected to an oxygen source, delivering FiO_2 of 30–80% at flow rates of 8–10 L/min (Fig. 10.6);
c. Trans-tracheal oxygen therapy – Hollow transtracheal catheter for long-term domiciliary oxygen therapy at flow rates of 0.5–4 L/min with FiO_2 40%.

10.6 Dosage and Monitoring of Patients on Oxygen

Monitoring during oxygen therapy includes arterial blood gas analyses, oxygen saturation charting, respiratory rate, end-tidal carbon dioxide monitoring, and clinical assessment of the patient for consciousness level, comfort, and dryness of upper airway mucosa [13]. Hemodynamic parameters and hematocrit can also be monitored. Pressure in the oxygen cylinders should not fall below 200 psi (pressure in a full oxygen cylinder is 2000 psi). The BTS (British Thoracic Society) guideline [14] recommends titrated supplementation of oxygen with a target of 94–98% for most acute ill patients or 88–92% for those at risk of hypercapnic respiratory failure. If there are no contraindications, conscious hypoxemic patients must be nursed in the upright position to improve oxygenation. Humidified oxygen remains the acceptable mode [15, 16].

10.7 Oxygen Targets for Oncology Patients in ICU

Oxygen desaturation can be alarming and is generally regarded as deleterious in critically ill patients. However, some studies have demonstrated increased mortality in patients with liberal oxygen strategy [17]. The optimum range of SpO_2 in them was 94–98%. A new, dimensionless variable, known as "*oxygen reserve index (ORI)*", is a continuous, non-invasive index, using multi-wavelength pulse co-oximetry [18]. The benefits of using oxygen must outweigh the disadvantages of cancer [19–22].

10.8 Side Effects

The possible disadvantages of supplemental oxygen therapy are related to decreases ambulation and its related concern, and discomfort associated with oxygen delivery devices [23]. Hazards associated with oxygen storage and delivery devices can be dangerous. Oxygen under high pressure (2000 psi) in full tanks, if punctured or breaking off of valve, can result in deadly projectiles or explosion. Hazards of oxygen therapy like atelectasis, oxygen-related free radicles formation, etc. should be noted while its use [24]. Since oxygen is a supporter of combustion, extreme care should be taken to avoid critical injuries or explosive accidents. Smoking should be avoided while using oxygen and in home-care settings, oxygen devices should be kept far away (more than 5 feet) from the kitchen, heaters, and flammable liquids. Administration of oxygen to COPD patients will suppress their hypoxic ventilatory drive, resulting in hypercapnia and sometimes, respiratory acidosis. Pulmonary fibrosis can occur due to potentiation of oxygen toxicity in cancer patients who have taken chemotherapy with bleomycin or in cardiac patients on amiodarone. Hyperoxia is a continuing risk in these patients, requiring controlled and titrated oxygen usage.

10.9 High-Frequency Nasal Oxygen Therapy in Cancer Patients

The recent usefulness of high-flow, warmed and humidified nasal oxygen has been reported in critically ill patients with reversible causes while the drugs and strategies are being administered for optimization [25]. Humidified, high-flow nasal oxygen has shown improved oxygenation and lower respiratory rate. A study by Kamei et al. [26] showed that HFNC may improve dyspnea in DNI (Do Not Intubate) patients with advanced cancer and sometimes improve quality of life (QOL).

10.10 Conventional Vs Conservative Oxygen Therapy in Oncology ICU

The conventional approach oxygen therapy has its own limitation and an conservative approach of oxygen supplementation has been found to be useful in critically care settings. This is especially true in cases of advanced or terminal cancer patients [27]. The oxygen therapy requires close collaboration between oncologists, intensivists, palliative care physicians, nutritionists, nursing staff, and physiotherapists.

10.11 Role of Hyperbaric Oxygen Therapy in Cancer Patients

Hyperbaric oxygen (HBO) therapy has also been indicated in the selected group of cancer patients who are critically ill [28–33]. HBO induces an anti-angiogenic effect, and overcomes chemotherapeutic resistance. There are two different clinical applications for use of HBO in combination with radiotherapy: (a) Therapeutic: to treat late radiation injury, and (b) Radiosensitizer: to increase the effect of radiotherapy. Hyperbaric oxygen can particularly be helpful in the healing of radiation-induced colitis.

10.12 Oxygen Therapy in Palliative Care Cancer Patients

Palliative care is an essential part of cancer therapy at any stage of their treatment. Oxygen therapy may be required in their course of management, not only for tiding over crises but also in end-of-life care. The typical indications for oxygen include hypoxia and dyspnea. In end-stage cancer patients, especially in lung cancer, the prime aim is to abolish dyspnoea and improve patient comfort [34]. Oxygen is neither the only management option nor is it the most efficacious treatment for relieving dyspnea [35–37].

10.13 Conclusions

Oxygen must be used cautiously in oncology patients and must be considered a medication with its side effects. The main indications are hypoxemia, dyspnea, acute conditions, and peri-operative situations. Adjuvant therapies like the use of appropriate antibiotics, nasal drops, inhalers, nebulization, chest physiotherapy, and deep breathing exercises should be advised concurrently to treat such patients. Treatment of the underlying cause should be done in case of reversible conditions like infections. In refractory cases with a terminal illness, prognostication with supportive care ensuring patient comfort should be attempted.

10.14 Future Prospects

Future research must focus on the development of oxygen conservation technology, miniaturization of storage and delivery devices, better portable systems with humidification, and methods to minimize hazards. The role of hyperbaric oxygen in cancer patients needs further studies in specific cancers with a way to avoid oxygen toxicity. The awareness regarding role of palliative care in advanced and terminally-ill cancer patients must be spread further and alternatives to oxygen must be searched in such patients to improve quality of life and provide comfort to these patients.

References

1. Corsonello A, Pedone C, Scarlata S, Zito A, Laino I, Antonelli-Incalzi R. The oxygen therapy. Curr Med Chem. 2013;20(9):1103–26.
2. Arora S, Tantia P. Physiology of oxygen transport and its determinants in intensive care unit. Indian J Crit Care Med. 2019;23(Suppl 3):S172–7.
3. Hantzidiamantis PJ, Amaro E. Physiology, alveolar to arterial oxygen gradient. [Updated 2020 Oct 11]. In: StatPearls [Internet]. Treasure Island, FL: StatPearls Publishing; 2020 Jan.
4. Muzumdar H, Arens R. Central alveolar hypoventilation syndromes. Central alveolar hypoventilation syndromes. Sleep Med Clin. 2008;3(4):601–15.
5. Shehabi Y, Collins DW. Arterial Hypoxemia. In: Vincent JL, Hall JB, editors. Encyclopedia of intensive care medicine. Heidelberg: Springer, Berlin; 2012.
6. Sarkar M, Niranjan N, Banyal PK. Mechanisms of hypoxemia. Lung India. 2017;34(1):47–60.
7. Collins JA, Rudenski A. Relating oxygen partial pressure, saturation and content: the haemoglobin-oxygen dissociation curve. Breathe (Sheff). 2015;11(3):194–201.
8. de la Fuente-Sancho I, Romeu-Bordas Ó, Fernández-Aedo I, De la Hoz GV, Ballesteros-Peña S. Microbiological contamination in high and low flow oxygen humidifiers: a systematic review. Med Intensiva. 2019;43(1):18–25.
9. Maunder RJ. JPM patient information. Oxygen therapy at the end of life. J Palliat Med. 2006;9(4):1030–1.
10. Igarashi H, Fukushi M, Nago N. Oxygen use and survival in patients with advanced cancer and low oxygen saturation in home care: a preliminary retrospective cohort study. BMC Palliat Care. 2020;19(1):3.
11. Batool S, Garg R. Appropriate use of oxygen delivery devices. The Open Anesthesiology Journal. 2017;11:35–8.
12. Srivastava U. Anaesthesia gas supply: gas cylinders. Indian J Anaesth. 2013;57(5):500–6.
13. Lellouche F, L'Her E. Usual and advanced monitoring in patients receiving oxygen therapy. Respir Care. 2020;65(10):1591–600.
14. O'Driscoll BR, Howard LS, Earis J, Mak V on behalf of the British Thoracic Society Emergency Oxygen Guideline Group. BTS guideline for oxygen use in adults in healthcare and emergency settings. Thorax. 2017;72:ii1–ii90.
15. Diaz-Lobato S, Perales JMC, Inigo JMA, Alises SM, Segovia B, et al. Things to keep in mind in high flow therapy: as usual the devil is in the detail. Int J Crit Care Emerg Med. 2018;4:048.
16. McCoy RW. Options for home oxygen therapy equipment: storage and metering of oxygen in the home. Respir Care. 2013;58(1):65–85.
17. Beasley R. Increased risk of mortality with liberal oxygen therapy compared with conservative oxygen therapy in critically ill adults. BMJ Evid Based Med. 2019;24(3):113–4.
18. Szmuk P, Steiner JW, Olomu PN, Ploski RP, Sessler DI, Ezri T. Oxygen reserve index: a novel non-invasive measure of oxygen reserve—a pilot study. Anesthesiology. 2016;124(4):779–84.
19. Clemens KE, Quednau I, Klaschik E. Use of oxygen and opioids in the palliation of dyspnoea in hypoxic and non-hypoxic palliative care patients: a prospective study. Support Care Cancer. 2009;17(4):367–77.
20. Girardis M. Effect of conservative vs conventional oxygen therapy on mortality among patients in an intensive care unit: the oxygen-ICU randomized clinical trial. JAMA. 2016;316(15):1583–9.
21. Chu DK, Kim LH-Y, Young PJ, Zamiri N, Almenawer SA, Jaeschke R, et al. Mortality and morbidity in acutely ill adults treated with liberal versus conservative oxygen therapy (IOTA): a systematic review and meta-analysis. Lancet. 2018;391(10131):1693–705.

22. Zhou D, Li Z, Zhou J. Time spent in oxygen saturation 95-99% is associated with reduced mortality in critically ill patients with mechanical ventilation. Crit Care. 2020;24:414.
23. Criner GJ. Ambulatory home oxygen: what is the evidence for benefit, and who does it help? Respir Care. 2013;58(1):48–64.
24. Tiep B, Carter R, Zachariah F, Williams AC, Horak D, Barnett M, Dunham R. Oxygen for end-of-life lung cancer care: managing dyspnea and hypoxemia. Expert Rev Respir Med. 2013;7(5):479–90.
25. Epstein AS, Hartridge-Lambert SK, Ramaker JS, Voigt LP, Portiock CS. Humidified high-flow nasal oxygen utilization in patients with cancer at Memorial Sloan-Kettering Cancer Center. J Palliative Med. 2011;14(7):835–9.
26. Kamei T, Okuma Y, Yomota M, Sone R, Tanaka K. High flow nasal cannula oxygen therapy for do-not-intubate patients with advanced cancer. Euro Resp J. 2017;50(61):PA1882.
27. Varela IP, del Portillo IP. Critical care admissions and discharge criteria in cancer patients. In: Nates J, Price K, editors. Oncologic Critical Care. Cham: Springer; 2020.
28. Howell RS, Criscitelli T, Woods JS, Gillette BM. Gorenstein S, et al. Hyperbaric oxygen therapy: indications, contraindications, and use at a tertiary care center. AORN J2018;107(4):442.
29. Granowitz EV, Tonomura N, Benson RM, Katz DM, Band V, et al. Hyperbaric oxygen inhibits benign and malignant human mammary epithelial cell proliferation. Anticancer Res. 2005;25:3833–42.
30. Mayer R, Hamilton-Farrell MR, Kleij AJ, Schmutz J, Granstrom G, Sicko Z, et al. Hyperbaric oxygen and radiotherapy. Strahlenther Onkol. 2005;181:113–23.
31. Stuhr EBL, Iversen VV, Oddbjorn S, Mahle B, Reed RK. Hyperbaric oxygen alone or combined with 5-FU attenuates growth of DMBA-induced rat mammary tumors. Cancer Lett. 2004;210(1):35–40.
32. Daruwalla J, Christophi C. The effect of hyperbaric oxygen therapy on tumor growth in a mouse model of colorectal cancer liver metastases. Eur J Cancer. 2006;42(18):3304–11.
33. Sahni T, Jain M, Hukku S, Jadhav GK. Role of hyperbaric oxygen therapy in oncology and radiation induced tissue damage. Apollo Medicine. 2004;1(2):186–9.
34. Khan FA, Akhtar SS, Sheikh MK. Cancer treatment – objectives and quality of life issues. Malays J Med Sci. 2005;12(1):3–5.
35. Tanaka K, Akechi T, Okuyama T, Nishiwaki Y, Uchitomi Y. Development and validation of the cancer dyspnea scale: a multidimensional, brief, self-rating scale. Br J Cancer. 2000;82(4):800–5.
36. Kako J, Morita T, Yamaguchi T, Kobayashi M, Sekimoto A, Kinoshita H, et al. Fan therapy is effective in relieving dyspnea in patients with terminally ill cancer: a parallel-arm, randomized controlled trial. J Pain Symptom Manag. 2018;56(4):493–500.
37. Wen-Yu H, Chiu T-Y, Cheng S-Y, Chen C-Y. Morphine for dyspnea control in terminal cancer patients: is it appropriate in Taiwan? J Pain Symptom Manag. 2004;28(4):356–63.

Mechanical Ventilation in Critically Ill Cancer Patient

11

Jyotsna Goswami and Sudipta Mukherjee

11.1 Introduction

Respiratory support in cancer patients can be very challenging and tricky. Irrespective of underlying acute pulmonary pathology, it depends on many other factors such as severity of underlying malignancy, ongoing treatment and/or further treatment plan, any treatment related cardiorespiratory dysfunction and its reversibility, current immune status and anticipated duration of immuno-suppressive state (if any), intent of therapy and anticipated life expectancy, wish of the patient and the family members and financial burden related to advance organ support. Invasive respiratory support like mechanical ventilation needs to be used judiciously, especially in the background of advanced pulmonary malignancy, metastatic disease, severe immunocompromised state and palliative intent of therapy. If the patients do not have enough reversible factors, they may be dependent on invasive respiratory support for prolonged duration without significant improvement in final outcome. On the contrary, not offering mechanical ventilation just because of underlying malignancy is also not a right clinical decision. So clear understanding of the cause of respiratory failure and current status of malignancy along with vision about long term outcome and expectation of the family members will guide us to take correct decision in terms of respiratory support.

a. Respiratory support strategies:

In past, respiratory failure in cancer patients used to have poor outcome. Presently because of advancement of cancer therapy, the anticipated life span of patients has been prolonged. Up to 20% admission of mixed medical-surgical ICU have underlying malignancy [1]. Respiratory failure is the most common cause of ICU admission along with major cause of death in this sub-group of patients [2]. Respiratory

J. Goswami (✉) · S. Mukherjee
Tata medical Center Kolkata, Kolkata, India

V. Kumar et al. (eds.), *Onco-critical Care*,
https://doi.org/10.1007/978-981-16-9929-0_11

failure can be related to malignancy (cancer related or chemo-radiotherapy related) or unrelated to it (decompensation of co-morbidities, pulmonary infection or other infection). It can be classified as acute, sub-acute and chronic (depending on onset of the disease) or type 1 to type 4 (pathophysiological classification). Type of respiratory support is decided based on pathophysiological changes in pulmonary system. Detailed clinical and radiological assessment will guide to identify the level and extent of pathology to airway (upper and lower), alveoli, interstitium, pulmonary circulation; or extra-pulmonary causes like pleural space, thoracic wall, diaphragm and accessory muscles; or systemic causes like cardiovascular, renal or central nervous system.

b. Non-invasive ventilation (NIV):

Historically, mechanical ventilation in cancer patients specially with haematological malignancy and post bone marrow transplant, had very poor outcome with high mortality rate. As invasive ventilation bypasses the upper airway immune protection, chance of micro-aspiration along the cuff of endotracheal tube (ETT) leading to ventilator associated pneumonia (VAP) is very high. Studies have shown that prevalence of silent aspiration of gastric contents in mechanically ventilated patients, confirmed by pepsin measurement in bronchoalveolar lavage (BAL), can be as high as 89% [3]. Additionally, there can be bleeding or bacterial transmigration through the eroded mucosa by ETT cuff. Recently significant improvement has been achieved in the outcome of cancer patients requiring mechanical ventilation, even for the patients with haematological malignancy. Therefore, avoiding invasive ventilation is not a current norm in cancer patients.

European Respiratory Society/American Thoracic Society (ERS/ATS) clinical practice guideline for use of NIV in acute respiratory failure has recommended NIV in indications like acute exacerbation of COPD with respiratory acidosis, cardiogenic pulmonary oedema, immunocompromised patients, palliative care patients, post-operative respiratory failure, chest trauma and prophylactic usage for weaning from mechanical ventilation [4]. But data for hypoxaemic respiratory failure due to pulmonary pathology is not available to make any recommendation, especially for de novo lung pathology. In most of the immunocompromised patient, the sub-group comprising of haematological malignancy and post bone marrow or solid organ transplant patients, NIV has been compared with supplemental oxygen [5–7]. Results are little heterogenous in terms of need for mechanical ventilation and mortality; even then it is difficult to extrapolate the positive outcomes in other sub-group of cancer patients.

Empirical NIV usage for all cancer patients admitted in ICU with acute respiratory failure may lead to high failure rate. Multifocal pulmonary infection/Acute respiratory Distress Syndrome (ARDS), progressive disease, newly diagnosed lung cancer, associated other organ failure, high disease severity score, male sex, prolonged NIV, high respiratory rate, NIV as first line therapy for respiratory failure and septic shock/concomitant use of vasoactive agents are main negative predictive risk factors [8, 9]. Hypoxaemic respiratory failure de novo is not immediately reversible and need prolonged respiratory support to reduce the work of breathing. High metabolic demand in sepsis leads to high inspiratory flow requirement.

Combination of large intra-pleural pressure swing because of spontaneous breathing effort with high inspiratory pressure in NIV lead to high and variable transpulmonary pressure and tidal volume, which may worsen early lung injury—self inflicting lung injury (SILI). High inspiratory pressure in NIV may lead to poor toleration, leak, gastric distension and aspiration [10, 11].

High Flow Nasal Cannula (HFNC)—HFNC can be an interesting modality for acute respiratory failure in cancer patients—specially with type 1 failure. It is a simple machine capable of delivering warm (37 °C) and humidified oxygen up to a flow rate of 60 l/min. It consists of oxygen compressor, specialised flowmeter capable of 60 l/min flow, humidifier, corrugated heated tube and nasal cannula at patient end. Along with delivery of high FiO_2, it also decreases dead space, develops certain amount of positive end-expiratory pressure (PEEP) (2–7 cm H_2O depending on flow rate and whether mouth is open or close) and improves patient's compliance. It has been used with good effect in cancer patients under palliative care [11]. But role of HFNC in cancer patients with acute respiratory failure need further evaluation.

In last decade, HFNC has been used extensively in hypoxaemic respiratory failure in general population. Frat et al. [12] in FLORALI trial, have compared HFNC with supplemental oxygen and NIV in ARDS patients. Even though the intubation rate is same, 90-days mortality was less with HFNC compared to the others. But study on immunocompromised patients [13] has shown that HFNC decreases intubation rate but does not affect mortality. So, if used judiciously, HFNC is non inferior to supplemental oxygen and NIV as per current literature.

The usage of NIV for acute respiratory failure has increased significantly over last 2 decades [14]. Even though the evidence is lacking, the use of NIV is significantly more for hypoxaemic respiratory failure (non-COPD) than patients with hypercarbic respiratory failure (COPD). Non—COPD patients have higher chance of NIV failure requiring invasive ventilation. Patients with failed NIV trial usually have poor outcome [15, 16], which may be due to delayed intubation/failure to pick up right time for invasive ventilation leading to progressive pulmonary damage due to volutrauma and barotrauma followed by emergency intubation because of rapid deterioration. So, patients having risk factors for NIV failure need more intense monitoring of their respiratory parameters.

There are different predictive scoring systems for anticipating NIV failure. Commonly used score is HACOR score [17]. HACOR score is an objective scoring system that comprises of heart rate, acidosis, consciousness, oxygenation, and respiratory rate. Maximum score is 25. Score more than 5 at 1 h of NIV trial predicts high chance of NIV failure (87%) and also mortality (65%), specifically if intubation is delayed more than 12 h. So, use of NIV should be conducted with strict monitoring of the objective criteria for identification of NIV failure to avoid undue delay in intervention such as invasive ventilation.

c. Invasive ventilation- Conventional & Non-conventional modes of ventilation (Biphasic- Bilevel, APRV, high frequency ventilation)

Proper selection of patients and improved critical care management have resulted into improved outcome of cancer patients requiring invasive ventilation. There are two challenges related to this—difficult airway & ventilatory strategies.

Airway: Airway management always requires special mention in critical care. Along with anatomical challenges, there are physiological compromises those make patient vulnerable to develop acute complications during intubation. Cancer patients can have anticipated difficult airway because of head neck tumour, acute or impending upper airway obstruction, anatomical distortion following surgery or radiotherapy around the airway. In addition to conventional assessment, objective scoring system like MACOCHA score [18] can be very helpful to assess difficult airway. It takes into consideration underlying pathology (coma, severe hypoxia) and the skill of the operator. With a cut off value of 3, it has a good sensitivity (76%) and negative predictive value (97%). Intubation difficulty scale (IDS) is a combination of objective and subjective scoring system to measure difficulty of intubation both qualitatively and quantitatively [19].

The complication data related to predictive score can be correlated clinically. Studies have shown that airway management related complication rate varies with different clinical setting. While intubation failure is a rarity in planned surgical procedures (1 in 2000); in emergency and ICU set up, it can be as high as 1 in 50 procedures [20]. Among standard anatomical airway assessments, few findings are common in head neck cancer patients like restricted mouth opening, restricted neck mobility, stiffened submental soft tissue, decreased space within oral cavity and overall distorted normal anatomy, especially after surgery or radiotherapy. Physiological challenges that make intubation difficult in this sub-group are hypoxaemia, hypotension and right heart dysfunction [21].

Ventilation: Among the cancer patients who require ICU admission, almost 50–70% need mechanical ventilation. About half of them need ventilatory support on admission and rest require ventilatory support during their ICU stay because of clinical deterioration. Incidence of invasive ventilation is higher in surgical patients compared to medical one, mostly because of less use of NIV in surgical patients; but the overall mortality is comparable (approximately 20%). Ventilatory management of respiratory failure including ARDS in cancer patients are same like any other non-cancer patients. More than 95% mechanically ventilated patients are managed with conventional mode on ventilator. Non-conventional modes like biphasic positive airway pressure (BiPAP) ventilation, airway pressure release ventilation (APRV), pressure regulated volume control (PRVC), neurally adjusted ventilatory assist (NAVA), proportional assist ventilation (PAV), high frequency oscillatory ventilation (HFOV) are used in a small proportion of cases, especially as rescue therapy in patients with ARDS [22]. Experience of using these non-conventional ventilatory modes in cancer patients is very limited.

Currently 'Low tidal volume ventilation' is the standard of care for all ICU ventilated patients with tidal volume 6 ml/kg (range 4–8 ml/kg) of ideal body weight. The original ARMA trial comparing tidal volume 6 vs. 12 ml/kg did not include bone marrow transplant patients or cancer patients with high 6-month mortality [23]. Seong et al. had shown that low tidal volume ventilation is associated with lower mortality (OR 0.37) in ARDS in haematological malignancy [24]. Though volume control mode or pressure control mode did not show any difference in outcome, most of the critical care unit is using volume control mode for its ease of use. Respiratory rate is to be adjusted to achieve targeted minute ventilation. In non paralysed patient, the set rate should be less than patient's triggered rate by 3–5, so that patient can continue to trigger and there is minimum chance of hyperventilation. FiO_2 should be titrated to achieve SpO_2 92–94%; even lower SpO_2 target of 88–90% is acceptable for patients with chronic obstructive pulmonary disease or ARDS. Setting up of optimal PEEP is challenging in ARDS patients. Routinely, PPEP usually set at 6–8 cm H_2O pressure. In ARDS, optimal titration of PEEP is needed to maintain 'Open lung ventilation' (OLV) strategy—i.e. open the collapsed alveoli with recruitment and keep them open by optimal PEEP. At one hand, suboptimal PEEP will fail to open up basal collapsed alveoli leading to hypoxaemia and atelectotrauma; on the other hand, disproportionately high PEEP will lead to hyperinflation of lung, barotrauma, hypoventilation, right ventricular dysfunction and haemodynamic instability. So, optimisation of PEEP is of paramount importance. There are different techniques that can be used for the same such as (1) by PEEP—FiO_2 contingency table, (2) pressure volume loop, (3) low inflation points, (4) point of maximum curvature or (5) trans-pulmonary pressure etc.

PRCC (Pressure regulated volume control) mode is a hybrid mode currently available in multiple brands of ventilator with different name (e.g. Autoflow in Dragger). It is a pressure regulated and has a decelerating flow pattern; patient ventilator dyssynchrony is apparently less as patient can decide his/ her own flow requirement. Besides, it ensures delivery of targeted tidal volume. It has been compared with volume control or synchronised intermittent mandatory ventilation (SIMV) mode in small trials in patients with ARDS, COPD and traumatic brain injury (TBI). PRVC has consistently shown to decrease peak inspiratory pressure with some improvement in oxygenation [25].

BiPAP & APRV are spectrum of biphasic ventilation. These are closed loop, partial support, time cycled, pressure-controlled mode with two pressure settings at two different level (P high & P low). The difference is in inspiratory to expiratory (I: E) ratio—T high & T low. BiPAP has normal I:E ratio, but APRV has reverse I:E ratio leading to generation of an auto-PEEP leading to some recruitment. These modes have some benefits. In experimental animal model, these have shown to reduce markers of inflammation, apoptosis, fibrinogenesis and epithelial/ endothelial damage compared to conventional modes. APRV reduces endothelial permeability and preserved surfactant proteins A and B concentrations. Other potential benefits are decreased intra-thoracic pressure, improved venous return, increased cardiac output and higher oxygen delivery. Biphasic modes have been compared with conventional modes and also with HFOV (specially in children) without any significant improvement in outcome [26].

Among high frequency ventilations (HFV), high frequency oscillatory ventilation (HFOV) was most widely used, which uses the respiratory frequency is >2 Hertz and provides low tidal volume less than the dead space. The proposed mechanisms for gas exchange are convective ventilation, Taylor dispersion, the Pendelluft effect, cardiogenic mixing, molecular diffusion and asymmetrical velocity profiles. Because of two large randomised control trials—OSCAR and OSCILLATE trial, use of HFOV has significantly decreased in ICU.

Like other ARDS patients, recommendation for prone ventilation is same for oncology patients; i.e., moderate to severe ARDS with PaO_2/FiO_2 ratio <150.

PROSEVA trial has shown 28- and 90-day mortality benefit with prolonged proning (>16 h a day) in severe ARDS patients [27].

d. ECMO: Cancer is not an absolute contraindication of extra corporeal life support. In patients with 'full code' management i.e., for patients with cancer in remission or under curative intent of therapy, ECMO can be considered for reversible cardiorespiratory failure like pneumonia, ARDS, pulmonary embolism, diffuse alveolar haemorrhage etc. Literatures for ECMO in cancer patients are very limited. ESLO registry [28] over 17 years period (1992–2008) had shown only 72 cases with 65% solid tumour and rest haematological malignancy and bone marrow transplant, with equal proportion of veno-venous and vino-arterial ECMO. Mortality is very high with haematological malignancy. In another multi-center trial (IDEA study) [29], out of 225 immuno-compromised patients 30% suffered from haematological malignancy and 19% are having solid tumour. Malignancy is associated with worse outcome compare to any immune-suppressed state. Elderly, prolonged mechanical ventilation, hypercapnia, and higher driving pressure prior to ECMO are associated with poor prognosis. Six-month mortality is around 80%. So appropriate selection of cases is of paramount importance.

11.2 Conclusion

Outcome of cancer patients is improving over time. With better chemotherapeutic agents and recent usage of immunotherapy, lots of cancer patients are coming to ICU with "full code". Acute deterioration because of reversible factors like infection should be treated with aggressive medical management including organ supports. Invasive ventilation should be offered, when indicated, as per clinical status of the patient.

Key Points

- Respiratory failure is the most common cause of ICU admission and major cause of death in cancer patients
- It can be related to malignancy per se and related therapy or absolutely unrelated to it.
- Besides underlying respiratory pathology, respiratory support may be needed depending on status of underlying malignancy, its treatment plan and anticipated outcome.
- Noninvasive ventilation or HFNC can be a good therapeutic option specially for haematological malignancy or post bone marrow transplant patients
- When indicated, invasive ventilation should not be delayed or denied as it can cause poor outcome
- Invasive ventilatory strategy in cancer patients is same like non cancer patients and no conventional or unconventional mode has shown any superiority over others.
- Role of extra corporeal support like ECMO in cancer patients need further research.

References

1. Taccone FS, Artigas AA, Sprung CL, Moreno R, Sakr Y, Vincent JL. Characteristics and outcomes of cancer patients in European ICUs. Crit Care. 2009;13:R15.
2. Pastores SM, Voigt LP. Acute respiratory failure in the patient with cancer: diagnostic and management strategies. Crit Care Clin. 2010;26:21–40.
3. Metheny NA, Clouse RE, Chang YH, Stewart BJ, Oliver DA, Kollef MH. Tracheobronchial aspiration of gastric contents in critically ill tube-fed patients: frequency, outcomes, and risk factors. Crit Care Med. 2006;34:1007–15.
4. Rochwerg B, Brochard L, Elliott MW, Hess D, Hill NS, Nava S, et al. Official ERS/ATS clinical practice guidelines: noninvasive ventilation for acute respiratory failure. Eur Respir J. 2017;50:1602426.
5. Hilbert G, Gruson D, Vargas F, Valentino R, Gbikpi- Benissan G, Dupon M, Reiffers J, Cardinaud JP, et al. Noninvasive ventilation in immunosuppressed patients with pulmonary infiltrates, fever, and acute respiratory failure. N Engl J Med. 2001;344:481–7.
6. Antonelli M, Conti G, Bufi M, Costa MG, Lappa A, Rocco M, et al. Noninvasive ventilation for treatment of acute respiratory failure in patients undergoing solid organ transplantation—a randomized trial. JAMA. 2000;283:235–41.
7. Wermke M, Schiemanck S, Höffken G, Ehninger G, Bornhäuser M, Illmer T. Respiratory failure in patients undergoing allogeneic hematopoietic SCT--a randomized trial on early non-invasive ventilation based on standard care hematology wards. Bone Marrow Transplant. 2012;47:574–80.
8. Ferreira JC, Medeiros P Jr, Rego FM, Caruso P. Risk factors for noninvasive ventilation failure in cancer patients in the intensive care unit: a retrospective cohort study. J Crit Care. 2015;30:1003–7.
9. Chen WC, Su VY, Yu WK, Chen YW, Yang KY. Prognostic factors of noninvasive mechanical ventilation in lung cancer patients with acute respiratory failure. PLoS One. 2018;13:e0191204.
10. L'Her E, Deye N, Lellouche F, Taille S, Demoule A, Fraticelli A, et al. Physiologic effects of noninvasive ventilation during acute lung injury. Am J Respir Crit Care Med. 2005;172:1112–8.
11. Kallet RH, Diaz JV. The physiologic effects of non- invasive ventilation. Respir Care. 2009;54:102–15.
12. Frat JP, Thille AW, Mercat A, Girault C, Ragot S, Perbet S, et al. FLORALI study group and the REVA network. High-flow oxygen through nasal cannula in acute hypoxemic respiratory failure. N Engl J Med. 2015;372:2185–96.
13. Azoulay E, Pickkers P, Soares M, Perner A, Rello J, Bauer PR, et al. Efraim investigators and the nine-I study group. Acute hypoxemic respiratory failure in immunocompromised patients: the Efraim multinational prospective cohort study. Intensive Care Med. 2017;43:1808–19.
14. Walkey AJ, Wiener RS. Use of noninvasive ventilation in patients with acute respiratory failure, 2000–2009: a population-based study. Ann Am Thorac Soc. 2013;10:10–7.
15. Chandra D, Stamm JA, Taylor B, Ramos RM, Satterwhite L, Krishnan JA, et al. Outcomes of noninvasive ventilation for acute exacerbations of chronic obstructive pulmonary disease in the United States, 1998–2008. Am J Respir Crit Care Med. 2012;185:152–9.
16. Molina R, Bernal T, Borges M, Zaragoza R, Bonastre J, Granada RM, et al. Ventilatory support in critically ill hematology patients with respiratory failure. Crit Care. 2012;16:R133.
17. Duan J, Han X, Bai L, Zhou L, Huang S. Assessment of heart rate, acidosis, consciousness, oxygenation and respiratory rate to predict noninvasive ventilation failure in hypoxemic patients. Intensive Care Med. 2017;43:192–9.
18. De Jong A, Molinari N, Terzi N, Mongardon N, Arnal JM, Guitton C, et al. AzuRéa network for the Frida-Réa study group: early identification of patients at risk for difficult intubation in intensive care unit: development and validation of the MACOCHA score in a multicenter cohort study. Am J Respir Crit Care Med. 2013;187:832–9.

19. Adnet F, Borron SW, Racine SX, Clemessy JL, Fournier JL, Plaisance P, et al. The intubation difficulty scale (IDS): proposal and evaluation of a new score characterizing the complexity of endotracheal intubation. Anesthesiology. 1997;87:1290–7.
20. Cook TM, MacDougall-Davis SR. Complications and failure of airway management. Br J Anaesth. 2012;109(Suppl 1):i68–85.
21. Mosier JM, Joshi R, Hypes C, Pacheco G, Valenzuela T, Sakles JC. The physiologically difficult airway. West J Emerg Med. 2015;16:1109–17.
22. Esteban A, Frutos-Vivar F, Muriel A, Ferguson ND, Peñuelas O, Abraira V, et al. Evolution of mortality over time in patients receiving mechanical ventilation. Am J Respir Crit Care Med. 2013;188:220–30.
23. Acute Respiratory Distress Syndrome Network, Brower RG, Matthay MA, Morris A, Schoenfeld D, Thompson BT, Wheeler A. Ventilation with lower tidal volumes as compared with traditional tidal volumes for acute lung injury and the acute respiratory distress syndrome. N Engl J Med. 2000;342:1301–8.
24. Seong GM, Lee Y, Hong S-B, Lim C-M, Koh Y, Huh JW. Prognosis of acute respiratory distress syndrome in patients with hematological malignancies. J Intensive Care Med. 2020;35:364–70.
25. Riverso P, Bernard PL, Corsa D, Morra MG, Pagannini G, Parigi F. A comparison of ventilation techniques in ARDS. Volume controlled vs pressure regulated volume control. Minerva Anesthesiol. 1998;64:339–43.
26. Zhou Y, Jin X, Lv Y, Wang P, Yang Y, Liang G. Early application of airway pressure release ventilation may reduce the duration of mechanical ventilation in acute respiratory distress syndrome. Intensive Care Med. 2017;43:1648–59.
27. Guérin C, Reignier J, Richard JC, Beuret P, Gacouin A, Boulain T, et al. PROSEVA study group. Prone positioning in severe acute respiratory distress syndrome. N Engl J Med. 2013;368:2159–68.
28. Gow KW, Lao OB, Leong T, Fortenberry JD. Extra- corporeal life support for adults with malignancy and respiratory or cardiac failure: the extracorporeal life support experience. Am J Surg. 2010;199:669–75.
29. Schmidt M, Schellongowski P, Patroniti N, Taccone FS, Reis Miranda D, Reuter J, et al. IDEA study group collaborators. Six-month outcome of immunocompromised patients with severe acute respiratory distress syndrome rescued by extracorporeal membrane oxygenation. An international Multicenter retrospective study. Am J Respir Crit Care Med. 2018;197:1297–307.

Respiratory Interventions in ICU

12

Vijay Hadda and Rahul Tyagi

12.1 Introduction

Cancer incidence and mortality is on the rise across the globe. The 2011 political declaration on prevention and control of non-communicable diseases aims to reduce the mortality due to non-communicable diseases by 25% till year 2025 [1]. Global Burden of Disease Cancer Collaboration has estimated that there were 24.5 million new cancer cases in the year 2017 [2]. In the same year, there were 9.6 million deaths and 233.5 Disability Adjusted Life Years (DALY) lost due to cancer [2]. In India also, deaths due to cancer have doubled from 1990 to 2016 [3]. It is estimated that there were 1.15 million new cancer cases in India in 2018 and this figure is likely to double by the year 2040 [3].

Over last few decades, the advances in management of cancer have resulted in a substantial increase in number of patients living with cancer. This has increased the number of patients with cancer requiring admission in intensive care unit (ICU). ICU admission contributes to a significant proportion of health care costs. In a study conducted at University of Texas, Anderson Cancer Centre, authors investigated the use of ICU care and outcomes among patients admitted to a comprehensive oncology care centre between 1st January 1994 and 31 Dec 2013 [4]. There were over 380,000 patient admissions during the study period and the ICU utilization rate was 12.9%. For all inpatients, sepsis, pneumonia and other infections were the cause for highest mortality (8.5%) [4]. Various studies have shown that 5–10% of cancer patients will develop a life threatening illness requiring ICU admission [5]. Patients with hematological malignancies have higher utilization of ICU [5]. The survival rates in cancer patients admitted to ICU have been meaningful in recent times, albeit higher than general population of critically ill patients [6]. Hospital mortality in mechanically ventilated cancer patient has also shown a decline from 90 to 60%

V. Hadda (✉) · R. Tyagi
All India Institute of Medical Sciences, New Delhi, New Delhi, India

V. Kumar et al. (eds.), *Onco-critical Care*,
https://doi.org/10.1007/978-981-16-9929-0_12

over time [6]. These improvements may be attributable to improved cancer care as well as improvement in supportive care such as availability of better drugs for management of neutropenia and fungal infections [6].

12.2 Requirement of ICU in Oncology Patients

Acute respiratory failure is a common and dreaded complication in both hematological and solid organ malignancies. Azoulay et al. [7] conducted a 5-year study at a teaching hospital in Paris. During the period, a total of 3782 patients with hematological or solid organ malignancies were admitted to the centre. Of these, 203 (5.4%) required ICU admission for Acute Respiratory Failure (ARF) and 97 (47.7%) of the patient with ARF died. The most common cause of ARF in this study was infectious pneumonia (58%). No cause could be identified in 21% patients [7]. This is relevant as the mortality in this subset noted in this study was 64% which was more than the overall mortality noticed in patients with ARF.

Anisoglou et al. studied the outcomes of 105 lung cancer patients admitted to ICU with ARF [8]. The authors noted an in hospital mortality of 56.1%. These studies show the seriousness of ARF in a patient with underlying hematological or solid organ malignancy. They also reflect that approximately one out of two patients requiring ICU admission with ARF and an underlying malignancy is likely to survive.

Causes of ARF in patient with underlying malignancy are variable [9]. ARF can be due to the underlying malignancy or drugs used for the treatment. The causes of ARF among patients with malignancy are summarized in Table 12.1.

Table 12.1 Causes of Acute Respiratory Failure (ARF) in patients with Malignancy

Compartment involved	Related to underlying malignancy	Related to treatment
Parenchymal	• Mass Lesion—large mass causing V/Q mismatch • Lymphangitis Carcinomatosis	• Pneumonitis or ARDS: due to infection, chemotherapy, or radiotherapy • HSCT: Peri-engraftment syndrome, diffuse Alveolar Haemorrhage, Bronchiolitis obliterans organizing pneumonia (BOOP) • Drugs—bleomycin, methotrexate etc.
Vascular	• Acute pulmonary thromboembolism • Tumour embolism	
Pleural	• Malignant pleural effusion	• Drug induced pleural Effusion—bleomycin, methotrexate, cyclophosphamide etc.
Chest wall disorders	• Chest wall tumor • Rib fractures	
Airway	• Endobronchial metastasis	
Respiratory Drive/ Neuro-Muscular Disorder Related	• CNS metastasis • Paraneoplastic syndromes • Lambert Eaton Syndrome, myasthenia gravis	• Overdose of narcotics

12.3 Respiratory Interventions in Oncology ICU

Respiratory interventions in patients with malignancy and admitted in ICU are important armamentarium for the diagnosis of the cause as well as the management of ARF. For example, bronchoscopic BAL is the investigation of choice for the microbiological diagnosis of pneumonia in these patients. Similarly, there are rigid bronchoscopic interventions which may be life-saving for the patients with malignant central airway obstruction (CAO). The summary of possible respiratory interventions in critically ill patients with solid organ or hematological malignancy is provided as Table 12.2.

12.3.1 Flexible Bronchoscopy

Flexible bronchoscopy (FB) has been used ICU, with a considerable success, for various diagnostic and therapeutic indications. However, use of FB in ICU has its own set of challenges. Therefore, it is important to know the indications and complications associated with bronchoscopy in critically ill patients.

Indications for bronchoscopy in oncology ICU may be diagnostic or therapeutic [10].

Diagnostic indications:

1. Evaluation of pulmonary infiltrates
2. Hemoptysis evaluation
3. Airway assessment in cases of suspected central airway obstruction (CAO) or bronchial obstruction
4. Suspicion of tracheo-esophageal Fistula (TEF)

Table 12.2 Respiratory interventions in the oncology ICU

Conditions	Diagnostic interventions	Therapeutic interventions
Pneumonia/ARDS	• Broncho alveolar lavage • Bronchial washings • Brush cytology • Trans bronchial lung biopsy	• High flow nasal cannula (HFNC) • Non-invasive ventilation (NIV) • Invasive mechanical ventilation (IMV)
Tracheal/endobronchial tumour/metastasis	• Flexible bronchoscopy	• Cryo-extraction • Diode laser • Argon plasma coagulation • Photodynamic therapy • Rigid bronchoscopy with mechanical debulking
Malignant Pleural Effusion	• Diagnostic pleurocentesis/pleuroscopy	• Small/large bore ICD placement • Indwelling pleural catheter • Pleurodesis (thoracoscopic or via ICD)

Therapeutic indications:

1. Lung/Lobar collapse not improving with physiotherapy
2. Management of CAO/bronchial obstruction
3. Bronchoscopic intubation
4. Percutaneous tracheostomy

Critically ill patients are at a higher risk of complications during bronchoscopic procedures [11]. The factors which predispose ICU patients to a higher complication rate include presence of hypoxemia, hypotension, renal failure, thrombocytopenia and use of anticoagulant/anti-platelet drugs. It should be noted that partial pressure of oxygen (PaO_2) usually falls by 10–20 mm Hg after bronchoscopy even in non-critically ill patients, hence, there is risk of pre-exiting hypoxemia [12]. In critically ill patients, FB is frequently performed on patients who are on invasive or non-invasive ventilation. There are general principles guiding the FB procedure in ICU [10, 11]. We suggest following step to minimize the complications—

1. Pre-oxygenation with 100% Oxygen for 5–10 min prior to procedure
2. Titrate FiO_2 and PEEP during the procedure to maintain $SpO_2 > 90\%$ during procedure and in the immediate post procedure period
3. Controlled mode should be preferred in patients on mechanical ventilation. Increase in PIP (Peak Inspiratory Pressure) alarm limits to allow adequate volume delivery is also recommended
4. Continuous monitoring of vital parameters (Heart rate, Blood pressure, SpO_2,ECG) is essential
5. In patients on Endotracheal/Tracheostomy tube the diameter of tube should be at least 2 mm more than the outer diameter of the bronchoscope. This helps in allowing delivery of tidal volume (V_T) and reduces development of auto PEEP.

It usually takes 24 h for the respiratory mechanics in critically ill patients to return to baseline after FB. Close monitoring for initial 24 h after procedure is essential [12]. It is important to note that although use of FB for removal of retained secretions (pulmonary toilet) is often practiced, it's routine use is not evidence based [12]. Respiratory therapy alone has performed equally well in randomized control trials and should be utilized before resorting to FB [11]. Routine use of BAL for diagnosis of VAP in critically ill patients is not recommended due to lack of mortality benefits as compared endotracheal aspirate ET aspirates.

12.3.2 Rigid Bronchoscopy

Rigid bronchoscopy is an invasive procedure that can visualize oropharynx, vocal cords, trachea and main bronchi and done under general anesthesia either in operation theatre or bronchoscopy suite. Rigid bronchoscopy provides a better airway control, hence is ideal tool for therapeutic purposes. The indications of rigid bronchoscopy include therapeutic interventions for management of CAO, hemoptysis, deeper biopsy etc.

Central airway obstruction (CAO) is defined as an obstruction involving trachea or main stem bronchus and can occur due to a primary or metastatic thoracic malignancy [13]. Primary endoluminal malignancies as cause of CAO are less common as compared to airway metastasis [14]. Common malignancies causing metastasis to airway include renal, breast, thyroid and colon [14]. CAO can be classified as endoluminal, extraluminal or mixed (having both endoluminal and extraluminal components) [14].

Usual symptoms of CAO include breathlessness, wheeze or stridor. Respiratory distress develops with advanced airway obstruction (usually tracheal lumen <5 mm) and majority of these patients present with acute respiratory failure without any significant previous symptoms [14]. Extent and location of CAO is important for choosing appropriate therapeutic modality. While a unilateral wheeze indicates focal airway obstruction, stridor is indicative of severe laryngeal or tracheal obstruction. Chest radiographs have limited utility for diagnosis, location and extent of lesion causing CAO [13]. Computerized tomography (CT) scan of the thorax is the imaging modality of choice for evaluation of CAO. Virtual bronchoscopic evaluation of the endoluminal airways and 3-D reconstruction of structures surrounding the airways can provide a comprehensive evaluation of CAO [13]. Also, CT scan can be helpful in determining minimum size of the airways, length and site of obstruction, and patency of airways distal to the obstruction [14].

The principles of CAO management follow the standard guidelines for any unstable patient with airway stabilization being the first priority. For patient with doubtful airway stability, rigid bronchoscopy is the procedure of choice; as it will help in securing the airway, provide excellent oxygenation and ventilation and also allow a therapeutic intervention such as "coring" or "debulking" of a tumor, dilatation of a stenosis, and placement of stent [14]. In patient deemed to have relatively stable airway with CAO, tracheostomy in proximal CAO and endotracheal intubation in patients with distal obstruction may be tried in a controlled environment with availability of intervention at a short notice. The various modalities employed for management of CAO could include "hot therapies" such as elecrocautery, Argon Plasma Coagulation, Laser therapy, Photodynamic therapy or "Cold therapies" such as cryotherapy [14].Although success rate of therapeutic bronchoscopy is high, there are significant complications—hypoxia, pneumothorax, bleeding, hypotension and increase in level of care [13]. Patient with poor ASA (3 or 4) and poor performance status (Karnofsky Performance Scale below 70) are at a higher risk of complications [13].

12.4 Tracheostomy in Oncology ICU

In oncology patients, apart from upper airway obstruction and airway protection, prolonged mechanical ventilation may be an indication for tracheostomy [15]. Tracheostomy may be performed via surgical or percutaneous methods [16]. Surgical tracheostomy in critically ill patients is a cumbersome process requiring transport to surgical operation theatre [16]. While surgical tracheostomy involves full dissection of pre tracheal tissues followed by insertion of tracheostomy tube under direct vision, percutaneous tracheostomy (PCT) utilizes Seldinger technique and blunt dissection of pretracheal tissues [17].

a. **Indications—**
    1. Upper airway obstruction
    2. Difficult weaning
    3. Management of trachea bronchial secretions
    4. Prevention of aspiration
b. **Absolute contraindication -**
    1. Uncontrolled coagulopathy
    2. Unstable cervical spine
    3. Infection at the planned site
c. **Procedure:**

Various procedures described to perform PCT include Ciaglia Blue Rhino, Blue dolphin, Grigg's Percu Twist or Fantoni technique. Among these, Ciaglia blue rhino technique is comparatively better than other techniques. There are commercially available PCT sets (Fig. 12.1). In blue rhino technique, a hydrophilic coated curved dilator is used for dilatation of stoma. The dilator is passed over a J-guide wire which is passed into the tracheal lumen through a cannula. Incision is made midway between cricoid and sternal notch [17]. Before initiating the procedure, patient should be placed in a position of neck extension and endotracheal tube (ET) should be

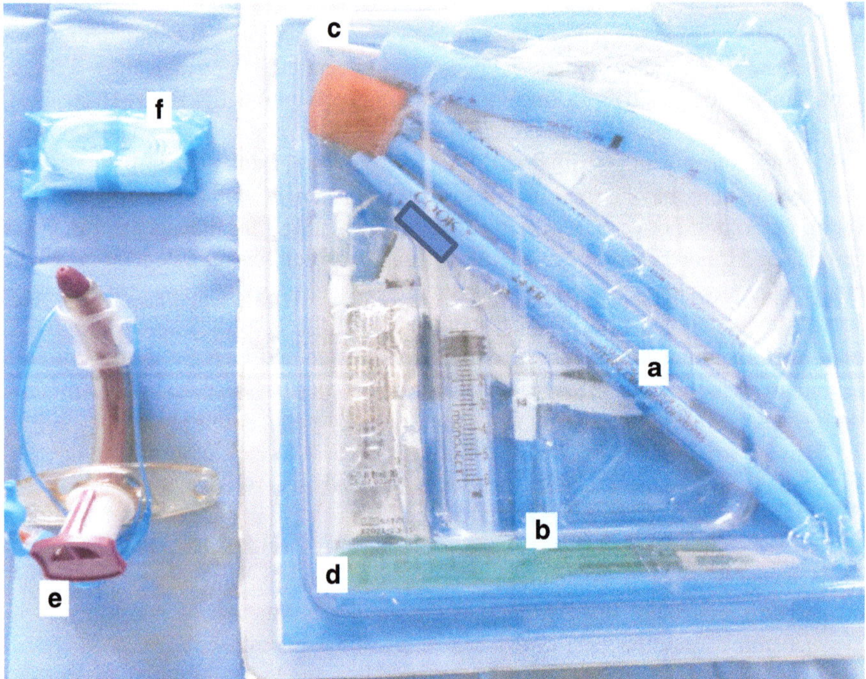

Fig. 12.1 Percutaneous tracheostomy set—various sizes of dilators (**a**), surgical blade with handle for incision (**b**), guide wire (**c**), introducer needle with sheath (**d**), tracheostomy tube (**e**), and tie (**f**)

withdrawn to a level just below the vocal cord. Ultrasonography (USG) should be used to screen the tracheostomy site to look for any blood vessel which may be injured during procedure. Bronchoscope should be passed through ET to visualize tracheal lumen during the procedure. Bronchoscope can also be used to confirm the position of tracheostomy tube once it is passed. The steps of the procedure are described below.

Box 1 Steps of Percutaneous Tracheostomy

1. Written informed consent must be obtained prior to the procedure
2. General anaesthesia is required for performing the procedure.
3. Correct neck position is essential for the procedure. Neck should be in full extension. Towels may be placed under shoulder blades to achieve neck extension
4. USG use is preferred to evaluate the neck anatomy and rule out any large vessels in the operative fields.
5. Sterile precautions must be followed during the procedure. Pre-procedure hand washing, use of sterile gloves and gowns, preparation of site and field with full aseptic measures must be done.
6. Identify the landmarks by palpation. Neck landmarks to be identified include thyroid cartilage, cricoid cartilage and second to third tracheal rings.
7. Make a horizontal incision approximately 2–3 cm between second and third tracheal ring.
8. Do a blunt dissection of pre-tracheal tissue till trachea is clearly palpable.
9. Flexible bronchoscope is introduced through the ET tube and kept inside just proximal to the tip of ET tube. This helps in visualization of the trachea while avoiding injury to bronchoscope during the procedure.
10. Deflate the cuff and withdraw the ET tube to a position where the cuff is just below the glottis. Re-inflate the cuff at this site while maintaining the position of bronchoscope inside the tube.
11. Puncture the anterior wall of trachea using the introducer needle under guidance of bronchoscope.
12. Withdraw the trocar while leaving the sheath in place. Introduce the guide wire through the sheath and visualise it going towards the carina. Once the guidewire is in position, remove the sheath over the guide wire.
13. Use the dilators over the guide wire to dilate the track to place tracheostomy tube.
14. Withdraw the dilator and gently pass the tracheostomy tube over guide wire. Once the tracheostomy tube is in place withdraw the ET tube and bronchoscope.
15. Bronchoscope may be passed through the tracheostomy tube to see the position and distance from carina.
16. Make sure hemostasis is achieved and there is no active bleed.
17. Tie the tracheostomy around the neck with help of tie. Make sure that the tie is not too tight as that may cause interruption of blood supply.

d. **Complications**

Complication of PCT are similar to surgical tracheostomy. Early complications include formation of false tract, iatrogenic trauma to airways leading to pneumothorax/pneumo-mediatinum/surgical emphysema, hemorrhage and injury to posterior tracheal wall.

Late complications may include displacement, trachea-esophageal fistula, subglottic stenosis, stromal infection and voice change [17].

12.5 Interventions for Malignant Pleural Effusion

Malignant pleural effusion is most commonly seen in lung cancer, breast cancer and lymphoma [18]. Patients usually present with breathlessness (fresh onset or worsening depending on underlying disease), cough and chest pain. Development of malignant pleural effusion usually portends worse prognosis; its presence shifts the treatment goals from curative intent to palliative intent [18].

a. **Modalities for management of malignant pleural effusion**

Various modalities available for the management of malignant pleural effusion include repeated thoracocentesis, placement of intercostal drain (ICD), pleurodesis and indwelling pleural catheter (IPC). The modalities for management of malignant pleural effusion and their indications [19] are as given in Table 12.3.

All pleural interventions in ICU should be carried out under USG guidance. All patients with MPE should initially undergo a therapeutic thoracocentesis to confirm relief of symptom and re-expansion of lungs after pleural drainage [19].

Both IPC and tube thoracostomy followed by pleurodesis have been used in patients in MPE. The advantages and disadvantages [20] of both are listed in Table 12.4.

Although VATS/thoracoscopy guided surgical pleurodesis is also possible, it is usually not feasible in ICU patients due to their poor performance status.

Placement of either large-bore chest drain (ICD) or small-bore chest drain (pig tail catheter) may be undertaken for cases with MPE for symptomatic relief and subsequent pleurodesis. Small bore tubes have equivalent success rates as compared to large tube thoracostomy [20, 21]. The advantages of small-bore tubes include lesser pain and better patient comfort.

Table 12.3 Modalities for management of malignant pleural effusion and their indications

MPE management modality	Indications
Repeated therapeutic thoracocentesis	• MPE with expected survival <3 month
Intercostal Drainage	• Therapeutic drainage and pleurodesis
Pigtail Catheter Drainage	• Outpatient management of MPE and pleurodesis
Indwelling Pleural Catheter	• Failed pleurodesis/symptomatic loculated effusion • Trapped Lung

Table 12.4 Comparison of pleurodesis with IPC

Procedure	Advantages	Disadvantages
Pleurodesis	• Rapid resolution of MPE	• More Invasive • Failure is common • Not possible in trapped lung
IPC	• Less invasive • Spontaneous pleurodesis may occur over time • Effective in patients with trapped lung • Less requirement of repeated pleural intervention • Less median hospitalization	• Prolonged drainage • Prolonged ongoing care • Costly

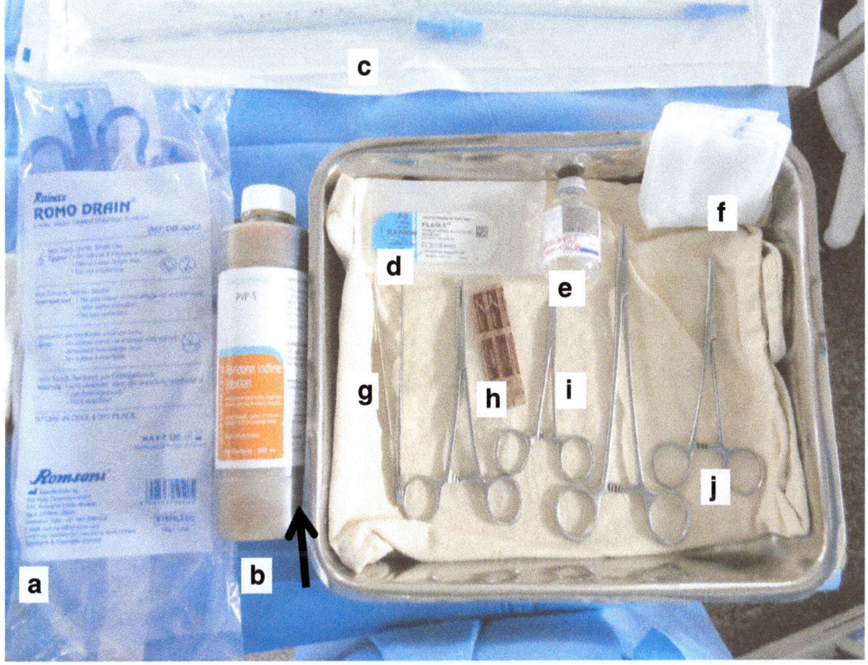

Fig. 12.2 The ICD-set showing various instruments required during the procedure—under water seal (**a**), povidone iodine (**b**), inter-costal tube (**c**), suture (**d**), lignocaine (**e**), gauze (**f**), non-tooth forceps (**g**), surgical blade (**h**), needle holder (**i**), and artery forceps

b. **Procedure**

Site of maximal effusion should be confirmed on USG and position marked on chest wall. Patient should preferably be in a sitting position, although it will not be possible in patients on mechanical ventilation; in that case patient can be kept in semi-recumbent. If on mechanical ventilation, PEEP should be reduced pre-procedure. We should check that the ICD set is complete (Fig. 12.2). The steps of ICD insertion are summarized in Box 2.

Box 2 Steps for Intercostal Drain Insertion (ICD) Insertion

1. Written informed consent must be obtained prior to the procedure
2. Use Ultrasonography (USG) to ascertain the site and size of effusion. It is essential that USG be used in these patients as localization of effusion on clinical basis will be difficult and to avoid complications related to trauma to vital organs during procedure.
3. Under USG guidance ascertain the depth of fluid from chest wall, site of maximum collection and approximate volume of effusion.
4. Sterile precautions must be followed during the procedure. Pre-procedure hand washing, use of sterile gloves and gowns, preparation of site and field with full aseptic measures must be done
5. Preferred patient position is patient lying at 45 degree with arm behind the head. However in ICU setting it may be required to place an ICD in supine position also.
6. Local infiltration with 2% lignocaine upto a maximum of 3 mg/kg may be used to provide pain relief during the procedure
7. Choose appropriate drain size. Intercostal drain are available in size varying from 12 FG to 34 FG. A small bore ICD may be used for pneumothorax and simple effusion while large bore tube may be used in hemothorax and empyema. Inter costal space available may also be a determining factor in deciding size of ICD. Patient with reduced intercostals space due to chronic collapse or pleural thickening may require a small bore ICD.
8. After adequate local anaesthesia insert a needle from above the lower rib at the site of maximum collection already ascertained. Aspirate fluid or air to confirm the correct position.
9. Make a skin and soft tissue incision using a sterile blade. Do blunt dissection of deeper tissues with forceps. Spread the intercostals muscles on the superior surface of ribs to avoid injury to intercostals bundle in the inferior rib surface.
10. After the track has been created insert the ICD through the track with help of forceps. After pleura is breached gush of air or fluid may be felt. Keep ICD closed till connected to underwater drain
11. Secure the ICD using 1/0 or 2/0 silk sutures
12. Connect the ICD to underwater drain and open the ICD.
13. Do sterile dressing around the tube. Change the dressing every 48 to 72 h.
14. Do a chest radiograph to confirm position of tube

c. **Complications**

Various complications which may occur during placement of intercostals drain include hemorrhage, lung injury resulting in alveolo-pleural fistula and hydropneumothorax, re-expansion pulmonary edema, vasovagal syncope.

Key Points

- Acute respiratory failure is a common cause for utilization of critical care in patients with haematological/solid organ malignancies. ARF can occur due to myriads of causes.
- Pulmonary interventions such as flexible and rigid bronchoscopy, placement of ICD, and tracheostomy may be very useful for immediate relief of symptoms and reversal of ARF. It is important to ensure correct indication and take adequate precautions while performing the procedure as chances of deterioration in 24 h of procedure are high
- Rigid bronchoscopy is the modality of choice for the management of CAO of malignant etiology.
- Tracheostomy may be required for patients having upper airway obstruction or requiring prolonged ventilation. Percutaneous tracheostomy is a relatively less invasive procedure than surgical tracheostomy and can be performed on bedside thus avoiding risking the transfer of a critically ill patient
- Management of MPE mainly depends on the status of underlying lung. Drainage and pleurodesis are preferable if the lung expands after drainage of fluid. However if the underlying lung is trapped repeated therapeutic thoracocentesis/ indwelling pleural catheter may be preferred.

References

1. United Nations. High level meeting onprevention and control of non-communicable diseases. 2011. http://www.un.org/en/ga/ncdmeeting2011/. Accessed 16 Sept 2011.
2. Global Burden of Disease Cancer Collaboration. Global, regional, and National Cancer Incidence, mortality, years of life lost, years lived with disability, and disability-adjusted life-years for 29 cancer groups, 1990 to 2017: a systematic analysis for the global burden of disease study. JAMA Oncol. 2019;5(12):1749–68. https://doi.org/10.1001/jamaoncol.2019.2996.
3. Smith RD, Mallath MK. History of the growing burden of cancer in India: from antiquity to the 21st century. J Glob Oncol. 2019 Jul;5:1–15. https://doi.org/10.1200/JGO.19.00048.
4. Wallace SK, Rathi NK, Waller DK, Ensor JE Jr, Haque SA, Price KJ, Piller LB, Tilley BC, Nates JL. Two decades of ICU utilization and hospital outcomes in a Comprehensive Cancer Center. Crit Care Med. 2016 May;44(5):926–33. https://doi.org/10.1097/CCM.0000000000001568.
5. Shimabukuro-Vornhagen A, Böll B, Kochanek M, Azoulay É, von Bergwelt-Baildon MS. Critical care of patients with cancer. CA Cancer J Clin. 2016;66(6):496–517. https://doi.org/10.3322/caac.21351.
6. Mokart D, Pastores SM, Darmon M. Has survival increased in cancer patients admitted to the ICU? Yes Intensive Care Med. 2014;40(10):1570–2. https://doi.org/10.1007/s00134-014-3433-2.
7. Azoulay E, Thiery G, Chevret S, et al. The prognosis of acute respiratory failure in critically ill cancer patients. Medicine (Baltimore). 2004;83:360–70.
8. Anisoglou S, Asteriou C, Barbetakis N, Kakolyris S, Anastasiadou G, Pnevmatikos I. Outcome of lung cancer patients admitted to the intensive care unit with acute respiratory failure. Hippokratia. 2013;17(1):60–3.
9. Martos-Benítez FD, Soler-Morejón CD, Lara-Ponce KX, Orama-Requejo V, BurgosAragüez D, Larrondo-Muguercia H, Lespoir RW. Critically ill patients with cancer: a clinical perspective. World J Clin Oncol. 2020;11(10):809–35.

10. Mohan A, Madan K, Hadda V, Tiwari P, Mittal S, Guleria R, et al. Guidelines for diagnostic flexible bronchoscopy in adults: joint Indian chest society/National College of chest physicians (I)/Indian association for bronchology recommendations. Lung India. 2019;36:S37–89.
11. Ergan B, Nava S. The use of bronchoscopy in critically ill patients: considerations and complications. Expert Rev Respir Med. 2018;12(8):651–63. https://doi.org/10.1080/17476348.2018.1494576.
12. Maitre B, Jaber S, Maggiore SM, Bergot E, Richard JC, Bakthiari H, Housset B, Boussignac G, Brochard L. Continuous positive airway pressure during fiberoptic bronchoscopy in hypoxemic patients. A randomized double-blind study using a new device. Am J Respir Crit Care Med. 2000;162(3 Pt 1):1063–7. https://doi.org/10.1164/ajrccm.162.3.9910117.
13. Mudambi L, Miller R, Eapen GA. Malignant central airway obstruction. J Thorac Dis. 2017;9(Suppl 10):S1087–110. https://doi.org/10.21037/jtd.2017.07.27.
14. Ernst A, Feller-Kopman D, Becker HD, Mehta AC. Central airway obstruction. Am J Respir Crit Care Med. 2004;169:1278.
15. El-Anwar MW, Nofal AA, Shawadfy MA, Maaty A, Khazbak AO. Tracheostomy in the intensive care unit: a University Hospital in a Developing Country Study. Int Arch Otorhinolaryngol. 2017;21(1):33–7. https://doi.org/10.1055/s-0036-1584227.
16. Delaney A, Bagshaw SM, Nalos M. Percutaneous dilatational tracheostomy versus surgical tracheostomy in critically ill patients: a systematic review and meta-analysis. Crit Care. 2006;10(2):R55. https://doi.org/10.1186/cc4887.
17. MehtaC,MehtaY.Percutaneoustracheostomy.AnnCardAnaesth.2017;20(Supplement):S19–25. https://doi.org/10.4103/0971-9784.197793.
18. Desai NR, Lee HJ. Diagnosis and management of malignant pleural effusions: state of the art in 2017. J Thorac Dis. 2017;9(Suppl 10):S1111–22. https://doi.org/10.21037/jtd.2017.07.79.
19. Feller-Kopman DJ, Reddy CB, DeCamp MM, Diekemper RL, Gould MK, Henry T, Iyer NP, Lee YCG, Lewis SZ, Maskell NA, Rahman NM, Sterman DH, Wahidi MM, Balekian AA. Management of malignant pleural effusions. An official ATS/STS/STR clinical practice guideline. Am J Respir Crit Care Med. 2018;198(7):839–49. https://doi.org/10.1164/rccm.201807-1415ST.
20. Ghoneim del HA, Elkomy HA, Elshora AE, Mehrez M. Usefulness of pigtail catheter in pleurodesis of malignant pleural effusion. Egyptian Journal of Chest Diseases and Tuberculosis. 2014;63(1):107–12. https://doi.org/10.1016/j.ejcdt.2013.11.004.
21. Fortin M, Tremblay A. Pleural controversies: indwelling pleural catheter vs. pleurodesis for malignant pleural effusions. J Thorac Dis. 2015;7(6):1052–7. https://doi.org/10.3978/j.issn.2072-1439.2015.01.51.

Deep Venous Thrombosis and Pulmonary Embolism

13

M. D. Ray

Learning Objectives: Introduction, Review of literature, pathophysiology of venous thromboembolism (VTE) with cancer and Incidence of VTE in malignancy, Diagnosis of VTE, Diagnostic value, Clinical features of VTE, Cancer surgical risk groups, Caprini Score Model and Preventive measures.

Introduction: To tell the truth that relationship between malignancy and thromboembolism has been well established fact but unfortunately pathophysiology is still not fully cleared. Troussau is the person who reported migratory thrombophlebitis in gastric cancer patients in 1865 [1]. Since then a large number of evidence has been identified to showing the relationship between venous thromboembolism (VTE) and cancer. Despite significant advancement in the prevention of VTE, however it remains the most common preventable cause of hospital death in surgical patients [2]. It is well known that Asian population is genetically quite different from US and European group. A large number of trails support that Asians have low risk for DVT [3].There is no Indian data from any major cancer centre reporting the incidence of post-operative cancer patients; hence there is no uniform policy to practice thromboprophylaxis in Onco Surgery patients.

The very few literature available in India only two RCTs showed very low incidence of DVT after major abdominal surgeries [4, 5]. A prospective observational study conducted in 250 patients at Surgical Oncology Department at IRCH, AIIMS from 2013 to 2016 showed none of the patients who underwent complete resection (RO) for various cancers, showed any evidence of VTE both clinically and radiologically. Post operatively patients were monitored closely for any signs of DVT. Bilateral Colour Doppler should be done by using all modes, on the post op day 7, 28 andearlier if VTE is suspected clinically. But without any doubt VTE is the captain of post surgical death worldwide. Effective and newer prophylactic methods are now available for high risks patients [6, 7] and different evidence based

M. D. Ray (✉)
Department of Surgical Oncology, AIIMS New Delhi, New Delhi, India

V. Kumar et al. (eds.), *Onco-critical Care*,
https://doi.org/10.1007/978-981-16-9929-0_13

guidelines have been showing the way of preventing VTE [8, 9]. But most audits demonstrated that appropriate thromboprophylaxis is not being offered to large number of cancer surgical patients [10, 11].

Review of literature: The complications of deep vein thrombosis (DVT), pulmonary embolism (PE) i.e. VTE and the post thrombotic syndrome are important not only as the most common preventable cause of post operative death in hospital but also important cause for long term morbidity [12]. Proper understanding of underlying epidemiology, pathophysiology, and natural history of VTE is important in guiding appropriate prophylaxis for cancer surgery patients. National Comprehensive Cancer Network (NCCN) guidelines divided venous thromboembolism (VTE) broadly into deep vein thrombosis (DVT), pulmonary embolism (PE), superficial vein thrombosis (SVT) and thrombosis in other vascular territories (portal vein, mesenteric vein, inferior vena cava and superior vena cava) [13].

A thrombus is a semisolid mass formed from the components of fibrin and red blood cells with a variable platelet and leukocyte component. A clot is nothing but blood which has coagulated in vitro (i.e. in a test tube). A DVT is a thrombus, which has formed in the deep veins beneath the deep fascia of the lower limb. Thrombus within the pelvic or abdominal veins that carry blood from the legs is also commonly classified as "deep vein thrombosis' and some would include thrombus in the communicating veins of the lower limb within the definition [12].

Pathophysiology of DVT: Over a period of time it has been realized that the formation of DVT is multifactorial, with components of Virchow's triad as depicted below

Virchow's triad is well-known for this regard. It consisting of (1) Stasis- abnormalities in blood flow such as immobilization, obesity, pregnancy, malignancies, paralysed patients (2) Vessel wall Injury-vascular endothelial injury due to surgery or venepuncture,hypertension,atherosclerosis,chronicinflammation,infectionetc and (3) Hypercoagulability-post operative period, malignancies,pregnancy etc.

Pathophysiology of VTE and cancer: Various studies suggest the prothrombotic pathways of cancer molecular biology [14].

The thrombus formation in cancer is involving of multiple complicated pathways [15].

The association between cancer and thrombosis is well known but pathophysiology remains poorly understood. Trousseau was first to recognize the association between thrombosis and malignancy and later his work was supported by Sack [14]. The genesis of thrombosis in onco-surgery is critical and reflects of multiple pathways including activation of procoagulants, inhibition of anticoagulant or fibrinolytic pathways and cytokine release [15].

Cell-cell interactions and procoagulants: It is known that cancer cells expresses important factors for platelet adhesion.Studies have shown that tumor cells express glycoprotein Ib and glycoproteinIIb/IIIa (GP IIb/IIIa), which are key platelet adhesions molecules likewise, cancer has been associated with high levels of von Willebrand factor. Platelet adhesion to tumor cells via GP IIb/IIIa could play a key function in tumour spread. The main pathway for activation of the coagulation involves Exposure of the tissue factor (TF) and endothelium. TF subsequently activates Coagulation factor VIIa, which leads to conversion of prothrombin to thrombin. It has been defined that tumour cells not only express TF, but also express normal cells, such as Vascular endothelial cells, monocyte and macrophages. Tumour cells also express a cysteine protease, cancer Procoagulants that directly splits factor X to Xa (34,35). Studies that used enzyme linked Immunoabsorbent assay have shown increased cancer procoagulants levels in 81% of malignant patients. Accordingly, cancer procoagulant has been identified as a Potential tumor marker.

Adhesions of platelet to tumour cells play an important role in tumour spreading. The main pathway for activation of coagulation pathway involves exposure of sub-endothelium and tissue factor (TF). Ultimately VIIa activated by this tissue factor which is responsible for the conversion of prothrombin to thrombin. Normal cells also can express TF. Tumour cells also express cancer procoagulants cystine protease which directly convert factor X to Xa (34,35). As per the literature around 81% of malignant patients having increased level of procoagulant in their blood and thus procoagulants have been acting as tumour markers.

Fibrinolysis: Fibrinolytic pathway playing the most important part in maintaining hemostatic balance. Tissue plasminogen activities and urokinase type pasminogen (UPA) activities converting plasminogen to plasmin. Plasminogen activities inhibitor(PAI) these enzymes. High levels of UPA (Urokinase type Plasminogen Activities) and its corresponding receptors (UPAR) and PAI are associated with malignancies. When the normal coagulation fibrinolytic balance in malignancy, bleeding in leukemia patients and VTE episode occur in solid organ tumours.

Cytokines and Angiogenesis: The role of cytokines in tumour genesis is well known. It is also established, angiogenesis plays very important role in tumour growth. These cytokines predispose to develop thrombosis.

VEGF, TNFα, IL_1 all stimulates the expression of tissue factor on vascular endothelium leading to formation of thrombosis. Both TNFα & IL_1 down regulate the expression of thrombomodulin. The thrombin and thrombomodulin complexes lead to activation of protein c, a strong anticoagulation!

Thus both the up regulation and down regulation of tissue factor produce a prothrombotic effect. On the other hand IL_1 and TNFα produce PAI by stimulating vascular endothelium, thereby there is increase propensity to form the clots.

Incidence of VTE in malignancy: To tell the truth true incidence of VTE in cancer patients is not well understood still.

Silvertein et al. estimated a yearly incidence of VTE of 117 per 100,000 population but as far as cancer patients are concerned VTE rate increased1, in 200 per year. It is more than four folds compared to non malignant patients [16]. Stein et al. showed that incidence of VTE is doubled in cancer patient (2 vs. 1%) [17].

A study in Natherlan of 66,329 patients showed the cumulative incidence of DVT is 12.3 per 1000 population in initial 6 months [18].

Certain tumours like haematological and metastatic diseases are more prone to develop VTE [19]. Mucin producing cancers like ovarian carcinoma, colorectal cancers and lung cancers are likely to be associated with VTE than other solid tumours [15].

Levitan et al. reported systematically the incidence of VTE with different cancers eg- Ovarian ca (12 per 1000 patiemts), lymphoma (9.8 per 1000), pancreatic ca (11 per 1000 pts), brain tumour (11.7 per 1000 patients). They described lowest rates of VTE in Ca breast (2.2 per 1000 pts), Ca bladder (2.2 per 1000 pts) and in head & neck malignancy (1.6 per 1000 pts).

Diagnosis of DVT: only 25% of patients of DVT present with compatible symptoms. Maximum patients may have minimal or atypical symptoms and clinical features.

Harmon's test itself 30% sensitive only. So, a proper clinical assessment, history of varieties of risk factors and sensitive diagnostic tests may confirm the diagnosis of DVT.

Symptoms: The symptoms that are commonly produced by deep vein thrombosis are pain, swelling, and a faint red blue discoloration of the skin. Profound cyanotic discoloration (phlegmasiaceruleadolens), or pallor (phlegmasiaalbadolens) and frank venous gangrene are much less common. The more proximal and occlusive thrombus leads to more marked symptoms and physical signs. Deep vein thrombosis may also present as pyrexia of unknown origin or with the symptoms of pulmonary embolism without any leg symptoms.

Signs: The physical signs of a deep vein thrombosis may be as ephemeral as thesymptoms, and often there are none. Diagnostic values of clinical features have beensummarized in Table 13.1 and shows that the clinical evaluation may imply the need forfurther evaluation but cannot, by itself, be relied on to confirm or exclude thediagnosis of DVT.

Table 13.1 Wells clinical probability score

Clinical features	Score
Active malignancy (On treatment, <6 months, or on palliative care)	1
Paralysis, paresis or recent plaster immobilization of the lower limbs	1
Recently bedridden more than 3 days or major surgery <12 weeks need general or regional anaesthesia	1
Localized tenderness along the deep Venous system	1
Swelling of Entire lower limb	1
Leg swelling >3 cm compare to contralateral side (Measured 10 cm below the tibial tuberosity)	1
Pitting edema of involving symptomatic leg	1
Collateral superficial veins (non-varicose)	1
Previous H/O DVT	1
Alternative diagnosis likely as DVT	-2

13.1 Diagnostic Value of Clinical Features of VTE

Clinical feature	Sensitivity (%)	Specificity
Calf pain	66–91	3–87
Calf tenderness	56–82	26–74
Homans'sign	13–48	39–84
Swelling of calf or leg	35–97	8–88

13.2 Wells Clinical Probability Score (Table 13.1)

This is a scoring method that categorizes patients into high, intermediate and low risk of DVT according to numerous defined criteria (outlined below). A score of ≥3 indicates high probability of DVT, 1 or 2 a moderate probability, and ≤0 indicates low probability.

13.2.1 Diagnostic Tests for DVT

1. Non-invasive Diagnostic Tests Includes Duplex Ultrasound,ImpedancePlethysmography, CT Venography, MRI/MR Venography.
2. Invasive diagnostic tests: Contrast Venography.
3. Fibrinogen Uptake Test.

Biomarkers for the diagnosis of deep vein thrombosis: Gold standard for DVT diagnosis is compression ultrasound. Biomarkers and making a serological diagnosis are desirable. D-dimer, a highly sensitive biomarker, is very useful to exclude VTE. But it lacks of specificity.

The upcoming plasma biomarkers in the diagnosis of VTE are selectins, microparticles, IL 10 and other inflammatory markers. These inflammatory markers may also predict recurrence rate, thrombi which resolve spontaneously and determine the therapy either standard anticoagulation or aggressive therapies.

13.3 Risk Factors for DVT

DVT occurring in the setting of a known risk factor is defined as secondary, where as that occurring in the absence of risk factors is defined as primary or idiopathic. Risk factors can be further classified into acquired or congenital risk factors. (Table 13.2).

13.3.1 Cancer Surgical Risk Groups Are

(i) Increasing age
(ii) Past history of VTE
(iii) Family h/o VTE

Table 13.2 Acquired and Congenital risk factors for DVT

Acquired risk factors for DVT
Acute spinal cord injury Laparoscopic surgery
Age Major Surgery
Central venous access Malignancy
Congestive heart failure Minor surgery
Elective major lower extremity arthroplasty Multiple trauma
Heparin-induced thrombocytopenia Myocardial infarction
Hip, pelvic, or proximal femur fracture Obesity
History of DVT or PE Oral contraceptives
Hormone replacement therapy Pregnancy
Homocysteinemia Sepsis
Immobilizing plaster casts Stroke
Inflammatory bowel disease Patient confined to bed .72 hours
Varicose veins
Congenital risk factors for DVT
Antiphospholipid antibody syndrome
Hyper viscosity syndromes
Ant thrombin III deficiency
Lupus anticoagulant
Disorders of plasminogen and plasmin activation
Myeloproliferative disorders
Dysfibrinogenemia
Protein C deficiency
Homocysteinemia
Protein S deficiency
Prothrombin 20210A allele

(iv) H/o inherited or acquired hyper coagulable state
(v) Obese patient
(vi) History of Chemotherapy 6.5 fold, Presence of mucin secreting cancer like ovary, colorectal, lung other like brain, pancreatic ca, pelvic malignancies three to five fold
(vii) More co-morbidities (like heart disease, infection, sepsis, chronic inflammatory disease, recent stroke etc. more prone to develop VTE)

The risk of developing post-operative VTE also depends upon degree of invasiveness type and duration of surgery, Anaesthesia and requirement for immobilization [20]. As per world literature, in the absence of appropriate prophylaxis incidence of asymptomatic DVT is widely varied from 10 to 80% and total pulmonary embolism is 0.1–0.8 percent after effective general surgery [21]. In high risk patient with Caprini score 5 or more and undergoing abdomino-pelvic surgery without prophylaxis, chance of VTE is approximately 6%.

13.4 Caprini Risk Scoring Method for the Risk Assessment (Table 13.3)

The Caprini score is calculated by adding the scores of all risk factors. The Caprini score is calculated in the following method:

- **Score 0–1**: Low risk
- **Score 2**: Moderate
- **Score 3–4**: High risk
- **Score ≥ 5**: Highest risk

13.4.1 Preventive Measures of VTE

Risk Assessment and Preventive Measures: Patients with gynaecological malignancies undergoing surgery needs to have a proper assessment and evaluation of the postoperative risk of VTE. The American College of Chest Physicians (ACCP) [22] has advised using various risk assessment tools to determines the level of risk of VTE like Caprini Score and Rogers Score.

Table 13.3 Caprini score model

Five points	Three points	Two points	One point
• Stroke (previous month) • Fracture of the hip, pelvis, or leg • Elective hip replacement surgery • Recent spinal cord injury (in the previous month)	• Age≥ 75 years • Previous H/O VTE • Positive F/H/O VTE • Prothrombin A • Factor V Leiden • Lupus anticoagulants • Anticardiolipin antibodies • Increased homocysteine in the blood • HIT • Other congenital or acquired thrombophilia	• Age: 61–74 years • THR surgery • Lap surgery lasting >45 min • General surgery lasting >45 min • Malignancy • Plaster cast • Bedridden for >72 h • Central venous catheter	• Age 41–60 years • BMI >25kg/m^2 • Minor procedures • Edema in the lower limb • Varicose veins • Pregnancy • Post-partum • OCP • HRT • Unexplained or recurrent abortion • Recent H/O Sepsis • H/O Pneumonia in previous month • Abnormal PFT • Acute MI • Congestive heart failure (in the previous month) • IBD

The different scores for the factors included in the Caprini score depicted in the table below
Score 0–1: Low risk, **Score 2**: Moderate, **Score 3–4**: High risk, **Score ≥5**: Highest risk

The Caprini Score has been validated for the use in patients with gynaecological malignancies [23]. The score is calculated by adding scores allotted to individual risk factors and is given as follows:

- **Score 0–1**: Low risk
- **Score 2**: Moderate risk
- **Score 3–4**: High risk
- **Score ≥ 5**: Highest risk

Wells Clinical Probability Score: is a scoring system used for prediction of DVT in patients with malignancies where the score indicates the probability of DVT.

There are two standard approaches to prevent VTE and PE (Table 13.4).

Table 13.4 Comparison

Warfarin	Heparin: UFH	Heparin: Low molecular weight heparin
Limitations: Dosing difficult Slow onset (the anticoagulant effect may not reach its peak until after 72–96 h) Slow clearance (Duration of action, 25 days). Recent guidelines recommend Effectiveness of therapy titrated to a target INR 2–3—requires frequent blood sampling Cost: Vol. 1 mg (10 Tabs)—Rs. 95 Vol. 2 mg (10 Tabs)—Rs. 115 Vol. 5 mg (10 Tabs)—Rs. 200	Mechanism of action—Pentasaccaride sequence binding to antithrombin which enhances its ability to inhibit both thrombin and factor Xa Route—S.c or Iv Antidote—Protamine sulfate Complication—HIT Cost: Rs. 100–150/dose (5000 IU)	Compared with UFH, LMWHs have more predictable pharmacokinetics and greater bioavailability. Weight adjusted dose once or twice daily Recommended for: Thromboprophylaxis in moderate and high risk surgical patients, For post-discharge thromboprophylaxis in high risk surgical patients Initial short term treatment of DVT in general population First 3–6 months for long term treatment of DVT and cancer Cost: Daltaparin Cost Rs 400–600/dose (5000 IU) Fondaparinox Rs1050–1300/dose (2.5 mg) Enoxaparin Cost 175–250/dose (40 mg)

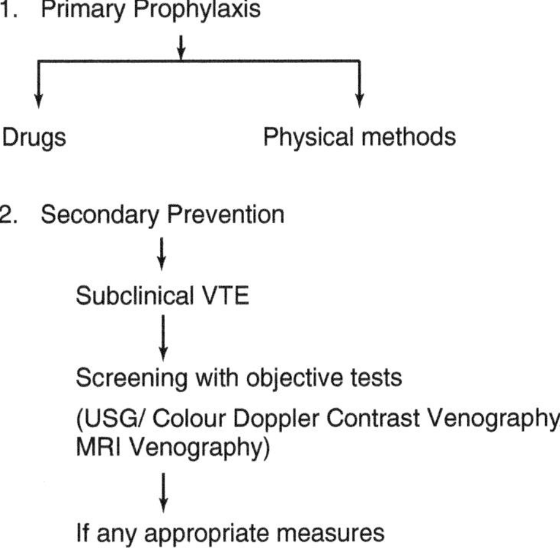

Primary prophylaxis is preferred method as it is safe, effective and no need or limited need for laboratory monitoring.

And the secondary prevention is advised for patients in whom primary prophylaxis is either contraindicated or ineffective.

13.4.2 Primary Prophylaxis

1. Early and frequent ambulation for all patients, maintenance of hydration and prevention of sepsis.
2. Mechanical methods are preferred in low risk group (Caprini score 1–2) and patients with a contraindication to pharmacologic prophylaxis.
3. Pharmacologic prophylaxis is preferred in surgical patients at moderate and high risk patients (Caprini score ≥3)
4. Combined pharmacologic and mechanical methods (usually intermittent pneumatic compression) are considered for very high risk patients (Caprini score ≥5).

Pharmacologic Agents for VTE Prevention—Various drugs are now available for VTE prevention, including unfractionated heparin, the LMW heparins, fondaparinux, the vitamin K antagonists, and the newer antithrombotic agents rivaroxaban, dabigatran, and apixaban. These will be discussed below. When available, meta-analyses of the comparative effectiveness among these various agents will also be discussed.

13.4.3 Pharmacological Agents Usually Used

1. **UFH**: LMW (Low Molecular Weight) heparins, Daltaparin and Fondaparinux, are preferred than UFH. UFH is safe in renal function derangement and cost is Rs 100–150/dose (5000 IU)

(a) **Daltaparin** (Fragmin) in moderate to in-high risk cancer patients—2500 IU subcutaneously 1–2 h. before surgery followed by 2500 IU 8–12 h later and then.

Once daily post operative dose of 5000 IU subcutaneously for 5–10 days or till the time of discharge depending upon the risk score. Contraindication: Renal Insufficiency.

Coagulation profiles like PT and APTT are relatively insensitive measures of Daltaparin therefore unsuitable for monitoring the anticoagulant effect. Creatinine clearance should be monitored and the Cost for single dose (5000 IU) is Rs 400–600/– in Indian currency.

(b) **Fondaparinux**: Prophylactic dose 2.5 mg s/c to be started 6–8 h after surgery. Once daily for 5–10 days or till discharge of the patient. Cost Rs1050–1300/ dose (2.5

(c) **Enoxaparin:** 30–40 mg s/c once daily starting 12 hours after surgery. Next time Low dose unfractionated Heparin (UFH) is used where LMW is contraindicated i.e. in renal insufficiency and where cost is an issue. Cost 175–250/dose (40 mg).

Thrombocytopenia to be monitored routinely.

(d) **Warfarin** may be advised as an alternative to LMWH and UFH when delayed prophylaxis is planned.

13.5 Comparison among all Type of Heparins (Table 13.3)

Comparison of agents—To Compare the agents across studies of hip or knee surgery have been difficult, since the drugs under investigation and the dosing schedules have varied between trials. Even in the similar clinical trial there can be considerable variability. In addition, bleeding rates have varied across the trails, at least in part because different definitions for bleeding have been used.

A number of randomized trials have compared LMW heparin with UFH, warfarin or acenocoumarol, or fondaparinux in patients undergoing total hip replacement (THR), and to a lesser extent total knee replacement (TKR). A meta-analysis compared vitamin K antagonists versus LMW heparin for the prevention of VTE in orthopaedic surgery revealed that the vitamin K antagonists are less effective than LMW heparin, without any remarkable difference in bleeding risk.

In general, LMW heparin has been shown to be superior to UFH or warfarin, but inferior to fondaparinux in terms of efficacy, with similar bleeding rates in patients undergoing THR OR TKR surgeries.

The use of LMW heparin enoxaparin differs between regions. Thus:

- In North America, enoxaparin at a dose of 30 mg twice daily started after 12 to 24 hours after surgery.
- In Europe, enoxaparin at a dose of 40 mg is started 12 hours after surgery and is then given once daily.
- Other LMW heparin preparations have usually been given in a once daily dose, started after surgical procedure.

A meta-analysis in patients underwent surgery for cancer concluded that there was no difference between LMWH and UFH in terms of efficacy, DVT location, or bleeding complications.

A Cochrane review of the use of LMW heparin to prevent VTE in surgical patients with lower immobilization concluded that LMW heparin in outpatients effectively reduced the VTE incidence. A further meta-analysis reviewed the use of intermittent pneumatic compression (IPC) with or without pharmacologic prophylaxis. It was shown that, compared with IPC alone, combined prophylactic methods reduced the VTE incidence.

In neurosurgical procedures, LMW heparin was shown to be effective then IPC. In major trauma management, LMW heparin was effective then UFH in the prevention of DVTs.

Timing of Prophylaxis: Recommended either before or immediately after surgical procedure and continued until the patient is mobile.

In moderate and high risk patients LMWH started either 12 hours before surgery or 18–24 h after surgery.

The term extended prophylaxis is used by ACCP & NCCN and ASCO—for a very high risk patients (Caprini score >5) where prophylaxis may be extended 10–35 days. It is recommended for a period of 5 weeks.

Other drugs used are—direct thrombin &Xa inhibitor, Rivaroxaban, DabigationXilate, Apixaban, Endoxaban etc.

13.5.1 Mechanical Methods

1. Intermittent Pneumatic compression (IPC)—It enhances blood flow in the deep veins in the leg, thereby preventing venous stasis.

   It reduces plasminogen activator inhibitor-1 (PAI-1) thereby increasing endogenous fibrinolytic activity [24]

   Among all mechanical devices, efficacy of IPC appears best [22]
2. A Graded compression stocking (GCS)—GCS when combined with other prophylactic modalities appears to improve rate of DVT prevention.
3. Venous foot pump (VFP)—Like GCS, it is used combined with other prophylactic methods.

   Inferior Vena Cava (IVC) filters: In general IVC filters should be avoided as primary prophylaxis. The indication for filter placement as a therapy for DVT (Figs. 13.1 and 13.2).

13.5.2 Summary and Recommendations

Every hospital may develop a formal strategy for the prevention of VTE for their surgical patients. Strategies should be developed with proper thromboprophylaxis recommendations, including authorized order sets, periodic audit, follow up with feedback.

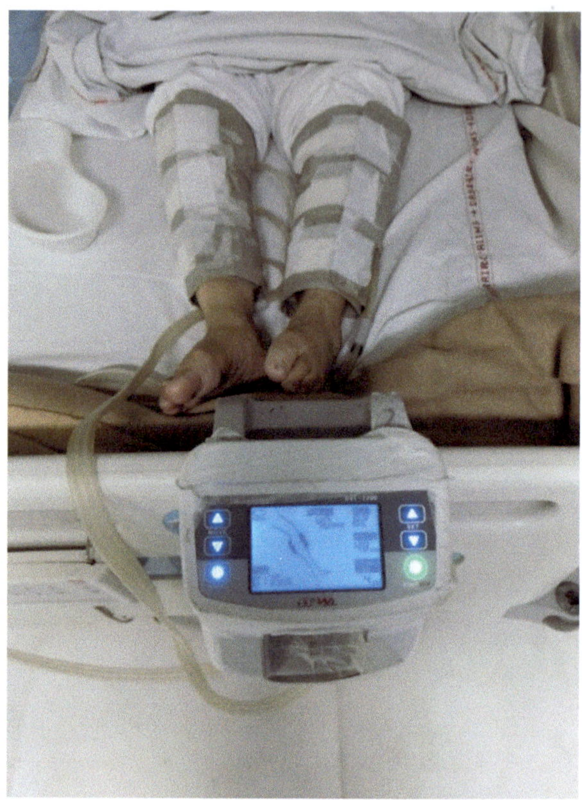

Fig. 13.1 DVT Pump used for DVT Prophylaxis

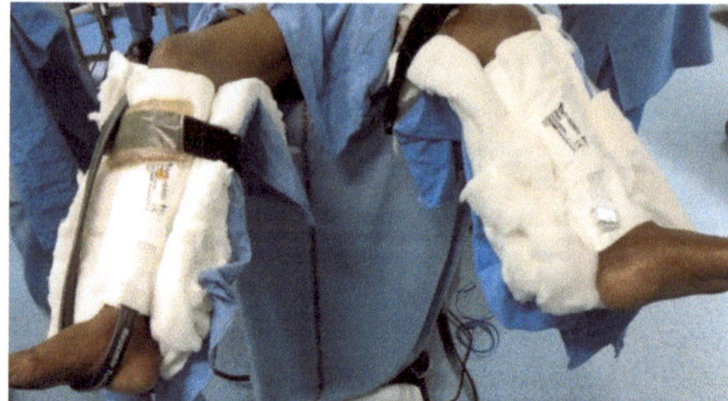

Fig. 13.2 DVT pump used intra operatively In Post-operative period in ICU

The article "Prevention of venous Thromboembolism" ACCP evidenced based clinical practice guidelines (eighth Edition) is a recommended guidelines for the prevention of VTE which may be useful in formulating these policies [25].

Number of attempt has been made to develop risk assessment models for VTE in individual patients. At this time, none of the risk stratification models has been validated in prospective trials, although this subject is under active study.

In patients with additional risk factors (eg, previous H/O VTE, advanced age particularly >75 years, active cancer or a history of cancer, a more extensive surgical procedure) consideration should be given to more aggressive prophylaxis in the form of increased intensity or duration of a pharmacologic agent, or the addition of Intermittent Pneumatic compression (IPC) [25].

In patients from specific ethnic groups in which the incidence of post-surgical venous thromboembolism is low (eg, Asian populations), consideration may be given to **less** aggressive prophylaxis.

Assignment of surgical risk groups: The risk of postoperative VTE depends upon the surgical procedure (eg, type and duration of anaesthesia and surgery, requirement for post-operative immobilization), as well as patient-related factors (eg, increasing age, prior VTE, presence of cancer or obesity, presence of an inherited or acquired hypercoagulable state). Patients have been generally divided into low, moderate, and high risk categories.

Low risk general and abdominal-pelvic surgery: For low risk surgery (Caprini score 1–2) the use of mechanical prophylaxis is preferred, over no prophylaxis or prophylactic anticoagulation.

Moderate risk general and abdominal-pelvic surgeries: For moderate risk general and abdominal-pelvic surgery (Caprini score 3–4) the recommend method is the use of prophylactic anticoagulation over no prophylaxis.

High risk general and abdominal-pelvic surgery: For high risk general and oncologic abdominal-pelvic surgery (Caprini score 5 or more) the use of prophylactic anticoagulation is recommended. Reasonable choices include LMW heparin, UFH in renal insufficiency, or Fondaparinux.

Length of treatment: For moderate risk patients undergoing major general and abdominal-pelvic surgeries, the recommendation is that continue thromboprophylaxis until hospital discharge, rather than for a shorter or longer period.

13.6 Timing of Regional Anaesthesia/Analgesia: (Cork University Hospital, Version 1 Guideline 2015)

13.6.1 UFC (Subcutaneous)

- Should Wait minimum 4 h after a dose prior to block or catheter removal
- Should Wait minimum 1 h prior to dosing after procedure (catheter insertion or withdrawal)

13.6.2 UFH (Intravenous)

- Infusion should be stopped 2–4 h prior to block
- Start infusion >1 h after block
- Remove epidural catheter not before 2–4 h after discontinuation of infusion

13.6.3 LMWH

- Should Wait minimum 12 h after a prophylaxis dose before block
- Should Wait minimum 24 h after a therapeutic dose before block
- Should Wait minimum 10 h after dose before removing catheter
- After catheter removal wait 2–4 h before next dose

13.6.4 Present Recommendation for Major Surgery like CRS and HIPEC

- Prophylaxis against thromboembolism to be started 12 h prior to CRS ± HIPEC should be performed
- Mechanical thromboprophylaxis until complete mobilisation in association with
- pharmacological thromboprophylaxis as an option
- Pharmacological thromboprophylaxis routinely Extended pharmacological thromboprophylaxis until 4 weeks after CRS ± HIPEC, as an option in Addition to in-hospital thromboprophylaxis should be performed routinely

Conclusion: For selected high risk general and abdominal-pelvic surgery patients, the suggestion that continuing thromboprophylaxis after hospitalization with LMW heparin for up to 4 weeks be considered, minimum till the patient discharges from the hospital and ask the patient to keep on moving at home, not to be at bed always.

Further trails involving various regional cancer centres with huge sample size may provide further epidemiological data related to VTE in onco-surgery patients. So continue efforts to be made to find the most effective and safest method to prevent and manage VTE.

References

1. Trousseau. Phlegmasiaalbadolens. In: Clinique Medicale de L'Hotel-Dieu Paris. London: New Sydenham society; 1865. p. 94–6.
2. Lindblad B, Eriksson A, Bergqvist D. Autopsy-verified pulmonary embolism in a surgical department: analysis of the period from 1951 to 1988. Br J Surg. 1991;78:849.
3. Klatsky AL, Baer D. What protects Asians from venous thromboembolism? Am J Med. 2004;116(7):493–5.
4. Murugesan A, Srivastava DN, Ballehaninna UK, Chumber S, Dhar A, Misra MC, et al. Detection and prevention of post-operative deep vein thrombosis [DVT] using nadroparin among patients undergoing major abdominal operations in India; a randomised controlled trial. Indian J Surg. 2010;72(4):312–7.
5. Shukla PJ, Siddachari R, Ahire S, Arya S, Ramani S, Barreto SG, et al. Postoperative deep vein thrombosis in patients with colorectal cancer. Indian J GastroenterolOff J Indian SocGastroenterol. 2008;27(2):71–3.
6. Clagett GP, Reisch JS. Prevention of venous thromboembolism in general surgical patients. Results of meta analysis. Ann Surg. 1988;208:227.

7. Nurmohamed MT, Rosendaal FR, Büller HR, et al. Low-molecular-weight heparin versus standard heparin in general and orthopaedic surgery: a meta-analysis. Lancet. 1992;340:152.
8. Geerts WH, Bergqvist D, Pineo GF, et al. Prevention of venous thromboembolism: American College of Chest Physicians Evidence-Based Clinical Practice Guidelines (8th edition). Chest. 2008;133:381S.
9. Lyman GH, Khorana AA, Falanga A, et al. American Society of Clinical Oncology guideline: recommendations for venous thromboembolism prophylaxis and treatment in patients with cancer. J ClinOncol. 2007;25:5490.
10. Cohen AT, Tapson VF, Bergmann JF, et al. Venous thromboembolism risk and prophylaxis in the acute hospital care setting (ENDORSE study): a multinational cross-sectional study. Lancet. 2008;371:387.
11. Muntz J. Duration of deep vein thrombosis prophylaxis in the surgical patient and its relation to quality issues. Am J Surg. 2010;200:413.
12. Rathbun S. The surgeon General's call to action to prevent deep vein thrombosis and pulmonary embolism. Circulation. 2009;119(15):e480–2.
13. National. Cancer-associated venous thromboembolic disease [Internet]. NCCN version 2.2014; [cited 2015 Apr 26]. http://www.nccn.org
14. Nijziel MR, van Oerle R, Hillen HFP, Hamulyák K. From Trousseau to angiogenesis: the link between the haemostatic system and cancer. Neth J Med. 2006;64(11):403–10.
15. Caine GJ, Stonelake PS, Lip GYH, Kehoe ST. The hypercoagulable state of malignancy: pathogenesis and current debate. Neoplasia N Y N. 2002;4(6):465–73.
16. Heit JA, Silverstein MD, Mohr DN, Petterson TM, O'Fallon WM, Melton LJ. Risk factors for deep vein thrombosis and pulmonary embolism: a population-based case-control study. Arch Intern Med. 2000;160(6):809–15.
17. Stein PD, Beemath A, Meyers FA, Skaf E, Sanchez J, Olson RE. Incidence of venous thromboembolism in patients hospitalized with cancer. Am J Med. 2006;119(1):60–8.
18. Blom JW, Vanderschoot JPM, Oostindiër MJ, Osanto S, van der Meer FJM, Rosendaal FR. Incidence of venous thrombosis in a large cohort of 66,329 cancer patients: results of a record linkage study. J ThrombHaemost JTH. 2006;4(3):529–35.
19. Barbui T, Finazzi G, Falanga A. The impact of all-trans-retinoic acid on the coagulopathy of acute promyelocyticleukemia. Blood. 1998;91(9):3093–102.
20. Donzé JD, Ridker PM, Finlayson SR, Bates DW. Impact of sepsis on risk of postoperative arterial and venous thromboses: large prospective cohort study. BMJ. 2014;349:g5334.
21. Geerts WH, Pineo GF, Heit JA, et al. Prevention of venous thromboembolism: the seventh ACCP conference on antithrombotic and thrombolytic therapy. Chest. 2004;126:338S.
22. Gould MK, Garcia DA, Wren SM, et al. Prevention of VTE in nonorthopedic surgical patients: antithrombotic therapy and prevention of thrombosis, 9th ed: American College of Chest Physicians Evidence-Based Clinical Practice Guidelines. Chest. 2012;141(2 Suppl):e227S–77.
23. Stroud W, Whitworth JM, Miklic M, Schneider KE, Finan MA, et al. Validation of a venous thromboembolism risk assessment model in gynecologic oncology. Gynecol Oncol. 2014;134:160–3.
24. Comerota AJ, Chouhan V, Harada RN, et al. The fibrinolytic effects of intermittent pneumatic compression: mechanism of enhanced fibrinolysis. Ann Surg. 1997;226:306.
25. Geerts WH, Bergqvist D, Pineo GF, et al. Prevention of venous thromboembolism: American College of Chest Physicians Evidence-Based Clinical Practice Guidelines (8th edition). Chest. 2008;133:381S.

Catheter-Related Blood Stream Infections (CRBSI) 14

Kingshuk Dasgupta

14.1 Introduction

Modern critical care medicine necessitates the placement of central venous catheters (either short or long term) for various indications. These include administration of intravenous fluids, medications, blood products, parenteral nutrition fluids, monitoring hemodynamic status, and providing hemodialysis.

Catheter-related bloodstream infections (CRBSI) are the most common nosocomial infections in intensive care units and causes significant morbidity and mortality in critically ill patients. CRBSI occur in an estimated 250,000–500,000 patients annually in the United States, has a 10–30% mortality rate, prolongs hospitalization and burdens the healthcare system with an additional $300 million–$2.3 billion a year [1].

14.2 Definitions

***Catheter-related bloodstream infection (CR-BSI)—Infectious Diseases Society of America (IDSA)* definition** [2]: Catheter-related bloodstream infection (CRBSI) is the preferred term used by the IDSA. CRBSI Is a clinical definition, used for diagnosing and treating patients and requires specific laboratory testing that identifies the catheter as the source of the Blood Stream Infection (BSI).

K. Dasgupta (✉)
Department of Pediatrics and Pediatric Critical Care, Avera McKennan Children's Hospital & University Health Center, Sanford School of Medicine of the University of South Dakota, Sioux Falls, SD, USA

V. Kumar et al. (eds.), *Onco-critical Care*,
https://doi.org/10.1007/978-981-16-9929-0_14

The definitive diagnosis of CRBSI requires either *ONE* of the following:

1. Isolation of the same pathogen from a quantitative blood culture drawn through the central line and from a peripheral vein with a single bacterial colony count (colony-forming units; CFU) at least threefold higher in the sample from the central line as compared to that obtained from the peripheral vein.
2. The same organism is recovered from percutaneous blood culture and quantitative (>15 colony-forming units; CFU) culture of the catheter tip.
3. A shorter time to positive culture (>2 h earlier) in the central line sample than the peripheral sample (differential time to positivity [DTP] [2])

CLABSI—Centers for Disease Control and Prevention (CDC) definition: CLABSI is a surveillance definition used by the CDC and is defined as recovery of a pathogen from blood culture (a single positive blood culture for organism not commonly present on the skin, and two or more blood cultures for organism commonly present on the skin) in a patient who had a central line at the time of infection or within 48 hours before the development of infection. The infection cannot be related to any other infection the patient might have and must not have been present or incubating when the patient was admitted to the facility [3]. However, since some bloodstream infections (BSIs) are from sources other than the central line (for example pancreatitis, mucositis) that may be difficult to recognize, the CDC CLABSI surveillance definition may overestimate the true incidence of CRBSI.

Exit site infection—Signs of inflammation confined to an area (typically <2 cm surrounding the catheter exit site and the presence of exudate that proves to be culture positive).

Tunnel infection—Inflammation extending beyond 2 cm from the exit site (along with the track or extending centrally towards the vein entry site or extending beyond the cuff), associated with pain and tenderness along the subcutaneous tract and culture-positive exudate from the exit site. (this may not be seen unless expressed by palpation).

1. **Epidemiology**

Worldwide, approximately 250,000 bloodstream infections occur annually, and most are related to the presence of intravascular devices. In the United States, the CLABSI rate in intensive care units (ICUs) is estimated to be 0.8 per 1000 central line days. International nosocomial infection control consortium (INICC) surveillance data from January 2010 through December 2015 (703 intensive care units in 50 countries) reported a CLABSI rate of 4.1 per 1000 central line days.

CLABSIs are an important cause of morbidity and mortality worldwide. However, the incidence of CLABSI associated with central lines among patients hospitalized in intensive care units appears to be decreasing in incidence in resource-rich countries. In the United States, the incidence of CLABSI decreased from 3.64

to 1.65 infections per 1000 central line days between 2001 and 2009 [4]. In contrast, the reported pooled incidence of CLABSI across 428 ICUs in 36 countries in countries in Latin America, Asia, Africa and Europe was substantially higher, 6.8 events per 1000 central line days [5].

14.3 Risk Factors

Host factors- the host factors commonly associated with nosocomial bloodstream infections include

1. Chronic illness (hemodialysis, gastrointestinal tract disorders, pulmonary hypertension)
2. Immune deficiency due to various reasons including malignancy, bone marrow transplantation, neutropenia, diabetes mellitus
3. Malnutrition, total parenteral nutrition administration.
4. Previous bloodstream infections
5. Extremes of age
6. Loss of skin integrity (burns).

Catheter factors:

1. Location: Femoral central venous catheters are associated with the highest risk of bloodstream infection and catheter colonization followed by the internal jugular and subclavian catheters [6]. The subclavian venous catheter is associated with the lowest risk of infection [6, 7].
2. Duration of catheterization.
3. Conditions during insertion (dirty or clean).
4. Catheter site care.
5. The skill of the catheter inserter.

- Neutropenic patients are at high risk for CRBSIs as well as other infections. Those with an absolute neutrophil count <100 cells/mm^3 are at the highest risk [8].
- Pseudomonas is commonly seen in association with neutropenia, severe illness and known prior colonization.
- Patients hospitalized with burns are also at high risk for nosocomial BSIs because of necrotic tissue in the burn wounds. The thermal injury sustained during the burn process decreases host resistance with a significant inflammatory response to the above [9].
- Candida is associated with the following risk factors; colonization with candida at multiple sites, prolonged exposure to broad-spectrum antibiotics, ICU stay >1-week, total parenteral nutrition, and immunosuppression (chemotherapy, neutropenia, haematological malignancy, solid organ or hematopoietic stem cell transplantation).

14.4 Pathophysiology

Central venous catheters are of two types.

- Temporary/non tunnelled catheters: Temporary central venous catheters are inserted percutaneously and account for most CRBSIs. The absence of a tunnel puts non-tunnelled catheters at high risk for CRBSIs.
- Long term/tunnelled catheters: These catheters are implanted surgically (by creating a subcutaneous tract before entering the vein) in the internal jugular, subclavian, or fair femoral vein for long term (weeks to months) usage. They are used for chemotherapy or hemodialysis. Typically, tunnelled catheters have a cuff that causes a fibrotic reaction around the catheter, keeping it in place and creates a barrier to bacterial migration.
- How do catheters get infected?

  There are 4 recognized routes for contamination of central venous catheters.

1. Migration of skin organisms along the exterior surface of the catheter.
2. Direct contamination of the catheter or the hub by manipulation without proper sterile procedures.
3. From hematogenous spread from a distant infection site.
4. Rarely from a contaminated infusate.

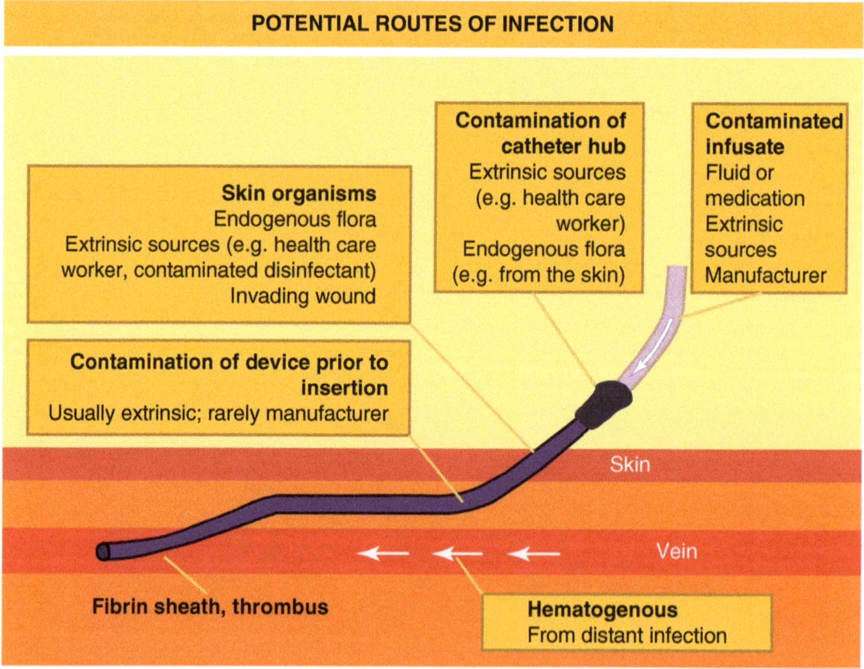

Potential sources of CRBSI from Gahlot et al. 2014 [10].

Time course of catheter-related infections

- **Early infections** (≤ 14 days) often arise from the skin:
  - (a) These may occur during line insertion by migration of skin organisms down the external surface of the catheter into the bloodstream.
  - (b) There may be gradual infection, beginning where the catheter exits the skin.
- **Later infections** (> 14 days) may arise from the catheter hub or luminal surface (fibrin sheath) [11]. Silastic catheters are at a higher risk than polyurethane catheters because of the higher tendency to form fibrin sheaths [12].

14.5 Microbiology

The vast majority of reported pathogens for CLABSI are gram-positive organisms (75%) and include Coagulase-negative *staphylococci*, *Staphylococcus aureus*, *Enterococcus* and *Candida* species (13%).

Coagulase-negative Staphylococcus are the most common cause of catheter-related infection. Gram-negative bacilli account for 14–20% of CLABSI reported to the CDC and the surveillance and control of pathogens of epidemiological importance (SCOPE) databases respectively. Recent global data has shown that the epidemiology of CRBSI has changed, with a predominance of gram-negative bacteria (GNB) such as *Pseudomonas aeruginosa*, *Klebsiella* spp., or *Acinetobacter* spp. as the causative organisms [13, 14].

Surveillance reports have also documented a trend towards more antibiotic microbial resistance among all the common pathogens causing CRBSI [15]. Although methicillin-resistant *Staphylococcus aureus* (MRSA) is not responsible for more than 50% of all *S. aureus* isolates obtained in the ICU, the incidence of MRSA CRBSI is steadily decreasing due to preventive efforts [15].

14.6 Diagnosis

Detection of CRBSI depends on both clinical examination as well as meticulous laboratory evaluation.

When to suspect a line infection?

1. Fever or septic shock in a patient in whom a central line has been present more than 48 h who has no other obvious cause of the fever. Patients may have subtle symptoms such as malaise and nausea or severe symptoms including fever with rigor, vomiting, and altered mental status.
2. Local signs of infection at the line site include erythema, pain and purulent exudate from the site. Unfortunately, this is often absent. Obvious evidence of infection at the line site is specific but poorly sensitive [16].
3. Malfunction of a previously working line may be due to an infected thrombus and supports the diagnosis of line infection.

Laboratory diagnosis of catheter-related bloodstream infections

- It is important to note that the positive predictive value of all laboratory tests for catheter-related bloodstream infections increases greatly with high pretest clinical probability.
- Catheters should not be cultured routinely but rather only if CRBSI is suspected clinically [6, 17].
- When a catheter infection is suspected, send at least two blood cultures obtained from peripheral veins (different sites) and one set of cultures from the distal port of the central line [2, 18].
- It is extremely important to ensure that equal volumes of blood (e.g., 10 ml) are obtained from each site.
- Some institutions draw blood cultures from each port of the central line which may increase the sensitivity of the blood culture [19]. However, obtaining more cultures will also increase the likelihood of false-positive results due to contamination.
- When sending paired blood cultures, ensure that they are either quantitative cultures or qualitative cultures with continuously monitored differential time to positivity (DTI) [18].
- A Differential Time to positivity (DTI) difference >2 h from the central venous catheter blood culture versus the peripheral blood or simultaneous quantitative paired blood culture with >5: 1 one ratio of Central venous catheter vs peripheral culture is highly suggestive of CRBSI [20]. The DTI method is simpler and is readily provided by currently used automated blood culture systems in hospitals.
- A positive semi-quantitative culture result is >15 CFU per catheter segment. A positive quantitative culture is $>10^3$ per catheter segment.

The clinician will be faced with one of the following four general patterns of blood culture results obtained via blood sampling.

1. The peripheral and central venous catheter cultures all turn positive with DTI 1 < 2 h. This suggests bacteremia due to another cause (for example endocarditis). It is important to note that this can also definitely occur with catheter infection, so clinical judgment has to be used. If after due diligence no other source of infection is ascertained then catheter infection may become increasingly likely [21]
2. The central venous line cultures turn positive >2 h earlier than the peripheral cultures. This method has a sensitivity of 91% and a specificity of 94% and is fairly diagnostic (85%) of CRBSI.
3. One of the peripheral blood cultures turned positive and none of the other cultures does. This suggests contamination with the caveat that gram-negative organisms and candida should still be taken seriously.
4. The central line culture turns positive but none of the peripheral blood cultures does. This is the most difficult pattern to evaluate. This may represent contamination, but it could equally represent early colonization of catheter infection. Removal of the catheter is the most prudent course but systemic antibiotics may or may not be necessary (depending on the clinical context).

The isolation of the following low-virulence skin organisms may be suggestive of line infection in the right clinical context and if confirmed from the culture of multiple sites.

- *Coagulase-negative staphylococci*
- *Micrococcus spp*
- *Propionibacterium* spp.
- *Corynebacterium jeikeium*
- *Bacillus* spp.
- *Malassezia furfur*

14.7 Management

(a) **General management**

(i) **Indications for catheter removal**

(a) Definite catheter infection

(i) The catheter needs to be removed if there is definite evidence of infection such as purulent exudate at the catheter insertion site or positive blood cultures from the catheter.

(ii) Possible catheter infection plus increased risk of "harm" with leaving the catheter in place.

1. Sepsis and septic shock
2. Neutropenic or immunosuppressed patients.
3. Presence of endovascular hardware (e.g., pacemaker), prosthetic valves.
4. Presence of concomitant endocarditis or evidence of disseminated infection.
5. Presence of suppurative thrombophlebitis
6. Presence of a propagating clot.
7. Persistent bacteremia after 72 h of appropriate antimicrobial therapy.
8. Tunnelled central venous catheter tunnel tract infection or subcutaneous port reservoir infection.

(iii) Additionally, catheter removal is also indicated in the setting of infection with the following pathogens:

1. *Staphylococcus aureus*
2. *Pseudomonas aeruginosa*
3. *Drug-resistant gram-negative bacilli*
4. *Candida* spp.

(b) **Definitive management**

(i) **Short term central venous CRBSI**

- When CRBSI is suspected, the initial choice of antibiotics should be based on the most likely organisms, the severity of the patient's illness, risk factors for infection and other pre-existing conditions.
- Empirical treatment should be instituted promptly after blood cultures are obtained. In general, coverage for gram-positive and gram-negative

organisms is necessary. The local prevalence and antimicrobial susceptibility patterns in institutional antibiograms should also be considered.

- Keeping all these in mind, the following general recommendations can be made.
- CRBSI due to gram-positive organisms
  (a) For CRBSI due to gram-positive organisms, empirical therapy consists of vancomycin [2]. If there is a high institutional prevalence of methicillin-resistant *S. aureus* (MRSA) isolates with vancomycin minimal inhibitory concentration(MIC) > 2 mcg/ml, an alternative agent such as daptomycin should be used [22].
  (b) Linezolid is not recommended for empirical treatment of CRBSI. In 2007, the FDA released a warning regarding the use of linezolid for CRBSI [23–25]. However, subsequent studies have shown that Linezolid is effective for bacteremia [26–28]. Currently, vancomycin remains the preferred drug of choice for gram-positive bacteremia.
- CRBSI due to gram-negative bacilli
  (a) Monotherapy with antipseudomonal beta-lactamase antibiotics such as piperacillin-tazobactam, cefepime, ceftazidime and meropenem is recommended in patients with neutropenia or severe burns. For patients with hemodynamic instability and settings where local resistance suggests <90% susceptibility to antipseudomonal beta-lactams, adding a second antipseudomonal agent such as an aminoglycoside may be considered while awaiting culture results. Once susceptibilities are available, the patient can be switched to appropriate monotherapy [29].
  (b) In the absence of hemodynamic instability, severe burn or neutropenia, monotherapy with ceftriaxone is appropriate and antipseudomonal coverage is unnecessary.
  (c) Patients known to be colonized with drug-resistant organisms should receive appropriate empiric antibiotic therapy.

(ii) **Long-term central venous CRBSI**

- Empirically treat hemodialysis patients suspected of having a CRBSI with intravenous vancomycin and ceftazidime.
- In stable patients, vancomycin can be administered during the last 60 min of the hemodialysis session and ceftazidime immediately after completion of the dialysis session. In hemodynamically unstable patients who are unable to get dialyzed, the antibiotics should be administered immediately after collection of blood cultures without waiting for a dialysis session.
- For patients with a documented vancomycin allergy or history of vancomycin-resistant enterococci, daptomycin should be used instead of vancomycin. The typical dose of daptomycin is 9 mg/kg among patients receiving hemodialysis with a high-flux dialyzer and 7 mg/kg among patients receiving hemodialysis with a low-flux dialyzer. This dose is administered during the last hour of dialysis [30].

- If the patient has a severe allergy to beta-lactam antibiotics, then aminoglycosides such as gentamicin or tobramycin may be used. For gentamicin, the typical dose is 1–2 mg/kg of ideal body weight with the dose not to exceed 100 mg in a single dose [31]. Gentamicin or tobramycin are typically administered in the last hour of dialysis.

(iii) **Specific management**

- All durations are calculated from the date of the first negative blood culture.
- **Uncomplicated CRBS:** Blood culture becomes negative and fever resolves ≤72 h and patient has no hardware and no evidence of suppurative thrombophlebitis or endocarditis and for *S. aureus* does not have active malignancy or immunosuppression)
- **Coagulase-negative Staphylococcus (CoNS)**:
  (a) For patients with no endovascular or orthopaedic hardware with CoNS CRBSI remove the catheter and continue systemic antibiotics for 5–7 days.
  (b) For patients with Intravascular implant or orthopaedic hardware and uncomplicated CoNS CRBSI who undergo catheter removal and have rapid clearance of bacteremia—systemic antibiotics are recommended for 14 days.
  (c) If the catheter is retained treat with systemic antibiotic therapy and ALT (described below) for 10–14 days.
  (d) If the organism is *S Lugadensesis*, systemic antibiotics are recommended for 2–6 weeks.
- **Staphylococcus aureus**
  (a) In general S aureus CRBSI consists of catheter removal and systemic antibiotic therapy for ≥14 days.
- **Enterococcus**
  (a) Management of CRSBI due to *Enterococcus* spp. is catheter removal and systemic antibiotics for 7–14 days.
- **Gram-negative organisms**
  (a) For patients with uncomplicated CRBSI due to gram-negative organisms who undergo catheter removal, systemic antimicrobial therapy is recommended for 7–14 days.
- **Candida spp**
  (a) Management of candida CRBSI includes catheter removal and systemic antifungal therapy with echinocandins (caspofungin or micafungin) for 14 days.
  (b) Consider getting a [1, 3] beta D-Glucan level (FUNGITELL) as well.
- **Complicated CRBSI**
  (a) If the patient has active malignancy, ongoing immunosuppression, suppurative thrombophlebitis, endocarditis, osteomyelitis etc. then remove the catheter and continue systemic antibiotics for 4–6 weeks.

(c) Antibiotic lock therapy -ALT
   (i) Refers to the installation of antibiotic solution into the catheter lumen. This is used in situations where the catheter cannot be removed and is most commonly used for the management of CRBSI due to CoNS and drug-susceptible *Enterobacteriaceae*. This always must be done in conjunction with systemic antimicrobial therapy. Infectious disease consult is strongly recommended if this course of action is entertained.

14.8 Prevention

(a) **CVC insertion bundles** incorporate evidence-based science and are recommended in CRBSI guidelines [6, 32, 33].
   (i) Potential CVC insertion bundle components [33]:
      - Strict adherence to hand hygiene protocols
      - Use full barrier precautions /personal protective equipment (PPE)
      - Chlorhexidine screen antisepsis.
      - Optimal catheter type selection.
      - Optimal catheter site selection.
      - Proper procedures four catheters addressing monitoring /changes.
      - Safe disposal of sharps.
      - Daily review of line necessity and prompt removal of unnecessary CVCs.
      - Health cares personnel education about CRBSI.
      - Availability of CVC carts that contain all necessary supplies.
      - Checklist to ensure adherence to proper sterile practices [34].
      - Procedures stopped in non-emergent situations when sterility is breached.
      - Feedback provided to healthcare personnel regarding the CRBSI rate and overall healthcare-associated infection (HAI) rates.
      - Proper documentation

14.9 Surveillance and Reporting

(a) Surveillance involves systematically collecting, analyzing, interpreting, and disseminating data to members of the health care team as a means to facilitate improvement in patient outcomes [35].
(b) Specific outcome measures (for tracking rates) and process measures (to determine adherence to recommended practices should be identified in individual institutions that have been earmarked for performance improvement.
(c) Public reporting of surveillance measures can promote transparency, engender trust, and provide an incentive to improve care. In many US states reporting of HAI rates including CRBSI rates are required by law.

References

1. jointcommission.org. clabsi_monograph.
2. Manian FA. IDSA guidelines for the diagnosis and management of intravascular catheter-related bloodstream infection. Clin Infect Dis. 2009;49(11):1770–1; author reply 1771–1772
3. Wright MO, Decker SG, Allen-Bridson K, Hebden JN, Leaptrot D. Healthcare-associated infections studies project: an American journal of infection control and National Healthcare Safety Network data quality collaboration: location mapping. Am J Infect Control. 2018;46(5):577–8.
4. Vital signs: central line-associated bloodstream infections--the United States, 2001, 2008, and 2009. MMWR Morb Mortal Wkly Rep. 2011;60(8):243–248.
5. Rosenthal D, Victor. Central line-associated bloodstream infections in limited-resource countries: a review of the literature. Clin Infect Dis. 2009;49(12):1899–907.
6. O'Grady NP, Alexander M, Burns LA, et al. Guidelines for the prevention of intravascular catheter-related infections. Clin Infect Dis. 2011;52(9):e162–93.
7. Parienti J-J, Mongardon N, Mégarbane B, et al. Intravascular complications of central venous catheterization by insertion site. N Engl J Med. 2015;373(13):1220–9.
8. Bodey GP, Buckley M, Sathe YS, Freireich EJ. Quantitative relationships between circulating leukocytes and infection in patients with acute leukemia. Ann Intern Med. 1966;64(2):328–40.
9. Church D, Elsayed S, Reid O, Winston B, Lindsay R. Burn wound infections. Clin Microbiol Rev. 2006;19(2):403–34.
10. Gahlot R, Nigam C, Kumar V, Yadav G, Anupurba S. Catheter-related bloodstream infections. Int J Crit Illn Inj Sci. 2014;4(2):162–7.
11. Mehall JR, Saltzman DA, Jackson RJ, Smith SD. Fibrin sheath enhances central venous catheter infection. Crit Care Med. 2002;30(4):908–12.
12. Mehall JR, Saltzman DA, Jackson RJ, Smith SD. Catheter materials affect the incidence of late blood-borne catheter infection. Surg Infect. 2001;2(3):225–9; discussion 229–230
13. Surapat B, Montakantikul P, Malathum K, Kiertiburanakul S, Santanirand P, Chindavijak B. Microbial epidemiology and risk factors for relapse in gram-negative bacteria catheter-related bloodstream infection with a pilot prospective study in patients with catheter removal receiving short-duration of antibiotic therapy. BMC Infect Dis. 2020;20(1):604.
14. Braun E, Hussein K, Geffen Y, Rabino G, Bar-Lavie Y, Paul M. Predominance of gram-negative bacilli among patients with catheter-related bloodstream infections. Clin Microbiol Infect. 2014;20(10):O627–9.
15. Weiner LM, Webb AK, Limbago B, et al. Antimicrobial-resistant pathogens associated with healthcare-associated infections: summary of data reported to the National Healthcare Safety Network at the Centers for Disease Control and Prevention, 2011–2014. Infect Control Hos Epidemiol. 2016;37(11):1288–301.
16. Rupp ME, Karnatak R. Intravascular catheter-related bloodstream infections. Infect Dis Clin N Am. 2018;32(4):765–87.
17. Safdar N, Fine JP, Maki DG. Meta-analysis: methods for diagnosing intravascular device-related bloodstream infection. Ann Intern Med. 2005;142(6):451–66.
18. Mermel LA, Allon M, Bouza E, et al. Clinical practice guidelines for the diagnosis and Management of Intravascular Catheter-Related Infection: 2009 update by the Infectious Diseases Society of America. Clin Infect Dis. 2009;49(1):1–45.
19. Guembe M, Rodríguez-Créixems M, Sánchez-Carrillo C, Pérez-Parra A, Martín-Rabadán P, Bouza E. How many lumens should be cultured in the conservative diagnosis of catheter-related bloodstream infections? Clin Infect Dis. 2010;50(12):1575–9.
20. Seifert H, Cornely O, Seggewiss K, et al. Bloodstream infection in neutropenic cancer patients related to short-term nontunnelled catheters determined by quantitative blood cultures, differential time to positivity, and molecular epidemiological typing with pulsed-field gel electrophoresis. J Clin Microbiol. 2003;41(1):118–23.

21. Bouzidi H, Emirian A, Marty A, et al. Differential time to positivity of central and peripheral blood cultures is inaccurate for the diagnosis of Staphylococcus aureus long-term catheter-related sepsis. J Hosp Infect. 2018;99(2):192–9.
22. Boucher HW, Sakoulas G. Perspectives on Daptomycin resistance, with emphasis on resistance in Staphylococcus aureus. Clin Infect Dis. 2007;45(5):601–8.
23. linezolidhcp_fdaletter.pdf.
24. Lentino JR, Narita M, Yu VL. New antimicrobial agents as therapy for resistant gram-positive cocci. Eur J Clin Microbiol Infect Dis. 2008;27(1):3–15.
25. Wilcox H, Mark TJ, Kenneth BE, et al. Complicated skin and skin-structure infections and catheter-related bloodstream infections: noninferiority of linezolid in a phase 3 study. Clin Infect Dis. 2009;48(2):203–12.
26. Chuang Y-C, Wang J-T, Lin H-Y, Chang S-C. Daptomycin versus linezolid for treatment of vancomycin-resistant enterococcal bacteremia: systematic review and meta-analysis. BMC Infect Dis. 2014;14(1)
27. Shorr AF, Kunkel MJ, Kollef M. Linezolid versus vancomycin for Staphylococcus aureus bacteraemia: pooled analysis of randomized studies. J Antimicrob Chemother. 2005;56(5):923–9.
28. Mancino P, Ucciferri C, Falasca K, Pizzigallo E, Vecchiet J. Methicillin-resistant Staphylococcus epidermidis (MRSE) endocarditis treated with linezolid. Scand J Infect Dis. 2008;40(1):67–73.
29. Safdar N, Handelsman J, Maki DG. Does combination antimicrobial therapy reduce mortality in gram-negative bacteraemia? A meta-analysis. Lancet Infect Dis. 2004;4(8):519–27.
30. Salama NN, Segal JH, Churchwell MD, et al. Intradialytic Administration of Daptomycin in end-stage renal disease patients on Hemodialysis. Clin J Am Soc Nephrol. 2009;4(7):1190–4.
31. Allon M. Treatment guidelines for dialysis catheter-related Bacteremia: an update. Am J Kidney Dis. 2009;54(1):13–7.
32. Marschall J, Mermel LA, Classen D, et al. Strategies to prevent central line-associated bloodstream infections in acute care hospitals. Infect Control Hos Epidemiol. 2008;29(S1):S22–30.
33. CLABSI_Toolkit_Tool_3-22_CVC_Maintenance_Bundlespdf.pdf.
34. CLABSI_Toolkit_Tool_3-23_Daily_Central_Line_Maintenance_Checklist_-_Templatepdf.pdf.
35. CLABSI_Toolkit_Tool_5-1_Examples_of_National_and_International_HAI_Surveillance_Systemspdf (1).pdf.

Sepsis in Cancer Patient

15

Dhruva Chaudhry, Lokesh Lalwani, and B. G. Manjunath

Sepsis is a well-known complication in immunocompromised cancer patients that relates to increased morbidity and mortality. In the era of antibiotic resistance, it has become a unique concern in these patients because any delay in administering effective empirical antibiotics will lead to poor outcomes. In this chapter, we address the most likely mechanism of sepsis and septic shock in these patients along with risk factors associated with poor prognosis. Impact of initial empirical antibiotic therapy and optimal management of sepsis with significance of control of the infection source is also stressed upon.

15.1 Introduction

Sepsis is a preventable life-threatening organ dysfunction caused by a dysregulated host response to infection. Septic shock is a subset of sepsis in which circulatory, cellular, and metabolic abnormalities are associated with a greater risk of mortality than with sepsis alone [1]. Sepsis and septic shock are significant problems affecting many people each year that put an extra cost on the health care system. The estimated cost to healthcare system is around 17 billion per year in the United States [2]. Indian data for the same are lacking. The number of sepsis patients has increased recently because of increasing age of the population and comorbidities like chronic organ failure, immunosuppressive diseases, and cancer.

D. Chaudhry (✉) · B. G. Manjunath
Department of Pulmonary & Critical Care Medicine, Pt. B.D.S PGIMS, Rohtak, Haryana, India

L. Lalwani
Department of Respiratory Medicine, Pt. B.D.S PGIMS, Rohtak, Haryana, India

V. Kumar et al. (eds.), *Onco-critical Care*,
https://doi.org/10.1007/978-981-16-9929-0_15

Cancer patients are at a ten-fold higher risk for sepsis than the general population, with slight variation according to the cancer subtype [3]. The prevalence of sepsis in cancer is around 16.4 cases per 1000 patients with cancer per year in the US population. Compared to the general population, cancer patients are more likely to be hospitalized (relative risk, 2.77; 95% confidence interval, 2.77–2.78) and also have severe sepsis (relative risk, 3.96; 95% confidence interval, 3.94–3.99). Overall, sepsis is present in 8.5% of total cancer-associated mortality at the cost of 3.4 billion dollars per year [4]. The overall mortality due to sepsis in cancer patients has decreased with time because of improved clinical management, general care, improved cancer therapies and changes in the intensive care unit admission policies for these patients. In recent years we have been facing the emergence of antibiotics resistance in the microorganisms, causing infection and sepsis in the general population as well as cancer and immunocompromised patients leading to poor outcomes.

Some of the microorganisms which are variant of concern are multidrug-resistant gram-negative bacteria (MDR-GNB). Several authors reported high rates of sepsis due to extended-spectrum β lactamase (ESBL)- producing Enterobacteria [5], MDR- pseudomonas aeruginosa (MDR-PA) [6], and carbapenem-resistant enterobacteria (CRE) [7]. Additional fungal and viral infection in cancer patients is also associated with poor outcomes. A well-known therapy with the β-lactamase inhibitors is effective and safe in treating some MDR infections [8]. Additionally, some of the advanced strategies can help to improve the prognosis of immunocompromised cancer patients, such as early identification of sepsis (scoring systems and biomarkers), extended infusion instead of bolus of β-lactamase antibiotics, improve source control, increase the quality of care, prompt diagnosis and aggressive ICU management.

15.2 Burden of Sepsis in Cancer Patients

Previously, Angus et al. reported that one out of 6 sepsis patients had underlying malignant pathology, and these patients had 30% extra mortality than other patients with sepsis [9]. Recently it has been found that ICU load is increased by 15–20% due to haematological and solid malignancies and mostly sepsis being a leading cause of ICU admission in these patients [10]. In recent decades sepsis-related mortality in cancer patients has decreased mainly due to improved sepsis diagnosis and management, cancer therapies, prompt and early ICU admission [11].

Currently, in-hospital death of cancer patients presenting with sepsis and septic shock is nearly 20 and 40%, respectively [12]. Sepsis-associated mortality depends not only on the early management of multiple organ failure but also on the number of days in ICU and other associated complications [13]. Higher rates of mortality were found in patients with pneumonia and bacteraemia than gastrointestinal and urinary tract infections. The long-term outcome of the cancer patients who survived after sepsis-related ICU admission depends upon the underlying disease and the degree of loss of functional status and continued organ dysfunction [14]. As mortality in the early sepsis patients has decreased, attention has been paid to late mortality after sepsis recovery. The exact cause of delayed mortality is unclear; some investigators presumed that advanced age, comorbidities, and continued organ injury are the leading causes of immune system dysfunction with persistent inflammation and catabolism [15].

15.3 Pathophysiology of Sepsis in Cancer Patients

Cytotoxic chemotherapy and cytotoxic radiation therapy cause destruction of hematopoietic precursor cells in the bone marrow, causing neutropenia that results in an elevation in the levels of IL6, IL8 and G-CSF. This therapy also leads to disruption of mucosal barriers, thus allowing entry of pathogens from these disrupted epithelial barriers. Because of neutropenia and overall pancytopenia, there is a deranged inflammatory response and no adaptive immune response against these pathogens, causing sepsis [16]. Sepsis and neutropenia result in elevated TLR2 and TLR4 and further the pathogenesis described in Fig. 15.1.

Sepsis-related immunosuppression- Sepsis is a complex process. It includes severe immunosuppression of innate and adaptative immune systems even after recovery from disease. It includes functionally active cells such as neutrophils, macrophages, monocytes, natural killer cells, dendritic cells, B and T lymphocytes. On the other side, sepsis induces complex immune dysfunction, including hyper inflammation (release of inflammatory cytokines, IL-1, TNF and IL-17), complement activation, mitochondrial dysfunction, molecular alterations and homeostatic dysfunction [17].

Cancer-related immunosuppression- Cancer-specific onco-haematological therapies are the most common cause of cancer-related immunosuppression, which lead to increased risk of infection and sepsis. Chemotherapy and radiotherapy used in the treatment of cancer decrease the phagocytic activity of monocytes and neutrophils by decreasing circulating counts and hindering the capacity of chemotaxis and phagocytosis [18]. The risk of infection and sepsis is directly associated with the duration and severity of neutropenia and monocytopenia [19]. Cytostatic chemotherapies mainly hamper the lymphocytes and NK cells, qualitatively and quantitatively. While other anti-lymphoproliferative drugs and monoclonal antibodies, e.g., fludarabine, rituximab, alemtuzumab, bendamustine, can cause B and/or T cell lymphopenia [20]. Corticosteroid use in cancer patients also increases the chances of immunosuppression. Similarly, treatment with HSCT delays the immune reconstitution because of low cell diversity, altered lymphocyte function and persistent lymphopenia. In addition to these facts, chemotherapy and radiotherapy may impair other organ and tissue functions, limiting their capacity to deal with initial aggression [21].

Some haematological malignancies or solid metastatic tumours may involve the bone marrow and lead to cytopenia with or without the altered phagocytic activity of neutrophils and monocytes.

The two-way interaction between cancer and sepsis: There are similarities between the pathophysiological pathway of cancer and sepsis. Some cancer-related

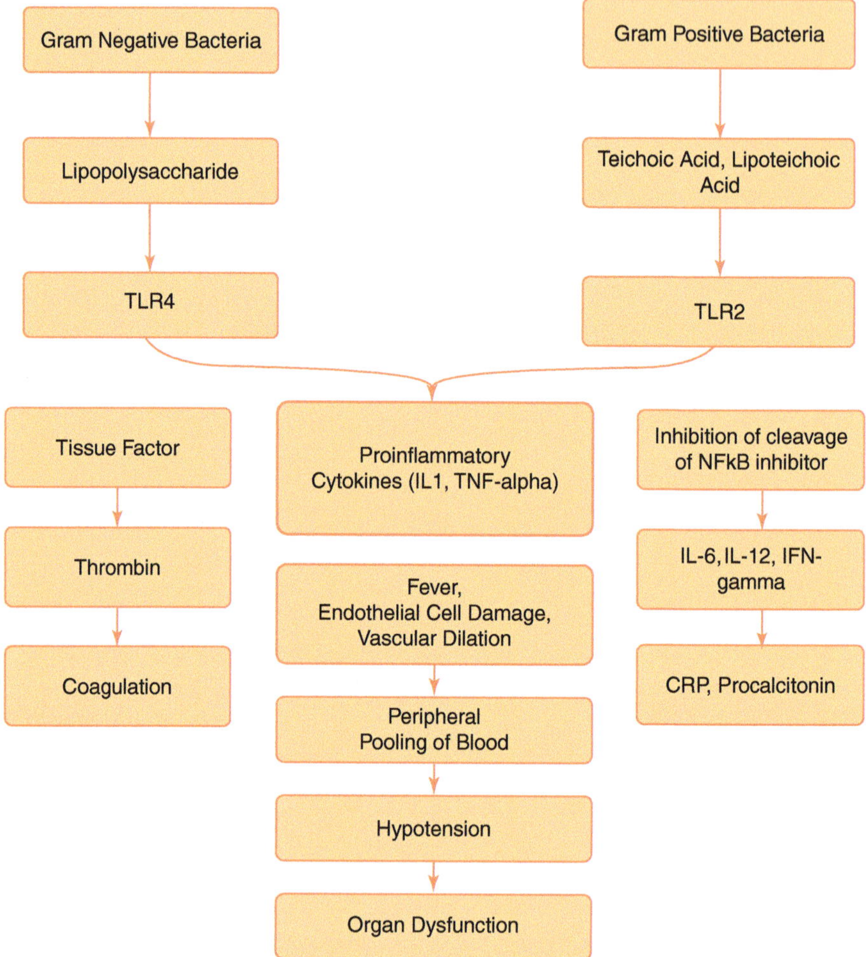

Fig. 15.1 Pathophysiology of sepsis in cancer patients. *TLR* Toll like receptor, *IL* Interleukin, *TNF* Tumor necrotic factor, *IFN* Interferon

conditions and a few unfavourable side effects of cancer drugs can present as sepsis and hinder the difference [22]. Remarkably, some haematological diseases like acute leukaemia or high-grade B-cell lymphoma may initially present as a multiple organ dysfunction using multiple pathways such as anatomical compression, direct infiltration of tissue by tumour cells, dysregulated coagulation and hemophagocytic lymphohistiocytosis [23]. Some anti-tumoral agents like monoclonal antibodies or all-trans-retinoic arsenic acid can stimulate acute systemic inflammatory syndrome that mimics sepsis [24]. The need of differentiating these entities is essential because the management of both entities is entirely different.

There are some similarities in immune dysfunction induced by cancer and sepsis. It has been observed that immune defects caused by the infectious agent can help grow tumour cells.

Many studies support that sepsis may increase the risk of cancer [25]. On the other hand, some studies have proven that sepsis has anti-tumoral activity [26], and even sepsis may induce tumour suppression [27].

15.4 Risk Factor of Sepsis in Cancer Patients

Increased prevalence of sepsis in cancer patients, although is primarily due to immunosuppression caused by cancer, is multifactorial. Specific onco-haematological treatment, including chemotherapy and/or radiotherapy, induces immunosuppression. Invasive procedures like urinary catheters, long term central venous catheters and indwelling drainages raise the risk of infection. However, there is significant variation in the severity of immunosuppression in the cancer patients. Those with acute leukaemia are at higher risk of infection and sepsis due to the presence of prolonged and profound neutropenia [4], one of the major risk factors for sepsis and mortality in the cancer patients.

Cancer patients with neutropenia, monocytopenia, indwelling catheters, defect in cellular and humoral immunity, defective phagocytic function, impaired lymphocytic function, mucositis are an ideal target for the development of fungal infections [28]. Apart from these, some opportunistic viral infections lead to morbidity and mortality mainly in bone marrow transplant patients and haematological malignancies [29].

Demographic and lifestyle risk factors are very similar to those of non-cancer patients who develop sepsis and include tobacco use, age more than 65 years, low-income level, poor dental hygiene and decreased level of exercise. Regional variation in the sepsis prevalence is also observed as a population from a defined geographical area has similar habits like tobacco use, patient income and comorbidities like diabetes or chronic obstructive pulmonary disease [30]. Patients with depression, anxiety or substance abuse have raised risk of developing sepsis.

In the patients of solid tumour, the most common underlying diseases which lead to sepsis are lung or gastrointestinal cancers, followed by other subtypes. In patients with solid cancers, the primary or metastatic cancer site primarily serves as the port of entry [4]. On the other hand, patients of multiple myeloma and hematopoietic stem cell transplant recipients (HSCT) are at a higher risk of sepsis than other haematological malignancies [12]. HSCT patients with graft vs host disease (GVHD) are more prone to sepsis and death than non-HSCT recipients and patients without GVHD, reaching mortality rates as high as 55% [31].

Febrile neutropenia (FN) is a well-known complication, cropping up in 20–30% of solid tumour patients and 80% of haematological malignancies patients who receive chemotherapy, but only 20–30% of these will develop bacteraemia. In a recent Brazilian study, it has been found that shock occurred in 3.2% of patients on the first day of FN, and early death occurred in 1.1% [32]. The leading cause for septic shock was bacterial infection due to Escherichia coli, Enterobacter species and Acinetobacter species.

Apart from this, one more critical risk factor associated with sepsis and septic shock in the patients who received radiotherapy and systemic chemotherapy is intestinal mucositis leading to disruption of the intestinal mucosal lining. Matrix metalloproteinase and release of pro-inflammatory cytokines trigger cellular and tissue death, resulting in ulceration in the intestinal mucosa and allow gut bacteria to enter from the intestinal tract causing bacteraemia and sepsis [33].

15.5 Etiology of Sepsis in Cancer Patients

The site for entry of organism is hardly described in the few series of sepsis in cancer. Infectious etiology associated with sepsis is described in Table 15.1. Rosolem et al. described the port of entry in 563 admitted cases of sepsis in ICU and found that most frequently sites are lung (44%) followed by abdomen (31%) and urinary tract (8%). 4% of patients had more than one site of entry for infectious agents [34]. Primary bloodstream infection has also been found to be common [35]. Mostly

Table 15.1 Infectious etiology of sepsis in cancer patients

Infectious Etiology of sepsis in cancer patients:
Skin
• Cellulitis • Burn • wound
CNS
• Meningitis
Chest
• Pneumonia • Indwelling catheter
Abdomen
• Pancreatitis • Intra-abdominal abscess
Genitourinary
• Urinary tract infection • Endometritis • Chorioamnitis • Indwelling catheter

gram-negative bacilli were responsible for sepsis, with E. coli (16%), P. aeruginosa (13%) and Klebsiella pneumonia (13%) being the commonest. Apart from bacteria, some fungal infections, viruses and protozoan are also associated with a severe infection in cancer patients [36]. Common organisms involved in causing sepsis in cancer patients are described in Table 15.2.

Table 15.2 Common pathological organisms causing sepsis in cancer patients

Gram negative bacteria
Escherichia coli
Klebsiella spp.
Enterobacteria
Pseudomonas aeruginosa
Acinetobacter
Proteus
Bacteroides fragilis
Gram positive bacteria
Staphylococcus aureus
Streptococcus
Enterococcus
Fungi
Candida
Histoplasma
Aspergillus
Fusarium
Scedosporium
Cryptococcus
Coccidiodomycosis
Virus
Varicella zoster virus
Herpes simplex virus
Cytomegalovirus
Respiratory syncytial virus
Adenovirus
Influenza virus
H1N1
West nile virus
Bocavirus
Norovirus
Protozoa
Entamoeba
Giardia
Cryptosporidium

15.6 Diagnosis of Sepsis in Cancer Patients

Although challenging, it is essential to diagnose early and provide prompt treatment to the patient when sepsis is suspected. Complete clinical history with thorough clinical examination is essential for diagnosis. Symptoms of sepsis are wide-ranging and can vary in a different population of patients. They include but are not limited to fever, decreased intake, altered mental status, chest pain, cough, dyspnea, dysuria, vomiting, pain abdomen or diarrhoea. Most of the patients with sepsis can have tachycardia, tachypnea, alterations in body temperature, altered blood pressure, cellulitis, infected catheters, changes in mental status, mottled skin or petechiae. Indications of decreased tissue perfusion include, but are not limited to, oliguria, altered mentation, delayed capillary refill, cool or clammy skin and extremities.

Clinical symptoms have minimal specificity, and initial bloodstream cultures mostly came out negative. Despite this, cultures from all the suspected sites before initiating empiric antimicrobial treatment are the mainstay of the diagnosis. Medical imaging like radiography, ultrasonography, computed tomography and radioisotope labelled imaging, including FDG-PET, can diagnose and monitor antimicrobial treatment response.

There should be a lookout on each patient elaborated medical history, sepsis risk factors and signs of sepsis after every cycle of radiotherapy or systemic chemotherapy and any other immunosuppressive therapy. The clinician should undertake a thorough general physical examination with systemic review including respiratory, gastrointestinal tract, neurological and cardiovascular system for a sign of infection. Any suspicion should be immediately evaluated for sepsis and provided early supportive care. In high-risk subjects, monitoring of sepsis and systemic inflammation should be framed at least weekly. Monitoring these patients should include clinical examination as blood pressure, heart rate, respiratory rate and blood oxygen level, and lab count of white blood cells.

It is not necessary that all patients with sepsis present with fever, although fever is the only sign of neutropenic sepsis. Cut off value to evaluate fever in neutropenic patients is if the patient has an oral temperature of 101° F or having a temperature of 100.4°F for at least 1 h or more. Patients who have sepsis without fever or hypothermia have a higher mortality rate than those with a fever. Patients without fever should be evaluated for the other signs of sepsis-like altered cognitive status, heart arrhythmias or change in urine output.

The quick sequential sepsis-related organ failure assessment (qSOFA) can be used if sepsis is suspected. It includes a Glasgow coma scale of less than 13 or altered mental status, systolic blood pressure less than 100 mm Hg or less, respiratory rate is of more than 22 breaths per minute. If the score of qSOFA is two or more, then the patient ought to be evaluated with detailed SOFA score. It has been observed that the SOFA and qSOFA scores are instrumental in the identification and prediction of severity, complications and mortality of sepsis. Therefore, these clinical scores should be applied to all cancer patients suspected of sepsis.

Lactate, procalcitonin and C-reactive protein levels should be tested. CRP levels of more than 17 mg/dL may be suggestive of sepsis. Levels of other laboratory parameters include lactate level more than 4 mmol/L, leukopenia (WBC <4000/mm^3), leucocytosis (WBC >11,000/mm^3), low platelet counts (<100,000/mm^3), bilirubin (>4 mg/dL) and increase in creatinine (>0.5 mg/dL). The role of recently available biomarkers in the diagnosis of sepsis in cancer patients needs to be further elucidated.

15.7 Management of Sepsis in Cancer Patients

The "Surviving Sepsis Campaign" published by Lat I et al. in 2021 [37], an international guideline, describes sepsis and septic shock management.

In the current age of antimicrobial resistance, a physician should evaluate some general considerations before starting empirical treatment for the sepsis-like presence of any risk factor for antibiotic resistance, previous history of infection with resistant pathogens, local epidemiological and resistance pattern of the bacteria according to the geographical area, hospital and ward and another patient dependent factor which can complicate the course of treatment, i.e. advanced age, systemic comorbidities, local infection or shock.

Urgent therapy with broad-spectrum anti-pseudomonal antibiotics with or without another agent effective for both suspected microorganism and site of infection is recommended [38]. Figure 15.2 is the flowchart summarizing the management of sepsis in cancer patients.

The issue of benefit after adding short course aminoglycosides and the broad-spectrum antibiotic in severely ill patients remains unsettled. A meta-analysis and prospective observational cohort study of 648 ICU patients failed to establish this association. The study by Ong et al., which was mainly done on the immunocompetent patients, was unable to prove speedy reversal of shock or increase 14 days survival by use of gentamycin along with broad-spectrum antimicrobial agents in sepsis. Surprisingly some previous studies have shown the beneficial role in improving 7 and 14 days mortality in the patients who received combination antibiotic therapy including aminoglycosides [39, 40]. In a prospective trial in 510 hospitalized patients with bacteraemia in connection with neutropenia due to haematological malignancies, there was improved 30 days survival in the patients who received combination therapy [41]. Other studies also demonstrated similar findings [42, 43]. Short course of aminoglycoside and a broad-spectrum antimicrobial may help those with neutropenia in the setting of higher prevalence multidrug resistance.

The empirical use of antifungal medications in patients at higher risk of infection despite providing broad-spectrum antibiotics has reduced invasive fungal infection and morbidity and mortality associated with them. Amphotericin-B, Azoles (Voriconazole, Posaconazole) and Echinocandins (Caspofungin, Micafungin, Anidulafungin) are recommended in fungal infections in cancer patients. The antifungal therapy should be continued during the period of neutropenia and until the manifestation of invasive aspergillosis have been entirely resolved or are reduced to residual scarring. Although with limited data, it has been proven that the response of liposomal amphotericin B is decreased by more than 20% in neutropenic patients

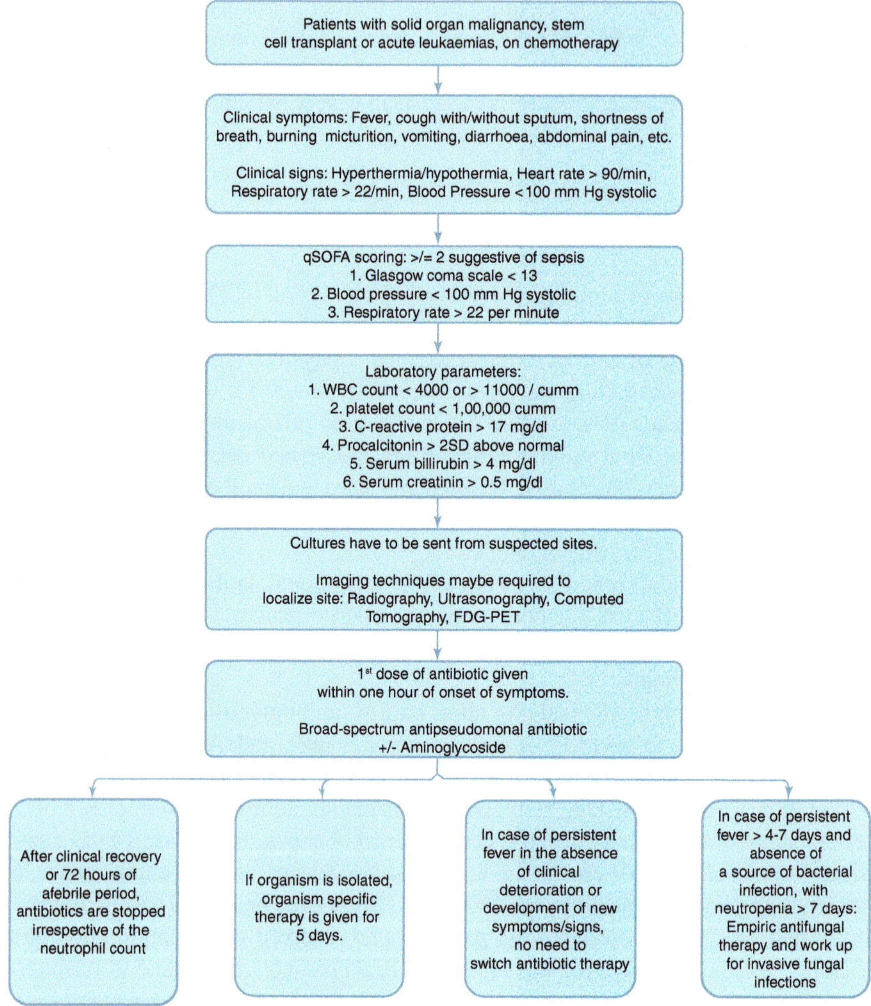

Fig. 15.2 Clinical evaluation and management of sepsis in cancer patients

with invasive aspergillosis, compared to voriconazole, where response rates were similar in patients with or without neutropenia [44].

An alternative strategy for treating resistant bacteria is to give an extended or continuous infusion of beta-lactamase antibiotics to increase their pharmacokinetics activity [45]. Severe and critically ill patients have specific changes in their pathophysiology, mainly as increased renal clearance and increased volume of distribution, making them a magnificent target for this strategy. Two meta-analyses have supported that prolonged antibiotic infusion can decrease mortality in critically ill patients [46, 47]. The pharmacokinetics of cancer patients with febrile neutropenia is considered like critically ill patients. Superior outcome of extended infusion in the patients with pneumonia have been observed.

With antimicrobial resistance increasing exponentially, antimicrobial stewardship has had extreme significance in decreasing the use of antibiotics and decreasing the spread of antimicrobial resistance. De-escalation or discontinuation of antibiotics in the initial few days after clinical improvement and resolution of infection and/or if there is a paucity of evidence to continue should be the strategy. In a recent randomized clinical trial, it has been noticed to be safe to stop empirical antibiotic therapy in neutropenic haematological patients after clinical recovery or 72 h of being afebrile disregarding of neutrophil count [48].

The other recommended strategies to decrease the course of sepsis are management of stress ulcers, infection-induced diabetes, adequate fluid management, appropriate choice of vasopressor agents in parallel with antimicrobial treatment [49].

The need for ICU management in cancer patients has increased profoundly over the past years though overall mortality has decreased. Some salient changes in the comprehensive management of cancer patients in critical illness can be the crucial factor of this improved outcome. These factors include less threshold for admission in ICU and early treatment of organ dysfunction. Similarly, so-called predictors of mortality in cancer (neutropenia, second-line therapy, need of blood transfusion) are no more extended hurdles in the therapeutic approach. The improved alliance between oncologists and critical illness providers, using specific therapy for ICU setting, upgraded management of sepsis in neutropenic patients including source control, specific antimicrobial use with improved strategies are associated with a significant survival benefit.

15.8 Conclusion

Advanced stage of cancer, treatment of cancer, neutropenia in these patients and many more factors lead to increased incidence of sepsis and associated mortality. Hence early detection and management of cancer, trying immunotherapies to avoid/reduce chemotherapy/radiotherapy whenever feasible and appropriate general care of these patients will help in reducing the incidence of sepsis in these patients. In spite of these sepsis and septic shock will continue to haunt cancer patients, and early detection and treatment will go long way in improving their survival chances.

References

1. Hotchkiss RS, Moldawer LL, Opal SM, Reinhart K, Turnbull IR, Vincent JL. Sepsis and septic shock. Nat Rev Dis Primers. 2016;2:16045.
2. Coopersmith CM, Wunsch H, Fink MP, Linde-Zwirble WT, Olsen KM, Sommers MS, et al. A comparison of critical care research funding and the financial burden of critical illness in the United States. Crit Care Med. 2012;40(4):1072–9.
3. Danai PA, Moss M, Mannino DM, Martin GS. The epidemiology of sepsis in patients with malignancy. Chest. 2006;129(6):1432–40.

4. Williams MD, Braun LA, Cooper LM, Johnston J, Weiss RV, Qualy RL, et al. Hospitalized cancer patients with severe sepsis: analysis of incidence, mortality, and associated costs of care. Crit Care. 2004;8(5):R291–8.
5. Liang T, Xu C, Cheng Q, Tang Y, Zeng H, Li X. Epidemiology, risk factors, and clinical outcomes of bloodstream infection due to extended-Spectrum Beta-lactamase-producing Escherichia coli and Klebsiella pneumoniae in hematologic malignancy: a retrospective study from central South China. Microb Drug Resist. 2021;27(6):800–8.
6. Trecarichi EM, Pagano L, Candoni A, Pastore D, Cattaneo C, Fanci R, et al. Current epidemiology and antimicrobial resistance data for bacterial bloodstream infections in patients with hematologic malignancies: an Italian multicentre prospective survey. Clin Microbiol Infect. 2015;21(4):337–43.
7. Satlin MJ, Cohen N, Ma KC, Gedrimaite Z, Soave R, Askin G, et al. Bacteremia due to carbapenem-resistant Enterobacteriaceae in neutropenic patients with hematologic malignancies. J Infect. 2016;73(4):336–45.
8. Bassetti M, Giacobbe DR, Robba C, Pelosi P, Vena A. Treatment of extended-spectrum β-lactamases infections: what is the current role of new β-lactams/β-lactamase inhibitors? Curr Opin Infect Dis. 2020;33(6):474–81.
9. Angus DC, Linde-Zwirble WT, Lidicker J, Clermont G, Carcillo J, Pinsky MR. Epidemiology of severe sepsis in the United States: analysis of incidence, outcome, and associated costs of care. Crit Care Med. 2001;29(7):1303–10.
10. Soares M, Bozza FA, Azevedo LC, Silva UV, Corrêa TD, Colombari F, et al. Effects of organizational characteristics on outcomes and resource use in patients with cancer admitted to intensive care units. J Clin Oncol. 2016;34(27):3315–24.
11. Pène F, Percheron S, Lemiale V, Viallon V, Claessens YE, Marqué S, et al. Temporal changes in management and outcome of septic shock in patients with malignancies in the intensive care unit. Crit Care Med. 2008;36(3):690–6.
12. Lemiale V, Pons S, Mirouse A, Tudesq JJ, Hourmant Y, Mokart D, et al. Sepsis and septic shock in patients with malignancies: a Groupe de Recherche Respiratoire en Réanimation Onco-Hématologique study. Crit Care Med. 2020;48(6):822–9.
13. Jamme M, Daviaud F, Charpentier J, Marin N, Thy M, Hourmant Y, et al. Time course of septic shock in immunocompromised and nonimmunocompromised patients. Crit Care Med. 2017;45(12):2031–9.
14. Lee DS, Suh GY, Ryu JA, Chung CR, Yang JH, Park CM, et al. Effect of early intervention on long-term outcomes of critically ill cancer patients admitted to ICUs. Crit Care Med. 2015;43(7):1439–48.
15. Boomer JS, To K, Chang KC, Takasu O, Osborne DF, Walton AH, et al. Immunosuppression in patients who die of sepsis and multiple organ failure. JAMA. 2011;306(23):2594–605.
16. Kochanek M, Schalk E, von Bergwelt-Baildon M, Beutel G, Buchheidt D, Hentrich M, et al. Management of sepsis in neutropenic cancer patients: 2018 guidelines from the infectious diseases working party (AGIHO) and intensive care working party (iCHOP) of the German Society of Hematology and Medical Oncology (DGHO). Ann Hematol. 2019;98(5):1051–69.
17. Delano MJ, Ward PA. The immune system's role in sepsis progression, resolution, and long-term outcome. Immunol Rev. 2016;274(1):330–53.
18. Mendonça MA, Cunha FQ, Murta EF, Tavares-Murta BM. Failure of neutrophil chemotactic function in breast cancer patients treated with chemotherapy. Cancer Chemother Pharmacol. 2006;57(5):663–70.
19. Schimpff S, Satterlee W, Young VM, Serpick A. Empiric therapy with carbenicillin and gentamicin for febrile patients with cancer and granulocytopenia. N Engl J Med. 1971;284(19):1061–5.
20. García Muñoz R, Izquierdo-Gil A, Muñoz A, Roldan-Galiacho V, Rabasa P, Panizo C. Lymphocyte recovery is impaired in patients with chronic lymphocytic leukemia and indolent non-Hodgkin lymphomas treated with bendamustine plus rituximab. Ann Hematol. 2014;93(11):1879–87.

21. Karvunidis T, Chvojka J, Lysak D, Sykora R, Krouzecky A, Radej J, et al. Septic shock and chemotherapy-induced cytopenia: effects on microcirculation. Intensive Care Med. 2012;38(8):1336–44.
22. Contou D, Roux D, Jochmans S, Coudroy R, Guérot E, Grimaldi D, et al. Septic shock with no diagnosis at 24 hours: a pragmatic multicenter prospective cohort study. Crit Care. 2016;20(1):360.
23. Moreau AS, Longline E, Seguin A, Lemiale V, Canet E, Raffoux E, et al. Respiratory events at the earliest phase of acute myeloid leukemia. Leuk Lymphoma. 2014;55(11):2556–63.
24. Brudno JN, Kochenderfer JN. Toxicities of chimeric antigen receptor T cells: recognition and management. Blood. 2016;127(26):3321–30.
25. Liu Z, Mahale P, Engels EA. Sepsis and risk of cancer among elderly adults in the United States. Clin Infect Dis. 2019;68(5):717–24.
26. Maywald O, Buchheidt D, Bergmann J, Schoch C, Ludwig WD, Reiter A, et al. Spontaneous remission in adult acute myeloid leukemia in association with systemic bacterial infection-case report and review of the literature. Ann Hematol. 2004;83(3):189–94.
27. Buzás K, Marton A, Vizier C, Gyukity-Sebestyén E, Harmati M, Nagy K, et al. Bacterial sepsis increases survival in metastatic melanoma: Chlamydophila pneumoniae induces macrophage polarization and tumor regression. J Invest Dermatol. 2016;136(4):862–5.
28. Walsh TJ, Lee JW. Prevention of invasive fungal infections in patients with neoplastic disease. Clin Infect Dis. 1993;17(Suppl 2):S468–80.
29. Holland HK, Wingard JR, Saral R. Herpesvirus and enteric viral infections in bone marrow transplantation: clinical presentations, pathogenesis, and therapeutic strategies. Cancer Investig. 1990;8(5):509–21.
30. Tavakoli A, Carannante A. Nursing Care of Oncology Patients with sepsis. Semin Oncol Nurs. 2021;37(2):151130.
31. Kumar G, Ahmad S, Taneja A, Patel J, Guddati AK, Nanchal R. Severe sepsis in hematopoietic stem cell transplant recipients*. Crit Care Med. 2015;43(2):411–21.
32. Guarana M, Nucci M, Nouér SA. Shock and early death in hematologic patients with febrile neutropenia. Antimicrob Agents Chemother. 2019;63(11)
33. Gustinetti G, Mikulska M. Bloodstream infections in neutropenic cancer patients: a practical update. Virulence. 2016;7(3):280–97.
34. Rosolem MM, Rabello LS, Lisboa T, Caruso P, Costa RT, Leal JV, et al. Critically ill patients with cancer and sepsis: clinical course and prognostic factors. J Crit Care. 2012;27(3):301–7.
35. Torres VB, Azevedo LC, Silva UV, Caruso P, Torelli AP, Silva E, et al. Sepsis-associated outcomes in critically ill patients with malignancies. Ann Am Thorac Soc. 2015;12(8):1185–92.
36. Islas-Muñoz B, Volkow-Fernández P, Ibanes-Gutiérrez C, Villamar-Ramírez A, Vilar-Compte D, Cornejo-Juárez P. Bloodstream infections in cancer patients. Risk factors associated with mortality. Int J Infect Dis. 2018;71:59–64.
37. Lat I, Coopersmith CM, De Backer D. The surviving sepsis campaign: fluid resuscitation and vasopressor therapy research priorities in adult patients. Crit Care Med. 2021;49(4):623–35.
38. Diana A, Christina O, Catherine C, David ML, Małgorzata M, Claudio V, et al. European guidelines for empirical antibacterial therapy for febrile neutropenic patients in the era of growing resistance: summary of the 2011 4th European conference on infections in Leukemia. Haematologica. 2013;98(12):1826–35.
39. Paul M, Lador A, Grozinsky-Glasberg S, Leibovici L. Beta lactam antibiotic monotherapy versus beta lactam-aminoglycoside antibiotic combination therapy for sepsis. Cochrane Database Syst Rev 2014;2014(1):Cd003344.
40. Ong DSY, Frencken JF, Klein Klouwenberg PMC, Juffermans N, van der Poll T, Bonten MJM, et al. Short-course adjunctive gentamicin as empirical therapy in patients with severe sepsis and septic shock: a prospective observational cohort study. Clin Infect Dis. 2017;64(12):1731–6.
41. Marín M, Gudiol C, Ardanuy C, Garcia-Vidal C, Jimenez L, Domingo-Domenech E, et al. Factors influencing mortality in neutropenic patients with hematologic malignancies or solid tumours with bloodstream infection. Clin Microbiol Infect. 2015;21(6):583–90.

42. Martínez JA, Cobos-Trigueros N, Soriano A, Almela M, Ortega M, Marco F, et al. Influence of empiric therapy with a beta-lactam alone or combined with an aminoglycoside on prognosis of bacteremia due to gram-negative microorganisms. Antimicrob Agents Chemother. 2010;54(9):3590–6.
43. Jacobs FM. Early combination antibiotic therapy yields improved survival compared with monotherapy in septic shock: a propensity-matched analysis. Crit Care Med. 2011;39(3):608. author reply 9
44. Herbrecht R, Denning DW, Patterson TF, Bennett JE, Greene RE, Oestmann JW, et al. Voriconazole versus amphotericin B for primary therapy of invasive aspergillosis. N Engl J Med. 2002;347(6):408–15.
45. Roberts JA, Webb S, Paterson D, Ho KM, Lipman J. A systematic review on clinical benefits of continuous administration of beta-lactam antibiotics. Crit Care Med. 2009;37(6):2071–8.
46. Roberts JA, Abdul-Aziz MH, Davis JS, Dulhunty JM, Cotta MO, Myburgh J, et al. Continuous versus intermittent β-lactam infusion in severe sepsis. A meta-analysis of individual patient data from randomized trials. Am J Respir Crit Care Med. 2016;194(6):681–91.
47. Vardakas KZ, Voulgaris GL, Maliaros A, Samonis G, Falagas ME. Prolonged versus short-term intravenous infusion of antipseudomonal β-lactams for patients with sepsis: a systematic review and meta-analysis of randomized trials. Lancet Infect Dis. 2018;18(1):108–20.
48. Aguilar-Guisado M, Espigado I, Martín-Peña A, Gudiol C, Royo-Cebrecos C, Falantes J, et al. Optimization of empirical antimicrobial therapy in patients with haematological malignancies and febrile neutropenia (how long study): an open-label, randomized, controlled phase 4 trial. Lancet Haematol. 2017;4(12):e573–e83.
49. Rhodes A, Evans LE, Alhazzani W, Levy MM, Antonelli M, Ferrer R, et al. Surviving sepsis campaign: international guidelines for Management of Sepsis and Septic Shock: 2016. Intensive Care Med. 2017;43(3):304–77.

Antibiotic Stewardship in Onco-Critical Patient

16

Ravi Jain, Monika Rajani, and Yash Javeri

16.1 Introduction

Antimicrobials are among one of the most crucial advances in the field of healthcare. These drugs are the mainstay of therapy in the management of infections and prompt initiation provides survival advantages in patients with sepsis and septic shock [1, 2]. Hence early and appropriate use has been promoted vigorously in recent times as a standard of care in sepsis management [2]. However many studies report that majority of hospitalized patients were exposed to broad-spectrum antimicrobials and this exposure is often unnecessary, suboptimal, and inadequate [3, 4]. these observations have also pointed out a significant scope of improvement in antimicrobial prescriptions and an urgent need for antimicrobial stewardship.

It is largely noticed that special patient populations (E.g. Cancer patients, immunocompromised patients, anti-cancer therapy patients) were excluded from antimicrobial stewardship program (ASP) research. On the contrary, this special population should have been the most important groups for ASP. The last updated guidelines make ASP mandatory across the spectrum of health care. However, no specific recommendations were made for this subset of patients [4].

R. Jain
Department of Critical Care Medicine, Mahatma Gandhi Medical College & Hospital, Mahatma Gandhi University of Medical Sciences and Technology, Jaipur, India

M. Rajani (✉)
Career Institue of Medical Sciences and Hospital, Lucknow, India

Y. Javeri
Convener-Indian Sepsis Forum, Head, Critical Care, Anaesthesia, and Emergency Medicine, Regency Super Specialty Hospital, Lucknow, India

V. Kumar et al. (eds.), *Onco-critical Care*,
https://doi.org/10.1007/978-981-16-9929-0_16

Although basic stewardship tenets (pre-authorization, prospective audit and feedback) are applicable, there are novel aspects in caring for oncology patients. In the present chapter, we make an attempt to evaluate that aspect of care of cancer patients.

16.2 Evolution of the Concept of Antimicrobial Stewardship

As with any other medication, antimicrobials also have serious adverse reactions, and the development of antimicrobial resistance(AMR) is one such emerging and disturbing public health issue [5, 6]. This concern was first raised by Sir Alexander Flemming when he pointed out that 'inappropriate use of Penicillin may lead to adaptation of bacteria against it'. [7] This was a reality soon after the discovery of penicillin when the first methicillin-resistant *Staphylococcus Aureus* (MRSA) isolate was discovered and reported in 1964 [8, 9]. During the following decades, several reports of antimicrobial discoveries and emerging infectious microbes were published in the medical literature. The first time in a futuristic article in the year 1996 it was finally identified that there is a causal relation between antimicrobial use and developing resistance and a robust large-scale method is urgently needed to address this problem [10]. "Stewardship" term was also coined in this context for the first time. This fight with microbes was a global crisis and the discovery of antimicrobials was not able to keep pace with new and emerging resistance [11, 12]. Resistant infection in patients causes a high risk of mortality and at least two times higher cost implications in comparison to susceptible isolates infections [13]. In fact, inappropriate use of antimicrobials can have an adverse effect on the health of patients who were not even exposed to antimicrobials, because of the emergence of resistant infections at the community and institutional level and pose a significant threat to lives [4, 5]. Citing these emerging concerns the Society for Healthcare Epidemiology of America (SHEA) and Infectious Diseases Society of America (IDSA) released guidelines for the prevention of antimicrobial resistance in hospitals [14]. Ten years later SHEA and IDSA formally adopted the "Antimicrobial Stewardship" term and released guidelines to develop Antimicrobial Stewardship programs (ASP) [15].

ASP formally described by IDSA, SHEA, and Pediatric infectious disease society (PIDS) as "Coordinated interventions designed to improve and measure the appropriate use of antimicrobial agents by promoting the selection of the optimal antimicrobial drug regimen including dosing, duration of therapy, and route of administration." [16] These societies strongly recommend the need for ASP at the institutional level and even advocate the need for a legislature for implementing ASP effectively. Last updated guidelines issued jointly by these societies for implementation of ASPs [4]. Similarly, ASP is strongly recommended in Joint Commission International (JCI) publication [17]. This document mandates ASP across all spectrum of healthcare, including cancer and transplant patients.

16.3 Focus of Antimicrobial Stewardship in Oncology Patients

ASP interventions are challenging in immunocompromised, complex oncology context, because of difficulty in accurate diagnosis and higher than usual rates of invasive infections [18]. And for the same obvious reasons, patients with cancer have higher frequency of infection, and antibiotics exposure than the general population. This leads to unusually high antimicrobial pressure on the patient's own normal microbial flora and surrounding environment. In past several years this immense antimicrobial pressure have grown up and led to emergence of resistant MDR microbes and high prevalence of CDI [19–22]. Antimicrobial resistance warrants empirical higher antimicrobials which further increases selection pressure. This vicious cycle is ultimately responsible for higher length of stay in Intensive care units and poor outcomes [23].

There are several opportunities to reduce unnecessary antimicrobial use and hence universal goals of providing timely, efficacious and safe antimicrobials to treat infection and limiting ecological impact of antimicrobials is applicable to oncology patient's population also [4, 23].

One interventional study demonstrated that antibiotics use, emergence of MDR organisms and *clostridium difficile* infections (CDI) emergence was reduced in cancer patients by adapting to ASP interventions with significant harm, and this ultimately can boost patient's health, and reduce medical cost and long term defects [24].

16.4 Summary of Core Elements of Antimicrobial Stewardship

CDC and IDSA have prescribed core elements that should be incorporated in institutional ASPs, a summary of these elements is provided in (Tables 16.1 and 16.2) [4, 25].

Apart from usual stewardship elements and interventions we could identify some specific elements related to stewardship in oncology patients. We shall elaborate on unique factors and interventions in practice of ASP for oncology patients.

16.5 Leadership Commitments

CDC guidelines for ASP suggest a crucial leadership commitment for implementation of the program. Extending the benefits of ASP to oncology patients is urgently needed [18]. The concept of ASP has been woven around the key role of Infectious disease expert and pharmacist; however integration of intensive care in leadership is vital in critical oncology patients for success of ASP.

Table 16.1 Core elements of antibiotic stewardship [4, 25]

Core element	Summary
Leadership commitment	To establish ASP, ensure close collaboration and adequate resource allocation for ASP, formulate strategy, and ensure feedback regulation
Accountability	ASP leader and co-leaders responsibilities to ensure activities and functioning
Pharmacy expertise	ASP trained physician and/or pharmacist to monitor the whole program
Action implementation	Interventions to promote appropriate antibiotics use (Table 2)
Tracking	Regular interval audits of interventions and outcome measures **Antibiotics use** measures: Maintaining and auditing pharmacy record systems data with benchmarks Outcome measures: CDI rates, antibiotics resistance patterns Process/quality measures: Compliance measures, preauthorization audits, adherence to local treatment guides
Reporting	Provide key stewardship updates and antibiograms to physicians, pharmacists, nurses, other key stakeholders and administrations
Education	One of the key components but not effective as an independent measure for stewardship Implement robust infection control and preventive strategy

Table 16.2 Action implementation

Elements	Summary
Priority interventions:	• **Pre-authorization**, • **Prospective audit and feedback** to limit the use, duration of restricted antibiotics, promote a prompt de-escalation • **Facility specific treatment guidelines**
Clinical pathways:	Mandatory selection of case definition and logical selection of antimicrobial, based on microbiology lab provided local antibiograms guidance
Provider-based interventions	• Antibiotics time outs • Assessing drug allergy
Pharmacy-based interventions	• Documentation of indications for antibiotics • Automatic changes from intravenous to oral antibiotic therapy • Dose adjustments: When needed, such as in cases of organ dysfunction, especially renal, or based on therapeutic drug monitoring • Dose optimization • Duplicative therapy alerts • Time-sensitive automatic stop orders • Detection and prevention of antibiotic-related drug-drug interactions
Microbiology based interventions	• Selective reporting of antimicrobial susceptibility testing results • Comments in microbiology reports • Rapid diagnostics and testing for galactomannan and 1–3-beta-D-glucan for rapid bacterial and fungal diagnosis aids
Nursing based interventions	• Optimizing microbiology cultures: a proper technique to reduce culture contaminations • Intravenous to oral transitions • Prompting antibiotic reviews ("timeouts")

16.6 Clinical Guidelines

ASP stakeholders and oncology clinicians should jointly develop clinical case definition based guidelines for a judicious approach towards an oncologic patient. Treatment pathways for febrile neutropenia, antifungal prophylaxis in neutropenia, cytomegalovirus treatment and prophylaxis guidance are few important clinical pathways.

Till date, data to support the above notion is not available and not studied in trials, but some studies suggest that implementing such integrative antifungal stewardship programs for selection of appropriate therapy in accordance with existing guidelines, improved efficacy, impact, and reduce toxicity and cost [26–28]. One study showed significant cost saving when an internal protocol to switch from Echinocandin to Fluconazole was followed in 70.3% patients based on clinical and susceptibility criteria [29]. Complete adherence to guideline is rarely possible, but even partial adherence can give improve outcomes [30, 31]. A closed integrated group approach (between various specialties E.g. infectious disease, Intensive care leadership, clinical microbiology, oncology, stem cell transplant teams and pharmacy) based guidance should be adopted for such a diverse group of patients who may have many mechanisms of immune paresis.

16.7 Antimicrobial Restriction

Antimicrobial restriction [pre authorization, prospective audit and feedback (PAF)] is one of the key components in ASP, and hence strongly recommended in IDSA guidelines [4]. Limited research data is available in this context as oncology patients are generally considered to be at high risk of resistant infections.

In a study ASP recommendations were able to reduce antimicrobial prescription (coefficient: −3.221; $P = 0.039$) during the intervention period, however consumption for same increased (pre-intervention: 84.58 defined daily doses [DDDs]/100 patient-days [PDs]; intervention: 102.52 DDDs/100 PDs) authors concluded that PAF implementation was based on culture reports and occurred at 72 h only [32]. Another study revealed decreased antimicrobial use (278 vs. 247 DDDs per 100 PDs; $P < 0.01$). They didn't noticed any differences in length of stay (LOS), in hospital mortality, or CDI rates [33]. One study using multimodal approach with antibiotics restriction at 48 h for febrile neutropenia, found that vancomycin discontinuation was increased from 31% (31/100) pre-intervention to 70% (70/100) post-intervention ($P < 0.0001$) [34]. One study focusing on carbapenem restriction based on extensive education, consultation and computerized clinical decision support found decreased carbapenem use post interventions (78.43 vs. 67.43 days of therapy [DOTs]; $P = 0.018$) demonstrating no differences in all-cause mortality (6.54 and 6.57 deaths per 1000 PDs; $P = 0.926$). However, reduction in resistance pattern was not observed during the study period [35].

Paucity of data, for the role of preauthorization in oncology patients has probably resulted from a likely increased risk of delaying antibiotics and high risk of resistant infection in this subset of patients. Similarly data for PAF was also not evaluated in large studies, hence not rendered reliable and should be adopted with due cautions as more research in the subject matter is needed. However antimicrobial restriction post administration can be adopted and considered for future research [36].

16.8 Antimicrobial Cycling

This strategy involves deliberate change of antimicrobial strategy to other effective regimens and form a part of formulary management in ASP. However IDSA and SHEA guidelines couldn't recommend it as an effective measure of Antimicrobial Stewardship due to conflicting data. A few studies demonstrated no change in mortality and resistance patterns, however raised concerns regarding gram positive resistance [37, 38]. Another study demonstrated that cycling preserved antibiotics susceptibility of gram negative bacteria but had increased resistance in *Enterococcus spp*.Vancomycin and Ampicillin resistance among Enterococci [39]. hence with the lack of sufficient evidence this aspect of intervention will require further research.

16.9 Intravenous to Oral Conversion (IV to Oral)

Many transplant centers use Intravenous-to-oral antimicrobial strategy, helping reduce cost, hospital length-of-stays, and the need for intravenous catheters [40]. Hence now it is strongly recommended in clinical practice guidelines [4].

Reducing the burden of invasive access in oncology patients is certainly one of the most crucial steps toward infection control and hence it should be considered even more strongly in oncology patients.

16.10 Biologic Markers as Stewardship Tool

Procalcitonin is a biomarker used to determine risk of sepsis and used as a tool for de-escalation of antibiotics. A review which included at least 30 publications concluded that due to limited production ability, delayed peak levels, and lower sensitivity, procalcitonin is unlikely to benefit in management of empirical therapy in neutropenic fever patients [41]. However serial measurements can be of help in reducing duration of therapy, as in non neutropenic patients [42, 43].

16.11 Stewardship of Antifungal Agents

Oncology patients, specifically neutropenic patients, are treated with prophylactic antifungal drugs during the high risk period, as they harbor a higher risk for developing invasive fungal infections(IFI) [44]. Many a times this prophylactic therapy is continued way beyond the high risk period and poses a significant threat for development of resistant fungal infections and toxicity from drugs.

Rapid diagnostic modalities like biomarkers (E.g Galactomannan, (1–3)-b-D-glucan levels), rapid candida detection panel (T2 Biosystems Inc), and imaging modality may enhance ability to diagnose IFIs early [44].

Systematic and standardized implementation of these diagnostics modalities along with antifungal therapies can contribute to successful implementation of antifungal stewardship. Some small studies indicated that ASP interventions can lead improvement in patient care and minimization of antifungal therapy use [45, 46].

16.12 Scope of Future Research

Literature search shows that most of the studies for stewardship in oncology patients are focused on institution specific clinical guidelines and further on de-escalation of antimicrobials. Hence even after there is enough proven benefits of stewardship interventions, there is still fair amount of scope exists for future research. Few specific recommendations have been enumerated in (Table 16.3). Key identified areas are diagnostic stewardship, pharmacological optimizations strategies and lastly audits feedbacks and application interventions.

Table 16.3 Scope of future research for antimicrobial stewardship in oncology patients

Diagnostic stewardship	– Development of oncology specific antibiograms [47] – Procalcitonin based differentiation of bacterial sepsis and de-escalation in oncology subset of patients – Rapid microbiological diagnostics and its impact
Pharmacological optimization	– Role for therapeutic drug monitoring of β-lactams – Safety of intravenous to oral switch of antibiotics in setting of bloodstream infections [48]
Prospective Audit, feedback, and application interventions	– Differences between syndrome-specific and drug-targeted intervention [49]. – Safety of preauthorization strategy [50] – Implementing clinical guidelines of non neutropenic infectious diseases – Antimicrobial Prophylaxis [51] – Oral Vancomycin prophylaxis for *Clostridioides difficile* infection [52, 53]

16.13 Conclusions

- Early and appropriate antimicrobial therapy can be life saving for the oncology patients. However non judicious use of antimicrobials leads to serious individual, institutional and ecological consequences.
- Oncology patients provide us with many novel opportunities for antimicrobial stewardship practice.
- Even in this high risk subset of patients, Antimicrobial stewardship program (ASP) interventions applied with due cautions can yield reasonably successful outcomes.
- Before embarking upon stewardship interventions one must ensure contemporary guidance for antimicrobial use in this subset of patients and also consider local pathogen flora and antibiograms.
- ASP in oncology patients requires a close interaction of infectious disease physicians, pharmacist, oncologist, hematologist and other practitioners.
- Adequate research data is still lacking for ASP in this subset of patients.
- ASP along with a robust infection control program can render sustained positive effect in this subset of patients.
- Even after proven benefits to ASP in oncology patients, there is scope of significant research and practice improvements.

References

1. Kumar A, Roberts D, Wood KE, Light B, Parrillo JE, Sharma S, et al. Duration of hypotension before initiation of effective antimicrobial therapy is the critical determinant of survival in human septic shock. Crit Care Med. 2006;34(6):1589–96.
2. Rhodes A, Evans LE, Alhazzani W, Levy MM, Antonelli M, Ferrer R, et al. Surviving sepsis campaign: international guidelines for management of sepsis and septic shock: 2016. Crit Care Med [Internet]. 2017 Mar [cited 2021 Jan 20];45(3):486–552. https://journals.lww.com/ccmjournal/Fulltext/2017/03000/Surviving_Sepsis_Campaign___International.15.aspx.
3. Fridkin S, Baggs J, Fagan R, Magill S, Pollack LA, Malpiedi P, et al. Vital signs: improving antibiotic use among hospitalized patients. MMWR Morb Mortal Wkly Rep. 2014;63(9):194–200.
4. Barlam TF, Cosgrove SE, Abbo LM, MacDougall C, Schuetz AN, Septimus EJ, et al. Implementing an antibiotic stewardship program: guidelines by the infectious diseases society of america and the society for healthcare epidemiology of America. Clin Infect Dis [Internet]. 2016 May 15 [cited 2021 Jan 21];62(10):e51–77. https://academic.oup.com/cid/article/62/10/e51/2462846.
5. Tamma PD, Avdic E, Li DX, Dzintars K, Cosgrove SE. Association of Adverse Events with Antibiotic use in hospitalized patients. JAMA Intern Med. 2017;177(9):1308–15.
6. Huttner A, Harbarth S, Carlet J, Cosgrove S, Goossens H, Holmes A, et al. Antimicrobial resistance: a global view from the 2013 world healthcare-associated infections forum. Antimicrob Resist Infect Control. 2013;2:31.
7. Tan SY, Tatsumura Y. Alexander Fleming (1881–1955): discoverer of penicillin. Singapore Med J [Internet]. 2015 Jul [cited 2021 Jan 21];56(7):366–7. https://www.ncbi.nlm.nih.gov/pmc/articles/PMC4520913/.
8. Moellering RC. MRSA: the first half century. J Antimicrob Chemother. 2012;67(1):4–11.
9. Cimolai N. Methicillin-resistant Staphylococcus aureus in Canada: a historical perspective and lessons learned. Can J Microbiol. 2010;56(2):89–120.

10. McGowan JE, Gerding DN. Does antibiotic restriction prevent resistance? New Horiz Baltim Md. 1996;4(3):370–6.
11. Boucher HW, Talbot GH, Bradley JS, Edwards JE, Gilbert D, Rice LB, et al. Bad bugs, no drugs: no ESKAPE! An update from the Infectious Diseases Society of America. Clin Infect Dis Off Publ Infect Dis Soc Am. 2009;48(1):1–12.
12. Boucher HW. Bad bugs, no drugs 2002–2020: progress, challenges, and call to action. Trans Am Clin Climatol Assoc [Internet]. 2020 [cited 2021 Jan 22];131:65–71. https://www.ncbi.nlm.nih.gov/pmc/articles/PMC7358500/.
13. Barrasa-Villar JI, Aibar-Remón C, Prieto-Andrés P, Mareca-Doñate R, Moliner-Lahoz J. Impact on morbidity, mortality, and length of stay of hospital-acquired infections by resistant microorganisms. Clin Infect Dis Off Publ Infect Dis Soc Am. 2017;65(4):644–52.
14. Shlaes DM, Gerding DN, John JF, Craig WA, Bornstein DL, Duncan RA, et al. Society for Healthcare Epidemiology of America and Infectious Diseases Society of America joint committee on the prevention of antimicrobial resistance: guidelines for the prevention of antimicrobial resistance in hospitals. Infect Control Hosp Epidemiol. 1997;18(4):275–91.
15. Dellit TH, Owens RC, McGowan JE, Gerding DN, Weinstein RA, Burke JP, et al. Infectious Diseases Society of America and the Society for Healthcare Epidemiology of America guidelines for developing an institutional program to enhance antimicrobial stewardship. Clin Infect Dis Off Publ Infect Dis Soc Am. 2007;44(2):159–77.
16. Society for Healthcare Epidemiology of America, Infectious Diseases Society of America, Pediatric Infectious Diseases Society. Policy statement on antimicrobial stewardship by the Society for Healthcare Epidemiology of America (SHEA), the Infectious Diseases Society of America (IDSA), and the Pediatric Infectious Diseases Society (PIDS). Infect Control Hosp Epidemiol. 2012;33(4):322–7.
17. New_antimicrobial_stewardship_standardpdf.pdf [Internet]. [cited 2021 Jan 24]. https://www.jointcommission.org/-/media/enterprise/tjc/imported-resource-assets/documents/new_antimicrobial_stewardship_standardpdf.pdf?db=web&hash=69307456CCE435B134854392C7FA7D76.
18. Robilotti E, Holubar M, Seo SK, Deresinski S. Feasibility and applicability of antimicrobial stewardship in immunocompromised patients. Curr Opin Infect Dis. 2017;30(4):346–53.
19. Rangaraj G, Granwehr BP, Jiang Y, Hachem R, Raad I. Perils of quinolone exposure in cancer patients: breakthrough bacteremia with multidrug-resistant organisms. Cancer. 2010;116(4):967–73.
20. Mihu CN, Rhomberg PR, Jones RN, Coyle E, Prince RA, Rolston KV. Escherichia coli resistance to quinolones at a comprehensive cancer center. Diagn Microbiol Infect Dis. 2010;67(3):266–9.
21. Ohmagari N, Hanna H, Graviss L, Hackett B, Perego C, Gonzalez V, et al. Risk factors for infections with multidrug-resistant Pseudomonas aeruginosa in patients with cancer. Cancer. 2005;104(1):205–12.
22. Worth LJ, Thursky KA, Seymour JF, Slavin MA. Vancomycin-resistant enterococcus faecium infection in patients with hematologic malignancy: patients with acute myeloid leukemia are at high-risk. Eur J Haematol. 2007;79(3):226–33.
23. Rolston KVI. The use of new and better antibiotics for bacterial infections in patients with leukemia. Clin Lymphoma Myeloma. 2009;9(Suppl 3):S357–63.
24. Mardani M, Abolghasemi S, Shabani S. Impact of an antimicrobial stewardship program in the antimicrobial-resistant and prevalence of clostridioides difficile infection and amount of antimicrobial consumed in cancer patients. BMC Res Notes [Internet]. 2020 Dec [cited 2021 Jan 24];13(1):246. https://bmcresnotes.biomedcentral.com/articles/10.1186/s13104-020-05085-3
25. The core elements of hospital antibiotic stewardship programs. https://www.cdc.gov/antibiotic-use/healthcare/pdfs/hospital-core-elements-H.pdf. Accessed 22 Jan 2021.
26. López-Medrano F, Juan RS, Lizasoain M, Catalán M, Ferrari JM, Chaves F, et al. A non-compulsory stewardship programme for the management of antifungals in a university-affiliated hospital. Clin Microbiol Infect Off Publ Eur Soc Clin Microbiol Infect Dis. 2013;19(1):56–61.

27. Micallef C, Aliyu SH, Santos R, Brown NM, Rosembert D, Enoch DA. Introduction of an antifungal stewardship programme targeting high-cost antifungals at a tertiary hospital in Cambridge. England J Antimicrob Chemother. 2015;70(6):1908–11.
28. Mondain V, Lieutier F, Hasseine L, Gari-Toussaint M, Poiree M, Lions C, et al. A 6-year antifungal stewardship programme in a teaching hospital. Infection. 2013 Jun;41(3):621–8.
29. Bal AM, Shankland GS, Scott G, Imtiaz T, Macaulay R, McGill M. Antifungal step-down therapy based on hospital intravenous to oral switch policy and susceptibility testing in adult patients with candidaemia: a single Centre experience. Int J Clin Pract. 2014;68(1):20–7.
30. Zuckermann J, Moreira LB, Stoll P, Moreira LM, Kuchenbecker RS, Polanczyk CA. Compliance with a critical pathway for the management of febrile neutropenia and impact on clinical outcomes. Ann Hematol. 2008;87(2):139–45.
31. Rosa RG, Goldani LZ, dos Santos RP. Association between adherence to an antimicrobial stewardship program and mortality among hospitalised cancer patients with febrile neutropaenia: a prospective cohort study. BMC Infect Dis. 2014;23(14):286.
32. Yeo C-L, Chan DS-G, Earnest A, Wu T-S, Yeoh S-F, Lim R, et al. Prospective audit and feedback on antibiotic prescription in an adult hematology-oncology unit in Singapore. Eur J Clin Microbiol Infect Dis [Internet]. 2012 Apr [cited 2021 Jan 24];31(4):583–90. http://link.springer.com/10.1007/s10096-011-1351-6.
33. So M, Mamdani MM, Morris AM, Lau TTY, Broady R, Deotare U, et al. Effect of an antimicrobial stewardship programme on antimicrobial utilisation and costs in patients with leukaemia: a retrospective controlled study. Clin Microbiol Infect Off Publ Eur Soc Clin Microbiol Infect Dis. 2018;24(8):882–8.
34. Perreault S, McManus D, Bar N, Foss F, Gowda L, Isufi I, et al. The impact of a multimodal approach to vancomycin discontinuation in hematopoietic stem cell transplant recipients (HSCT) with febrile neutropenia (FN). Transpl Infect Dis Off J Transplant Soc. 2019;21(2):e13059.
35. Ko J-H, Kim S-H, Kang C-I, Cho SY, Lee NY, Chung DR, et al. Evaluation of a carbapenem-saving strategy using empirical combination regimen of piperacillin-tazobactam and amikacin in hemato-oncology patients. J Korean Med Sci [Internet]. 2019 Jan 4 [cited 2021 Jan 24];34(2). https://www.ncbi.nlm.nih.gov/pmc/articles/PMC6327090/.
36. Tverdek FP, Rolston KV, Chemaly RF. Antimicrobial stewardship in patients with cancer. Pharmacotherapy [Internet]. 2012 Aug [cited 2021 Jan 24];32(8):722–34. http://doi.wiley.com/10.1002/j.1875-9114.2012.01162.x.
37. Craig M, Cumpston AD, Hobbs GR, Devetten MP, Sarwari AR, Ericson SG. The clinical impact of antibacterial prophylaxis and cycling antibiotics for febrile neutropenia in a hematological malignancy and transplantation unit. Bone Marrow Transplant. 2007;39(8):477–82.
38. Dominguez EA, Smith TL, Reed E, Sanders CC, Sanders WE. A pilot study of antibiotic cycling in a hematology-oncology unit. Infect Control Hosp Epidemiol. 2000;21(1 Suppl):S4–8.
39. Cadena J, Taboada CA, Burgess DS, Ma JZ, Lewis JS, Freytes CO, et al. Antibiotic cycling to decrease bacterial antibiotic resistance: a 5-year experience on a bone marrow transplant unit. Bone Marrow Transplant [Internet]. 2007 Jul [cited 2021 Jan 24];40(2):151–5. https://www.nature.com/articles/1705704.
40. Seo SK, Lo K, Abbo LM. Current state of antimicrobial stewardship at solid organ and hematopoietic cell transplant centers in the US. Infect Control Hosp Epidemiol [Internet]. 2016 Oct [cited 2021 Jan 24];37(10):1195–200. https://www.ncbi.nlm.nih.gov/pmc/articles/PMC5466005/.
41. Sakr Y, Sponholz C, Tuche F, Brunkhorst F, Reinhart K. The role of procalcitonin in febrile neutropenic patients: review of the literature. Infection. 2008;36(5):396–407.
42. Liew YX, Chlebicki MP, Lee W, Hsu LY, Kwa AL. Use of procalcitonin (PCT) to guide discontinuation of antibiotic use in an unspecified sepsis is an antimicrobial stewardship program (ASP). Eur J Clin Microbiol Infect Dis Off Publ Eur Soc Clin Microbiol. 2011;30(7):853–5.
43. Hayashi Y, Paterson DL. Strategies for reduction in duration of antibiotic use in hospitalized patients. Clin Infect Dis Off Publ Infect Dis Soc Am. 2011;52(10):1232–40.

44. Hamdy RF, Zaoutis TE, Seo SK. Antifungal stewardship considerations for adults and pediatrics. Virulence. 2017;8(6):658–72.
45. Micallef C, Aliyu SH, Santos R, Brown NM, Rosembert D, Enoch DA. Introduction of an antifungal stewardship programme targeting high-cost antifungals at a tertiary hospital in Cambridge. England. J Antimicrob Chemother. 2015;70(6):1908–11.
46. Mondain V, Lieutier F, Hasseine L, Gari-Toussaint M, Poiree M, Lions C, et al. A 6-year antifungal stewardship programme in a teaching hospital. Infection. 2013;41(3):621–8.
47. Smith ZR, Tajchman SK, Dee BM, Bruno JJ, Qiao W, Tverdek FP. Development of a combination antibiogram for Pseudomonas aeruginosa bacteremia in an oncology population. J Oncol Pharm Pract [Internet]. 2016 Jun 1 [cited 2021 Feb 15];22(3):409–15. https://doi.org/10.1177/1078155215586081.
48. Yan LZ, Herrington JD. Outcomes of hospitalized neutropenic oncology patients with *Pseudomonas aeruginosa* bloodstream infections: focus on oral fluoroquinolone conversion. J Oncol Pharm Pract [Internet]. 2016 Aug [cited 2021 Feb 15];22(4):584–90. http://journals.sagepub.com/doi/10.1177/1078155215591389.
49. Mediwala KN, Kohn JE, Bookstaver PB, Justo JA, Rac H, Tucker K, et al. Syndrome-specific versus prospective audit and feedback interventions for reducing use of broad-spectrum antimicrobial agents. Am J Infect Control. 2019;47(11):1284–9.
50. Paskovaty A, Lucarelli CD, Patel P, Ryan M, Seyboth B, Thackray J, et al. Antimicrobial stewardship efforts to manage a pentamidine shortage. Am J Health-Syst Pharm AJHP Off J Am Soc Health-Syst Pharm. 2014;71(23):2014–8.
51. Mikulska M, Averbuch D, Tissot F, Cordonnier C, Akova M, Calandra T, et al. Fluoroquinolone prophylaxis in haematological cancer patients with neutropenia: ECIL critical appraisal of previous guidelines. J Infect. 2018;76(1):20–37.
52. Ganetsky A, Han JH, Hughes ME, Babushok DV, Frey NV, Gill SI, et al. Oral vancomycin prophylaxis is highly effective in preventing Clostridium difficile infection in allogeneic hematopoietic cell transplant recipients. Clin Infect Dis Off Publ Infect Dis Soc Am. 2019;68(12):2003–9.
53. Morrisette T, Van Matre AG, Miller MA, Mueller SW, Bajrovic V, Abidi MZ, et al. Oral vancomycin prophylaxis as secondary prevention against Clostridioides difficile infection in the hematopoietic stem cell transplantation and hematologic malignancy population. Biol Blood Marrow Transplant J Am Soc Blood Marrow Transplant. 2019;25(10):2091–7.

Management of Fluids and Electrolytes in Onco-Critical Patient

17

Muhanad Aboud, Waiel Al-Moustadi, Virendra K. Arya, and Rajeev Chauhan

17.1 Introduction

Fluid and electrolyte abnormalities are a common manifestation in critically ill oncologic patients. Often these abnormalities are associated with either the underlying disease itself or the therapeutics used during treatment. The critically ill patient often experiences alterations in absorption, distribution, and excretion of fluids and electrolytes. Significant complications can result from fluid and electrolyte imbalances, and the severity of which parallels the magnitude of the underlying disorder.

Fluid and electrolyte derangements occurring acutely and rapidly are often associated with increased symptoms and complications relative to chronically occurring abnormalities. Critically ill cancer patients often require frequent monitoring and evaluation of fluid status and serum electrolyte concentrations throughout their treatment, especially in an acute state. An actual example of an oncologic emergency is tumour lysis syndrome (TLS). TLS most commonly occurs after initiation of cytotoxic chemotherapy; rapid breakdown of tumour cells leaves the patient in a metabolically chaotic state which requires immediate management [1].

M. Aboud
University of Winnipeg, Winnipeg, Canada

W. Al-Moustadi
Max Rady College of Medicine, University of Manitoba, Saint Boniface Hospital, Winnipeg, Canada

V. K. Arya (✉)
Max Rady College of Medicine, University of Manitoba, Saint Boniface Hospital, Winnipeg, Canada

Department of Anaesthesia & Intensive Care, PGIMER, Chandigarh, India

R. Chauhan
Department of Anaesthesia & Intensive Care, PGIMER, Chandigarh, India

V. Kumar et al. (eds.), *Onco-critical Care*,
https://doi.org/10.1007/978-981-16-9929-0_17

Drug-related complications do not only include tumour lysis syndrome; anticancer drugs cause many side effects that deteriorate a patient's state; among them, electrolyte disturbances are relatively frequent and could be life-threatening if not recognized promptly and treated appropriately. Platinum-based chemotherapy used in lymphomas and various solid tumours are commonly associated with Fanconi's syndrome, a rare disorder causing a generalized defect in reabsorption at the proximal renal tubules [2]. Vinca alkaloids and tyrosine kinase inhibitors cause hyponatremia [3]. Currently, an array of anticancer drug types are frequently prescribed; thus, recognizing the cause of electrolyte abnormalities is important when managing a critically ill oncologic patient. Table 17.1 summarises the fluid and electrolyte abnormalities induced by certain oncological conditions and anticancer drugs used to treat them.

Fluid overload is another challenge facing oncologic patients, and management of this complication is not always straightforward because many perpetrators can cause fluid retention. For example, differentiation syndrome in acute promyelocytic leukemia patients undergoing induction therapy causes fluid retention and renal failure, which consequently progresses to respiratory failure [4]. Fluid overload is also a complication for patients who may have undergone Allogenic Hematopoietic

Table 17.1 Fluid and electrolyte anomalies in oncological conditions and anticancer therapy

Condition/drug	Electrolyte or fluid abnormality	Mechanism
Tumour Lysis Syndrome	Hyperkalemia Hyperphosphatemia Hypercalcemia Hyperuricemia	Post cytotoxic chemotherapy initiation
Allogenic Hematopoietic Cell Transplantation	Fluid overload	Veno-occlusive disease
Acute Promyelocytic Leukemia	Fluid retention/overload	Differentiation Syndrome *[induced by ATRA and ATO induction therapy]*
Cisplatin and other Platinum based drugs	Hypomagnesmeia	Gastrointestinal and renal loss
	Hypocalcemia	Hypomagnesemia mediated resistance to PTH
	Hyponatremia	SIADH
	Hypokalemia	Hypomagnesemia mediated renal loss
Cyclophosphamide	Hyponatremia	SIADH
Vincristine, Vinblastine	Hyponatremia	SIADH
Imatinib, Dasatinib, Axitinib, Nilotinib, Bosutinib	Hyponatremia	SIADH
Axitinib	Hypocalcemia	Unknown
Dacomitinib, Afatinib, Erlotinib, and Gefitinib	Hypochloremia	Diarrhea

SIADH syndrome of inappropriate antidiuretic hormone secretion, *ATRA* all-trans retinoic acid, *ATO* arsenic trioxide, *PTH* parathyroid hormone

Cell Transplantation (AHSCT). Even though the survival rate in these patients has improved over time, a Veno-oclusive disease (VOD) may develop by which hepatic venules and sinusoids are narrowed or occluded; potentiating fluid overload that could ultimately lead to liver failure, ascites, progressive cardiac, pulmonary, and renal failure [5–7]. VOD occurs likely due to the post-transplantation regimens involving cyclophosphamide and alkylating agents such as busulfan [8, 9]. Fluid and electrolyte management is critical in these patients as the amount and rate of weight gain is directly correlated with mortality risk [10].This chapter aims to present the contemporary evidence regarding the management of fluid and electrolyte abnormalities attributed to various oncologic emergencies.

17.2 Tumour Lysis Syndrome

Tumour Lysis Syndrome (TLS) is a constellation of metabolic derangement characterized by the tetrad of *hyperkalemia, hyperphosphatemia, hypercalcemia, and hyperuricemia* [1]. TLS commonly occurs after cytotoxic chemotherapy initiation in patients with high-grade lymphomas and acute lymphoblastic leukemia (ALL) [1]. The clinical signs and symptoms of TLS reflect the underlying metabolic imbalance. Malignant cells, for example, have a higher concentration of phosphorus, and thus hyperphosphatemia develops relative to the degree of tumour cell lysis [2].

The prevention of tumour lysis syndrome relies fundamentally on careful monitoring of fluids and hypouricemic therapy [3]. Exogenous sources of both potassium and calcium should be stopped to prevent further derangement of the metabolic imbalance. Urine output and volume status should also be closely monitored.

Hydration is the essential factor in preventing TLS. Intravenous crystalloid therapy should be tailored to the individual patient. If the patient is hypovolemic or hyponatremic, isotonic saline solution should be the initial hydration fluid used [1]. Volume repletion is a critical factor in reducing the risk of TLS because it maintains both renal blood flow and urine flow, thus promoting urinary excretion of potassium, phosphate, and uric acid [4]. Intravenous fluids should be started 24–48 h prior to induction therapy and should be twice the usual maintenance requirement to preserve urine output at 80–100 mL/m^2/h. in adults [4]; 2 mL/kg h. for both pediatric and adult patients and 4–6 mL/kg/h. if weight $\leq$10 kg [5].

Oncologic patients, particularly the elderly, may have underlying cardiovascular and renal diseases, that would limit volume expansion. This is of specific importance as pre-existing conditions may increase their risk of heart failure and volume overload [4]. A nephrologist should immediately evaluate patients who are unresponsive to volume expansion efforts or with oliguria not due to volume depletion. This will help ascertain the potential presence of acute kidney injury and the most appropriate therapeutic options for the patient based on their volume status and clinical and laboratory parameters [4]. An evaluation is also beneficial in identifying the role of diuretic drug boluses or infusions and the potential benefit of changing a patient's status from oliguric AKI to non-oliguric as a means of short-term management before initiating renal replacement therapy [4].

Sodium retention and hypertension are concomitant morbidities commonly seen in those receiving steroid therapy; thus, choosing the appropriate IV fluid solution is an essential component of management. Isotonic saline solution (5% dextrose) should be considered for patients on high-dose steroid therapy. In these patients, diuretics are not required if renal function is within the normal range [1]. Intravenous fluids should be continued until serum LDH levels return to normal or the tumour burden has resolved [1, 4]. In managing TLS, daily administration of IV crystalloids is 2–3 L/m^2; this is dependent on the volume status of the patient and the presence of any comorbidities [1, 4]. Urine output, serum electrolytes (potassium, calcium, phosphorus), uric acid, and creatinine must be vigilantly monitored, especially in high-risk patients [1, 4].

17.3 Fluid Management in Veno-Occlusive Disease as a Consequence of Allogenic Hematopoietic Cell Transplantation

Allogenic hematopoietic cell transplantation (AHSCT) is a well-established treatment for various hematologic disorders. Veno-occlusive disease (VOD), also referred to as a sinusoidal obstructive syndrome, is a potentially fatal complication associated with AHSCT and involves the desquamation of hepatic cells from the sinusoidal endothelium. These cells occlude the microvascular lamina and cause a pro-inflammatory response and subsequent collagen deposition in hepatic venules, potentiating the risk of liver failure, ascites, progressive cardiac, pulmonary, and renal failure [6–8]. Fluid overload is another consequence of VOD and commonly occurs during hospitalization for AHSCT. VOD presumably is due to the treatment itself. Early VOD usually occurs within the first 20 days post-transplantation in regimens containing cyclophosphamide [9]. Late VOD may occur after myeloablative chemotherapy for more than 30 days. Typically, this form of therapy includes several alkylating agents such as busulfan, melphalan, and thiotepa [10].

Diagnosing VOD is difficult primarily because it is challenging to differentiate VOD from severe sepsis, hemolysis, and Acute Graft versus Host Disease. Also, medications used during AHSCT treatment can cause cholestasis, which also mimics the symptoms of VOD. These differentials should be excluded, and great care must be taken to correct fluid and electrolyte imbalances; because patients suffering from VOD inevitably have fluid overload [11].

The survival rate of AHSCT patients has gradually improved, significant fluid overload remains a frequent occurrence. Up to 20% of patients experience a weight gain of ≥20 percent of their baseline [12]. Rondón and colleagues found that this grade of fluid overload, when diagnosed by Day 30 post-transplantation, accounted for most non-relapse mortality and was the strongest predictor of non-relapse mortality in AHSCT patients [12].

Treatment of VOD includes mainly supportive measures. Ascites is treated using a combination of sodium restriction, diuretics, and paracentesis [13]. Fluid management should be adjusted to the patient's baseline weight, especially during a state of acute fluid overload [11]. Usually, patients experience a weight increase of roughly 5% above their baseline [14]. Fluid and electrolyte management is critical in AHSCT patients as the amount and rate of weight gain due to fluid overload have been identified as predictors of high mortality risk [15]. Total fluid intake may need to be restricted to 50–75% of the normal maintenance fluids, and controlled diuresis may also prove to be critical in these patients [11].

Once veno-occlusive disease is diagnosed, diuresis may be indicated to restore euvolemia [11]. It is not uncommon for patients with VOD to have capillary leak syndrome (CLS), as this also plays a role in the pathophysiology of fluid overload seen in AHSCT patients [8]. In addition to the concurrence of capillary leak syndrome (CLS), VOD patients also have a "portal hypertension-like complication," which further exacerbates peritoneal leakage [11]. In the instance that patients whose daily maintenance fluid requirements are met by blood product transfusions and medication volumes alone, diuresis may prove crucial in establishing euvolemia in these situations [11].

Mahadeo and colleagues suggest that an incremental approach to diuretic administration should be considered, and diuresis may be increased for scheduled diuresis or for continuous infusion for worsening fluid overload. Adjunctive therapy may include Chlorothiazide, Bumetanide, Metolazone, Spironolactone. In the event of abdominal compartment syndrome, paracentesis should be considered [11]. Restoration of a euvolemic state requires strict monitoring of fluid intake and urine output. Monitoring hemodynamic and renal function parameters is also imperative during diuresis. Patients who suffer worsening weight gain and fluid overload despite medical management, have uncontrolled electrolyte abnormalities, or those who have progressive oliguria/anuria should undergo renal replacement therapy. Lastly, continuous renal replacement therapy may be indicated in those patients with unremitting oliguria and worsening renal function [11].

17.4 Acute Promyelocytic Leukemia

All-trans retinoic acid (ATRA) has revolutionized the treatment outcomes of patients with Acute Promyelocytic Leukemia (APL). Not only did it increase the cure rate to over 80%, but it also decreased the induction mortality rate to less than 10% [16]. Further improvements to survival outcomes occurred after introducing arsenic trioxide (ATO), resulting in a 95% complete remission rate and a 5-year disease-free survival rate of 96% [16]. Even though there has been significant progress, a small subset of patients (<5%) still experience early induction mortality or require admission to the intensive care unit during induction therapy [16]. A significant complication during APL induction therapy is Differentiation Syndrome (DS). A hallmark of DS is Fluid retention and renal failure, amongst other complications. Fluid overload due to IV fluid administration and transfusion of blood products has received little attention in the literature; this is alarming because the signs and symptoms of fluid overload can be subtle and often overlooked. Consequently, patients with fluid overload can develop concomitant complications such as respiratory failure and require intensive observation [16].

A high total volume of transfusions and older age are the only factors associated with fluid overload during induction therapy [16]. For patients with weight gain or dyspnea due to DS, cautious diuresis is given as tolerated by their hemodynamic and renal status. Approximately 87 percent of patients with DS require diuretic therapy; in some cases, this has led to rapid improvement [17]. In the PETHEMA protocols, furosemide is usually administered to treat signs or symptoms of fluid overload. Some cases with refractory acute renal failure and fluid overload may need renal replacement therapy. In patients at risk for fluid overload and high blood product requirements to control the coagulopathy, the use of cryoprecipitate, fibrinogen concentrate, and other coagulation-factor concentrates like Prothrombin complex concentrate (factor II, VII, IX, X and proteins C & S) also called Octaplex or Beriplex instead of fresh-frozen plasma may be considered. These supportive measures are frequently needed in patients with severe DS relative to moderate DS. Moreover, many patients will develop prerenal failure and hypotension in the context of CLS. In these cases, careful fluids and vasopressor agents should be implemented in conjunction with empirical therapy with intravenous antibiotics [17].

Temporary discontinuation of ATRA and ATO is indicated on APL patients experiencing woxrsening clinical conditions or severe organ failure due to DS, such as those who develop renal failure or require admission into the ICU with respiratory distress. Otherwise, these agents could be maintained [17]. In a few cases, dexamethasone has successfully resolved early episodes of DS. However, DS may relapse. In such cases, dexamethasone should be continued until the complete disappearance of signs and symptoms, and then ATRA and ATO therapy should be resumed [17]. Otherwise, ATRA or ATO could be maintained unless a lack of response to dexamethasone is observed [17].

17.5 Anticancer Therapy Related Fluid and Electrolyte Abnormalities

Anticancer drug therapy is a staple of managing critically ill oncologic patients, but these drugs are frequently associated with electrolyte disorders, many of which can be fatal. Platinum chemotherapy, particularly cisplatin, is commonly associated with *hypomagnesemia, hypokalemia, hypophosphatemia, hypocalcemia and hyponatremia* [18]. These drugs also cause Fanconi's syndrome (*hypophosphatemia, aminoaciduria, hypouricemia, and glucosuria*). Alkylating agents have been associated with hyponatremia due to SIADH. Vinca alkaloids also cause hyponatremia due to SIADH [19]. Tyrosine kinase inhibitors induce hyponatremia and hypophosphatemia. Thus, the prevention of electrolyte abnormalities would not only be a lifesaving decision, but it may also lead to a reduction in adverse events during the anticancer drug therapy itself.

17.5.1 Platinum-Based Chemotherapy

Cisplatin, the model platinum agent, and its derivatives carboplatin and oxaliplatin have traditionally been first-line agents in treating numerous malignancies, including lung, colorectal, bladder, breast, ovarian, and testicular cancers, among others. A side effect of these widely used drugs, particularly cisplatin, is *low magnesium* [20]. Magnesium loss occurs through two primary mechanisms, gastrointestinal and renal excretion [18]. It is relatively common for oncologic patients to have a magnesium deficiency even in the absence of platinum therapy [21]; however, this symptom frequently goes undetected, making it difficult to manage. Serum magnesium concentration significantly influences the serum levels of other electrolytes such as calcium, potassium, and phosphate [22], suggesting that magnesium concentration plays a central role in electrolyte abnormalities in oncologic patients.

Traditionally, the National Cancer Institute (NCI) grading criteria have been the standard used in managing hypomagnesemia; however, measurement of serum levels lacked accuracy [18]. Thus, the decision to treat hypomagnesemia should be based on clinical judgment, factoring in any comorbidities such as heart disease or diabetes, both of which may lead to dangerous arrhythmias. Clinicians should also factor in concomitant medications predisposing a patient to magnesium loss, such as diuretics, bisphosphates, beta-2 agonists, proton pump inhibitors, and steroids [18]. As previously stated, hypomagnesemia leads to other electrolyte abnormalities such as hypocalcaemia and hypokalemia; therefore, calcium and potassium levels should be measured as they are essential diagnostic clues to the presence of hypomagnesemia [18].

The two preferred repletion agents are intervenors magnesium sulphate (2–4 g) and magnesium oxide [23]. Additional oral preparations that may be used include magnesium sulphate, magnesium gluconate, and sustained-release preparations such as Slow-Mag and Mag-Table SR [18]. Oral replenishment of magnesium typically requires a daily dose of 400–800 mg, although a dose greater than 400 mg likely causes diarrhea, a magnesium loss mechanism due to excretion [18]. Patients in a critical state may require additional magnesium doses, especially in the presence of vomiting and diarrhea [18].

Interestingly, intravenous magnesium supplementation has been related to a significantly decreased risk for cisplatin-induced nephrotoxicity. Even though hypermagnesemia (> 2.6 mg/dL) is a possible consequence of management, it is uncommon except in the setting of renal insufficiency, which is the most common acute toxicity of platinum-based drugs [18] Also, excess magnesium is efficiently excreted by the kidneys allowing for plasma levels to remain between 1.5 and 2.1 mEq/L [18] In addition to hypomagnesemia, platinum agents have been known to cause other electrolyte abnormalities including, hypokalemia, hypocalcemia, and hypophosphatemia. *Hypokalemia, hypocalcemia, and hypophosphatemia resulting from magnesium deficiency are considered together because their refractoriness to correction depends on correcting the magnesium imbalance* [18]. Although renal potassium, calcium, and phosphate wasting may also occur independent of low magnesium due to platinum drug-related tubular damage [18].

17.5.2 Alkylating Agents

Alkylating agents are used in numerous treatments, including leukemias, lymphomas, and various solid tumours such as breast, ovaries, and small cell lung cancer. These agents have been reported to include the central release of ADH leading to *hyponatremia* [19]. Amongst the various alkylating agents, cyclophosphamide is the main culprit behind the development of hyponatremia. This occurs with high intravenous doses (30–50 mg/kg of cyclophosphamide). However, there are cases where hyponatremia was observed with lower doses (10–15 mg/kg) also. Cyclophosphamide is given with a high volume of hypotonic fluids to prevent hemorrhagic cystitis; this volume expansion further exacerbates the hyponatremia.

Hyponatremia can be associated with different volume states: hypovolemia, euvolemia or hypervolemia, and therefore an accurate assessment of the patient's volume status is critical to determine the appropriate treatment strategy [24]. The management approach to hyponatremia depends mainly on its etiology (volume status), speed of onset (acute vs. chronic), and symptomatology. Hypovolemic hyponatremia should be treated with isotonic saline. In a state of acute hyponatremia, correction of sodium should not exceed 1–2 mmol/h. and 8 mmol/day on any given day of treatment. The aim should not be to normalize a patient's sodium level entirely but instead, raise the concentration to a safe level (>120 mmol/L). After a safe level is reached, conservative management such as fluid restriction can be utilized. As for euvolemic or hypervolemia patients presenting with acute hyponatremia, hypertonic saline (3% normal saline) can be used in their management [24, 25].

17.5.3 Vinca Alkaloids

Vincristine and, less frequently, vinblastine is associated with the occurrence of *hyponatremia* [19]. Vincristine is administered via intravenous infusion for use in various chemotherapeutic regimens. Vincristine is mainly used in the treatment of non-Hodgkin's lymphoma, Hodgkin's lymphoma, acute lymphoblastic leukemia (ALL) and nephroblastoma (Wilms tumour, a renal tumour common in children) [26].

Vinca Alkaloid drugs induce SIADH since they directly affect the neurohypophysis and hypothalamic system [19]. The incidence of SIADH is 1.3/100,000 treated patients with these agents (Hammond et al., 2002). However, the incidence of vincristine-related SIADH linked with hyponatremia is up to 44% when the drug is given with antifungal azoles (ketoconazole, itraconazole, posaconazole, and voriconazole). *Clinicians should be aware that antifungal agents inhibit the metabolism of vincristine, leading to increased vincristine levels and neurotoxicity* [19]. Treating Vincristine-associated SIADH is mainly based on fluid restriction supplemented with 3% hypertonic saline solution and diuresis with intravenous furosemide [26].

17.5.4 Tyrosine Kinase Inhibitors

Imatinib, dasatinib, nilotinib, bosutinib and axitinib have been dose-dependently linked to *hyponatremia*. The primary underlying mechanism is the induction of SIADH. Imatinib, apart from hyponatremia, can also induce *hypophosphatemia* through tubular damage and inappropriate phosphaturia. Another contributing factor to the occurrence of hypophosphatemia is *secondary hyperparathyroidism* due to diminished calcium levels.

Tyrosine kinase inhibitors (**TKIs**) targeting the epidermal growth factor receptor (**EGFR**) are common in the therapeutic armentarium of lung cancer today. Fluid management needs to be top of mind for patients on TKI EGFR therapy because one of the most common side effects observed during treatment is diarrhea. A possible case for this side-effect could be the TKI EGFR induced chloride secretion into the intestine lumen or impairment of the intestinal absorption. Consequently, this can perpetuate electrolyte losses, hypochloremia resulting in dehydration, acid-base imbalance, and extreme cases of renal insufficiency. Diarrhea associated with a molecularly targeted therapy appears mainly in the first 2 weeks of treatment [27].

During TKI EGFR treatment, diarrhea appears in 20–90% of patients. Most patients report Common Terminology Criteria for Adverse Events (CTCAE) grade 1 or 2 diarrhea intensity, which may also develop fluid and electrolyte imbalances that may downgrade a patient's quality of life over a long period. Clinicians should be mindful that not all tyrosine kinase inhibitor agents are created equal. It is essential to recognize that second-generation *irreversible* TKI EGFR agents such as dacomitinib and afatinib have a greater incidence of diarrhea regardless of the CTCAE grade. Phase III clinical trials have shown that these agents cause diarrhea in 70% of patients, 10% of which have CTCAE grade 3 or higher [27]. In patients being treated with *reversible* TKI EGFR agents (erlotinib and gefitinib), diarrhea was observed in 33–47%. Only 2% of patients suffered grade 3 or higher [28], suggesting that patients on erlotinib and gefitinib may require less stringent fluid and electrolyte management.

Fluid and electrolyte management in these patients centers around reducing the onset and duration of diarrhea; this includes discontinuation of the offending agent. For example, 3% of patients treated with the irreversible TKI EGFR discontinued their therapy due to diarrhea [29]. In cases of CTCAE grades 1 and 2, Loperamide should be used at an initial dose of 4 mg, followed by 2 mg every 4 h. If diarrhea persists longer than 1 day, Loperamide may be given every 2 h. Loperamide should then be discontinued after 12 hours of the last episode of diarrhea.

Patients presenting with grade 3 or 4 diarrhea will require hospitalization, and parenteral fluid supplementation should be provided to prevent dehydration [27]. Loperamide use, like in those with CTCAE grade 1 and 2, is also indicated in more severe cases [27]. Furthermore, TKI EGFR therapy should be discontinued until symptoms regress to grade 1 or subside completely [27]. Then, TKI EGFR treatment may be continued at the current or reduced dose. If severe diarrhea recurs, treatment may require a further dose reduction or temporary withdrawal of TKI EGFR therapy [27].

17.6 Conclusion

Fluid and electrolyte disorders are a common complication befalling critically ill cancer patients. Apart from general principals of fluid and electrolyte therapy, timely recognition and management of these tumour and chemotherapy specific disorders are vital in the prevention of serious complications. Oncologic emergencies are often diverse in their etiology and often manifest in acute settings. This chapter has outlined several significant complications and their appropriate management to achieve the desired goals of care. Without question, management of the critically ill oncologic patient is complex, and their treatment often includes restoration of normal fluid status and electrolyte levels and a multidisciplinary team approach. Understanding the underlying cause for the specific chemical imbalance is essential for the clinician to establish an effective treatment plan. Moreover, clinicians should be aware that the administration of anticancer drugs comes with a high probability for the development of electrolyte abnormalities, and if not managed appropriately, these electrolyte derangements may prove to be harmful and, in many cases, fatal.

References

1. Puri I, Sharma D, Gunturu KS, Ahmed AA. Diagnosis and management of tumor lysis syndrome. J Commun Hosp Intern Med Perspec. 2020;10(3):269–72.
2. Brown RB, Razzaque MS. Phosphate toxicity and tumorigenesis. Biochimica Et Biophysica Acta Bba - Rev Cancer. 2018;1869(2):303–9.
3. He P, Mann-Collura O, Fling J, Edara N, Razzaque MS. Elevated phosphate mediates extensive cellular toxicity: from abnormal proliferation to excessive cell death. Biorxiv. 2020; https://doi.org/10.1101/2020.01.02.892638.
4. Abu-Alfa AK, Younes A. Tumor lysis syndrome and acute kidney injury: evaluation, prevention, and management. Am J Kidney Dis. 2010;55(5):S1–13.
5. Coiffier B, Altman A, Pui C-H, Younes A, Cairo MS. Guidelines for the Management of Pediatric and Adult Tumor Lysis Syndrome: an evidence-based review. J Clin Oncol. 2008;26(16):2767–78.
6. McDonald GB, Sharma P, Matthews DE, Thomas ED, Shulman H. Venocclusive disease of the liver after bone marrow transplantation: diagnosis, incidence, and predisposing factors. Hepatology (Baltimore, Md). 1984;4(1):116–22.
7. Retter A. Oxford textbook of critical care. In: Webb A, Angus D, Finfer S, Gattinoni L, Singer M, editors. 2 ed. Oxford University Press; 2016. p. 1795–7.
8. Vion A-C, Rautou P-E, Durand F, Boulanger C, Valla D. Interplay of inflammation and endothelial dysfunction in bone marrow transplantation: focus on hepatic Veno-occlusive disease. Semin Throm Hemos. 2015;41(06):629–43.
9. McDonald GB, Hinds MS, Fisher LD, Schoch HG, Wolford JL, Banaji M, Hardin BJ, Shulman HM, Clift RA. Veno-occlusive disease of the liver and multiorgan failure after bone marrow transplantation: a cohort study of 355 patients. Ann Intern Med. 1993;118(4):255.
10. Lee JL, Gooley T, Bensinger W, Schiffman K, McDonald GB. Veno-occlusive disease of the liver after busulfan, melphalan, and thiotepa conditioning therapy: incidence, risk factors, and outcome. Biol Blood Marrow Tr. 1999;5(5):306–15.
11. Mahadeo KM, McArthur J, Adams RH, Radhi M, Angelo J, Jeyapalan A, Nicol K, Su L, Rabi H, Auletta JJ, Pai V, Duncan CN, Tamburro R, Dvorak CC, Bajwa RPS. Consensus report by the Pediatric acute lung injury and sepsis investigators and Pediatric blood and marrow trans-

plant consortium joint working committees on supportive care guidelines for Management of Veno-Occlusive Disease in children and adolescents: part 2—focus on ascites, fluid and electrolytes, renal, and transfusion issues. Biol Blood Marrow Tr. 2017;23(12):2023–33.
12. Rondón G, Saliba RM, Chen J, Ledesma C, Alousi AM, Oran B, Hosing CM, Kebriaei P, Khouri IF, Shpall EJ, Popat UR, Champlin RE, Ciurea SO. Impact of fluid overload as new toxicity category on hematopoietic stem cell transplantation outcomes. Biol Blood Marrow Tr. 2017;23(12):2166–71.
13. Senzolo M, Germani G, Cholongitas E, Burra P, Burroughs A-K. Veno occlusive disease: Update on clinical management. World J Gastroentero. 2007;13(29):3918.
14. Jones R, Lee KS, Beschorner WE, Vogel VG, Grochow LB, Braine HG, Vogelsang GB, Sensenbrenner LL, Santo GW, Saral R. Venoocclusive disease of the liver following bone marrow transplantation. Transplantation. 1987;44(6):778–83.
15. Bearman SI, Anderson GL, Mori M, Hinds MS, Shulman HM, McDonald GB. Venoocclusive disease of the liver: development of a model for predicting fatal outcome after marrow transplantation. J Clin Oncol. 1993;11(9):1729–36.
16. Chamoun K, Kantarjian HM, Wang X, Naqvi K, Aung F, Garcia-Manero G, Borthakur G, Jabbour E, Kadia T, Daver N, DiNardo CD, Jain N, Konopleva M, Cortes J, Ravandi F, Yilmaz M. Unrecognized fluid overload during induction therapy increases morbidity in patients with acute promyelocytic leukemia. Cancer. 2019;125(18):3219–24.
17. Sanz MA, Montesinos P. How we prevent and treat differentiation syndrome in patients with acute promyelocytic leukemia. Blood. 2014;
18. Oronsky B, Caroen S, Oronsky A, Dobalian VE, Oronsky N, Lybeck M, Reid TR, Carter CA. Electrolyte disorders with platinum-based chemotherapy: mechanisms, manifestations and management. Cancer Chemoth Pharm. 2017;80(5):895–907.
19. Liamis G, Filippatos TD, Elisaf MS. Electrolyte disorders associated with the use of anticancer drugs. Eur J Pharmacol. 2016;777:78–87.
20. Blachley JD. Renal and electrolyte disturbances associated with cisplatin. Ann Intern Med. 1981;95(5):628.
21. Chaudhary DP, Sharma R, Bansal DD. Implications of magnesium deficiency in type 2 diabetes: a review. Biol Trace Elem Res. 2010;134(2):119–29.
22. Rasmussen HS, Cintin C, Aurup P, Breum L, McNair P. The effect of intravenous magnesium therapy on serum and urine levels of potassium, calcium, and sodium in patients with ischemic heart disease, with and without acute myocardial infarction. Arch Intern Med. 1988;148(8):1801–5.
23. Martin KJ, González EA, Slatopolsky E. Clinical consequences and Management of Hypomagnesemia. J Am Soc Nephrol. 2009;20(11):2291–5.
24. Baker M, Markman M, Niu J. Cyclophosphamide-induced severe acute Hyponatremic encephalopathy in patients with breast cancer: report of two cases. Case Reports Oncol. 2014;7(2):550–4.
25. Biswas M, Davies JS. Hyponatraemia in clinical practice. Postgrad Med J. 2007;83(980):373.
26. Nagappa M, Bhat RR, Sudeep K, Mishra SK, Badhe A, Hemavathi B. Vincristine-induced acute life-threatening hyponatremia resulting in seizure and coma. Indian J Critical Care Medicine. 2009;13(3):167–8.
27. Płużański A, Piórek A. Side effects of tyrosine kinase inhibitors — management guidelines. Oncol Clin Pract. 2016;4(12)
28. Soria J-C, Felip E, Cobo M, Lu S, Syrigos K, Lee KH, Göker E, Georgoulias V, Li W, Isla D, Guclu SZ, Morabito A, Min YJ, Ardizzoni A, Gadgeel SM, Wang B, Chand VK, Goss GD. Investigators L-L 8. Afatinib versus erlotinib as second-line treatment of patients with advanced squamous cell carcinoma of the lung (LUX-lung 8): an open-label randomised controlled phase 3 trial. Lancet Oncol. 2015;16(8):897–907.
29. Park K, Tan E-H, O'Byrne K, Zhang L, Boyer M, Mok T, Hirsh V, Yang JC-H, Lee KH, Lu S, Shi Y, Kim S-W, Laskin J, Kim D-W, Arvis CD, Kölbeck K, Laurie SA, Tsai C-M, Shahidi M, Kim M, Massey D, Zazulina V, Paz-Ares L. Afatinib versus gefitinib as first-line treatment of patients with EGFR mutation-positive non-small-cell lung cancer (LUX-lung 7): a phase 2B, open-label, randomised controlled trial. Lancet Oncol. 2016;17(5):577–89.

Transfusion Therapy: When to Give It and how to Minimize It

18

Prashant Sirohiya and Vinod Kumar

Change can be for good if you combine audacity with safety – Pedro Sánchez.

18.1 Introduction

From the discovery of the circulation system by William Harvey in the 1600s to the production of synthetic blood products in the laboratory, medical science has come a long way [1]. The ability to transfuse blood products to save lives is as important as the responsibility of safely transfusing it. As the demands of transfusion therapy are increasing day by day, various guidelines are being developed on choosing donors as well as indications and the art of administering products. Transfusion therapy aims to balance the risks of serious hemorrhages and decreased oxygen transport versus the complications of transfusion [2]. For clinicians to be able to make the right clinical decision about transfusion, they should be aware of the transfusion immunobiology, complications, practical aspects as well as controversial areas which are still under research.

18.2 Blood Group Systems

All blood cells like red blood cells (RBC), Leukocytes, platelets, and plasma proteins are antigenic and lead to the production of various alloantibodies which form the basis of various transfusion reactions. The antibodies against RBC antigens

P. Sirohiya
Onco-anesthesia & Palliative Medicine, All India Institute of Medical Sciences, New Delhi, India

V. Kumar (✉)
Department of Onco-Anesthesia and Palliative Medicine, Dr. B.R.A. Institute Rotary Cancer Hospital, All India Institute of Medical Sciences, New Delhi, India

V. Kumar et al. (eds.), *Onco-critical Care*,
https://doi.org/10.1007/978-981-16-9929-0_18

(ABO antigens, Rhesus {Rh} antigens, H substance, etc.) lead to major hemolytic reactions. Alloantibodies against platelets, plasma proteins, and leukocytes can lead to various non-hemolytic reactions. Apart from the most important ABO blood group systems, thirty-six other RBC group systems which are known in the medical literature (e.g., Lewis, Duffy, Kell, etc.) [3, 4].

18.3 Pretransfusion Testing

The pretransfusion tests consist of various processes and tests that must be performed before releasing any blood component and broadly consists of three tests: [5].

1. Typing

Typing is used to determine the ABO and Rh phenotype of the recipient using the antisera against A, B, and Rh antigens.

2. Screening

The screening process identifies any alloantibodies in the patient's serum against other RBC antigens which can cause hemolysis.

3. Cross-matching

Before the release of packed RBCs, the chosen donor Packed Red blood cells (PRBC) and the recipient's serum is mixed to find out any potential antibodies against the PRBC unit which is potentially chosen to be transfused.

In case of an emergency or life-threatening bleeding, an O type, and Rh-negative blood can be released without pretransfusion testing. This decision is taken by assessing the clinical situation on a case-by-case basis.

18.4 Blood Components

Blood components are separated by centrifugation. The various characteristics and storage conditions of different blood components are summarized in Table 18.1 [6, 7].

18.4.1 Modified Blood Products

Blood products are modified to decrease the adverse reactions of transfusion.

1. Leukocyte reduction

Leukocyte reduction decreases the risk of alloimmunization, febrile non-hemolytic reactions as well as transfusion-transmitted Cytomegalovirus transmission.

Table 18.1 Characteristics and storage conditions of different blood components

BLOOD COMPONENT	STORAGE temperature in degree celsius (°C)	VOLUME (ml)	CONTENT	CLINICAL RESPONSE	Indication
Whole blood	1–6 °C from 21 to 35 days	500 ml	RBCs, platelets, and plasma		Massive bleeding
PRBC	1–6 °C for 42 days	350 ml	RBCs	Increase of hemoglobin by ~1grams/decilitres (g/dL) by one unit of PRBC	Anemia, bleeding
FFP	−18 to −30 °C for a year Thawed plasma at 1–6 degrees for 5 days	200-300 ml	All plasma proteins and clotting factors	Increase coagulation factors by 2% 10-20 mg/kg dose increase any factor by 30%	Coagulopathy, Massive transfusion protocol
Platelets/RDP(from whole blood)	20–24 °C under a constant motion for 5–7 days under permanent motion	50-70 ml	Platelets	Increase platelet count by 5000/micro L	Thrombocytopenia
PLATELETS (from apheresis)	20–24 °C under constant motion for 5–7 days	200-400 ml	Platelets	Increase platelet counts by 30,000/microL	Thrombocytopenia
CRYOPRECIPITATE	−18 °C or colder for a year. After thawing, it can be stored at 20–24 °C for up to 6 hours.	10-20 ml	Fibrinogen factor, Von Willebrand factor (VWF), factor VIII, and FactorXIII	Increase fibrinogen by 50 mg/dl	**Disseminated intravascular coagulation** (DIC), hypofibrinogenemia,
GRANULOCYTES (by apheresis)	20–24 °C for 24 h	Variable	Variable	Increase fibrinogen by 50 mg/dl	Neutropenia

2. Irradiation

It inactivates T lymphocytes avoiding the ability to replicate in the marrow of the recipient and hence preventing graft versus host disease.

3. Washing

Washing gets rid of plasma proteins which decrease the risk of a severe allergic reaction to plasma components.

4. Pathogen inactivation

The lipid enveloped viruses are inactivated by solvent or detergent and nucleic acids are damaged hence making the blood product safer by eliminating infectious organisms like Zika virus, malaria, etc.

18.5 Blood Products Administration

Before administering the blood products there are a few practical points that are to be followed for safe transfusion [8, 9].

1. It is mandatory to take informed consent from the patient.
2. The patient should be identified and the unit of blood to be transfused is manually checked.
3. Adequate venous access should be taken before infusion. No pressure bags should be applied to push the blood.
4. The blood components should be transfused through a 170–270-micron filter.
5. If warming is required, the blood components should not be warmed more than 40 °C to avoid hemolysis.
6. Only 0.9 percent normal saline, albumin, or ABO compatible plasma should be administered through the same tubing. Avoid any medications or calcium-containing isotonic solutions.
7. Use of any premedication is not recommended before transfusion.
8. The patient should be monitored for any adverse effects or transfusion reactions.

18.6 Blood Transfusion Reactions and other Complications

The various transfusion reactions are classified in Table 18.2 [10–13].

18.7 Indications of Blood Transfusion in Oncology Patients

The indications of blood transfusion in oncology can be broadly divided into four scenarios [14, 15].

Table 18.2 Complications of Blood Product Transfusion

		Type of reaction	Cause/ etiology	Prevention
A	Acute transfusion reactions (within 24 h)			
I	Immunological reactions	Intravascular and extravascular hemolysis	Red cell incompatibility (antigen against RBCs)	Pre transfusion testing proper checking of products before transfusing
		Allergic reactions	Immunoglobulin E (IgE) antibody to donor plasma proteins	Washing
		Febrile non-hemolytic reactions (FNHTR)	Alloantibodies to donor white blood cells (WBC), platelets Cytokines in stored blood products	Leukocyte reduction
		Transfusion-associated acute lung injury (TRALI)	Human leukocyte antibodies (HLA) or HNA (human neutrophil antibodies) in plasma of the donor	Leukoreduction Avoid multiparous female donors Washing of RBCs
II	Non-immunological reactions	Transfusion-associated sepsis (TAS)	Bacterial contamination (mainly with platelets)	Visual inspection for bubbles or discoloration
		Hypotensive transfusion reaction	Angiotensin-converting enzyme (ACE) inhibitors prevent degradation of bradykinin in recipient blood leading to hypotension	Withdraw ACE inhibitors
		Air embolism	From central or intravenous (IV) cannulation	Administration of blood products with caution via IV accesses
		Transfusion-associated circulatory overload (TACO)	Fluid overload	Slow blood transfusion in high-risk patients
		Hypothermia	Rapid transfusion of cold or frozen blood	Employ warmer no more than 39 (°C)
		Hyperkalemia	Massive transfusion Potassium accumulation in stored blood	Washing Using fresh blood
		Citrate toxicity/ hypocalcemia	Rapid transfusion of citrated blood	Slow transfusion
		Non-immune hemolysis	Physical or chemical destruction of stored blood (heating, freezing)	Use fresh blood Avoid using warmers or excess freezing

(continued)

Table 18.2 (continued)

		Type of reaction	Cause/ etiology	Prevention
B	Delayed transfusion reactions			
I	Immunological reactions	Delayed hemolytic and serologic reactions	Immunoglobulin G (IgG) antibodies against red cell antigens	Transfuse compatible RBCs
		Transfusion-associated graft versus host disease (TA-GVHD)	Donor lymphocytes engraft in marrow and attack on host tissues	Irradiation
		Post transfusion purpura	Alloantibody against platelet antigens	–
II	Non-immunological reactions	Iron overload	Multiple chronic transfusions	–
		Transfusion transmitted diseases	Various blood transmitted infections	Pathogen activation Testing for diseases in blood products

1. A perioperative oncology patient with curative intent
2. Anemia in a patient with hematological or solid organ malignancy with curative intent
3. Acute massive hemorrhage/emergency
4. Chronic severe anemia in a patient with palliative intent of care

18.7.1 Causes of Anemia in Cancer Patients

1. Intra-tumoral bleeding, intraluminal bleeding, generalized bleeding
2. Anemia due to chronic inflammation, nutritional deficiencies
3. Hemolysis, Disseminated Intravascular Coagulation (DIC)
4. Hematological malignancy
5. Anemia due to chemotherapy and radiation therapy
6. Perioperative blood loss

18.7.2 Causes of Thrombocytopenia and Coagulopathy in Cancer Patients

1. Chemotherapy and radiotherapy
2. Hematological malignancy
3. DIC

18.8 Guidelines and Controversies

There are various guidelines on recommendations and indications of various blood components. The guidelines and recommendations are summarized in Table 18.3: [16–19].

18.9 Massive Blood Transfusion Protocols in Cancer Patients

Massive transfusion is defined as transfusion of ten or more units of PRBCs in 24 h or five or more units in 3 h or four units in one hour with ongoing blood loss of more than 150 ml/min [20, 21]. While the majority of guidelines for massive transfusion are based on the management of hemorrhage in the setting of acute trauma, oncology patients can have a massive hemorrhage in perioperative settings or after chemotherapy. A massive transfusion protocol (MTP) should be established locally as per blood bank capabilities. Setting an institutional protocol as well as goals of resuscitation for massive transfusion is important because it leads to various transfusion complications like hyperkalemia, coagulopathy, hypocalcemia, hypothermia, and metabolic alkalosis. The 1:1:1 ratio blood component (the damage control approach) is recommended in trauma patients although the exact ratio in oncology patients is still controversial [22]. The coagulation system should be frequently monitored during the activation of MTP. Various point-of-care viscoelastic tests like thromboelastography (TEG), Rotational thromboelastometry (ROTEM) can be used for the same [23].

Table 18.3 Guidelines for Blood Product Transfusion

Guidelines	Component	Recommendations
AABB practice guidelines for RBC transfusion and storage 2016	RBCs	Hospitalized stable anemia – 7 g/dL Patient undergoing major surgery- 8 g/dL Patient with history of cardiovascular disease- 8 g/dL Patient with ACS (acute coronary syndrome) or transfusion-dependent anemia- clinical decision
AABB practice guidelines for platelet transfusion 2015 ASCO guidelines for platelet transfusion in patients with cancer 2018	Platelets	Patient with hematological malignancy, undergoing stem cell transplant, solid tumors <10,000/microL Lumbar puncture, major surgery<50,000/microL Bone marrow aspiration and biopsies, insertion and removal of central venous catheters <20,000/microL
Evidence-based guidelines on plasma transfusion 2010	Plasma	Bleeding patients with coagulation deficiencies Massive transfusion protocol Guidelines based on strong recommendations are still not available

18.10 Alternatives to Transfusion

The term Patient Blood Management (PBM) was first used in 2005 by Professor James Isbister, an Australian hematologist. PBM is a multimodal, multidisciplinary patient-centered strategy aimed at minimizing the use of blood products and improving patient outcomes. PBM has three main objectives: (1) improving cell production in the body (2) minimizing blood loss (3) optimizing the tolerance of anemia by promoting maximum pulmonary and cardiac function and the use of a restrictive transfusion threshold. PBM aims to adopt alternative options to decrease transfusion requirements in patients [24].

There are various alternatives to minimize transfusions which will be summarized below.

1. **Modifications of transfusion Thresholds**
   The decision to transfuse is should be clinical and on a case-by-case basis. The restrictive strategy of transfusion is supported lately in the literature. The higher thresholds or triggers are supported for blood products by the American Association of Blood Banks (AABB).

   The threshold for RBCs is <7 g/dl and may be lower for patients with the acute coronary syndrome (ACS) but the latest randomized controlled trial suggests restricted therapy even for ACS patients.

   The threshold for platelets is less than 10,000 even for oncology patients as suggested by the American Society of Clinical Oncology (ASCO) guidelines.

   Plasma transfusion is guided by laboratory values of international normalized ratio (INR) > 1.5 though many point-of-care testing like visco-elastic tests may be used for a goal-directed approach.
2. **Improving cell production**
   Asymptomatic anemia due to chronic inflammatory processes in oncology patients can be corrected by Iron, folate, and vitamin B12 supplementation.

   Erythropoietin stimulating agents (ESAs) can be used in adjusted doses with caution in oncology patients to increase hemoglobin production. However, ESAs might have some side effects like increased thrombotic incidents, stroke, and tumor progression or recurrence. Whether ESAs cause tumor progression is still controversial. Granulocyte colony-stimulating factors may be offered to critically ill patients with neutropenia to increase leukocyte production.
3. **Minimizing blood loss**
   Antifibrinolytics (Epsilon-aminocaproic acid, tranexamic acid), desmopressin, recombinant coagulation factors (prothrombin complex concentrates), vitamin K and topical fibrin sealants are various pharmacological options that can be used instead of blood products to decrease blood loss. All these agents increase the risk of thrombosis. Cancer is a procoagulant state and there are no specific guidelines that mention specific indications, amount, and risk of thrombosis in oncology patients. The risk of thrombosis has to be balanced with the risk of bleeding before prescribing these agents.

4. **Maximizing tolerance of anemia**
   Tolerance of anemia can be increased by decreasing oxygen demand by sedation as well as supplementing oxygen. The concept of using synthetic blood for increasing oxygen-carrying capacity is very alluring but still under research and no product is available on market till now.
5. **Extracorporeal techniques of blood conservation**
   Various techniques can be used for intraoperative blood conservation if the patient undergoes some major surgical procedure with anticipated blood loss >1000 ml. Intraoperative cell salvage (ICS) is a method of separating, washing, and centrifuging (concentrating) blood aspirated from the surgical field and mixed with an anticoagulant. The result is a salvaged red blood cell (RBC) product with a Hemoglobin >17 g/dL. This autologous blood can be re-transfused. Postoperatively also the blood can be salvaged from drains and transfused. Acute normovolemic hemodilution (ANH) involves the removal of blood (shortly after induction of anesthesia, with the maintenance of normovolemia using crystalloid and/or colloid replacement fluid. The aim is to decrease hemoglobin (Hgb) concentration during the period when most surgical blood loss is occurring, thereby minimizing the effects of loss of red blood cells (RBCs) and then Reinfusing the patient's own fresh whole blood when it is needed during or shortly after the surgical procedure.
6. **Other Measures**
   Preoperative autologous blood donation, avoidance of hypothermia to avoid coagulopathy, and minimizing phlebotomies are other measures of minimizing blood loss and transfusions [25].

18.11 Conclusion

Cancer patients often require blood transfusion therapy during the course of their illness. The decision for transfusion of blood products should be based on correct physiological knowledge and principles, and an assessment of the patient's risk factors. Safe transfusion practices must be chosen to ensure good outcomes in these patients.

References

1. Highlights of transfusion medicine history [Internet]. Default. [cited 2021 Dec 2]. Available from: https://www.aabb.org/news-resources/resources/transfusion-medicine/highlights-of-transfusion-medicine-history
2. Blood safety and availability [Internet]. [cited 2021 Dec 2]. Available from: https://www.who.int/news-room/fact-sheets/detail/blood-safety-and-availability
3. Dean L. Blood transfusions and the immune system [Internet]. Blood Groups and Red Cell Antigens [Internet]. National Center for Biotechnology Information (US); 2005 [cited 2021 Dec 2]. Available from: https://www.ncbi.nlm.nih.gov/books/NBK2265/

4. Mitra R, Mishra N, Rath GP. Blood groups systems. Indian J Anaesth. 2014;58(5):524–8.
5. Pre-transfusion testing [Internet]. Professional education. [cited 2021 Dec 2]. Available from: https://professionaleducation.blood.ca/en/transfusion/clinical-guide/pre-transfusion-testing
6. Basu D, Kulkarni R. Overview of blood components and their preparation. Indian J Anaesth. 2014;58(5):529–37.
7. Garraud O, Tissot J-D. Blood and blood components: from similarities to differences. Front Med. 2018 Apr 9;5:84.
8. Doyle GR, McCutcheon JA. 8.7 Transfusion of blood and blood products. 2015 Nov 23 [cited 2021 Dec 2]; Available from: https://opentextbc.ca/clinicalskills/chapter/blood-and-blood-product-administration/
9. Ltd TIS. JPAC - Transfusion guidelines [Internet]. [cited 2021 Dec 2]. Available from: https://transfusionguidelines.org.uk/
10. Dasararaju R, Marques MB. Adverse effects of transfusion. Cancer Control J Moffitt Cancer Cent. 2015 Jan;22(1):16–25.
11. Sahu S, Hemlata null, Verma A. Adverse events related to blood transfusion. Indian J Anaesth. 2014 Sep;58(5):543–51.
12. Hatayama Y, Matsumoto S, Hamada E, Kojima N, Hara A, Hino N, et al. Analysis of acute transfusion reactions and their occurrence times. Yonago Acta Med. 2018 Mar 28;61(1):87–90.
13. Suddock JT, Crookston KP. Transfusion reactions. In: StatPearls [Internet]. Treasure Island (FL): StatPearls Publishing; 2021 [cited 2021 Dec 2]. Available from: http://www.ncbi.nlm.nih.gov/books/NBK482202/
14. Watkins T, Surowiecka MK, McCullough J. Transfusion indications for patients with cancer. Cancer Control J Moffitt Cancer Cent. 2015 Jan;22(1):38–46.
15. Blood Transfusions for People with Cancer [Internet]. [cited 2021 Dec 2]. Available from: https://www.cancer.org/treatment/treatments-and-side-effects/treatment-types/blood-transfusion-and-donation/what-are-transfusions.html
16. Carson JL, Guyatt G, Heddle NM, Grossman BJ, Cohn CS, Fung MK, et al. Clinical practice guidelines from the AABB: red blood cell transfusion thresholds and storage. JAMA. 2016 Nov 15;316(19):2025–35.
17. Kaufman RM, Djulbegovic B, Gernsheimer T, Kleinman S, Tinmouth AT, Capocelli KE, et al. Platelet transfusion: a clinical practice guideline from the AABB. Ann Intern Med. 2015 Feb 3;162(3):205–13.
18. Schiffer CA, Bohlke K, Delaney M, Hume H, Magdalinski AJ, McCullough JJ, et al. Platelet transfusion for patients with cancer: American Society of Clinical Oncology clinical practice guideline update. J Clin Oncol Off J Am Soc Clin Oncol. 2018 Jan 20;36(3):283–99.
19. Roback JD, Caldwell S, Carson J, Davenport R, Drew MJ, Eder A, et al. Evidence-based practice guidelines for plasma transfusion. Transfusion (Paris). 2010 Jun;50(6):1227–39.
20. Patil V, Shetmahajan M. Massive transfusion and massive transfusion protocol. Indian J Anaesth. 2014;58(5):590–5.
21. Jennings LK, Watson S. Massive Transfusion. [Updated 2021 Aug 30]. In: StatPearls [Internet]. Treasure Island (FL): StatPearls Publishing; 2022 Jan-. Available from: https://www.ncbi.nlm.nih.gov/books/NBK499929/.
22. Holcomb JB, Tilley BC, Baraniuk S, Fox EE, Wade CE, Podbielski JM, et al. Transfusion of plasma, platelets, and red blood cells in a 1:1:1 vs a 1:1:2 ratio and mortality in patients with severe trauma: the PROPPR randomized clinical trial. JAMA. 2015 Feb 3;313(5):471–82.
23. Shaydakov ME, Sigmon DF, Blebea J. Thromboelastography. In: StatPearls [internet]. Treasure Island (FL): StatPearls Publishing; 2021 [cited 2021 Dec 2]. Available from: http://www.ncbi.nlm.nih.gov/books/NBK537061/
24. Franchini M, Marano G, Veropalumbo E, Masiello F, Pati I, Candura F, et al. Patient blood management: a revolutionary approach to transfusion medicine. Blood Transfus. 2019 May;17(3):191–5.
25. Perioperative blood management: Strategies to minimize transfusions - UpToDate [Internet]. [cited 2021 Dec 2]. Available from: https://www.uptodate.com/contents/perioperative-blood-management-strategies-to-minimize-transfusions

Nutrition in Oncology ICU

19

Anju Gupta and Sarath Kumar

19.1 Introduction

Non communicable diseases estimated to be cause for 63% of deaths, in India and cancer was one of the leading cause [1]. The number of patients with cancer in India is 1.3 million for the year 2020 (as calculated from hospital-based cancer registries) and the common 5 leading sites are breast, lung, mouth, cervix uteri, and tongue [1]. Prevalence of Malnutrition in Oncology (PreMiO) study identified nutritional impairment of 51% in patients coming for first medical oncology visit [2].

Timely identification of malnutrition in patients with malignancy is important as it helps in early intervention by nutrition supplementation which improves patient outcome. These patients usually present with classic signs of malnutrition like weight loss along with wasting of muscle and fat, leading to higher mortality and morbidity. So, if such patients get admitted to critical care unit, early initiation of feeding, increased nutritional needs to meet the higher goals and demands, complications of feeding should be taken care well to have best patient outcome and survival.

19.2 Goals of Nutrition in Malignancy

As malignancy itself a catabolic state, which is aggravated during an acute critical illness, goals of nutrition lies in identifying patients at risk or who have already developed malnutrition and optimizing nutrition with appropriate intervention, promoting early recovery and shorter hospitalization, improves survival, wound

A. Gupta (✉) · S. Kumar
Department of Anaesthesiology, Pain and Critical Care, AIIMS, New Delhi, India

V. Kumar et al. (eds.), *Onco-critical Care*,
https://doi.org/10.1007/978-981-16-9929-0_19

healing, muscle mass, immune function, gastrointestinal function, skeletal growth in children [3].

19.3 Effect of Nutrition on Clinical and Oncological Outcomes

Critical illness is associated with weight loss, cachexia, sarcopenia, increased catabolic response, stress due to changes in hormonal milieu and cytokine storm (systemic inflammation) following major physiological insults [4] which is exacerbated during malignancy. This increased metabolic response is followed by tissue healing phase. Both these phases lead to increased nutritional requirements. Malignancy perse is a hypermetabolic state that further increases nutritional requirements. So, early initiation of nutritional therapy (enteral preferred than parenteral) reduces harmful deleterious effects of patients hyperdynamic responses, reduces complications, decreases mortality and the length of stay [5].

19.4 Importance of Nutrition in Malignancy

The risk of malnutrition and its severity are affected by the tumor type, stage of disease and the antineoplastic therapy used [6]. Intensivist face various challenges in replacing nutrition in critical ill patient due to unstable hemodynamics, poor acceptance of feeds, malabsorption, communication gap, aspiration risk etc. [7]. Patients with malignancy adds to the above risk due to increased demands, loss of weight, massive bowel resection, perioperative nil per oral situation and nutritive needs are poorly understood.

Nutrition is an important factor in determining tolerance, morbidity and outcomes associated with specific treatment for malignancy [4]. Old age, chronic illness (inflammation), loss of appetite, nausea and vomiting, decreased oral intake, fatigue, chronic starvation & less care by relatives, utilization by cancer cells, chemotherapy & vomiting, coexisting illness are usually associated with malignancy. So, identification of those with preexisting malnutrition and persons at risk of developing it is crucial so that nutritional interventions can be implemented to prevent developing or worsening of malnutrition in high risk cases [4] artificial nutrition is indicated if patients are not able to take orally [8] Cancer cachexia [9] defined by ongoing loss of skeletal muscle mass (with or without loss of fat mass) that cannot be fully reversed by conventional nutritional support and leads to progressive functional impairment.

19.5 Definition and Risk Assessment Tools for Nutrition

As per ASPEN guidelines nutrition is defined as "An acute, subacute or chronic state of nutrition, in which a combination of varying degrees of overnutrition or undernutrition with or without inflammatory activity have led to a change in body composition and diminished function".

Clinically nutritional risk can be assessed by acute weight loss, muscle bulk, skin thickness in posterior arm, BMI and lean body weight.

Various commonly used scoring systems that help in objective assessment of nutrition include

- Nutrition Risk Score (NRS 2002) [10], involves BMI, weight loss, dietary intake, and severity of illness scored from 0 to 3 with increasing severity
- NUTRIC Score [11], includes 6 variables -age, APACHE II, SOFA, comorbidities, IL 6 levels, days from hospital to ICU admission. High scores [6–9, 12] associated with worse clinical outcomes and low score (0–5) with low malnutrition risk

Some validated screening tools specific for oncological population [4], however less commonly used clinically:

- Malnutrition screening tool (MST), involving weight loss and change in appetite (both inpatients and outpatients)
- Malnutrition screening tool for cancer patients (MSTC), involves change in dietary intake, weight loss, performance status, BMI (only inpatients)
- Patient-Generated Subjective global assessment (PG-SGA) focusing weight, food intake, nutrition-related symptoms, function & activities
- Malnutrition Universal screening tool (MUST), includes BMI, unintentional weight loss >5%, reduced oral intake (only for inpatients).
- Mini Nutritional Assessment (MNA),
- Mini Nutritional Assessment—Short Form (MNA-SF)

None of the above scoring systems accurately assess patients the nutritional requirements [13], so nutritional requirements should always be individualized and patient specific nutritional plan is made.

Nutrition therapy: provision of either enteral nutrition (by enteral access device), and or parenteral nutrition (by central venous access).

Standard therapy: provision of intravenous fluids, no enteral or parenteral nutrition.

19.6 Components of Nutritional Therapy and Daily Requirements Calculation

Indirect calorimetry: The best method in determining energy needs in critically ill is Indirect calorimetry [14]. In its absence, weight-based equation of 25-30 kcal/kg/day used to determine energy requirements, 1.2–2 gm/kg/day for proteins can be used [15].

Resting energy expenditure(kcal/day) [16] = ((3.9×VO2) + (1.1×VCO2)-61)× 1440.

Substrate requirement for a normal adult patient:

- Carbohydrates—70% of caloric requirements.
- Proteins—1–1.5 gm/kg/day.
- Lipids—30% of energy requirements.
- Fluids—30 ml/kg + replacement of abnormal loses.
- Vitamins and micronutrients if needed.
- Note: requirements should be individualized.

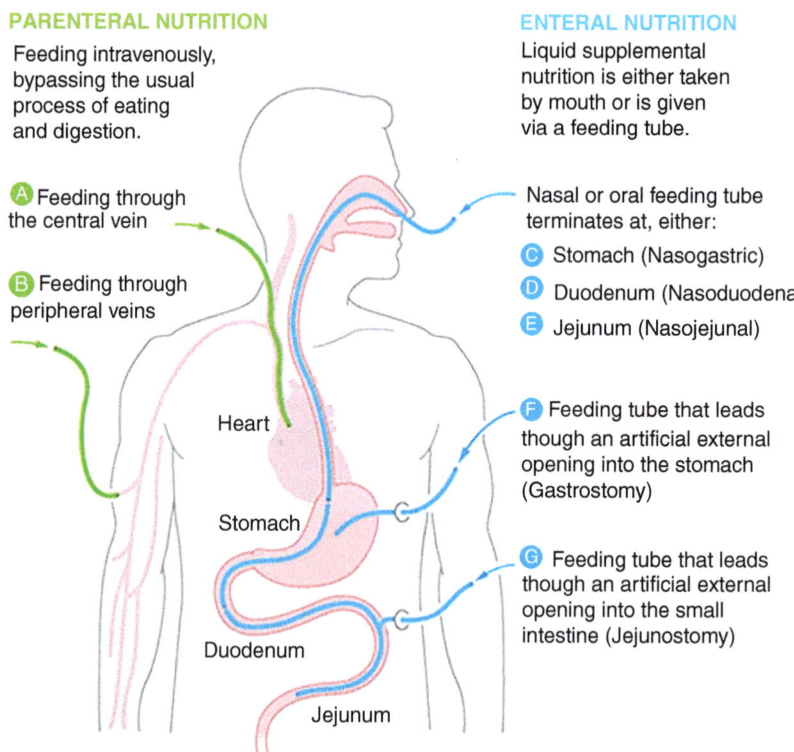

Fig. 19.1 Various routes of nutritional therapy [17]

19.7 Routes of Administration (Fig. 19.1)

19.7.1 Enteral Nutrition

Nutrition therapy in the form of early enteral nutrition is the preferred form and should be initiated within 24–48 h in a critically ill patient unless contraindicated [18].

Providing nutrition via a tube, catheter, or stoma delivering nutrients to GI tract distal to oral cavity.

Advantages:

- More physiological,
- less invasive and less costly.
- lower hyperglycemia risk and blunt hyperdynamic response.
- improved nitrogen balance,
- improved wound healing,
- maintenance of gut integrity.
- Reduced infective complications specifically central line associated infections and pneumonia.

Disadvantages:

- Requires functional GI tract.
- Increased risk of gut related complication.
- May need more time to reach goal calories.
- Avoided in patients with hemodynamic instability requiring high vasopressor support/inadequately resuscitated, severe diarrhea, and enteral nutritional intolerance.

Complications:

- Pulmonary aspiration.
- Diarrhea.
- Hyper/hypoglycemia.
- Dyselectrolytemia.
- Hyperhydration.
- Dumping syndrome.
- Refeeding syndrome.

Even though high fat/low carbohydrate formulations reduce co2 production, still it's not recommended as per recent study results.

Dosing of enteral nutrition-

- Energy needs: http://www.surgicalcriticalcare.net/Guidelines/ICU%20nutrition%202017.pdf – couldnt quote reference

  - Normal adult: 25 kcal/kg/day.
  - Cancer: Inactive, non ambulatory: 25–30.
    Weight gain, nutritional repletion: 30–35.
    Hypermetabolic, stressed: 35
- Protein needs:
  - Normal adult: 0.8–1.2 gm/kg/day.
  - Cancer: 1.2–2 gm/kg/day.

Composition of enteral nutrition:

- Caloric density: 1–2 kcal/L of feeding solution.
- Osmolality: 280–1100 mosm/kg H2O.
- Protein: 35–40 gm/L of feeding solution.
- Lipids: long chain triglycerides derived from vegetable oil.
- Fiber content.

The enteral feed need to be modified as per need (Table 19.1).

Key points in enteral nutrition:

- Polymeric feeds (whole protein) and Soluble fiber are preferred
- Fluid restricted, calorically dense formulations considered in acute respiratory failure without hypernatremia
- No change in protein intake in case of AKI
- Periodic glucose monitoring in diabetic patients
- Standard enteral formulations should be used in acute and chronic liver disease

Tolerance of enteral nutrition should be monitored daily (passage of flatus, stool, absence of abdominal pain or abdominal distension), and avoid inappropriate cessation of enteral nutrition. Withhold enteral feeds in case of vomiting, abdominal

Table 19.1 Commercially prepared enteral feeds [19]

Polymeric feeds	Elemental feeds	Disease specific feeds
• Suitable for those with a normal or near normally functioning bowel. • Contain whole protein as the nitrogen source—Most provide 500 g/l of nitrogen and energy of 1 kcal/ml, • Commonly used commercial feeds are now clinically lactose and gluten-free and contain enough vitamins, trace elements, and essential fatty acids to prevent deficiencies.	• Contain either pure amino acids or predigested protein and provide oligopeptides and amino acids. • Taste unpleasant and are relatively expensive, • Unless there is extensive impairment of gastrointestinal digestive and absorptive functions, they appear to offer little additional benefit.	• Used in severely ill patients, such as those with multiple burns or trauma, respiratory failure, advanced cirrhosis, or acute renal failure. • Renal specific diets can be useful in chronic renal failure. • Little part in long term enteral nutrition.

Table 19.2 Gastrostomy versus nasogastric tube versus oral support

	Oral feeding	Nasogastric feeding	Gastrostomy
Duration of feeding	Longer	Shorter	Longer (>4 weeks)
Indications	Early stages of any systemic malignancies, no risk of aspiration	Any esophageal or head and neck malignancy with reduced mouth opening or difficulty in swallowing,	Esophageal stenosis, after esophageal resections
Advantages	More physiological Less risk of infection Less invasive	Less invasive compared to gastrostomy, easy to insert, useful in intubated patients	Useful in intubated patients, less risk of aspiration, less tube displacement
Disadvantages	Loss of taste, not possible in intubated patients, risk of aspiration if GCS poor	Tip of tube position to be confirmed every time after placement, prone for tube blockade, mucositis, ulceration, esophagitis or esophageal perforation	High cost [22], invasive technique, need special person for insertion, risk of infection Need trained care giver

distension, high NG output, high gastric residual volume, abdominal radiographs suggestive of obstruction.

Trophic feeding [20] (10–20 kcal/hr. or up to 500 kcal/day) can be tried in case of bowel intolerance instead of stopping enteral feeds completely.

Absolute contraindications for enteral feeds include intestinal perforation, ischemia and obstruction.

Gastric residual volume, not a part of routine care to monitor enteral nutrition (either for initiation or for stopping) [21]. In patients with high risk of aspiration-post pyloric enteral feeding, continuous infusion (preferred than intermittent boluses), head end elevation, prokinetic agents (metoclopramide or erythromycin) can be helpful in such situations. The feed can be given via oral cavity, nasogastric tube and gastrostomy. (Table 19.2).

Other modes of enteral nutrition include: nasogastric, naso jejunal, percutaneous endoscopic gastrostomy, percutaneous endoscopic jejunostomy, radiologically inserted gastrostomy, surgical gastrostomy/jejunostomy.

19.8 Parenteral Nutrition

Providing nutrition via central or peripheral intravenous access.

Indications:

- Short term: interactable vomiting,
  - non-compliant to enteral nutrition.
- Long term: inflammatory bowel resection,
  - radiation enteritis,

– chronic malabsorption.

Components: dextrose, amino acids (50% essential & 50% non-essential/semi essential amino acids), lipids, electrolytes, minerals and trace elements [23]. Composition varies with various preparation.

Complications: catheter related infections, carbohydrate related (hyperglycemia, fatty liver), lipid related (oxidation induced cell injury), GI complications (mucosal atrophy & acalculous cholecystitis), volume overload, and other metabolic complications.

Refeeding syndrome: can occur in both enteral and parenteral nutrition. Patients who had very little nutritional intake for >5 days are at risk of refeeding syndrome [23]. Metabolic derangements and clinical symptoms due to fluid shifts and electrolyte imbalance in already malnourished patient. Characterized by low phosphate, low magnesium, low potassium, low sodium deranged sugars and water imbalance. Can also be associated with respiratory, cardiac, and neuromuscular complications. NICE guidelines recommend commencing nutritional support at 50% of estimated energy requirements for 2 days in patients at risk of refeeding syndrome, thereafter increasing by 200–400 kcal every day [24] and close monitoring of electrolytes needed.

19.8.1 Assessment of Adequacy of Nutrition

Commonly assessed *by nutrition-related health indicators, nutritional intake, and energy expenditure* [25]. Nutrition-related health indicators include body mass index (BMI) and serum levels of albumin, prealbumin, hemoglobin, magnesium, and phosphorus. Serum albumin is most commonly used substance to assess protein nutritional status. Low levels of albumin reflects both nutritional status and prolonged physiological stress associated with the critical illness. Conversely, however, Gluck [26] found that albumin levels were not predictive of weaning success.

Nutritional adequacy [27] was defined as energy intake (kilocalories received on the basis of physician' orders) divided by energy required (determined by indirect calorimetry or physician orders).

Resting energy demand usually calculated by Harris-Benedict equation based on weight, height and age of the patient. But these formulas have unpredictable errors when used to estimate energy demand in individual subjects [28]. The recommended method of measurement of resting energy expenditure in critically ill patients is indirect calorimetry [28].

19.9 Role of Immunotherapy in Malignancy

Immunotherapy was assumed to be crucial in fighting against cancer [29]. Recent systematic review and meta-analysis demonstrated [30] immunonutrition to improve outcome in surgical patients in perioperative period, by reducing postoperative infectious complications (moderate quality of evidence) and shortens the period of hospitalization (low quality) but does not reduce all-cause mortality. Formulas containing arginine and/or glutamine, ω-3 fatty acids, and ribonucleic acids modulate inflammatory and immune response in these patients [29]. Further research with larger patient samples and better study designs are still needed to give valuable conclusion.

19.10 Specific Concerns in Critically Ill Oncological Patients

19.10.1 Perioperative Period in Gastrointestinal and Head & Neck Malignancy

Patients with GI and head & neck malignancies are high risk of malnutrition because of dysphagia, odynophagia, reduced mouth opening, recurrent vomiting, malabsorption, loss of appetite, radiotherapy treatment like painful mucositis, altered taste, etc.

Enteral nutrition being first choice, feeding tube placement necessary prophylactically with inadequate oral intake [31]. Preoperative nutritional support in Head and Neck malignancy for 7 days decreases postoperative complications by approximately 10% in malnourished patients with weight loss of >10% [32].

In preoperative period, carbohydrate loading is safer, fasting can be limited to 6 h for solids and 2 h for liquids in patients without risk factors [33]. Early initiation of feeding recommended in postop period whenever possible [9].

Fluid and sodium intake need to be monitored in abdominal malignancies (causing peritoneal carcinomatosis), with obstruction or ascites, as excess sodium intake in such cases leads to fluid overload [8].

Hematopoietic stem cell transplant- There is high risk for malnutrition on HSCT treatment [34]. Immunonutrients did not show significant beneficial effects and therefore are not recommended for routine use. Neutropenic diets did not show a benefit over safe food handling approaches [34].

Feeding tube placement with thrombocytopenia(4)- thrombocytopenia(<1,50,000/μL) a common complication in critically ill patients with cancer either due to disease process or due to chemotherapy. It was earlier assumed invasive feeding tube access has the risk of increased bleeding tendencies. But few recent studies [35] concluded critically ill patients with cancer and thrombocytopenia are not at increased risk for bleeding complications after feeding tube placement than those without thrombocytopenia.

19.11 Other Special Conditions

- ARDS—trophic feeds in first week of hospitalization.

- AKI—standard ICU recommendations of protein 1.2–2 gm/kg and 25-30 kcal/kg/day followed (if receiving HD or CRRT increased protein up to maximum of 2.5 gm/kg/day.
- Hepatic failure—avoid restricting protein in liver failure, energy and supplementation based on dry weight rather than actual weight.
- Trauma—high protein polymeric diet preferably within 24–48 h of injury, immune modulating formulations (arginine) can be considered.
- TBI—early enteral feeding preferred
- Open abdomen—in absence of bowel injury, early enteral feeding preferred.
- Burns—protein of 1.5–2 gm/kg/day, early enteral feeding (4–6 h of injury).
- Severe sepsis—early enteral nutrition within 24–48 h of diagnosis, as soon as resuscitation complete and hemodynamically stable,
- Severe pancreatitis—enteral preferred over parenteral
- Hemodynamic instability—withhold till the patient is fully resuscitated, Can be continued with stable low dose vasopressors

19.12 Summary of Other Key Recommendations as per ASPEN Guidelines [18]

- Immune modulating enteral formulations should not be routinely used in medical ICU (can be considered in Surgical ICU patients)
- No recommendations for routine use of probiotic in ICU patients
- Antioxidant vitamins (C & E) and trace minerals (selenium, zinc, copper) not recommended routinely, but may improve outcome in burns, trauma, and critical illness with mechanical ventilation.
- Enteral or parenteral glutamine supplementation not recommended routinely
- In patients with low nutritional risk, exclusive parenteral nutrition can be withheld or delayed for first 7 days of ICU admission if early enteral nutrition not feasible or inability to maintain adequate oral intake in ICU
- In patients with high or low nutritional risk (enteral alone provides <60% of energy & protein requirements), supplemental parenteral nutrition considered after 7–10 days of ICU admission.
- In patients with high nutritional risk, exclusive parenteral nutrition initiated as soon as possible.

19.13 Conclusion

Malnutrition adversely affects outcome by increasing duration of mechanical ventilation, infection rates, gastric atrophy, growth reduction in children. Even though supplemental nutrition in critically ill patient with malignancy, may not reverse malnutrition, it may prevent progression and improve quality of life and survival.

References

1. Mathur P, Sathishkumar K, Chaturvedi M, Das P, Sudarshan KL, Santhappan S, et al. Cancer Statistics, 2020: report from national cancer registry programme, India. JCO Glob Oncol [Internet]. 2020 Jul 16 [cited 2021 Mar 7];6. Available from: https://www.ncbi.nlm.nih.gov/pmc/articles/PMC7392737/
2. Muscaritoli M, Lucia S, Farcomeni A, Lorusso V, Saracino V, Barone C, et al. Prevalence of malnutrition in patients at first medical oncology visit: the PreMiO study. Oncotarget. 2017 Aug 10;8(45):79884–96.
3. Allison SP. What is the goal of nutrition in the intensive care unit? In: Cynober L, Moore FA, editors. Nestlé nutrition workshop series: clinical & performance program [Internet]. Basel: KARGER; 2003 [cited 2021 Feb 14]. p. 119–32. Available from: https://www.karger.com/Article/FullText/72751
4. Lach. Nutrition support for critically Ill patients with cancer - Lach - 2017 - nutrition in clinical practice - Wiley Online Library [Internet]. [cited 2021 Jan 31]. Available from: https://onlinelibrary.wiley.com/doi/abs/10.1177/0884533617712488
5. Seron-Arbeloa C, Zamora-Elson M, Labarta-Monzon L, Mallor-Bonet T. Enteral nutrition in critical care. J Clin Med Res. 2013 Feb;5(1):1–11.
6. Davies M. Nutritional screening and assessment in cancer-associated malnutrition. Eur J Oncol Nurs. 2005 Jan 1;9:S64–73.
7. Mehta Y, Sunavala JD, Zirpe K, Tyagi N, Garg S, Sinha S, et al. Practice guidelines for nutrition in critically ill patients: a relook for Indian scenario. Indian J Crit Care Med Peer-Rev Off Publ Indian Soc Crit Care Med. 2018 Apr;22(4):263–73.
8. Arends J, Bachmann P, Baracos V, Barthelemy N, Bertz H, Bozzetti F, et al. ESPEN guidelines on nutrition in cancer patients. Clin Nutr Edinb Scotl. 2017 Feb;36(1):11–48.
9. Perioperative nutrition: Recommendations from the ESPEN expert group | Elsevier Enhanced Reader [Internet]. [cited 2021 Mar 14]. Available from: https://reader.elsevier.com/reader/sd/pii/S0261561420301795?token=AAED95E54069AAC948D45CE385A55B3364E9DB20C8BE93D843D44E422F298CF3CC5213D02CF3CBC9DF1CB485F8C56AA0
10. Kondrup J, Allison SP, Elia M, Vellas B, Plauth M. Educational and clinical practice committee, European Society of Parenteral and Enteral Nutrition (ESPEN). ESPEN guidelines for nutrition screening 2002. Clin Nutr Edinb Scotl. 2003 Aug;22(4):415–21.
11. Heyland DK, Dhaliwal R, Jiang X, Day AG. Identifying critically ill patients who benefit the most from nutrition therapy: the development and initial validation of a novel risk assessment tool. Crit Care Lond Engl. 2011;15(6):R268.
12. ASPEN | Definitions [Internet]. [cited 2021 Mar 7]. Available from: https://www.nutritioncare.org/Guidelines_and_Clinical_Resources/Toolkits/Malnutrition_Toolkit/Definitions/
13. Reber E, Gomes F, Vasiloglou MF, Schuetz P, Stanga Z. Nutritional risk screening and assessment. J Clin Med [Internet]. 2019 Jul 20 [cited 2021 Mar 14];8(7). Available from: https://www.ncbi.nlm.nih.gov/pmc/articles/PMC6679209/
14. Cooney RN, Frankenfield DC. Determining energy needs in critically ill patients: equations or indirect calorimeters. Curr Opin Crit Care. 2012 Apr;18(2):174–7.
15. Mtaweh H, Tuira L, Floh AA, Parshuram CS. Indirect calorimetry: history, technology, and application. Front Pediatr [Internet]. 2018 Sep 19 [cited 2021 Mar 7];6. Available from: https://www.ncbi.nlm.nih.gov/pmc/articles/PMC6157446/
16. Kagan I, Zusman O, Bendavid I, Theilla M, Cohen J, Singer P. Validation of carbon dioxide production (VCO2) as a tool to calculate resting energy expenditure (REE) in mechanically ventilated critically ill patients: a retrospective observational study. Crit Care. 2018 Dec;22(1):186.
17. Feeding methods – healthcare nutrition council [Internet]. [cited 2021 Mar 7]. Available from: https://healthcarenutrition.org/methods-of-nutrition/
18. McClave SA, Taylor BE, Martindale RG, Warren MM, Johnson DR, Braunschweig C, et al. Guidelines for the provision and assessment of nutrition support therapy in the adult critically

ill patient: Society of Critical Care Medicine (SCCM) and American Society for Parenteral and Enteral Nutrition (a.S.P.E.N.). JPEN J Parenter Enteral Nutr. 2016 Feb;40(2):159–211.
19. Pearce CB, Duncan HD. Enteral feeding. Nasogastric, nasojejunal, percutaneous endoscopic gastrostomy, or jejunostomy: its indications and limitations. Postgrad Med J. 2002 Apr 1;78(918):198–204.
20. Phan KA, Dux CM, Osland EJ, Reade MC. Effect of hypocaloric normoprotein or trophic feeding versus target full enteral feeding on patient outcomes in critically ill adults: a systematic review. Anaesth Intensive Care. 2017 Nov;45(6):663–75.
21. Yasuda H, Kondo N, Yamamoto R, Asami S, Abe T, Tsujimoto H, et al. Monitoring of gastric residual volume during enteral nutrition. Cochrane Database Syst Rev [Internet]. 2019 May 14 [cited 2021 Mar 7];2019(5). Available from: https://www.ncbi.nlm.nih.gov/pmc/articles/PMC6514529/
22. Jr CAG, Andriolo RB, Bennett C, Lustosa SA, Matos D, Waisberg DR, et al. Percutaneous endoscopic gastrostomy versus nasogastric tube feeding for adults with swallowing disturbances. Cochrane Database Syst Rev [Internet]. 2015 [cited 2021 Mar 7];(5). Available from: https://www.cochranelibrary.com/cdsr/doi/10.1002/14651858.CD008096.pub4/full
23. Macdonald K, Page K, Brown L, Bryden D. Parenteral nutrition in critical care. Contin Educ Anaesth Crit Care Pain. 2013 Feb 1;13(1):1–5.
24. Mehanna HM, Moledina J, Travis J. Refeeding syndrome: what it is, and how to prevent and treat it. BMJ. 2008 Jun 28;336(7659):1495–8.
25. Higgins PA, Daly BJ, Lipson AR, Guo S-E. Assessing nutritional status in chronically critically ill adult patients. Am J Crit Care. 2006 Mar;15(2):166–77.
26. Gluck EH. Predicting eventual success or failure to wean in patients receiving long-term mechanical ventilation. Chest. 1996 Oct;110(4):1018–24.
27. McClave SA, Lowen CC, Kleber MJ, Nicholson JF, Jimmerson SC, McConnell JW, et al. Are patients fed appropriately according to their caloric requirements? JPEN J Parenter Enteral Nutr. 1998 Dec;22(6):375–81.
28. Flancbaum L, Choban PS, Sambucco S, Verducci J, Burge JC. Comparison of indirect calorimetry, the Fick method, and prediction equations in estimating the energy requirements of critically ill patients. Am J Clin Nutr. 1999 Mar;69(3):461–6.
29. Prieto I, Montemuiño S, Luna J, de Torres MV, Amaya E. The role of immunonutritional support in cancer treatment: current evidence. Clin Nutr. 2017 Dec 1;36(6):1457–64.
30. Yu K, Zheng X, Wang G, Liu M, Li Y, Yu P, et al. Immunonutrition vs standard nutrition for cancer patients: a systematic review and meta-analysis (part 1). J Parenter Enter Nutr. 2020;44(5):742–67.
31. Evidence-Based Support for Nutrition Therapy in Head and Neck Cancer | SpringerLink [Internet]. [cited 2021 Mar 14]. Available from: https://link.springer.com/article/10.1007/s40137-017-0179-0
32. Bertrand PC, Piquet M-A, Bordier I, Monnier P, Roulet M. Preoperative nutritional support at home in head and neck cancer patients: from nutritional benefits to the prevention of the alcohol withdrawal syndrome. Curr Opin Clin Nutr Metab Care. 2002 Jul;5(4):435–40.
33. Melloul E, Lassen K, Roulin D, Grass F, Perinel J, Adham M, et al. Guidelines for perioperative Care for Pancreatoduodenectomy: enhanced recovery after surgery (ERAS) recommendations 2019. World J Surg. 2020 Jul 1;44(7):2056–84.
34. Baumgartner A, Schuetz P. Nutritional Support. In: Carreras E, Dufour C, Mohty M, Kröger N, editors. The EBMT handbook: hematopoietic stem cell transplantation and cellular therapies [Internet]. 7th ed. Cham (CH): Springer; 2019 [cited 2021 Mar 15]. Available from: http://www.ncbi.nlm.nih.gov/books/NBK553969/
35. Bleeding associated with feeding tube placement in critically ill oncology patients with thrombocytopenia - Patel - 2016 - nutrition in clinical practice - Wiley Online Library [Internet]. [cited 2021 Mar 15]. Available from: https://aspenjournals.onlinelibrary.wiley.com/doi/abs/10.1177/0884533615598964

Critical Care Issues in Post Stem Cell Transplant Patient

20

Vinod Sharma and Atul Sharma

20.1 Introduction

Hematopoietic stem cell transplant (HSCT) remains a viable life saving therapeutic option in the management of the various malignant (hematologic, solid), and non-malignant disorders (bone marrow failures, storage disorders, immune disorders). The donor hematopoietic stem cells and progenitor cells help in the reconstitution of the two important biological functions: hematopoiesis (high dose chemotherapy-induced myeloablation) and the immune function (graft versus host disease, GVHD). The sources of stem cells are peripheral blood (most common), bone marrow, and umbilical cord. The two major forms of transplant include Autologous (use of own stem cells) and Allogenic (use of stem cells from healthy related or unrelated donors) [1]. The most common reason for autologous transplants and allogeneic transplants worldwide are multiple myeloma and acute myeloid leukemia respectively [2]. Globally the most common form of transplant is autologous. Approximately 50% of allogeneic transplant donors are unrelated matched donors followed by a matched related donor, other relatives. Unrelated donor transplants using cord blood are only sizeable. Finding a donor for an allogenic transplant remained a major issue in the past. However, with the development of successful strategies using unrelated donor, haploidentical and umbilical blood as a donor source, the donor needs being addressed increasingly.

Increased availability of transplant services, use of reduced-intensity regimens (RIC; elderly, co-morbidities), and haploidentical transplant are some of the various contributing factors. Critical care remains an integral part of hematological oncology care because of associated life-threatening complications [3, 4]. From the initial

V. Sharma · A. Sharma (✉)
Department of Medical Oncology, Dr B R A Irch, All India Institute of Medical Sciences, New Delhi, New Delhi, India
e-mail: Atul.sharma@aiims.edu

V. Kumar et al. (eds.), *Onco-critical Care*,
https://doi.org/10.1007/978-981-16-9929-0_20

clinical successful transplant way back in the 1970s, we have moved a lot in the last half-century. In a report by WBMT (Worldwide Network for Blood and Marrow Transplantation, 2016) report, 1.3 million transplants had happened in 87 countries, with a rising rate of 7% per year (84,000/year). Nearly half of them were allogenic and unrelated HSCT [5]. With the increased availability of transplant services across the world, the number of the patient requiring critical care are rising day by day. Transplant is a major intervention event and put a patient at significant risk of both acute and long term life-threatening complications with frequent visit to the critical care unit. Most of the case burden is from allogenic and unrelated hematopoietic transplants. The use of the hematopoietic transplant comorbidity index helps in predicting and counseling the patient and relatives about the transplant-related mortality (TRM) and post-transplant outcome [6].

20.2 Pathophysiology and Burden of ICU Care

Transplant patients are at increased risk of infectious and non-infectious complications (organ dysfunction) [7]. Allogenic transplant forms the most common cohort of the patient who requires intensive care. HSCT-related therapies affect both the innate and adaptive immunity [8]. The two major factors responsible for high TRM and morbidity are delivery of high-dose chemotherapy and organ damage due to alloimmunization (donor immune cells). The latter is unique to allogeneic transplants. The adverse effects of high dose chemotherapy are myeloablation (neutropenia, lymphopenia, monocytopenia, and thrombocytopenia) which resolves with marrow recovery, mucosal barrier disruption (mucositis), and change in body microbiome system (lung, gut, etc). In allogeneic HSCT, the picture is further complicated by donor T cell-mediated alloimmunization, tissue injury, use of immune suppressants leading to prolonged myelosuppression. These key factors differentiate transplant patients from other ICU patients who lack myelosuppression and immune-mediated organ injury. As a result, allogeneic HSCT carries a substantially increased risk of TRM and morbidity compared to autologous transplants. The altered microbiota is a risk factor for increased TRM post allogenic transplant [9]. The use of RIC has helped in the reduction of TRM though with increased risk of relapse [10, 11].

The existing literature suggests variable ICU admission rates (range, 9–57%, average 20%) [12]. One out of every 4–5 patients planned for an allogenic transplant need intensive care. Nearly half of these succumb despite aggressive management. Observational studies suggest a higher rate of ICU admission with allogenic (matched; umbilical cord, 57%) compared to autologous transplant (6%) [13, 14].

20.3 Etiology of Causes Requiring ICU Care

The life-threatening complications can happen anytime from the start of the conditioning regimen to few years after HSCT. There are two subcategories of life-threatening complications: Infectious and non-infectious complications. These complications follow a chronological pattern. Infections remain the most common reasons for non-relapse mortality and morbidity. The transplant time is divided into three phases: peri-transplant (conditioning regimen, pre-engraftment), post engraftment, and late phase. These phases predisposes to different characteristic infectious and non-infectious complications (Tables 20.1 and 20.2). This knowledge helps physicians in the diagnosis and management of these complications. The

Table 20.1 Timeline of different infectious agents requiring ICU care following allogenic HSCT

	Conditioning regimen (−7 to day 0), Pre-Engraftment (day 1–30)	Post Engraftment (day 30–60)	Late phase (Post 60 days)
Bacterial	Gram Negative bacilli, Gram positive organisms, GIT streptococcal bacilli	Gram Negative bacilli, Encapsulated bacteria	Gram Negative bacilli, Encapsulated bacteria
Viral	HSV, RSV, BKV, Enteric	HSV, CMV, RSV, BKV virus	HSV, CMV, VZV, PTLD
Fungal	Aspergillus, Candida	Aspergillus, Candida, PCP	Aspergillus, PCP

HSV herpes simplex virus, *RSV* Respiratory syncytial virus, *BK* Polyomavirus hominis 1, *CMV* Cytomegalovirus, *VZV* Varicella Zoster Virus, *PTLD* Post-transplant lymphoproliferative disorder, *RSV* Respiratory syncytial virus, *virus* Enteric viruses (Adenovirus, Enterovirus, Norovirus, Hepatovirus, Rotavirus), *PCP* Pneumocystis pneumonia

Table 20.2 Timeline of different non-infectious agents requiring ICU care following allogenic HSCT

	Pre-Engraftment (day 1 to up-to 30 days)	Post Engraftment (day 30–60)	Late phase (Post 60 days)
All organs	aGVHD, Hemorrhage, drug toxicity, relapse	aGVHD, Hemorrhage, drug toxicity, Relapse, Iron overload	aGVHD, CGVHD, Drug toxicity, Disease relapse, Iron excess
Pulmonary	DAH, Capillary leak syndrome	DAH, IPS, Bronchiolitis, COP	IPS, Bronchiolitis, COP
Cardiac	Cardiac dysfunction, Pericardial effusion, Arrhythmia	Arrhythmia, CAD, CVD	Cardiac edema, CAD, CVD
Neurologic	Seizure, PRES, Metabolic encephalopathy	Seizure, PRES, Metabolic encephalopathy	Leukoencephalopathy
Hepatic	VOD, Transaminitis	VOD	–
Renal	ATN, septic AKI	ATN, Thrombotic microangiopathy, Calcineurin inhibitors	Thrombotic microangiopathy, Calcineurin inhibitors

PRES posterior reversible encephalopathy syndrome, *ATN* acute tubular necrosis, *AKI* acute kidney injury, *aGVHD* acute graft versus host disease, *cGVHD* chronic graft versus host disease, *DAH* diffuse alveolar hemorrhage, *VOD* veno occlusive disease, *COP* cryptogenic organized pneumonia, *CVD* cerebrovascular disease, *CAD* coronary artery disease, *IPS* idiopathic pulmonary syndrome

peri-transplant period is characterized by neutropenia and mucosal barrier breaks, providing a suitable environment to microorganism to invade and infect the human body. The most common infections during this time period are bacterial and candidal infections, less common ones are Aspergillus. Both autologous and allogeneic transplants face similar infection patterns during the peri-transplant period. The empirical anti-bacterial strategy remains the same in both types of transplant. However, post engraftment the allogeneic transplant patient is at higher risk of developing infection including bacteremia, invasive aspergillus, and cytomegalovirus (CMV) viremia [15]. Post allogeneic transplant immune recovery occurs in a phased manner, the first to recover is innate immunity followed by cell-mediated and later humoral immunity [16]. The recovery of cell-mediated immunity is influenced by GVHD and immune suppressants. This in-turn defines the infections during the post engraftment period (CMV, Aspergillus, Pneumocystis jiroveci—PCP). During the late phase of allogeneic HSCT, the common infection is viral, tuberculosis, and encapsulated bacteria (Haemophilus influenza, streptococcus pneumonia) [15].

20.4 Reasons for ICU Care

The primary purpose of ICU care is to support and closely monitor the deranged organ till recovery. The common forms include hemodynamic support (vasopressors), respiratory support (mechanical ventilation, non-invasive ventilation), renal support—(renal replacement therapies, dialysis), fluid resuscitation, electrolytes, etc. (Table 20.3). The most common reason are an acute respiratory failure (60%) and septic shock (Table 20.4).

20.4.1 Neutropenic Fever, Sepsis, and Septic Shock

Neutropenia (2–3 weeks) is the universal phenomenon during the transplant. It puts patients at significant risk of blood-borne bacterial sepsis, fungal infections, septic shock, and mortality. Neutropenia is frequently associated with febrile neutropenia (60–80%) [17]. The rate of septic shock, severe sepsis, and sepsis in patients with neutropenic fever is 5–10, 20–30, and >50% respectively [18]. Blood-borne infections are more common in recipients of allogenic (20–50%) than autologous transplant (5–10%) [19]. They are frequent in the pre-engraftment period and are an important cause of TRM and morbidity. Both gram negative bacilli (GNB) and gram positive cocci (GPC) infections are prevalent. However, the relative

Table 20.3 Use of various modalities in ICU care

Mechanical ventilation	20–70%
Non-invasive ventilation	30–40%
Vasopressors agents	50–70%
Renal Replacement Therapy	20–40%

Table 20.4 Reasons for ICU admission and associated etiology

Common		Less common	
Syndromes	Causes	Syndromes	Causes
Acute respiratory failure (60%)	Pulmonary hemorrhage, Infections (bacterial, fungal, viral), Fluid overload, Acute cardiac failure, Intra-alveolar hemorrhage	Cardiac dysfunction	Arrythmia, Fluid overload, pericardial effusion, tamponade, myocardial infarction
Acute Kidney Injury	Sepsis, Shock, Nephrotoxic drugs (vancomycin, amphotericin, foscarnet, acyclovir, aminoglycosides, cyclosporine, engraftment syndrome, VOD, Thrombotic angiopathy	Neurological failure	PRESS, Drugs (cyclosporine, beta-lactams, carbapenems, infection, hemorrhage, infarct), Metabolic disturbance, infections, radiologic abnormalities, intracranial hemorrhage
Severe sepsis, Septic shock	Gram negative bacilli, Fungal, Viral	Liver dysfunction	VOD, Hepatitis (CMV, EBV, Hepatitis A, B, C, E)

VOD veno-occlusive disorders, *PRESS* posterior reversible encephalopathy syndrome, *CMV* cytomegalovirus, *EBV* Epstein bar virus

proportion varies significantly around the world [20]. The former remains the major health concern. Aggressive workup to detect the source of infection and timely administration of empirical antibiotics is the key. Different antibiotic strategies (escalation, de-escalation) are part of management based on institutional and physician preferences [7]. The empirical antibiotic of choice is guided by local culture positivity reports and sensitivity, hemodynamic status at presentation, presence of specific signs and symptoms (mucositis, seizures, neck rigidity), past infection, colonization with resistant bacteria. The primary aim is to target commonly encountered bacteria that are associated with life-threatening sepsis and mortality. The commonly used drugs active against pseudomonas are cefoperazone and sulbactam, ceftazidime, carbapenems [21]. Non-specific use of aminoglycosides is not recommended. Indications for coverage of gram-positive bacteria include the presence of hemodynamic instability, pneumonia, and severe mucositis. The risk factors for bloodstream infection and pneumonia during transplant are male gender, acute myeloid leukemia, unrelated donor allogeneic transplant etc. [22]. The outcome of severe sepsis is better in patients undergoing autologous transplant, allogenic transplant without GVHD than allogeneic transplant with GVHD [23]. The increased incidence of MDR bacteria (multi-drug-resistant) is associated with high mortality [24, 25].

20.4.2 Respiratory System

Pulmonary complications develop in nearly 60% of cases of allogeneic transplant patients. Nearly 15% of them will require ICU care and have a mortality rate of 50% [26, 27]. Infectious complications (bacterial, viral, PCP, fungal) are the most common cause of acute respiratory failure. Post HSCT, patient are at risk of developing various from of pneumonia; bacterial pneumonia (20–50%), nocardia (1.75%), mycobacterium (0.25%) and fungal infections (allogenic 5–30%, autologous 1–5%) [28]. Viral infections (respiratory, non-respiratory) are not uncommon, and are associated with significant morbidity [29]. The acute and late non-infectious complications include acute pulmonary edema, transfusion-related acute lung injury, capillary leak syndrome, diffuse pulmonary hemorrhage, idiopathic pneumonia syndrome, and bronchiolitis obliterans syndrome, cryptogenic organizing pneumonia, acute fibrinous and organizing pneumonia etc. [30, 31]. A high rate of hospital mortality (50%) is seen among patients with acute respiratory failure [27]. Patients who required invasive ventilation for more than 96 h are at maximum risk of mortality [26]. The risk of death is similar in both autologous and allogenic transplants [32]. Pretransplant assessment of pulmonary function test (DLCO <60%, FEV1 < 60%) may help in identifying patients at high risk of development of acute respiratory failure [33]. A non-invasive method of ventilation is the preferred modality among hematologic patients due to the high frequency of concomitant thrombocytopenia and risk of bleeding, neutropenia, and better outcome than following mechanical ventilation [34–36]. However, the role of non-invasive ventilation (NIV) over the standard oxygen therapy remains unproven [37]. The early result of high flow oxygen cannula (HFO) appear are promising [38, 39]. The outcome of HFO appears similar to NIV [40]. The use of invasive mechanical ventilation should follow standard operative procedures. Etiological diagnosis is key to the success and includes timely use of computed tomography, bronchoalveolar lavage (BAL), culture, and occasionally biopsy.

20.4.3 Cardiovascular System and Hemodynamic System

Hemodynamic instability with shock may account for 20–80% of ICU admissions [41, 42]. The two major risk factors are sepsis and hypovolemia. Uncontrolled gram-negative sepsis is the primary reason for septic shock. Hypovolemia is often attributed to volume loss (diarrhea associated with GVHD, massive gastrointestinal bleeding, poor oral intake from severe mucositis). The less common reason is a cardiac failure. Cardiac dysfunction precipitated by the use of high dose cyclophosphamide, arrhythmia like atrial fibrillation, pericardial effusion, cardiac arrest, myocardial infarction is the common reasons for cardiac failure and hypotension [43]. Patients undergoing allogenic transplants, thrombocytopenia, graft versus host disease increases the risk of bleeding complications. Cardiac issues constitute 5–15% of causes for ICU admission and care [43–45]. General cardiac principles of management are used for managing these cases.

20.5 Neurologic Problems

Neurologic issues is also an important reason for ICU admission and encompass both infectious and non-infectious etiologies [46]. The incidence of neurologic complications in patients undergoing allogeneic transplants is approximately

5–20% [43–45, 47]. The common reasons are bleeding consequences, encephalopathy, seizures, posterior reversible encephalopathy syndrome (PRES), infections, metabolic, cerebrovascular events, thrombotic micro-angiopathy, neuropathies, etc. Few risk factors are associated with neurologic complications include age, female gender, donor type other than matched sibling donor (MSD), high dose total body irritation, use of umbilical cord blood (UCB) transplantation, transfusion-dependent thrombocytopenia, severe acute GVHD, extensive chronic GVHD and reported to have poor outcome [47–51]. Transplant patients exhibit a high incidence of radiological CNS abnormalities (11–60%), and even higher in autopsy studies (>90%) [52]. Bacterial infection is usually seen during the neutropenia period only, following which fungal and viral infections predominate. The use of a reduced-intensity conditioning regimen and umbilical cord blood transplantation does not appear to reduce the incidence of neurologic complications (14%) [49, 53]. Most complications are central and occur during the first 100 days. A significant proportion (up to 70%)of early complications are attributed to drug toxicity (cyclosporine, tacrolimus) and metabolic [48, 49, 53]. Limbic encephalopathy is unique to UCB transplantation [48]. Patients who develop neurologic complications do poorly (non-relapse mortality, progression-free survival, overall survival) [47–49, 51, 53]. An early study evaluated transplant during 1990–1996 showed a higher risk of neurologic complications with allogenic than autologous transplant [54]. A timely integrated approach in conjunction with a neurology specialist (physician, intensive care experts) is needed for exact diagnosis and treatment.

20.6 Acute Kidney Injury

Both acute and chronic renal injuries follow HSCT with quite distinct etiologies. The occurrence of acute kidney failure and chronic kidney failure is 30–80 and 16% respectively [33, 55, 56]. Transplant done with umbilical cord are at increased risk of AKI (83%) [57, 58]. The early acute kidney injury (AKI) could be due to the use of nephrotoxic drugs (conditioning regimen, antibiotics—amphotericin, aminoglycosides, vancomycin-piperacillin, colistin, immune suppressants—calcineurin inhibitors), volume depletion (mucositis, diarrhea, nausea, vomiting), sepsis and septic shock, part of multiorgan dysfunction syndrome (MODS), veno-occlusive disease (VOD) [59]. Risk factors for AKI include UCB transplantation, critical illness, use of nephrotoxic drugs, low pretransplant albumin [57]. The risk of death is directly proportional to the severity of AKI [4]. The onset of AKI may affect the management of GVHD by altering the administration of immune suppressants. This leads to a cascade of poor control of GVHD with the risk of hypotension and further aggravation of the renal injury. Minimizing the use of drugs with nephrotoxic potential with close monitoring of fluid balance, electrolytes are critical in the prevention of renal injury. Acute kidney injury carries potential for the development of chronic kidney disease on long term. AKI carries risk for poor outcome [55, 56].

20.7 Liver Complications

Liver issues are common following HSCT, and the incidence with allogenic transplants (84%) is double compared to autologous transplants (44%) [60, 61]. The common reason include drugs (conditioning regimen) and GVHD (acute, chronic) for allogenic and drugs, sepsis, viral hepatitis for autologous transplant [62]. However, the presence of liver complications does not lead to an increased risk of liver dysfunction over the long term and death. The complications are in form of VOD, drug-induced injury, GVHD, cirrhosis, hepatic malignancies. Pretransplant liver function assessment of stem cell recipients and use of ursodeoxycholic acid (UDCA) is important in the reduction of the incidence of liver complications [63]. Approximately 15% of TRM can be attributed to liver dysfunction. The mortality rate shows a direct correlation with serum bilirubin level, with the level above 10 mg/dl, the mortality is 80% [64]. Severe liver injury defined as AST level > 1500/l, occur in 1% of cases; the common reasons are hypoxic hepatitis and VOD [65]. The veno-occlusive disease is common in first month following the HSCT, characterized by endothelial injury, hypercoagulation state, sinusoidal obstruction, and necrosis. Diagnosis is based on clinical features, using modified Seattle and Baltimore diagnostic criteria [66, 67]. Advanced age, poor functional status, pre-existing liver disease, history of abdominal RT, allogenic transplant, use of cyclophosphamide, melphalan, gemtuzumab ozogamicin, inotuzumab ozogamicin, busulfan are among the various risk factors for the development of VOD [61, 66, 67]. The mean incidence is 37%, with a mortality rate up to >80% [68]. Defibrotide (oligodeoxyribonucleotide) and UDCA help in the prevention and treatment of VOD [67, 69].

20.8 Outcome and Prognosis

Transplantation is a complex and expensive process and a life-long commitment of follow-up. It requires a significant amount of expertise at each level of care (physicians, nursing, rehabilitation, supportive care). The outcome can vary significantly from center to center and transplant centers with high turnover per year have shown lower mortality [70]. Several observational cohort studies have reported the outcome of transplant patients admitted to intensive care units (Table 20.5). The majority of a patient in these studies show a higher incidence of 30-day mortality, varying 50–90%. Growing evidence shows improvement in ICU outcome over the last 3 decades, with the mortality rate decreasing from 90% to nearly 50% in recent studies [75, 82]. Literature suggests a similar outcome among cancer patients admitted to ICU patients with or without a history of HSCT (50%) [82]. In an analysis over two successive time periods (1997–2003, 2004–2011), the ICU and 1-year mortality were 52 versus 30% and 67 versus 48% respectively [76]. The improved outcome could be due to advances in supportive care (defibrotide), early transfer to ICU facility, use of prognostic models for ICU admission, increased use of RIC transplant, use of colony-stimulating factors, better control of infectious complications, less number of organ failure, advances in donor selection, refined HLA

Table 20.5 Selected studies describing the outcome of transplant patients requiring intensive care facilities over the last 4 decades

Study	Study year, n	%, Allogenic Transplant	ICU admission rate	Mortality
Torrecilla [71]	1981–1987, 23	100%	40%	30 day—96%
Jackson [72]	1988–1993, 116	63%	80%	Hospital—77%
Scales [73]	1992–2002, 504	60%	19%	1 year—87%
Pene [74]	1997–2003, 209	85%	20%	ICU—52%
Benz [44]	1998–2007, 33	100%	13%	6 month—85%
Townsend [75]	1996–2007, 164	100%, RIC 22%	30%	1 year—40%
Allareddy [26]	2004–2010, 6074	68%	–	Hospital—28%
Lengline [76]	1997–2003, 2004–2011, 497	Allogenic	20% 23%	52% 30%
Mokart [77]	2003–2011, 102	RIC	17%	ICU 40%, hospital 60%
Nakamura [78]	2008–2014, 39	100%	15%	1 year—88%
Azoulay [79]	2010–2011 Allogenic 145 Autologous 107	57%	–	Hospital 52% 38%
Platon [80]	2009–2013, 73	100%	23%	40%
Bayraktar [81]	2001–2020, 377	100%	13%	Hospital—64%

RIC reduced intensity conditioning.

matching, increased use of peripheral blood stem cells leading to early bone marrow recovery or due to selection bias in form of selective admission of patients with expected favorable outcome [83]. The high mortality rate in initial studies had probably created hesitance in the admission of critically sick post-transplant patients [84]. The observation of improved outcomes over time is further evidenced by the fact that the proportion of transplant patients with advanced age, advanced disease, increased number of co-morbidities have increased [76]. The common reason for admission in ICU are acute respiratory failure (30–70%), sepsis and shock (10–40%), neurologic (20%), and cardiac (8–20%) issues [44, 72, 79].

Several factors predict the outcome of transplant patients following ICU admission and can be broadly classified into three categories based on their relation; pre-transplant factors, transplant-related and ICU-related [11]. The pre-transplant include the age of the patient (>60 years), performance status, HSCT-CI score, disease type, remission status, time from diagnosis to HSCT. The factors related to transplant include the type of transplant (autologous, allogenic, myeloablative, RIC), donor stem cell source (cord blood, bone marrow or peripheral blood cells), conditioning regimen, GVHD. ICU related factors include the number of organ failures at the time of admission, time to ICU admission, presence of neutropenia at admission, critical illness severity, the reason for ICU admission, vasopressor use, mechanical ventilation, high bilirubin, low platelet count, bacterial sepsis, APACHE II, SOFA, SAPS II score, renal replacement therapy, neurological dysfunction [12]. However, the most consistent ones are the use of mechanical ventilation, GVHD, number of organ failures at the time of admission, vasopressor use, type of conditioning regimen (RIC or MAC) [10–13, 41, 42, 51, 73, 75, 77]. Prognostic factors like (age, low platelet count, bacterial infections) were found significant only in few studies.

20.9 Triage during the ICU Admission

From a hematologist/oncologist perspective, every patient who has opted and underwent a curative therapeutic modality treatment (bone marrow transplant) should be offered ICU care, especially during the early and acute period. However, the goals of care can vary between the hematologist/oncologist and the intensivist physician. Well, the treating physician has followed the patient through the entire course, and is well versed with the outcome of the underlying disease, and might be a better person to judge the importance of ICU admission. The intensive care play an important and vital part of the patient care, but they are not experienced with the long term disease outcome. The intensivist decision is usually affected by the comparative poor outcome of cancer and hematologic patients than non-cancer patients [85]. The high mortality associated with allogeneic HSCT puts intensivists in a challenging situation especially when resources are limited. For an intensivist, there is a continuous challenging task for the decision making of ICU admission, optimal resource utilization and to give beneficial care [86]. This is highlighted in a prospective study where the two physicians differed in 50% of ICU care triage decision [87]. Out of 206 patients requested for admission by the referring oncologist, only 51% got the admission. An equal percentage of patients were considered too sick (26%) and too well (23%) for the ICU admission. However, the 30-day mortality among patients admitted to the ICU care was labeled too sick and too well was 54, 74, and 22% respectively. The study highlights the importance of using a more conservative approach for ICU admission. Also, highlight the inclusion of treating physicians as part of the decision-making for ICU admission. However, welcome to all should not be the conclusion. There is a need to draft and prospective evaluate policy evaluating the triage for ICU admission. In the prospective ICU trial, palliative care patients and bedridden patients were denied ICU care. All newly diagnosed patients (<30 days) were given ICU admission [88].

20.10 Conclusion

HSCT is getting common day by day and will increase further in the near future. Many patients develop complications after the transplant and critical care remains vital for the short and long-term survival. The outcome has improved substantially over the past four decades, still, 50% die during ICU admission. Further improvement is required in form of triage decision-making for ICU admission, optimal use of supportive care, and improvement of outcome. There is a need to continue work in further increasing the outcome after HSCT. Prospective evaluation of the policies targeting to provide beneficial ICU care is in need of time.

References

1. Niederhuber JE. Abeloff's clinical oncology. 6th ed. Philadelphia, PA: Elsevier; 2019.
2. CIBMTR summary slides—HCT trends and survival data [Internet]. [cited 2021 Jul 6]. https://www.cibmtr.org/ReferenceCenter/SlidesReports/SummarySlides/pages/index.aspx.
3. Nates JL, Price KJ, editors. Oncologic Critical Care [Internet]. Cham: Springer International Publishing; 2020 [cited 2021 Jul 11]. https://link.springer.com/10.1007/978-3-319-74698-2.
4. Hall JB, Schmidt GA, Kress JP. Principles of critical care [Internet]. 2015 [cited 2021 Jul 7]. http://www.vlebooks.com/vleweb/product/openreader?id=none&isbn=9780071753272.
5. Niederwieser D, Baldomero H, Atsuta Y, et al. One and Half Million Hematopoietic Stem Cell Transplants (HSCT). Dissemination, Trends and Potential to Improve Activity By Telemedicine from the Worldwide Network for Blood and Marrow Transplantation (WBMT). Blood 2019;134(Supplement_1):2035–2035.
6. Sorror ML, Maris MB, Storb R, et al. Hematopoietic cell transplantation (HCT)-specific comorbidity index: a new tool for risk assessment before allogeneic HCT. Blood. 2005;106(8):2912–9.
7. The EBMT handbook: hematopoietic stem cell transplantation and cellular therapies. New York, NY, Berlin, Heidelberg: Springer; 2018.
8. Matulis M. Immune reconstitution after hematopoietic stem-cell transplantation and its influence on respiratory infections1. Semin Respir Infect. 2002;17(2):130–9.
9. Peled JU, Gomes ALC, Devlin SM, et al. Microbiota as predictor of mortality in allogeneic hematopoietic-cell transplantation. N Engl J Med. 2020;382(9):822–34.
10. Fornwalt RA, Brigham EP, Scott SR. Critical Care of Hematopoietic Stem Cell Transplant Patients. Crit Care Clin. 2021;37(1):29–46.
11. Afessa B, Azoulay E. Critical Care of the Hematopoietic Stem Cell Transplant Recipient. Crit Care Clin. 2010;26(1):133–50.
12. Saillard C, Blaise D, Mokart D. Critically ill allogeneic hematopoietic stem cell transplantation patients in the intensive care unit: reappraisal of actual prognosis. Bone Marrow Transplant. 2016;51(8):1050–61.
13. Naeem N, Eyzaguirre A, Kern JA, et al. Outcome of adult umbilical cord blood transplant patients admitted to a medical intensive care unit. Bone Marrow Transplant. 2006;38(11):733–8.
14. Trinkaus MA, Lapinsky SE, Crump M, et al. Predictors of mortality in patients undergoing autologous hematopoietic cell transplantation admitted to the intensive care unit. Bone Marrow Transplant. 2009;43(5):411–5.
15. Ninin E, Milpied N, Moreau P, et al. Longitudinal study of bacterial, viral, and fungal infections in adult recipients of bone marrow transplants. Clin Infect Dis Off Publ Infect Dis Soc Am. 2001;33(1):41–7.
16. Ogonek J, Kralj Juric M, Ghimire S, et al. Immune reconstitution after allogeneic hematopoietic stem cell transplantation. Front Immunol. 2016;7:507.
17. Signorelli J, Liewer S, Zimmer A, Freifeld AG. Incidence of febrile neutropenia in autologous hematopoietic stem cell transplant (HSCT) recipients on levofloxacin prophylaxis at a single-center Midwest cancer Center. Open forum Infect Dis. 2017;4(suppl_1):S713.
18. Kochanek M, Schalk E, von Bergwelt-Baildon M, et al. Management of sepsis in neutropenic cancer patients: 2018 guidelines from the infectious diseases working party (AGIHO) and intensive care working party (iCHOP) of the German Society of Hematology and Medical Oncology (DGHO). Ann Hematol. 2019;98(5):1051–69.

19. Tomblyn M, Chiller T, Einsele H, et al. Guidelines for preventing infectious complications among hematopoietic cell transplantation recipients: a global perspective. Biol Blood Marrow Transplant. 2009;15(10):1143–238.
20. Mikulska M, Viscoli C, Orasch C, et al. Aetiology and resistance in bacteraemias among adult and paediatric haematology and cancer patients. J Infect. 2014;68(4):321–31.
21. Taplitz RA, Kennedy EB, Flowers CR. Antimicrobial prophylaxis for adult patients with cancer-related immunosuppression: ASCO and IDSA clinical practice guideline update summary. J Oncol Pract. 2018;14(11):692–5.
22. the ONKO-KISS Study Group, Meyer E, Beyersmann J, et al. Risk factor analysis of blood stream infection and pneumonia in neutropenic patients after peripheral blood stem-cell transplantation. Bone Marrow Transplant. 2007;39(3):173–8.
23. Kumar G, Ahmad S, Taneja A, Patel J, Guddati AK, Nanchal R. Severe sepsis in hematopoietic stem cell transplant recipients*. Crit Care Med. 2015;43(2):411–21.
24. Satlin MJ, Jenkins SG, Walsh TJ. The global challenge of Carbapenem-resistant Enterobacteriaceae in transplant recipients and patients with hematologic malignancies. Clin Infect Dis. 2014;58(9):1274–83.
25. Forcina A, Lorentino F, Marasco V, et al. Clinical impact of Pretransplant multidrug-resistant gram-negative colonization in autologous and allogeneic hematopoietic stem cell transplantation. Biol Blood Marrow Transplant J Am Soc Blood Marrow Transplant. 2018;24(7):1476–82.
26. Allareddy V, Roy A, Rampa S, et al. Outcomes of stem cell transplant patients with acute respiratory failure requiring mechanical ventilation in the United States. Bone Marrow Transplant. 2014;49(10):1278–86.
27. Yadav H, Nolan ME, Bohman JK, et al. Epidemiology of acute respiratory distress syndrome following hematopoietic stem cell transplantation. Crit Care Med. 2016;44(6):1082–90.
28. Chi AK, Soubani AO, White AC, Miller KB. An update on pulmonary complications of hematopoietic stem cell transplantation. Chest. 2013;144(6):1913–22.
29. Vakil E, Evans SE. Viral pneumonia in patients with hematologic malignancy or hematopoietic stem cell transplantation. Clin Chest Med. 2017;38(1):97–111.
30. Haider S, Durairajan N, Soubani AO. Noninfectious pulmonary complications of haematopoietic stem cell transplantation. Eur Respir Rev. 2020;29(156):190119.
31. Ahya VN. Noninfectious acute lung injury syndromes early after hematopoietic stem cell transplantation. Clin Chest Med. 2017;38(4):595–606.
32. Munshi L, Darmon M, Soares M, et al. Acute respiratory failure outcomes in patients with hematologic malignancies and hematopoietic cell transplant: a secondary analysis of the EFRAIM study. Transplant Cell Ther. 2021;27(1):78.e1–6.
33. Parimon T, Madtes DK, Au DH, Clark JG, Chien JW. Pretransplant lung function, respiratory failure, and mortality after stem cell transplantation. Am J Respir Crit Care Med. 2005;172(3):384–90.
34. LUNG SAFE Investigators and the ESICM Trials Group, Cortegiani A, Madotto F, et al. Immunocompromised patients with acute respiratory distress syndrome: secondary analysis of the LUNG SAFE database. Crit Care 2018;22(1):157.
35. Wang T, Zhang L, Luo K, et al. Noninvasive versus invasive mechanical ventilation for immunocompromised patients with acute respiratory failure: a systematic review and meta-analysis. BMC Pulm Med. 2016;16(1):129.
36. Hilbert G, Gruson D, Vargas F, et al. Noninvasive ventilation in immunosuppressed patients with pulmonary infiltrates, fever, and acute respiratory failure. N Engl J Med. 2001;344(7):481–7.
37. Lemiale V, Mokart D, Resche-Rigon M, et al. Effect of noninvasive ventilation vs oxygen therapy on mortality among immunocompromised patients with acute respiratory failure: a randomized clinical trial. JAMA. 2015;314(16):1711.
38. Frat J-P, Thille AW, Mercat A, et al. High-flow oxygen through nasal cannula in acute hypoxemic respiratory failure. N Engl J Med. 2015;372(23):2185–96.
39. Azoulay E, Lemiale V, Mokart D, et al. Effect of high-flow nasal oxygen vs standard oxygen on 28-day mortality in immunocompromised patients with acute respiratory failure: the HIGH randomized clinical trial. JAMA. 2018;320(20):2099.

40. Frat J, Coudroy R, Thille AW. Non-invasive ventilation or high-flow oxygen therapy: when to choose one over the other? Respirology. 2019;24(8):724–31.
41. Kew AK, Couban S, Patrick W, Thompson K, White D. Outcome of hematopoietic stem cell transplant recipients admitted to the intensive care unit. Biol Blood Marrow Transplant. 2006;12(3):301–5.
42. Karagiannis P, Sänger L, Alsdorf W, et al. Intensive care outcomes of patients after high dose chemotherapy and subsequent autologous stem cell transplantation: a retrospective, single Centre analysis. Cancers. 2020;12(6):E1678.
43. Naeem N, Reed MD, Creger RJ, Youngner SJ, Lazarus HM. Transfer of the hematopoietic stem cell transplant patient to the intensive care unit: does it really matter? Bone Marrow Transplant. 2006;37(2):119–33.
44. Benz R, Schanz U, Maggiorini M, Seebach JD, Stussi G. Risk factors for ICU admission and ICU survival after allogeneic hematopoietic SCT. Bone Marrow Transplant. 2014;49(1):62–5.
45. Soubani AO, Kseibi E, Bander JJ, et al. Outcome and prognostic factors of hematopoietic stem cell transplantation recipients admitted to a medical ICU. Chest. 2004;126(5):1604–11.
46. Maffini E, Festuccia M, Brunello L, Boccadoro M, Giaccone L, Bruno B. Neurologic complications after allogeneic hematopoietic stem cell transplantation. Biol Blood Marrow Transplant. 2017;23(3):388–97.
47. Siegal D, Keller A, Xu W, et al. Central nervous system complications after allogeneic hematopoietic stem cell transplantation: incidence, manifestations, and clinical significance. Biol Blood Marrow Transplant. 2007;13(11):1369–79.
48. Kishi Y, Miyakoshi S, Kami M, et al. Early central nervous system complications after reduced-intensity stem cell transplantation. Biol Blood Marrow Transplant. 2004;10(8):561–8.
49. Narimatsu H, Miyamura K, Iida H, Hamaguchi M, Uchida T, Morishita Y. Early central nervous complications after umbilical cord blood transplantation for adults. Biol Blood Marrow Transplant. 2009;15(1):92–100.
50. Balaguer-Rosello A, Bataller L, Piñana JL, et al. Noninfectious neurologic complications after allogeneic hematopoietic stem cell transplantation. Biol Blood Marrow Transplant. 2019;25(9):1818–24.
51. Dowling MR, Li S, Dey BR, et al. Neurologic complications after allogeneic hematopoietic stem cell transplantation: risk factors and impact. Bone Marrow Transplant. 2018;53(2):199–206.
52. Nishiguchi T, Mochizuki K, Shakudo M, Takeshita T, Hino M, Inoue Y. CNS complications of hematopoietic stem cell transplantation. Am J Roentgenol. 2009;192(4):1003–11.
53. Barba P, Piñana JL, Valcárcel D, et al. Early and late neurological complications after reduced-intensity conditioning allogeneic stem cell transplantation. Biol Blood Marrow Transplant. 2009;15(11):1439–46.
54. Denier C, Bourhis J-H, Lacroix C, et al. Spectrum and prognosis of neurologic complications after hematopoietic transplantation. Neurology. 2006;67(11):1990–7.
55. Kagoya Y, Kataoka K, Nannya Y, Kurokawa M. Pretransplant predictors and Posttransplant sequels of acute kidney injury after allogeneic stem cell transplantation. Biol Blood Marrow Transplant. 2011;17(3):394–400.
56. Parikh CR, Yarlagadda SG, Storer B, Sorror M, Storb R, Sandmaier B. Impact of acute kidney injury on long-term mortality after Nonmyeloablative hematopoietic cell transplantation. Biol Blood Marrow Transplant. 2008;14(3):309–15.
57. Gutgarts V, Sathick IJ, Zheng J, et al. Incidence and risk factors for acute and chronic kidney injury after adult cord blood transplantation. Biol Blood Marrow Transplant. 2020;26(4):758–63.
58. Xue E, Chotivatanapong J, Pao EC, et al. High incidence of acute kidney injury after cord blood transplant. Biol Blood Marrow Transplant. 2020;26(3):S137–8.
59. Clemmons AB, Bech CF, Pantin J, Ahmad I. Acute kidney injury in hematopoietic cell transplantation patients receiving vancomycin and piperacillin/Tazobactam versus vancomycin and Cefepime. Biol Blood Marrow Transplant. 2018;24(4):820–6.
60. Kim B, Chung K, Sun H, et al. Liver disease during the first post-transplant year in bone marrow transplantation recipients: retrospective study. Bone Marrow Transplant. 2000;26(2):193–7.

61. Norvell JP. Liver disease after hematopoietic cell transplantation in adults. Transplant Rev. 2015;29(1):8–15.
62. Abdelbary H, Magdy R, Moussa M, Abdelmoaty I. Liver disease during and after hematopoietic stem cell transplantation in adults: a single-center Egyptian experience. J Egypt Natl Cancer Inst. 2020;32(1):11.
63. Ruutu T, Juvonen E, Remberger M, et al. Improved survival with Ursodeoxycholic acid prophylaxis in allogeneic stem cell transplantation: long-term follow-up of a randomized study. Biol Blood Marrow Transplant. 2014;20(1):135–8.
64. Gooley TA, Rajvanshi P, Schoch HG, McDonald GB. Serum bilirubin levels and mortality after myeloablative allogeneic hematopoietic cell transplantation. Hepatology. 2005;41(2):345–52.
65. Sakai M, Strasser SI, Shulman HM, McDonald SJ, Schoch HG, McDonald GB. Severe hepatocellular injury after hematopoietic cell transplant: incidence, etiology and outcome. Bone Marrow Transplant. 2009;44(7):441–7.
66. Corbacioglu S, Jabbour EJ, Mohty M. Risk factors for development of and progression of hepatic Veno-occlusive disease/sinusoidal obstruction syndrome. Biol Blood Marrow Transplant. 2019;25(7):1271–80.
67. Dalle J-H, Giralt SA. Hepatic Veno-occlusive disease after hematopoietic stem cell transplantation: risk factors and stratification, prophylaxis, and treatment. Biol Blood Marrow Transplant. 2016;22(3):400–9.
68. Coppell JA, Richardson PG, Soiffer R, et al. Hepatic Veno-occlusive disease following stem cell transplantation: incidence, clinical course, and outcome. Biol Blood Marrow Transplant. 2010;16(2):157–68.
69. Richardson PG, Riches ML, Kernan NA, et al. Phase 3 trial of defibrotide for the treatment of severe veno-occlusive disease and multi-organ failure. Blood. 2016;127(13):1656–65.
70. Loberiza FR, Zhang M-J, Lee SJ, et al. Association of transplant center and physician factors on mortality after hematopoietic stem cell transplantation in the United States. Blood. 2005;105(7):2979–87.
71. Torrecilla C, Cortés JL, Chamorro C, Rubio JJ, Galdos P, Dominguez de Villota E. Prognostic assessment of the acute complications of bone marrow transplantation requiring intensive therapy. Intensive Care Med. 1988;14(4):393–8.
72. Jackson S, Tweeddale M, Barnett M, et al. Admission of bone marrow transplant recipients to the intensive care unit: outcome, survival and prognostic factors. Bone Marrow Transplant. 1998;21(7):697–704.
73. Scales DC, Thiruchelvam D, Kiss A, Sibbald WJ, Redelmeier DA. Intensive care outcomes in bone marrow transplant recipients: a population-based cohort analysis. Crit Care. 2008;12(3):R77.
74. Pène F, Aubron C, Azoulay E, et al. Outcome of critically ill allogeneic hematopoietic stem-cell transplantation recipients: a reappraisal of indications for organ failure supports. J Clin Oncol. 2006;24(4):643–9.
75. Townsend WM, Holroyd A, Pearce R, et al. Improved intensive care unit survival for critically ill allogeneic haematopoietic stem cell transplant recipients following reduced intensity conditioning. Br J Haematol. 2013;161(4):578–86.
76. Lengliné E, Chevret S, Moreau A-S, et al. Changes in intensive care for allogeneic hematopoietic stem cell transplant recipients. Bone Marrow Transplant. 2015;50(6):840–5.
77. Mokart D, Granata A, Crocchiolo R, et al. Allogeneic hematopoietic stem cell transplantation after reduced intensity conditioning regimen: outcomes of patients admitted to intensive care unit. J Crit Care. 2015;30(5):1107–13.
78. Nakamura M, Fujii N, Shimizu K, et al. Long-term outcomes in patients treated in the intensive care unit after hematopoietic stem cell transplantation. Int J Hematol. 2018;108(6):622–9.
79. Azoulay E, Mokart D, Pène F, et al. Outcomes of critically ill patients with hematologic malignancies: prospective Multicenter data from France and Belgium—a Groupe de Recherche Respiratoire en Réanimation Onco-Hématologique study. J Clin Oncol. 2013;31(22):2810–8.

80. Platon L, Amigues L, Ceballos P, et al. A reappraisal of ICU and long-term outcome of allogeneic hematopoietic stem cell transplantation patients and reassessment of prognosis factors: results of a 5-year cohort study (2009–2013). Bone Marrow Transplant. 2016;51(2):256–61.
81. Bayraktar UD, Shpall EJ, Liu P, et al. Hematopoietic cell transplantation–specific comorbidity index predicts inpatient mortality and survival in patients who received allogeneic transplantation admitted to the intensive care unit. J Clin Oncol. 2013;31(33):4207–14.
82. Azoulay E, Soares M, Darmon M, Benoit D, Pastores S, Afessa B. Intensive care of the cancer patient: recent achievements and remaining challenges. Ann Intensive Care. 2011;1(1):5.
83. Gooley TA, Chien JW, Pergam SA, et al. Reduced mortality after allogeneic hematopoietic-cell transplantation. N Engl J Med. 2010;363(22):2091–101.
84. Faber-Langendoen K, Caplan AL, McGlave PB. Survival of adult bone marrow transplant patients receiving mechanical ventilation: a case for restricted use. Bone Marrow Transplant. 1993;12(5):501–7.
85. Puxty K, Kinsella J, McLoone P, Quasim T, Morrison D. 644: comparison of cancer and non-cancer patients admitted to ICU with a non-surgical diagnosis. Crit Care Med. 2013;41:A157–8.
86. Darmon M, Azoulay E. Critical care management of cancer patients: cause for optimism and need for objectivity. Curr Opin Oncol. 2009;21(4):318–26.
87. Thiéry G, Azoulay É, Darmon M, et al. Outcome of cancer patients considered for intensive care unit admission: a hospital-wide prospective study. J Clin Oncol. 2005;23(19):4406–13.
88. Lecuyer L, Chevret S, Thiery G, Darmon M, Schlemmer B, Azoulay É. The ICU trial: a new admission policy for cancer patients requiring mechanical ventilation*. Crit Care Med. 2007;35(3):808–14.

Febrile Neutropenia

21

Rupak Kumar Giri and Ranjit Kumar Sahoo

21.1 Definition

A single oral temperature of 101'F/38.3'C or a temperature of 100.4'F/38'C sustained over 1 h in a patient with absolute neutrophil count (ANC) < 500/mcl or expected to become <500/mcl in next 48 h is known as febrile neutropenia (IDSA) [1].

21.2 Incidence: [1, 2]

Incidence of febrile neutropenia in cancer patients receiving chemotherapy is higher in haematological cancer patients compared to solid tumors which are roughly as follows:

- Solid tumors: 5–10% of patients
- Non-leukemic haematological cancers: 20–25% of patients
- Acute leukemia: 85–95% of patients

21.3 Neutropenic Fever Syndromes

Neutropenic fever syndromes can be classified into following based on clinical presentation [2]:

1. First episode of neutropenic fever
2. Persistent neutropenic fever

R. K. Giri · R. K. Sahoo (✉)
Department of Medical Oncology, Dr.B.R.A.I.R.C.H, AIIMS, New Delhi, India

V. Kumar et al. (eds.), *Onco-critical Care*,
https://doi.org/10.1007/978-981-16-9929-0_21

3. Recrudescent neutropenic fever
4. Fever after resolution of neutropenia

1. *First episode of neutropenic fever:*

The first neutropenic fever is the first febrile episode occurring during a given period of chemotherapy-induced neutropenia. The International Immunocompromised Host Society has classified initial neutropenic fever syndromes into the following three categories [2, 3]:

- Microbiologically documented infection (10–20%): Neutropenic fever with a clinical focus of infection and an associated pathogen
- Clinically documented infection (20–30%): Neutropenic fever with a clinical focus (eg, cellulitis, pneumonia) but without the isolation of an associated pathogen
- Unexplained fever (50–60%): Neutropenic fever with neither a clinical focus of infection nor an identified pathogen

2. *Persistent neutropenic fever:*

A persistent neutropenic fever syndrome is a febrile episode without defervescence after at least 5 days of initial empiric broad-spectrum antibacterial therapy in high-risk neutropenic patients or after at least 2 days in low-risk neutropenic patients

Causes:
- Invasive fungal infections (IFI)
- Resistant bacterial infections

3. *Recrudescent neutropenic fever:*

A recrudescent neutropenic fever syndrome is a febrile episode that recurs following initial defervescence during a course of broad-spectrum antibacterial therapy while the patient remains neutropenic

Causes:
- Breakthrough bacterial infections
- Invasive fungal infections

4. *Fever after resolution of neutropenia:*

It refers to appearance of or worsening of fever at the time of recovery of neutrophil counts

Causes:
- Superinfection
- Myeloid reconstitution syndrome
- Engraftment syndrome
- Drug fever
- Deep vein thrombosis
- Transfusion reactions

21.4 Risk Stratification of Febrile Neutropenia

All patients with febrile neutropenia are initially evaluated clinically for risk of serious complications. Validated risk scoring systems (eg. MASCC score [4], CISNE score [5]) helps in predicting risk of serious complications. Approach to treatment including need for in-patient admission, intravenous antibiotics etc. is decided based upon the risk scores.

Multinational association for supportive care in cancer (MASCC) score:
It includes following parameters

- Burden of illness:
  - No/Mild symptoms (5 points)
  - Moderate symptoms (3 points)
  - Severe symptoms (0 points)
- Comorbidities:
  - No hypotension (systolic blood pressure > 90 mmHg) (5 points)
  - No chronic obstructive pulmonary disease (4 points)
  - Solid tumor or hematologic malignancy with no history of previous fungal infections (4 points)
  - No dehydration requiring parenteral fluids (3 points)
- Status:
  - Outpatient status at the time of onset of the neutropenic fever syndrome (3 points)
- Age:
  - <60 years (2 points)
  - ≥60 years (0 points)
- Interpretation of MASCC scores:
  - MASCC score 21–26: Low risk for complications, Patient can be managed on OPD basis with oral empiric antibiotics
  - MASCC score 0–20: High risk for complications, Patient requires hospitalisation for IV antibiotics

Most adult febrile neutropenia guidelines endorse the use of MASCC score. The pediatric guidelines support the concept of risk stratification but emphasize the importance of using strategies that have been validated locally.

Clinical Index of Stable Febrile Neutropenia (CISNE) score:

Dr BRA-IRCH, AIIMS High risk febrile neutropenia antibiotic protocol

DIAGNOSTIC EVALUATION

- History specially previous antibiogram
- Physical examination: oral cavity, paranasal sinuses, perineal region
- Routine investigations
- Blood cultures baseline
- Chest X ray
- S Procalcitonin (optional)
- S Galactomannan (optional)

FIRST LINE ANTIBIOTICS

Patients is clinically stable & previously not exposed to multipleantibiotics
1. Cefoperazone + Sulbactam
2. Amikacin

Patient is clinically unstable, heavily treated with antibiotics & resistant organisms suspected
1. Carbapenem
2. Amikacin

Indications for upfront G (+) antibiotics
1. Hemodynamic stability
2. Pneumonia
3. Severe mucositis
4. Skin or soft tissue infections
5. Clinically evident catheter related infections
6. Known colonisation with MRSA
7. Vancomycin is the glycopeptide of choice
8. Teicoplanin to be used if other nephroto xic drugs are being used
9. Linezolid is to be used if VRE is isolated or suspected

AFTER 48 HRS

Clinically stable
- No danger signs
- ANC recovering trend

Continue same antibiotic therapy till count recovery

Clinical worsening
Upgradation of antibiotics
- Add Carbapenem if patient was started on Cefoperazone + Sulbactam
- Add Colistin if patient was started on Carbapenem
- Do not add 2 nephrotoxic drugs together
- If culture reports are available, change antibiotics accordingly
- Add G(+) antibiotics

IF FEVER PERSISTS AFTER 48 HRS

- Look for focus of infection
- HRCT Chest
- S Galactomannan
- Empirical pre-emptive antifungal therapy
- AmphoB/Caspofungin/Voriconazole are preferred as pre-emptive therapy
- Dual antifungals are to be used in case of proven/probable fungal infection not responding to single agent

Risk stratification by using risk scores and other clinical parameters:

1. *Low risk febrile neutropenia:*

   Presence of all of the following is considered as low risk febrile neutropenia

- Expected duration of severe neutropenia (ANC < 500/mcl) is ≤7 days
- MASCC score ≥21 or CISNE score 0
- No comorbidities
- No evidence of hepatic or renal dysfunction

2. *High risk febrile neutropenia:*

   Presence of any of the following is considered as high risk

- Expected duration of severe neutropenia (ANC < 500/mcl) is >7 days
- MASCC score <21 or CISNE score ≥3
- Ongoing medical comorbidities
- Evidence of hepatic or renal dysfunction

21.5 Pathogenesis

The majority of documented infections during neutropenia are caused by the patient's own endogenous bacterial flora [6]. Chemotherapy induced mucositis leads to seeding of the blood stream from endogenous flora in the gastrointestinal tract which results in neutropenic fever. Immunosuppressive effects of chemotherapy and immune-dysfunctions associated with haematological malignancies are also contributing factors for neutropenic fever.

Bacterial infections in neutropenic patients:

- Bacteria are the most common infectious causes of neutropenic fever [7]
- Gram-negative bacteria (eg, *P. aeruginosa*) usually cause the most serious infections [8].
- *S. epidermidis* is the most common gram-positive pathogen, accounting for approximately one-half of all infections due to gram-positive infections. However, it is much less virulent than other bacterial pathogens [9]
- Among gram-positive bacteria, *S. aureus* (particularly methicillin-resistant strains), some viridans streptococci, and Enterococci (particularly vancomycin-resistant strains) can cause serious infections [10]
- Although anaerobic bacteria are abundant in the alimentary tract, they are infrequent pathogens isolated from patients with neutropenic fever. However, they can contribute to the pathogenesis of necrotizing mucositis, sinusitis, periodontal cellulitis, perirectal cellulitis, intra-abdominal or pelvic infection, and neutropenic enterocolitis (typhlitis) and can cause anaerobic bacteremia.

- Polymicrobial infections are infrequent, but their frequency appears to be rising [11]

Fungal infections:

- Fungal infections are rarely the cause of first febrile episode in neutropenic patients. More commonly, they are identified as causes of persistent or recurrent fever beyond the first week of neutropenia [12, 13].
- Fungal infections are commonly seen in high risk febrile neutropenia while they are rarely seen in low risk cases [12, 13].
- Prolonged duration of severe neutropenia is the major risk factor for invasive fungal infections [12, 13].
- *Candida* spp. and *Aspergillus* spp. account for most invasive fungal infections during neutropenia.
- Candida infections are usually acquired through gastrointestinal tract colonization and translocation across damaged intestinal epithelial surface [14].
- Fever is often the sole manifestation of candidemia. Erythematous macronodular skin nodules may occur in some patients with candidemia [14].
- Median time of candidemia following standard remission-induction therapy for acute myelogenous leukemia (AML) is about 16 days (range 13 to 25 days) from the first day of the cytotoxic regimen, coincident with the time of maximum cytotoxic therapy-induced intestinal epithelial damage [14].
- *Candida albicans* accounts for the majority of candidemias; *C. glabrata*, *C. tropicalis*, and other *Candida* spp. account for the remainder [15].
- However, higher proportions of candidemias are due to non-albicans *Candida* species when Fluconazole prophylaxis has been administered [15].
- *Candida* spp. are also commonly found as fungal causes of central venous catheter-associated infections and can cause disseminated candidiasis as well.
- Aspergillus infections are acquired by inhalation of airborne spores (conidia) into the upper and lower respiratory tract followed by germination and invasive hyphal growth [16].
- *Aspergillus infections* primarily affect the lower respiratory tract (pneumonia) and upper respiratory tract (sinusitis) but may also involve the central nervous system, bones, and skin [16].
- Mucormycosis can cause life-threatening rhino-orbital-cerebral, pulmonary, and disseminated infections in immunocompromised hosts, particularly those with prolonged neutropenia, uncontrolled hyperglycemia due to pre-existing diabetes mellitus or administration of glucocorticoids [17].
- *Fusarium* spp. have been increasingly reported to cause invasive fungal infections in patients with hematologic malignancies with prolonged severe neutropenia or significant glucocorticoid exposure.

Viral infections:

- Viral infections, particularly human herpes virus infections, are commonly seen in high risk febrile neutropenia
- Most herpes simplex virus (HSV-1 and -2) and varicella zoster virus infections in adults are due to reactivation of latent infections in seropositive patients [18].
- Infections caused by community-acquired respiratory viruses (CARVs) are a significant threat to patients with hematologic malignancies and stem cell transplantation.

21.6 Treatment

Fever in neutropenic patients should be considered as a medical emergency. It is critical to identify neutropenic fever early and to initiate empiric systemic antibacterial therapy promptly after blood cultures have been obtained in order to avoid progression to a sepsis syndrome and possibly death.

The aim of empiric therapy is to cover the spectrum of the most likely and most virulent pathogens that may rapidly cause serious or life-threatening infection in neutropenic patients. The following general principles apply: [19–21]

- Though antibiotics are usually started empirically but they should possess appropriate coverage for suspected or known infections. Even when the pathogen is known, a broad spectrum antibiotic regimen must be chosen for empiric coverage for the possibility of copathogens, unlike the treatment strategy adopted in many immunocompetent hosts.
- Initial antibiotic selection should be guided by the patient's history, allergies, symptoms, signs, recent or concurrent antibiotic use and culture data, and awareness of the susceptibility patterns of institutional nosocomial pathogens
- In high-risk patients, antibiotics should generally be administered intravenously (IV) in a hospital setting while low risk patients can be managed by oral antibiotics in out-patient setting
- Ideally, antibiotics should be bactericidal.
- Antibiotics should be started within 60 min of initial presentation.
- Clinical response and culture and susceptibility results should be monitored closely; therapy should be adjusted in a timely fashion in response to this information.

A. Low risk febrile neutropenia: [19, 22, 23]

*Low risk febrile neutropenia patients who are **not** receiving prophylactic Fluoroquinolones:*

- These patients are usually managed on an out patient basis with oral antibiotics
- Commonly used oral antibiotic regimen for low risk febrile neutropenia is a combination of β-lactam agent eg. Amoxycillin-Clavulunate (500 mg/125 mg orally three times daily or 875 mg/125 mg orally twice daily) with a fluoroquinolone (Ciprofloxacin 750 mg twice daily)
- Levofloxacin 750 mg once daily (in combination with Amoxycillin-Clavulunate) is an alternative to Ciprofloxacin but Ciprofloxacin is preferred as added gram positive coverage of Levofloxacin is not required when Amoxicillin-Clavulanate is used.
- Alternative regimens:
    1. Levofloxacin (750 mg OD) /Moxifloxacin (400 mg OD) monotherapy is a reserved option for patients who are allergic to penicillin and who also cannot take cephalosporins.
    2. Clindamycin (300 mg QID) is also an option in penicillin allergic patients
    3. Cefixime (400 mg OD) can be given in patients allergic to penicillin but deemed fit for cephalosporin

Low risk febrile neutropenia patients who are receiving prophylactic Fluoroquinolones:

- Such patients should receive one of the IV regimens recommended for high-risk patients in order to provide adequate activity against *P. Aeruginosa*
- It is reasonable to give an IV antibiotic regimen on an outpatient basis provided that the patient meets all the criteria for being at low risk for complications.

Monitoring:

- Patients should be monitored frequently at least in the initial 3 days; monitoring parameters include vital signs, oral intake, complete blood counts, fluid and electrolyte status etc.
- Defervescence of fever and resolution of foci of infection present at baseline are the primary goals while treating low risk as well as high risk febrile neutropenia.
- The observed median times to defervescence for patients with low risk febrile neutropenia is about 2 days
- Persistence of fever beyond the expected median time to defervescence of 2–3 days should mandate a reassessment and consideration of modification of the initial empiric regimen and hospital admission.
- The need to modify the regimen should be driven by clinical and/or microbiologic evidence for resistant organisms and evidence of ongoing and progressive infection.

Duration of anti-microbial therapy: [24]

- Optimal duration of antibiotics in febrile neutropenia is a matter of debate; however, antibiotics is usually continued until myeloid recovery i.e. recovery of ANC $\geq$ 500/mcl
- Low risk febrile neutropenia patients without any microbiological or clinical evidence of infection: Antibiotics are to be given until documentation of at least 2 afebrile days after ANC has recovered (ANC $\geq$ 500/mcl)
- Low risk febrile neutropenia patients without any microbiological or clinical evidence of infection: Most documented infections, such as pneumonia or bloodstream infection, require 10–14 days of therapy, which may extend well beyond the time of myeloid reconstitution

B. High risk febrile neutropenia:

Patients with high risk febrile neutropenia should ideally be managed with IV antibiotics in a in-patient setting.

1. Choosing the initial antibiotic regimen: [19]

- The initial antibiotic of choice is monotherapy with an anti-pseudomonal β-lactam antibiotic (, Piperacillin-Tazobactam, Meropenem, Imipenem, Cefepime)
- Cefoperazone-Sulbactam and Ceftazidime monotherapy should usually be avoided because of rising resistance among gram negative organisms to these agents and their comparatively lesser gram positive coverage compared to other alternatives.
- Some form of combination therapy should be chosen in patients who are clinically unstable or if there is high risk of infection caused by resistant gram negative organisms (second antibiotic with gram negative coverage is added) or if there is some evidence of infection by gram positive organisms (second antibiotic with gram positive coverage is added).
- In our institute, all patients with high risk febrile neutropenia are started with combination of two antibiotics with gram negative coverage as follows:
  - Patients is clinically stable & previously not exposed to multiple antibiotics: A combination of Cefoperazone-Sulbactam and Amikacin is started
  - Patient is clinically unstable, heavily treated with antibiotics & resistant organisms suspected: A combination of Meropenem and Amikacin or Meropenem and Cefoperazone-Sulbactam is started
- Initial empiric regimen options in penicillin allergic patients:
- Aztreonam + Vancomycin (Preferred)
- Ciprofloxacin + Clindamycin

- Gram positive antibiotics are not routinely given in initial empiric antibiotic regimen except in certain situations. Indications for addition of antibiotics with gram positive coverage at initial presentation include
  - Hemodynamic instability
  - Known colonisation with MRSA
  - Pneumonia
  - Severe mucositis
  - Skin or soft tissue infections
  - Clinically evident catheter related infection
- Vancomycin is the glycopeptide antibiotic of choice for gram positive coverage. However, due to its lower nephrotoxicity potential, Teicoplanin is more popular in our setting. Linezolid is to be used if VRE is isolated or suspected.
- Daptomycin is another alternative to vancomycin, but it has been less well studied and should **not** be used for pulmonary infections because it is inactivated by surfactant and therefore does not achieve sufficiently high concentrations in the respiratory tract

2. Modification of the initial antimicrobials regimen: [19]

The observed median times to defervescence for patients with high risk febrile neutropenia is about **4 to 5** days in case of patients with haematologic malignancies or haematopoietic stem cell recipients while it is about **2 days** in solid cancer patients. However, those patients with persistence of fever beyond expected time and those with clinical deterioration may require modification of the initial antimicrobial regimen. Modifications to the antimicrobial regimen during the course of neutropenic fever can be made based upon the following principles

- The initial treatment regimen should be modified based upon clinical and microbiologic data.
- Patients with persistent fever who become hemodynamically unstable after initial doses of a standard antimicrobial regimen for neutropenic fever should have their regimen broadened to include coverage for resistant gram-negative, gram-positive, and anaerobic bacteria as well as fungi.
- Unexplained persistent fever in a patient who is otherwise stable rarely necessitates an empiric adjustment to the initial antibacterial regimen.
- Documented infections (based on clinical findings and/or microbiologic data) should be treated with antibiotics that are appropriate for the site and susceptibility patterns of organisms that are isolated.
- If vancomycin or other gram-positive coverage was started initially, it may be stopped after 2–3 days if there is no evidence of a gram-positive infection. Vancomycin overuse has been associated with the development of resistance (eg, vancomycin-resistant *Enterococcus* spp).
- Empiric antifungal coverage should be considered in high-risk patients who have persistent fever after 4–7 days of a broad-spectrum antibacterial regimen and no identified source of fever.

- Oral ulcerations may be due to herpes simplex virus or *Candida* spp. Thus, addition of acyclovir and/or Fluconazole may be warranted if these findings are present.
- In patients with diarrhea, if there are abdominal signs, empiric therapy of *C. difficile* can be instituted while assays are pending

Persistent fever

- Key factors in the management of patients with persistent fever include whether the patient is clinically stable, whether there is an identified site of infection, and when the patient is expected to recover from neutropenia.
- Unexplained persistent fever in a patient who is otherwise stable rarely necessitates an empiric adjustment to the initial antibacterial regimen.
- Patients with persistent fever should be re-evaluated eg. Clinical examination, chest/abdomen imaging for focus of infection, blood cultures etc.
- Antibiotic resistance: [25–28]
- The following antibiotics can be used when resistant infections are suspected:
  - MRSA: Vancomycin, linezolid, or daptomycin; daptomycin should be avoided in patients with pneumonia
  - VRE: Linezolid or daptomycin.
  - ESBL-producing gram-negative bacilli: A Carbapenem (eg, Imipenem, meropenem).
- Carbapenemase-producing bacteria, including *K. pneumoniae* carbapenemase: Colistin or tigecycline
- Anti-fungal therapy: [29, 30]
- An empiric antifungal agent should be added after 4–7 days in high-risk febrile neutropenia patients with persistent fever. The rationale for this approach is that undiagnosed fungal infection is seen in many patients with prolonged neutropenia. In patients who are clinically unstable or have a suspected fungal infection, antifungal therapy should be considered even earlier.
- Choice of anti-fungal agent:
- The 2010 IDSA guidelines for empiric antifungal therapy recommend Amphotericin B deoxycholate, Liposomal Amphotericin B, Caspofungin, Voriconazole, or Itraconazole as suitable options for empiric antifungal therapy in neutropenic patients

Patient clinical profile	*Preferred antifungal*	*Additional information*
– Persistent febrile neutropenia – No evidence of fungal infection eg. Pulmonary nodules, sinusitis – No h/o antifungal prophylaxis	Caspofungin Any other Echinocandin	Candida sp. is likely cause in such cases and Echinocandins have very good activity against Candida

Patient clinical profile	*Preferred antifungal*	*Additional information*
– Persistent febrile neutropenia – Nodular pulmonary infiltrates – Not on anti-fungal prophylaxis	Voriconazole Amphotericin B (Preferably Liposomal formulation) Other options: Posaconazole Isavuconazole	Nodular pulmonary infiltrates suggest mold infection Aspergillosis is the most common mold infection in neutropenic patients
– Persistent febrile neutropenia – Nodular pulmonary infiltrates – H/O anti-fungal prophylaxis	A different mold active antifungal to be used	
Suspected Mucormycosis	Amphotericin B	Echinocandins and Azoles are less active

- Institutional practice:
  1. Anti-fungal prophylaxis: Voriconazole (Preferred) or Itraconazole
  2. Empiric antifungal in persistent febrile neutropenia: Amphotericin B; Echinocandins are sometimes added later in refractory cases
- Central venous catheter removal: [19]
- If blood cultures drawn from the CVC become positive at least 120 min before peripheral blood cultures drawn at the same time, then the CVC is likely to be the source of the bacteremia.
- In addition to antibiotics, CVC removal is recommended for patients with catheter-related bloodstream infections caused by any of the following organisms:
  1. *S. aureus*
  2. *P. Aeruginosa*
  3. *Candida* species
  4. Rapidly growing Non-tuberculous mycobacteria
- Other indications for CVC removal are
  1. Bloodstream infection that persists despite ≥72 h of therapy with appropriate antibiotics
  2. Tunnel infection, Port pocket infection
  3. Septic thrombosis
  4. Endocarditis
  5. Sepsis with hemodynamic instability
- Antibiotics should be administered for a minimum of 14 days following catheter removal **and** clearance of blood cultures.
- A prolonged duration of treatment of 4–6 weeks is recommended for patients with complicated CVC-associated infections, such as those with deep tissue infection, endocarditis, septic thrombosis, or persistent bacteremia or fungemia occurring >72 h following catheter removal in a patient receiving appropriate antimicrobial therapy

Duration of antimicrobial therapy: [31]

- If the patient has been afebrile for at least 3 days and the ANC is ≥500 cells/microL and is showing a consistent increasing trend, antibiotics are generally stopped.
- If an infectious source of fever is identified, antibiotics should be continued for at least the standard duration indicated for the specific infection (eg, 14 days for *E. coli* bacteremia)

Dr. BRA-IRCH, AIIMS High risk febrile neutropenia antibiotic protocol

Sl no	Antibiotic name	Adult dose	Pediatric dose
1	Cefoperazone-Sulbactam	Cefoperazone = 100 mg/kg day in 2–3 div doses	Cefoperazone = 100 mg/kg day in 2–3 div doses
2	Amikacin	15 mg/kg day single dose	15 mg/kg day single dose
3	Meropenem	60–120 mg/kg day in 2–3 div doses	60–120 mg/kg day in 2–3 div doses
4	Imipenem	500 mg QID	20 mg/kg dose QID
5	Teicoplanin	400 mg BD for 3 doses f/b OD	10 mg/kg dose BD for 3 doses f/b OD
5	Piperacillin-tazobactam	Piperacillin = 100 mg/kg dose TDS/QID	Piperacillin = 100 mg/kg dose TDS/QID
6	Colistin	1.5 mIU/kg loading f/b 0.5mIU/kg dose TDS	1.5 mIU/kg loading f/b 0.5mIU/kg dose TDS
7	Tigecycline	100 mg loading f/b 50 mg BD	1.5–3 mg/kg loading f/b 1–2 mg/kg dose BD
8	Clindamycin	600–2700 mg/day in 2–4 div doses	20–40 mg/kg day in 3–4 div doses
9	Daptomycin	6–8 mg/kg OD	6–8 mg/kg OD
10	Linezolid	600 mg BD	20–30 mg/kg day 2–3 div doses
11	Vancomycin	500 mg TDS	15 mg/kg dose TDS
12	Levofloxacin	750 mg IV	10 mg/kg dose OD
13	Aztreonam	30 mg/kg dose TDS	30 mg/kg dose TDS

Sl no	Antifungal name	Adult dose	Pediatric dose
1	Voriconazole	200 mg BD	9 mg/kg/dose BD
2	Amphotericin B Conventional	1 mg/kg OD	1 mg/kg OD
3	Amphotericin B Liposomal	3–5 mg/kg OD	3–5 mg/kg OD
4	Caspofungin	70 mg loading f/b 50 mg OD	70 mg/m^2/dose loading f/b 50 mg/m^2/dose (max: 70 mg)

21.7 Case Vignettes

Case 1: 20 year old male with therapy related AML, developed febrile neutropenia on day +14 following consolidation HiDAC chemotherapy. On examination, he was hemodynamically stable and systemic examination was normal. There was evidence of PICC line site thrombophlebitis.

Qu. 1: What should be the initial antibiotic regimen for this patient?

Ans: This is a case of high risk febrile neutropenia as the expected duration for recovery of neutrophil counts is more than 7 days. So, this patient must be managed with IV antibiotics with anti-pseudomonal coverage ideally in an in-patient setting. Since, there is a focus of catheter site infection, a gram positive coverage should also be given to this patient. So, a combination of antibiotics with anti-pseudomonal activity and an antibiotic with gram positive coverage should be started.

Qu.2 Should the PICC line be removed at this point?

Ans: No; there is no indication to remove the PICC line at this point. However, if the patient remains febrile 72 h after starting the antibiotic or if blood culture grows organisms like S aureus, Pseudomonas sps, Candida sps and Non-Tuberculous Mycobacteria or there is hemodynamic instability, catheter removal can be considered.

This patient was started on Inj Cefoperazone + Sulbactam, Inj Levofloxacin and Inj Teicoplanin. Patient became afebrile within 24 h of starting the antibiotics. PICC line site had also improved. But, the patient again developed fever after 72 h. On examination, patient was hemodynamically stable and there were no new clinical focus of infection. Blood c/s was sterile.

Qu.3 Does the antibiotic regimen needs to be changed?

- Ans: Yes; In view of breakthrough fever despite administration of anti-pseudomonal antibiotics, antibiotic resistance should be suspected. Carbapenems can be started at this point.
- Qu. 4 Are any other investigations required at this point?

Ans: Since, the patient is having prolonged neutropenia with breakthrough fever, possibility of fungal infections must be suspected at this point. Thus, HRCT- Chest to rule out fungal pneumonia and serum Galactomannan level must be done.

Inj Levofloxacin was changed to Inj Meropenem first {Magnex + Meropenem + Teicoplanin} and then, Inj Magnex was changed to Inj Piperacillin-Tazobactam {Pip-Taz + Meropenem + Teicoplanin} as fever persisted. HRCT-Chest was done which revealed patchy areas of consolidation with surrounding GGOs in bilateral lungs suggestive of fungal infection. Voriconazole dose is increased to 300 mg BD {Earlier patient was on prophylactic Voriconazole @ 200 mg BD}. Gradually, the fever spikes came down and there was no breakthrough fever until recovery of the ANC to ≥500/mcL.

Case 2: A 26 year housewife, newly diagnosed case of AML presented with fever along with left submandibular cellulitis. On examination, she was frail but hemodynamically stable. Local examination revealed left sub-mandibular tender swelling with overlying redness. USG revealed only inflammatory changes with no evidence of abscess. She was chemotherapy naive at the time of presentation.

Qu 1 What should be the initial antibiotic regimen for this patient?

Ans: This is a case of high risk febrile neutropenia as this patient is having disease related febrile neutropenia with no chance of recovery of neutrophil count without chemotherapy. With chemotherapy, there will be further neutropenia as well before final recovery of normal blood cell elements. Along with these factors, she is also frail and burden of disease is high. So, ideally this patient should be managed with IV antibiotics with anti-pseudomonal coverage. Since, there is a focus of soft tissue infection, a gram positive coverage should also be given to this patient. So, a combination of antibiotics with anti-pseudomonal activity and an antibiotic with gram positive coverage should be started.

This patient was started on combination of Cefoperazone-Sulbactam and Amoxycillin-Clavulanate. As the general condition deteriorated, Inj Meropenem was added and Amoxycillin-Clavulanate was changed to Inj Teicoplanin. Patient became afebrile within 48 h of this antibiotic modification. After a total 14 days of antibiotic therapy, induction 3 + 7 chemotherapy was started and antibiotics stopped.

Qu 2: After starting the 3 + 7 chemotherapy, on day +9, patient again developed neutropenic fever. On examination, vitals were stable and there were no obvious focus of infection other than the healing submandibular soft tissue infection. What should be done?

Ans: This should be considered as a fresh episode of febrile neutropenia {high risk}. After sending routine investigations like blood culture and sensitivity, chest x ray, serum procalcitonin and Galactomannan levels, patient should be started on empirical antibiotics with anti-pseudomonal activity.

This patient was started on Magnex and Amikacin. In view of persistent fever and a healing soft tissue focus, gram positive coverage was added early. Later, Amikacin was stopped and Meropenem was started as infection by ESBL producing organisms is suspected clinically.

Qu 3: Despite above treatment, patient continued to be febrile and by day 4 of starting the antibiotic therapy, patient developed diarrhea and right sided abdominal pain. On examination, she was hypotensive and there was tenderness at right iliac fossa. What should be done now?

Ans: Clinically, it looks like patient is having gram negative sepsis with shock. The likely focus of infection is neutropenic enterocolitis {Typhlitis}. For hemodynamic part, patient should be started on IV fluid support along with inotropes with appropriate titration. Repeat chest x ray, blood culture, serum procalcitonin level and serum Galactomannan level must be done. USG-abdomen must be done to look for evidence of typhlitis. From antibiotics point of view, colistin must be started at this point as there was progression of infection leading to septicaemia despite administration of Meropenem which indicates infection by carbapenemase producing organisms. Also, simulataneous fungal infections must be suspected at this point. HRCT-Chest and serum Galactomannan levels can help in identifying Aspergillus sps infections. Blood culture for fungal elements may help in identifying systemic candidiasis. Therapeutic antifungals like Amphotericin B/ Echinocandins/Azoles must be started as well.

This patient was started on Colistin and Caspofungin. Magnex was stopped but Meropenem and Teicoplanin were continued. Inotropes started. Patient was kept NPO and Ryles' tube drain was placed. Abdominal imaging confirmed typhlitis. Blood culture grew Klebsiella Pneumoniae which was sensitive to Colistin only. This confirmed our clinical suspicion of an infection by carbapenemase producing organism. Chest imaging revealed a patch of consolidation at RUL of lung {? fungal}. In view of no defervescence of fever after 24 h of starting colistin, meropenem was stopped and Tigecycline was added which is also active against carbapenemase producing organisms.

Qu 4; Despite 72 h of antibiotic therapy with a combination of Colistin + Tigecycline + Teicoplanin along with anti-fungal Caspofungin, patient remained febrile along with increasing requirement of inotropes. What should be done?

Ans: Reserve antibiotics are the options in this situation. Inj Linezolid can be started instead of Inj Teicoplanin which has coverage for VRSA/VRE. Inj Aztreonam can be added for carbapenemase producing organism coverage. Cefepime, 5th generation Cephalosporins and Phosphomycin are some other options as well. Piperacillin-Tazobactam can also be tried since patient was yet to be exposed to it but provided the clinical situation, it may not be a prudent step. Granulocyte transfusions can also be considered at this point to tide over the crisis. G-CSF can also be tried to hasten the neutrophil recovery.

This patient was switched to Aztreonam + Colistin + Linezolid. Blood culture also grew Enterococcus faecium sensitive to both Vancomycin and Linezolid. Later, Patient developed NEC related intestinal perforation which was managed conservatively. An enterocutaneous fistula also formed later. Multiple granulocyte transfusions, TPN support and G-CSF were given. Patient finally recovered by day 32 of 3 + 7 chemotherapy. Enterocutaneous fistula was surgically managed later.

References

1. Freifeld AG, Bow EJ, Sepkowitz KA, Boeckh MJ, Ito JI, Mullen CA, Raad II, Rolston KV, Young JA, Wingard JR. Clinical practice guideline for the use of antimicrobial agents in neutropenic patients with cancer: 2010 update by the infectious diseases society of America., Infectious Diseases Society of America SO. Clin Infect Dis. 2011;52(4):e56.
2. Bow EJ. Neutropenic fever syndromes in patients undergoing cytotoxic therapy for acute leukemia and myelodysplastic syndromes. Semin haematol. 2009;46:259–68.
3. From the Immunocompromised Host Society. The design, analysis, and reporting of clinical trials on the empirical antibiotic management of the neutropenic patient. Report of a consensus panel. J Infect Dis. 1990;161(3):397.
4. Klastersky J, Paesmans M, Rubenstein EB, et al. The multinational Association for Supportive Care in cancer risk index: a multinational scoring system for identifying low-risk febrile neutropenic cancer patients. J Clin Oncol. 2000;18:3038–51.
5. Carmona-Bayonas A, Jiménez-Fonseca P, Virizuela Echaburu J, et al. Prediction of serious complications in patients with seemingly stable febrile neutropenia: validation of the clinical index of stable febrile neutropenia in a prospective cohort of patients from the FINITE study. J Clin Oncol. 2015;33(5):465–71.

6. Schimpff SC, Young VM, Greene WH, Vermeulen GD, Moody MR, Wiernik PH. Origin of infection in acute nonlymphocytic leukemia. Significance of hospital acquisition of potential pathogens. Ann Intern Med. 1972;77(5):707.
7. Pagano L, Caira M, Nosari A, Rossi G, Viale P, Aversa F, Tumbarello M. Etiology of febrile episodes in patients with acute myeloid leukemia: results from the Hema e-chart registry; Hema e-chart group, Italy. Arch Intern Med. 2011;171(16):1502–3.
8. Bodey GP, Jadeja L, Elting L, Pseudomonas bacteremia. Retrospective analysis of 410 episodes. Arch Intern Med. 1985;145(9):1621.
9. Mikulska M, Viscoli C, Orasch C, Livermore DM, Averbuch D, Cordonnier C. Akova M; aetiology and resistance in bacteraemias among adult and paediatric haematology and cancer patients; fourth European conference on infections in Leukemia group (ECIL-4), a joint venture of EBMT, EORTC, ICHS, ELN and ESGICH/ESCMID. J Infect. 2014;68(4):321. Epub 2013 Dec 24.
10. Holland T, Fowler VG Jr, Shelburne SA 3rd. Invasive gram-positive bacterial infection in cancer patients. Clin Infect Dis. 2014:59.
11. Pagano L, Caira M, Nosari A, Rossi G, Viale P, Aversa F, Tumbarello M, Hema e-Chart Group, Italy. Etiology of febrile episodes in patients with acute myeloid leukemia: results from the Hema e-chart registry. Arch Intern Med. 2011;171(16):1502–3.
12. Chang HY, Rodriguez V, Narboni G, et al. Causes of death in adults with acute leukemia. Medicine (Baltimore). 1976;55:259–68.
13. Gardner A, Mattiuzzi G, Faderl S, Borthakur G, Garcia-Manero G, Pierce S, Brandt M, Estey E. Randomized comparison of cooked and noncooked diets in patients undergoing remission induction therapy for acute myeloid leukemia. J Clin Oncol. 2008;26(35):5684.
14. Bow EJ, Meddings JB. Intestinal mucosal dysfunction and infection during remission-induction therapy for acute myeloid leukaemia. Leukemia. 2006;20(12):2087–92. Epub 2006 Nov 02.
15. Messer SA, Jones RN, Fritsche TR. International surveillance of Candida spp. and aspergillus spp.: report from the SENTRY antimicrobial surveillance program (2003). J Clin Microbiol. 2006;44(5):1782.
16. Reichenberger F, Habicht JM, Gratwohl A, Tamm M. Diagnosis and treatment of invasive pulmonary aspergillosis in neutropenic patients. Eur Respir J. 2002;19
17. Petrikkos G, Skiada A, Lortholary O, Roilides E, Thomas J, Dimitrios P. Epidemiology and clinical manifestations of Mucormycosis. Clin Infect Dis. 2012;54(suppl_1):S23–34.
18. Saral R, Burns WH, Laskin OL, Santos GW, Lietman PS, Engl N. Acyclovir prophylaxis of herpes-simplex-virus infections. J Med. 1981;305(2):63.
19. Freifeld AG, Bow EJ, Sepkowitz KA, et al. Clinical practice guideline for the use of antimicrobial agents in neutropenic patients with cancer: 2010 update by the Infectious Diseases Society of America. Clin Infect Dis. 2011;52:e56.
20. National Comprehensive Cancer Network (NCCN) Clinical Practice Guidelines in Oncology. Prevention and treatment of cancer-related infections. Version 1.2018. http://www.nccn.org. Accessed 1 Aug 2018.
21. Taplitz RA, Kennedy EB, Bow EJ, et al. Outpatient management of fever and neutropenia in adults treated for malignancy: American Society of Clinical Oncology and Infectious Diseases Society of America clinical practice guideline update. J Clin Oncol. 2018;36:1443.
22. Taplitz RA, Kennedy EB, Bow EJ, Crews J, Gleason C, Hawley DK, Langston AA, Nastoupil LJ, Rajotte M, Rolston K, Strasfeld L, Flowers CR. Outpatient Management of Fever and Neutropenia in adults treated for malignancy: American Society of Clinical Oncology and Infectious Diseases Society of America clinical practice guideline update. J Clin Oncol. 2018;36(14):1443. Epub 2018 Feb 20.
23. Kern WV, Marchetti O, Drgona L, Akan H, Aoun M, Akova M, de Bock R, Paesmans M, Viscoli C, Calandra T. Oral antibiotics for fever in low-risk neutropenic patients with cancer: a double-blind, randomized, multicenter trial comparing single daily moxifloxacin with twice daily ciprofloxacin plus amoxicillin/clavulanic acid combination therapy--EORTC infectious diseases group trial XV. J Clin Oncol. 2013;31(9):1149. Epub 2013 Jan 28.

24. de Naurois J, Novitzky-Basso I, Gill MJ, Marti FM, Cullen MH, Roila F. Management of febrile neutropenia: ESMO clinical practice guidelines; ESMO guidelines working group. Ann Oncol. 2010;21(Suppl 5):v252.
25. Averbuch D, Cordonnier C, Livermore DM, Mikulska M, Orasch C, Viscoli C, Gyssens IC, Kern WV, Klyasova G, Marchetti O, Engelhard D, Akova M. Targeted therapy against multi-resistant bacteria in leukemic and hematopoietic stem cell transplant recipients: guidelines of the 4th European conference on infections in Leukemia (ECIL-4, 2011), ECIL4, a joint venture of EBMT, EORTC, ICHS, ESGICH/ESCMID and ELN. Haematologica. 2013;98(12):1836.
26. Rolston KV. Challenges in the treatment of infections caused by gram-positive and gram-negative bacteria in patients with cancer and neutropenia. Clin Infect Dis. 2005;40(Suppl 4):S246.
27. Sipsas NV, Bodey GP, Kontoyiannis DP. Perspectives for the management of febrile neutropenic patients with cancer in the 21st century. Cancer. 2005;103(6):1103.
28. Satlin MJ, Jenkins SG, Walsh TJ. The global challenge of carbapenem-resistant Enterobacteriaceae in transplant recipients and patients with hematologic malignancies. Clin Infect Dis. 2014;58(9):1274. Epub 2014 Jan 23.
29. Kibbler CC. Empirical antifungal therapy in febrile neutropenic patients: current status. Curr Top Med Mycol. 1997;8(1–2):5.
30. Wingard JR, Leather HL. Empiric antifungal therapy for the neutropenic patient. Oncology (Williston Park). 2001;15(3):351.
31. Aguilar-Guisado M, Espigado I, Martín-Peña A, Gudiol C, et al. Optimisation of empirical antimicrobial therapy in patients with haematological malignancies and febrile neutropenia (how long study): an open-label, randomised, controlled phase 4 trial. Lancet Haematol. 2017;4:e573–83.

Graft Versus Host Disease (GHVD) in Critically Ill Oncologic Patients

22

Neha Ganju, Sahitya Sri Krishna, and Mukul Aggarwal

22.1 Introduction

Allogeneic hematopoietic stem cell transplantation (Allo SCT) is an important therapeutic option for various malignant and non-malignant conditions. Graft-versus-host-disease (GVHD) is one of the most common life-threatening complications of Allo SCT. Despite immunosuppression, 30–70% of patients will develop GVHD [1]. Prevalence of grade II–IV acute GVHD and chronic GVHD is 15 and 28%, respectively, in Allo SCT patients admitted to ICU [2, 3]. Up to 70% of mortality rates are reported in acute GVHD patients requiring life-sustaining therapies [4, 5]. Patients with grade 3–4 acute GVHD had a 2-year survival of 20% and 5-year survival of only 8% [6].

Widespread use of alternate stem cell sources, including haploidentical donors in recent years, has seen an increase in GVHD prevalence. Management of GVHD in acutely ill patients is challenging. On the one hand, GVHD often affects vital organs, thus compromising their function, and on the other hand, GVHD therapy leads to further immunosuppression, predisposing patients to fatal infections.

Classically, GVHD is defined as acute or chronic depending on the time of onset using a cut-off of 100 days. However, this definition has been rechallenged given the varied presentations of GVHD outside their predefined time-period. To differentiate between acute and chronic GVHD, clinical manifestations and diagnostic criteria are being increasingly used rather than the time of onset [7].

N. Ganju · S. S. Krishna · M. Aggarwal (✉)
Department of Haematology, AIIMS, New Delhi, New Delhi, India

V. Kumar et al. (eds.), *Onco-critical Care*,
https://doi.org/10.1007/978-981-16-9929-0_22

22.2 Pathophysiology

The pathophysiology of GVHD is attributed to three phases:

1. Activation of antigen-presenting cells (APCs).
2. Donor T cell activation, proliferation, differentiation, and migration.
3. Target tissue destruction.

There is an activation of host antigen-presenting cells due to underlying disease and conditioning regimen (a combination of chemotherapeutic drugs given before SCT). Damage to host tissues leads to the secretion of proinflammatory cytokines, such as TNF- α and IL-1, and chemokines, such as CCL2–5 and CXCL9–11, increased expression of adhesion molecules, MHC antigens, and costimulatory molecules on host APCs. The intensity of the conditioning regimen and the degree of tissue injury appear to be associated with the risk of GVHD. Donor lymphocytes infused into the recipient profoundly damage tissues from the effects of the underlying disease, prior infections, and the transplant conditioning regimen. This leads to the activation of donor T lymphocytes and target organ damage [8].

22.3 Risk Factors and Prevention for GVHD

1. **Degree of major/minor histocompatibility disparity**: It is the most critical determinant of GVHD risk, with the lowest GVHD incidence seen in syngeneic transplants [9–11]. Allo SCT types can be sorted in order of GVHD risk as follows: syngeneic < HLA matched related (sibling) < HLA-matched unrelated < HLA-mismatched unrelated similar to the haploidentical donor.
2. **Gender disparity**: Female donor to male recipient transplants bears the higher risk of GVHD [12, 13].
3. **Graft source**: Peripheral blood grafts have a significantly high number of T cells than those in bone marrow grafts, and hence peripheral blood grafts carry a higher risk of GVHD compared to those from bone marrow grafts [14]. Umbilical cord grafts cause less GVHD [15].
4. **Conditioning regimen intensity**: Reduced-intensity conditioning regimens are associated with a lower risk of GVHD than myeloablative regimens [9, 16].
5. **Prior acute GVHD** increases the risk of developing chronic GVHD [12, 17].
6. **Prophylaxis type and intensity**: Calcineurin inhibitors (CNI) with/without methotrexate [18, 19] or mycophenolate mofetil (MMF) [20] are the most used GVHD prophylaxis regimens for Allo SCT from HLA-matched donors. Ex vivo T cell depletion of the graft [21], Anti thymocyte globulin (ATG), and high dose posttransplant cyclophosphamide [22] are commonly used strategies to mitigate the risk of GVHD in mismatched and haploidentical SCT.

Case 1: A 42-year-old female, a case of acute myeloid leukemia, presented on day + 40 post matched sibling stem cell transplantation with complaints of skin rash that started initially over palms and sole and progressed rapidly to involve

the whole body. There were areas of bullae formation and desquamation over the trunk. She was on prophylactic immunosuppression with cyclosporine post-transplant. On evaluation, her complete blood count was normal; the liver function test showed bilirubin of 2.5 mg/dl with SGOT and SGPT 3 times the upper limit of normal, and her renal function was normal.

First Line Therapy: This patient has stage IV skin GVHD, stage I liver GVHD, and stage 0 gut GVHD with an overall Glucksberg grade IV GVHD (Refer to Table 22.1 for stages and grades of GVHD). She was started on methylprednisolone 1 mg/kg twice a day along with skin-directed therapy. Since she had skin desquamation, wound dressings were done regularly, and due precautions were taken to prevent skin infections. Also, since extensive skin involvement can cause increased insensible water loss, strict intake output balance was maintained.

DISCUSSION: Choice of initial therapy for acute GVHD depends on organs involved, the severity of the disease, and the prophylactic regimen used. In grade II-IV acute GVHD cases, CNI levels should be optimized [9] to maintain trough cyclosporine level in the range of 200–400 ng/mL [23]. Standard first-line agents include corticosteroids, particularly methylprednisolone, initiated at a dose of 2 mg/kg day intravenously [24]. If the patient responds, oral steroids are continued at high doses for 1–2 weeks and then tapered gradually over several weeks. Most centres consider steroid-refractory patients as those who have progressive symptoms after 3 days or do not respond to 5–7 days of intravenous methylprednisolone 2 mg/kg in conjunction with CNIs. Despite being the standard therapy, the response rate to systemic steroids in acute GVHD is limited to 30–40%, and steroid-refractory patients are at an increased risk of transplantation related-mortality due to increased immunosuppression and infections.

Table 22.1 Glucksberg grading of acute GVHD

<table>
<tr><td colspan="2">I—Stage 1 or 2 skin involvement; no liver or gut involvement; ECOG PS 0</td></tr>
<tr><td colspan="2">II—Stage 1 to 3 skin involvement; grade 1 liver or gut involvement; ECOG PS 1</td></tr>
<tr><td colspan="2">III—Stage 2 or 3 skin, liver, or gut involvement; ECOG PS 2</td></tr>
<tr><td colspan="2">IV—Stage 1 to 4 skin involvement; stage 2 to 4 liver or gut involvement; ECOG PS 3</td></tr>
<tr><td>Organ</td><td>Stage</td></tr>
<tr><td>Skin</td><td>1—A maculopapular rash over <25% of body area</td></tr>
<tr><td></td><td>2—A maculopapular rash over 25–50% of body area</td></tr>
<tr><td></td><td>3—Generalised erythroderma</td></tr>
<tr><td></td><td>4—Generalized erythroderma with the bullous formation and often with desquamation</td></tr>
<tr><td>Liver</td><td>1—Bilirubin 2.0–3.0 mg/dL; SGOT 150 to 750 IU</td></tr>
<tr><td></td><td>2—Bilirubin 3.1–6.0 mg/dL</td></tr>
<tr><td></td><td>3—Bilirubin 6.1–15 mg/dL</td></tr>
<tr><td></td><td>4—Bilirubin >15 mg/dL</td></tr>
<tr><td>Gut</td><td>1—Diarrhoea >30 mL/kg or > 500 mL/day</td></tr>
<tr><td></td><td>2—Diarrhoea >60 mL/kg or > 1000 mL/day</td></tr>
<tr><td></td><td>3—Diarrhoea >90 mL/kg or > 1500 mL/day</td></tr>
<tr><td></td><td>4—Diarrhoea >90 mL/kg or > 2000 mL/day; or severe abdominal pain with or without ileus</td></tr>
</table>

In addition to systemic therapy, local skin directed therapy include:

For intact skin: Topical therapies like steroids, emollients, tacrolimus are prescribed. Topical steroids of mid-high potency like clobetasol are generally applied to moist skin and covered with warm wet towels as an occlusive measure (wet wraps). Topical tacrolimus is reserved for second-line therapy.

Antihistamines and moisturizers are used for pruritis [25].

Non-intact skin: Patients are prone to super-added infections (bacterial, viral, fungal). The wound dressings should be done regularly and treated with an adequate antibiotic if deemed necessary. Extensive skin involvement can cause third-spacing, thus increasing fluid requirement [26]. These management strategies, at times, parallels that in patients with extensive burns.

Prophylaxis: Antimicrobial prophylaxis, with antibacterial, antiviral, and antifungal therapy, is widely used during GVHD treatment. Commonly used agents include:

- Penicillin V as antibacterial prophylaxis.
- Posaconazole or voriconazole are commonly used for antifungal prophylaxis due to their activity against invasive mold infections [27].
- Pneumocystis prophylaxis with trimethoprim-sulfamethoxazole [28].
- Acyclovir or valacyclovir are used for herpes simplex and varicella-zoster prophylaxis.

Primary prophylaxis with valganciclovir/ganciclovir for cytomegalovirus (CMV) did not improve outcomes when compared to pre-emptive therapy. Therefore, strict vigilance is needed with regular monitoring for CMV viremia with DNA PCR and end-organ damage with CMV and other pathogens.

Continue case 1: After receiving steroids, her skin rash gradually improved. Her CMV PCR remained negative. Her Cyclosporine dose was optimized. On day 50, post-transplant, she developed fever, chills, and hypotension. She was shifted to the Intensive care unit. Broad-spectrum antibiotics were started along with vasopressors after taking appropriate blood cultures. Blood culture grew carbapenem-resistant Klebsiella, for which antibiotics were modified according to the culture sensitivity report, and steroids were tapered gradually. After receiving appropriate antibiotics, fever and hypotension settled in 3–4 days. But she developed acute kidney injury. All antibiotics were modified according to creatinine clearance, cyclosporine adjusted according to trough levels, and intake output was monitored. Gradually acute kidney injury(AKI) settled, and she was shifted back to the ward.

Infections are an important cause of mortality in GVHD patients. These patients are at high risk of bacterial, viral, and fungal infections due to immunosuppression. They can develop invasive mold fungal infections and uncommon viral infections like cytomegalovirus, adenovirus, BK polyoma virus. Hemodynamic instability can occur in 12–75% of patients requiring ICU care. Of the infectious causes, most common are bacterial (13%) followed by fungal (7%) and viral (4%) infections respectively [29]. The chance of acquiring an infection with multi-resistant organism increases with the duration of hospital stay, as well as due to previous antibiotics use during therapy prior to transplant.

AKI is an important cause of morbidity and mortality in sepsis. In addition to sepsis and systemic hypoperfusion secondary to shock, other factors that impair kidney function further include nephrotoxic antibiotics and antivirals. AKI is present in 65% of patients, with almost all patients being exposed to a median of three nephrotoxic drugs, such as aminoglycosides, cyclosporine/tacrolimus, vancomycin, acyclovir, contrast agents, renin-angiotensin-aldosterone system inhibitors, liposomal amphotericin, foscarnet etc. [30].

Continue case 1: After tapering steroids, she was started on second-line therapy with ruxolitinib as her skin rashes flared up again. LFT was normal. Her skin erythema stabilized after 7–10 days of treatment. After 1 month of ruxolitinib, she presented to the emergency with fever, cough, and respiratory distress. She was managed in ICU with non-invasive ventilation. CT chest showed bilateral ground-glass opacities. All infective work-up was negative except CMV PCR of 6 log copies/ml. In view of suggestive lung finds on CT Scan and increased CMV PCR, diagnosis of CMV pneumonitis was made. She was treated with ganciclovir and CMV immunoglobulin for 3 weeks. With the improvement of her clinical status, she was shifted to the ward, where maintenance with Valganciclovir was continued, as she required prolonged immunosuppression.

Second-line treatment for both acute and chronic graft-versus-host disease remains a challenge. In this context, many agents have been tried alone or in combination with, but none has convincing results. Table 22.2 summarises the list of available second-line agents.

Ruxolitinib is an effective and safe treatment option in steroid-refractory GVHD (SR GVHD). The overall response rate is 69.5% after a median of 2 weeks of treatment, and 21.7% reached complete remission [31]. In a retrospective study, 95 patients with moderate-severe GVHD refractory to steroids were treated with ruxolitinib. The overall response rate (ORR) was 81% and 85% for acute and chronic GVHD, respectively, with rates of up to 46% of CR in acute and 7.3% in chronic GVHD [32]. Common ruxolitinib-related side effects are infections, thrombocytopenia, and hepatic impairment. CMV reactivation is observed in both SR-acute GVHD (33.3%) and SR-chronic GVHD (14.6%) patients. Hence infectious surveillance is critical, and particularly CMV needs to be monitored carefully [32].

Her CMV pneumonia improved after 2–3 weeks of antiviral therapy. Meanwhile, she had a recurrence of skin GVHD (grade III). Because of repeated infections, she was started on twice-weekly Extracorporeal photopheresis.

CASE 2: A 37-year-old man was admitted to our department with abdominal pain, bloody diarrhoea, and vomiting on day 27 of his transplant. He had undergone myeloablative conditioning followed by haploidentical transplantation for acute lymphoblastic leukaemia. His complete blood count and renal functions were normal. LFT showed total bilirubin of 7 mg/dL, with conjugated bilirubin being 5.1 mg/dL. Infectious work was initiated. He underwent an urgent upper gut endoscopy and sigmoidoscopy that showed hyperaemic

Table 22.2 Second line agents for GVHD

Drugs	Renal modification	Hepatic modification	Comment
Antithymocyte globulin	Nil	Nil	Steroid sparing, durable effects are infrequent, considerable acute toxicity during administration, infections
Alemtuzumab	Not studied	Not studied	Infusion reactions, Reactivations of infections like CMV. Rarely durable responses
Daclizumab	Nil	Pre-existing hepatic disease, ALT/AST >2 times ULN/ history of autoimmune condition involving liver—Contraindicated	Limited availability
Infliximab	Nil	Pre-existing—Dose adjustment not studied On therapy liver injury (>5 ULN of liver enzymes)—discontinue	Preferable in Gut Disease, considerable risk of infection
Etanercept	Not studied	Not studied	Increased infection risk
Extracorporeal photopheresis	Nil	Nil	Optimal dosing not established. Excellent safety profiles, needs venous access, Min platelet count of 30 × 10^9/l. Costly, limited availability
Mycophenolate mofetil	Nil	Nil	Spares steroids. May mimic gut GVHD. Can cause nausea and diarrhoea but usually well tolerated
Sirolimus	No adjustment. But should be considered when using with cyclosporine and increased creatinine.	Loading dose: No dose adjustment Maintenance dose: Child Pugh class A/B—Reduce dose by 33% Child Pugh class C—Reduce dose by 50%	Risk of thrombotic microangiopathy, hyperlipidemia, myelosuppression, seizure, renal dysfunction
Mesenchymal stem cells	Not studied	Not studied	Preferable in gut GVHD, less side effects, repetitive application required. Costly and difficult to procure

Table 22.2 (continued)

Drugs	Renal modification	Hepatic modification	Comment
Ruxolitinib	Cr Cl 15–59 and any platelet count>5 mg once daily ESRD (Cr Cl <15) on dialysis and any platelet count>5 mg once after dialysis ESRD (Cr cl < 15) not on dialysis> avoid	Pre-existing hepatic impairment: Mild to severe impairment (NCI)and any platelet count—No adjustment Stage III/IV liver GVHD and any platelet count >5 mg once a day and close monitoring	Increased risk of viral reactivation

Table 22.3 Mimics of gastrointestinal GVHD

Upper gut GVHD	Medicines, Conditioning regimen related side effects (<20 days), Herpes virus infections, H pylori infection with ulcer, Increased intracranial pressure
Lowe Gut GVHD	Residual effect of conditioning chemotherapy (<20 days), Viral infections like CMV, Bacterial infections and parasitic infections, Side effects of drugs like MMF/ brincidofovir etc
Hepatic GVHD	**Early jaundice**: Cholangitis lenta, Drug induced liver injury(DILI), Residual effect of sinusoidal obstruction syndrome **Cholestatic pattern**: Cholangitis lenta, Drug induced liver injury, Biliary obstruction(sludge,stones) **Hepatitis pattern**: Hepatitis due to HBV/HCV, DILI, Hypoxic injury secondary to respiratory failure or shock

mucosa. Rectal and duodenal biopsies were taken and sent for histopathological examination and CMV inclusions. With a high pretest probability of GVHD, he was diagnosed with grade IV Gut GVHD andgrade III Liver GVHD. Methylprednisolone 1 mg/kg twice a day was started as 1st line therapy along with oral budesonide. Mycophenolate was continued, and the tacrolimus dose was optimized to target a trough of 5–15 ng/ml. He was on antiviral, antimold as well as pneumocystis prophylaxis. CMV was monitored as per schedule. After 1 week of steroids and optimal tacrolimus dose, there was an improvement of his clinical parameters.

This patient was at high risk for GVHD as he underwent a myeloablative haploidentical stem cell transplantation. In this case scenario, there was a high pretest probability of GVHD and lesser possibility of infection. There should be a low threshold to pursue histological diagnosis of GVHD by endoscopy and biopsy. Various limitations to histological diagnosis include sampling error, patchiness of GVHD-related abnormalities, and absence of early histologic abnormalities in both gut and liver GVHD [33]. Also, the correlation between severity on biopsy and clinical grading is limited to mostly stage IV disease. The differential diagnosis of diarrhoea with abdominal pain in an allograft recipient is given in Table 22.3.

Definite first line therapy include steroid which should be started on the basis of clinical suspicion, and biopsy should be planned urgently. Along with intravenous steroids, oral non-absorbable steroids like beclomethasone or budesonide addition to systemic therapy have been shown to increase response rates and decrease systemic steroid exposure [34].

Monitoring stool volume, consistency, and frequency and abdominal girth daily help the clinician dynamically stage the GVHD and take the appropriate and timely therapeutic decision. Blood in stools and increasing abdominal girth are indicators of grade IV GVHD, which has an abysmal prognosis with high mortality. Stool consistency is usually liquid with or without blood, and volume can be more than 2 L/day. Fluid resuscitation and electrolytes management can be extremely challenging in these settings and oral intake is usually restricted. An accurate intake-output measurement along with frequent electrolyte assessment is required for appropriate supplementation. Opioids should be used cautiously for abdominal pain due to the risk of ileus [26]. Octreotide use can reduce the amount of diarrhea, but early discontinuation should be ensured to avoid ileus development and tachyphylaxis [35–37]. Lower GI GVHD can cause malnutrition, protein-losing enteropathy, and nutrient deficiencies [38]. Malnutrition is associated with decreased overall survival and increased infection risk. Maintaining nutritional status in these patients can be very demanding, and they should be carefully assessed by a dietician [26]. In the peri-transplant period, enteral nutrition is preferable to parenteral nutrition. Nasogastric feeding is associated with less systemic infection and significantly less GVHD, if started early before the onset of mucositis [39]. Parenteral nutrition with oral glutamine is reserved for severely ill patients [40].

Hepatic dysfunction can lead to coagulopathy, increased risk of bleeding, drug toxicity requiring dose modifications, and avoidance of hepatotoxic drugs. Supportive measures include ursodeoxycholic acid, diuretics, albumin infusions, with careful fluid balance monitoring [26].

Continue Patient 2: His rectal biopsy was consistent with GVHD and no evidence of viral infections. CMV was not detectable by quantitative PCR. After 2 weeks of steroids, he again had severe abdominal pain along with bloody diarrhoea. His bilirubin level also started to rise again. He was shifted to the critical care unit because of a gastrointestinal bleed. He was advised for ruxolitinib, but due to low platelet counts, it could not be given. Etanercept 25 mg subcutaneously twice weekly for 4 weeks was added as a second-line agent and tapering schedule of steroids given steroid refractoriness. However, his GVHD did not respond and he succumbed to his illness.

Grade IV gut GVHD with GI bleed requires a lot of supportive care e.g., blood transfusions, fluid management, intake output balance, and antibiotics. This patient also needed a second agent for GVHD treatment. There are 4 categories of therapy that are in wide use for prednisone-refractory gut GVHD, but none achieves >30–50% sustained responses or >20% survival: anti–T-cell antibodies (ATG, alemtuzumab); additional T-cell suppressive drugs (mycophenolic acid, or sirolimus); anti-cytokine biological agents (TNF-a, IL-6); and a variety of other therapies (pulse cyclophosphamide, ECP, psoralen plus ultraviolet light therapy, Janus kinase inhibitors, autologous transplants, allogeneic transplants from different donors) [41]. Patients in early post-transplant period can have cytopenia, commonly thrombocytopenia due to poor graft function, drug toxicity, microangiopathic anemia, infections etc. This further complicates the management of these sick patients, as drugs like ruxolitinib, mycophenolate mofetil are best avoided in patients with platelet counts below 50,000/μL.

Case 3: 30-year-old male with B cell acute lymphoblastic leukaemia underwent a match sibling transplant for relapse disease after achieving measurable residual disease negative remission. He was relatively well till day + 45 when he developed grade II skin GVHD which was managed with topical therapy and optimization of cyclosporine as per trough levels with which he improved. His posttransplant bone marrow was also MRD negative. On day + 126, he presented to emergency with progressive breathlessness over the past 2 weeks. He had morphea like lesions on forehead. Cardiac and infectious causes were ruled out on OPD work up and pulmonary function testing (PFT) showed restriction with markedly reduced FEV1 and FVC.

This young patient has chronic skin and oral mucosa GVHD which responded to topical therapy and optimization of cyclosporine. His history, negative infectious work up and restrictive pattern on PFT were suggestive of lung GVHD.Lungs are involved in up to half of patients with chronic GVHD and are of significant consequence for patients in ICU. It is characterized by small airways inflammation and narrowing due to fibrous scarring leading to Bronchiolitis obliterans (BOS). It is diagnosed after excluding infectious causes and with the aid of computerized tomography imaging and, occasionally, histological examination [42]. The current definition of BOS includes: (1) FEV1 < 75% predicted and an irreversible ≥10% decline in <2 years, (2) FEV1-to-vital capacity (VC) ratio < 0.7 or the lower limit of the 90% confidence interval of the ratio, (3) absence of infection, and (4) either: (a) pre-existing diagnosis of cGVHD, (b) air trapping by expiratory CT, or (c) air trapping on PFTs by residual volume (RV) >120% or RV/total lung capacity (TLC) exceeding the 90% confidence interval [43].

These patients are predisposed to recurrent infections and respiratory failure requiring intensive care management. The condition can deteriorate and lead to chronic damage to lung parenchyma, to the extent that patients may require lung transplant as well.

Continue case 3: His CT chest was done which showed reticulonodular pattern and expiratory air trapping. He was already started on FAM regimen (Formoterol, Azithromycin, and Montelukast) on OPD basis. After few days he was admitted to ICU for worsening hypoxia and breathlessness with SPO2 of 82% on room air. He was managed with non-invasive ventilation alongwith empirical broad-spectrum antibiotics and work up was done for infectious causes of acute exacerbation. He was started on steroids and other immunosuppressive therapies were optimised considering bronchiolitis after ruling out pneumonia. BAL was done to rule out other infectious causes including Pneumocystis jirovecii, nocardia infection as well as routine respiratory viruses. All the infections work-up was negative. Ruxolitinib was added as a

steroid sparing agent. He was monitored for CMV reactivation and received mold and PCP prophylaxis in view of high dose steroids. He gradually improved but required BIPAP which was continued at home with the plan of tapering steroids over the next few weeks.

22.4 Conclusions

Majority of the transplant patients with GVHD seek intensive care management for bleeding, sepsis, shock, viral or fungal pneumonia with respiratory failure, acute kidney injury and altered mentation. These complications arise from GVHD and its consequences. Patients with GVHD are on immunosuppressive drugs, hence at higher risk for viral infections, fungal infections, and sepsis. Grade IV GVHD has a > 80% mortality rate, hence early suspicion of GVHD, prompt work up to rule out other causes and immediate treatment are essential factors for improved survival.

References

1. Zeiser R, Blazar BR. Acute graft-versus-host disease—biologic process, Prevention, and therapy. N Engl J Med. 2017;377(22):2167–79.
2. Bayraktar UD, Nates JL. Intensive care outcomes in adult hematopoietic stem cell transplantation patients. World J Clin Oncol. 2016;7(1):98–105.
3. Bayraktar UD, Milton DR, Shpall EJ, Rondon G, Price KJ, Champlin RE, et al. Prognostic index for critically ill allogeneic transplantation patients. Biol Blood Marrow Transplant. 2017;23(6):991–6.
4. Lengliné E, Chevret S, Moreau A-S, Pène F, Blot F, Bourhis J-H, et al. Changes in intensive care for allogeneic hematopoietic stem cell transplant recipients. Bone Marrow Transplant. 2015 Jun;50(6):840–5.
5. Saillard C, Blaise D, Mokart D. Critically ill allogeneic hematopoietic stem cell transplantation patients in the intensive care unit: reappraisal of actual prognosis. Bone Marrow Transplant. 2016 Aug;51(8):1050–61.
6. Jamani K, Russell JA, Daly A, Stewart D, Savoie L, Duggan P, et al. Prognosis of grade 3–4 acute GVHD continues to be dismal. Bone Marrow Transplant. 2013;48(10):1359–61.
7. Pavletic SZ, Vogelsang GB, Lee SJ. 2014 National Institutes of Health consensus development project on criteria for clinical trials in chronic graft-versus-host disease: preface to the series. Biol Blood Marrow Transplant J Am Soc Blood Marrow Transplant. 2015 Mar;21(3):387–8.
8. Choi SW, Levine JE, Ferrara JLM. Pathogenesis and Management of Graft versus host disease. Immunol Allergy Clin N Am. 2010 Feb;30(1):75–101.
9. Jagasia M, Arora M, Flowers MED, Chao NJ, McCarthy PL, Cutler CS, et al. Risk factors for acute GVHD and survival after hematopoietic cell transplantation. Blood. 2012;119(1):296–307.
10. Martin PJ, Levine DM, Storer BE, Warren EH, Zheng X, Nelson SC, et al. Genome-wide minor histocompatibility matching as related to the risk of graft-versus-host disease. Blood. 2017;129(6):791–8.
11. Santos N, Rodríguez-Romanos R, Nieto JB, Buño I, Vallejo C, Jiménez-Velasco A, et al. UGT2B17 minor histocompatibility mismatch and clinical outcome after HLA-identical sibling donor stem cell transplantation. Bone Marrow Transplant. 2016 Jan;51(1):79–82.

12. Carlens S, Ringdén O, Remberger M, Lönnqvist B, Hägglund H, Klaesson S, et al. Risk factors for chronic graft-versus-host disease after bone marrow transplantation: a retrospective single Centre analysis. Bone Marrow Transplant. 1998 Oct;22(8):755–61.
13. Gratwohl A, de Elvira CR, Gratwohl M, Greinix HT, Duarte R. Gender and graft-versus-host disease after hematopoietic stem cell transplantation. Biol Blood Marrow Transplant. 2016;22(6):1145–6.
14. Chang Y-J, Weng C-L, Sun L-X, Zhao Y-T. Allogeneic bone marrow transplantation compared to peripheral blood stem cell transplantation for the treatment of hematologic malignancies: a meta-analysis based on time-to-event data from randomized controlled trials. Ann Hematol. 2012;91(3):427–37.
15. Rocha V, Wagner JE, Sobocinski KA, Klein JP, Zhang M-J, Horowitz MM, et al. Graft-versus-host disease in children who have received a cord-blood or bone marrow transplant from an HLA-identical sibling. N Engl J Med. 2000;342(25):1846–54.
16. Mielcarek M, Martin PJ, Leisenring W, Flowers MED, Maloney DG, Sandmaier BM, et al. Graft-versus-host disease after nonmyeloablative versus conventional hematopoietic stem cell transplantation. Blood. 2003;102(2):756–62.
17. Przepiorka D, Anderlini P, Saliba R, Cleary K, Mehra R, Khouri I, et al. Chronic graft-versus-host disease after allogeneic blood stem cell transplantation. Blood. 2001;98(6):1695–700.
18. Ratanatharathorn V, Nash RA, Przepiorka D, Devine SM, Klein JL, Weisdorf D, et al. Phase III study comparing methotrexate and tacrolimus (prograf, FK506) with methotrexate and cyclosporine for graft-versus-host disease prophylaxis after HLA-identical sibling bone marrow transplantation. Blood. 1998;92(7):2303–14.
19. Storb R, Deeg HJ, Whitehead J, Appelbaum F, Beatty P, Bensinger W, et al. Methotrexate and cyclosporine compared with cyclosporine alone for prophylaxis of acute graft versus host disease after marrow transplantation for Leukemia. N Engl J Med. 1986;314(12):729–35.
20. Perkins J, Field T, Kim J, Kharfan-Dabaja MA, Fernandez H, Ayala E, et al. A randomized phase II trial comparing tacrolimus and mycophenolate mofetil to tacrolimus and methotrexate for acute graft-versus-host disease prophylaxis. Biol Blood Marrow Transplant. 2010;16(7):937–47.
21. Aversa F, Terenzi A, Tabilio A, Falzetti F, Carotti A, Ballanti S, et al. Full haplotype-mismatched hematopoietic stem-cell transplantation: a phase II study in patients with acute Leukemia at high risk of relapse. J Clin Oncol. 2005;23(15):3447–54.
22. Luznik L, Jalla S, Engstrom LW, Iannone R, Fuchs EJ. Durable engraftment of major histocompatibility complex–incompatible cells after nonmyeloablative conditioning with fludarabine, low-dose total body irradiation, and post-transplantation cyclophosphamide. Blood. 2001;98(12):3456–64.
23. Rogosheske JR, Fargen AD, DeFor TE, Warlick E, Arora M, Blazar BR, et al. Higher therapeutic cyclosporine levels early post-transplantation reduces risks of acute graft-versus-host disease and improves survival. Bone Marrow Transplant. 2014 Jan;49(1):122–5.
24. Ruutu T, Gratwohl A, de Witte T, Afanasyev B, Apperley J, Bacigalupo A, et al. Prophylaxis and treatment of GVHD: EBMT-ELN working group recommendations for a standardized practice. Bone Marrow Transplant. 2014 Feb;49(2):168–73.
25. Dignan FL, Clark A, Amrolia P, Cornish J, Jackson G, Mahendra P, et al. Diagnosis and management of acute graft-versus-host disease. Br J Haematol. 2012 Jul;158(1):30–45.
26. Bayraktar U. Graft versus host disease (GHVD) in critically ill oncologic patients. 2019. p. 1–17.
27. Ullmann AJ, Lipton JH, Vesole DH, Chandrasekar P, Langston A, Tarantolo SR, et al. Posaconazole or fluconazole for prophylaxis in severe graft-versus-host disease. N Engl J Med. 2007;356(4):335–47.
28. Guidelines for preventing infectious complications among hematopoietic cell transplantation recipients: a global perspective—biology of blood and marrow transplantation [Internet]. [cited 2021 Feb 24]. https://www.tctjournal.org/article/S1083-8791(09)00300-0/fulltext.

29. Escobar K, Rojas P, Ernst D, Bertin P, Nervi B, Jara V, et al. Admission of hematopoietic cell transplantation patients to the intensive care unit at the Pontificia Universidad Católica de Chile hospital. Biol Blood Marrow Transplant. 2015;21(1):176–9.
30. Acute kidney injury in critically ill allo-HSCT recipients | Bone Marrow Transplantation [Internet]. [cited 2021 Feb 19]. https://www.nature.com/articles/bmt2014100.
31. Escamilla Gómez V, García-Gutiérrez V, López Corral L, García Cadenas I, Pérez Martínez A, Márquez Malaver FJ, et al. Ruxolitinib in refractory acute and chronic graft-versus-host disease: a multicenter survey study. Bone Marrow Transplant. 2020;55(3):641–8.
32. Zeiser R, Burchert A, Lengerke C, Verbeek M, Maas-Bauer K, Metzelder SK, et al. Ruxolitinib in corticosteroid-refractory graft-versus-host disease after allogeneic stem cell transplantation: a multicenter survey. Leukemia. 2015;29(10):2062–8.
33. Shulman HM, Sharma P, Amos D, Fenster LF, McDonald GB. A coded histologic study of hepatic graft-versus-host disease after human bone marrow transplantation. Hepatol Baltim Md. 1988;8(3):463–70.
34. Hockenbery DM, Cruickshank S, Rodell TC, Gooley T, Schuening F, Rowley S, et al. A randomized, placebo-controlled trial of oral beclomethasone dipropionate as a prednisone-sparing therapy for gastrointestinal graft-versus-host disease. Blood. 2007;109(10):4557–63.
35. Ippoliti C, Neumann J. Octreotide in the management of diarrhea induced by graft versus host disease. Oncol Nurs Forum. 1998;25(5):873–8.
36. Ippoliti C, Champlin R, Bugazia N, Przepiorka D, Neumann J, Giralt S, et al. Use of octreotide in the symptomatic management of diarrhea induced by graft-versus-host disease in patients with hematologic malignancies. J Clin Oncol Off J Am Soc Clin Oncol. 1997;15(11):3350–4.
37. Beckman RA, Siden R, Yanik GA, Levine JE. Continuous octreotide infusion for the treatment of secretory diarrhea caused by acute intestinal graft-versus-host disease in a child. J PediatrHematol Oncol. 2000;22(4):344–50.
38. van der Meij BS, de Graaf P, Wierdsma NJ, Langius JAE, JJWM J, van Leeuwen PAM, et al. Nutritional support in patients with GVHD of the digestive tract: state of the art. Bone Marrow Transplant. 2013;48(4):474–82.
39. Seguy D, Berthon C, Micol J-B, Darré S, Dalle J-H, Neuville S, et al. Enteral feeding and early outcomes of patients undergoing allogeneic stem cell transplantation following myeloablative conditioning. Transplantation. 2006;82(6):835–9.
40. Murray SM, Pindoria S. Nutrition support for bone marrow transplant patients. Cochrane Database Syst Rev. 2008;4:CD002920.
41. Pidala J, Anasetti C. Glucocorticoid-refractory acute graft-versus-host disease. Biol Blood Marrow Transplant J Am Soc Blood Marrow Transplant. 2010;16(11):1504–18.
42. Williams KM. How I treat bronchiolitis obliterans syndrome after hematopoietic stem cell transplantation. Blood. 2017;129(4):448–55.
43. National institutes of health consensus development project on criteria for clinical trials in chronic graft-versus-host disease: I. The 2014 diagnosis and staging working group report—science direct [Internet]. [cited 2021 Feb 24]. https://www.sciencedirect.com/science/article/pii/S1083879114013780.

Carcinoid Crisis in ICU

23

Raja Pramanik and Aparna Sharma

23.1 Introduction

Carcinoid tumours are neuroendocrine tumours of enterochromaffin cell origin. They usually arise from the gastrointestinal system (67.5%) followed by the bronchopulmonary system (25.3%) [1]. Carcinoid tumours are usually slow growing and asymptomatic. These tumours may be functional or non-functional. The functional tumours secrete substances like histamine, 5-hydroxytryptamine (serotonin), and 5-hydroxytryptophan. Carcinoid syndrome is characterized by episodic flushing, diarrhea, dyspnea, wheezing, palpitations and right heart disease. Carcinoid syndrome is most commonly seen in neuroendocrine tumours of midgut and foregut origin. Carcinoid crisis is defined as a severe manifestation of carcinoid syndrome characterized by fluctuations in blood pressure, flushing, dyspnoea, pruritus and confusion. Carcinoid crisis can be life threatening. The most common triggers of carcinoid crisis are anaesthesia and surgery. This is why it becomes important to recognise and be familiar with the management of this syndrome.

23.2 Pathophysiology of Carcinoid Syndrome

The functional carcinoid tumours secrete mediators like histamine, serotonin and 5-hydroxytryptophan. Normally these substances get metabolized in the liver after passing through the portal circulation. However, tumour spread to the liver circumvents the liver metabolism of these substances and predisposes to carcinoid syndrome. During carcinoid crisis, mediators such as serotonin, histamine, 5-hydroxytryptophan and kallikreins are secreted in large quantities from the tumour. Serotonin causes both vasoconstriction and vasodilatory effects depending

R. Pramanik (✉) · A. Sharma
Department of Medical Oncology, AIIMS Delhi (Both), New Delhi, India

V. Kumar et al. (eds.), *Onco-critical Care*,
https://doi.org/10.1007/978-981-16-9929-0_23

on the type of receptor to which it is bound. Increase in kallikreins leads to increased level of bradykinin. This leads to increase in capillary permeability causing flushing, vasodilation, oedema and hypotension.

The predisposing factors for carcinoid crisis are not well defined. In some studies, presence of symptoms of carcinoid syndrome, heavy burden of disease, presence of liver metastases, high serum chromogranin A levels, high urine 5 HIAA levels and presence of carcinoid heart disease have been postulated as risk factors of carcinoid crisis [2–4]. In a study by Massimino et al., presence of liver metastases was the only factor in multivariate analysis predictive of carcinoid crisis [5]. In a study by Condron et al., advanced age was found to be predictive of carcinoid crisis [6].

23.3 Signs and Symptoms of Carcinoid Syndrome

Carcinoid syndrome is characterized by episodic flushing, loose motions, pruritus, palpitations, dyspnoea, wheezing and heart disease. The diarrhoea in carcinoid syndrome is secretory, watery in nature and can sometimes be explosive. It can lead to electrolyte disturbances and dehydration. Diarrhoea can have a significant impact on the quality of life of patients. Flushing is usually sudden in onset, pink or red in colour, involving face or trunk, multiple episodes in a day lasting few minutes. Alcohol, exercise and tyramine containing foods (e.g. banana, chocolate, walnuts) can be the triggering factors [7]. Flushing is usually not associated with sweating. Sometimes flushing can present atypically on the limbs with a purplish colour lasting several hours. Wheezing is due to bronchoconstriction produced due to the release of bradykinin. The most common complication of carcinoid syndrome is carcinoid heart disease. It is characterized by fibrotic degeneration of heart valves. The most common manifestation of carcinoid heart disease is tricuspid regurgitation.

Fibrosis can also affect extracardiac sites like mesentery and peritoneum leading to small bowel obstruction and bowel ischemia [8]. Massive fibrosis can lead to mesenteric vessel occlusion and small bowel infarction [9]. Carcinoid tumours can also be associated with retroperitoneal fibrosis resulting in ureteric stenosis and hydronephrosis [10]. Rarely, cutaneous scleroderma could also be associated with carcinoid syndrome [11]. The essential amino acid tryptophan is a precursor of both serotonin and niacin production. Uncontrolled production of serotonin leads to diversion of tryptophan away from niacin production resulting in niacin deficiency [12]. Niacin deficiency can lead to pellagra, characterised by diarrhoea, dermatitis, hypoalbuminemia, swelling, hair loss, angular stomatitis, glossitis and encephalopathy [13]. Carcinoid syndromes is also linked to cognitive disorders affecting all cognitive domains, most specifically verbal memory, delayed verbal recall and visual perceptual function [14]. Another potential complication of carcinoid syndrome is muscle wasting and proximal myopathy as a result of malabsorption related to chronic diarrhoea [15].

Carcinoid crisis is characterized by severe manifestations of symptoms of carcinoid syndrome. The risk of occurrence of a carcinoid crisis varies between 3.4% and 24% as per different reports [5, 16, 17]. It is characterized by flushing of skin, bronchospasm and severe dyspnoea, pruritus, chest pain, tachycardia, palpitations, arrhythmia, hemodynamic instability, peripheral cyanosis, metabolic acidosis, abdominal cramps, paraesthesia, hyperesthesia and confusion. Rarely carcinoid crisis can be fatal [6, 18]. The clinical manifestations of carcinoid crisis can mimic anaphylactoid reaction. Certain factors, most notably surgery, anaesthesia and biopsy can serve as triggers of carcinoid crisis. Mechanical stimulation of the tumour, e.g., needle biopsy, intraoperative palpation of the tumour, abdominal ultrasound, bronchoscopy in the presence of a bronchial carcinoid, may also serve as a trigger factor. Other factors like stress, anxiety, excess alcohol intake, hypertension or hypotension, hypercapnia, peptide radionuclide therapy, hypothermia, drugs causing histamine release and catecholamines can also lead to precipitation of carcinoid crisis.

23.4 Diagnosis

The typical clinical features of carcinoid syndrome are flushing (90%), diarrhoea (70%), and wheezing (15%) [19, 20]. 24-h urine 5-hydroxyindoleacetic acid (5-HIAA) is the initial lab test of choice. The serotonin secreted by the carcinoid tumours is metabolized to 5-HIAA by monoamine oxidases in the liver, lungs and brain. 24-h Urine 5-HIAA level has a 73% sensitivity and 100% specificity for diagnosing carcinoid [21]. 24 h urine 5-HIAA level can be elevated in persons having tryptophan rich food. Hence, such food items should be avoided for at least 72 h prior to sample collection [22]. Serum chromogranin A has got high sensitivity but low specificity for the diagnosis of carcinoid. It is used to assess disease progression and response to treatment [23, 24]. Imaging with 68-Gallium DOTA peptides is a single day procedure, higher spatial resolution, improved dosimetry and ability to semi-quantify the activity in terms of standard uptake value (SUV) [25]. Transthoracic 2D Echocardiography should be done in all patients of carcinoid tumours specifically to look for cardiac valve abnormalities. Tricuspid valve is affected most commonly.

The signs and symptoms of carcinoid crisis closely mimic anaphylactic reaction. The predominant symptom is wide blood pressure fluctuations with a predominance of hypotension. It is generally encountered in a known case of mid-gut neuroendocrine tumour undergoing a procedure or surgery.

23.5 Differential Diagnosis

The closest differential diagnosis is anaphylactic shock.

23.6 Prevention of Crisis

Carcinoid crisis should be anticipated by the treating team in any mid-gut NET who is being planned for tumour manipulation, biopsy, surgery, hepatic artery embolization, radionuclide therapy etc.

Administration of octreotide prior to resection (300–500 mcg intravenously or subcutaneously) is recommended for patients with a history of carcinoid syndrome who require surgical procedures as it reduces the incidence of carcinoid crisis. It is not clear if prophylactic octreotide is needed prior to surgical resection in a patient without carcinoid syndrome. Many experts recommend that urinary 5-HIAA levels should be assayed before surgery in all patients with metastatic midgut NETs, even those who do not have symptoms consistent with carcinoid syndrome. Prophylactic and intraoperative octreotide should be administered to all patients with carcinoid syndrome and/or elevated urinary 5-HIAA levels. Patients with tumours that do not produce serotonin (e.g., rectal NETs, most pancreatic NETs, or localized midgut NETs) do not require prophylactic octreotide.

There are various schedules pertaining to the dose and timing of somaostatin analogues mentioned in different publications. 250–500 mcg bolus short acting octreotide dose is recommended for patients with carcinoid syndrome in whom minor intervention is planned. 100–150 mcg/h. infusion of octreotide is used in addition to the bolus dose in case a major intervention is planned [5, 26, 27]. Condron et al. used a similar bolus octreotide dose but the dose of intraoperative infusion was 500 mcg/h [6]. UK guidelines and some other publications have used 50–100 mcg/h. infusion of octreotide to be started 2 h before the surgery and continue the infusion till 48 h after the procedure [5, 28]. In patients who are using octreotide for the treatment of carcinoid syndrome, higher dose of this agent may be needed in case of carcinoid crisis as compared to those patients who did not use octreotide before. The North American Neuroendocrine Tumor Society (NANETS) consensus guidelines recommend a preoperative bolus of octreotide 250–500 μg IV with extra doses available throughout the procedure in patients with suspected carcinoid syndrome who undergo major procedures.

To top it all, prior to any interventional procedure that will trigger the carcinoid crisis, dehydration or vitamin deficiency should be avoided. Electrolyte disorders, dehydration, and hypoproteinemia should be corrected.

23.7 Management

Severe carcinoid crisis is accompanied by hypotension or shock. The main aim of treatment in carcinoid crisis is to block the secretion as well as the effect of mediators by the tumour. Somatostatin analogues are the cornerstone of treatment. Intraoperative complications can still occur despite the administration of preoperative prophylactic octreotide. Octreotide should be readily available and should be repeated as needed.

Hypotension will generally be refractory to fluid resuscitation alone. Adrenergic agents to support blood pressure should BE AVOIDED as first line. Catecholamines and calcium actually provoke the release of mediators from the tumour and worsen the crisis. The blood pressure should be supported by infusion of octreotide as an intravenous drip at the rate of 50–200 mcg/h. Vasopressin may be used to treat hypotension. The patient should be carefully monitored for rapid changes in blood pressure.

Another drug useful in the treatment of carcinoid crisis is methylene blue. It competitively blocks the binding of nitric oxide synthase to guanylate synthase. This inhibits the activation of cyclic GMP in the downstream pathways and associated smooth muscle relaxation. Hence, methylene blue is used in the treatment of shock and non-cardiogenic pulmonary oedema seen in carcinoid crisis. The dose of methylene blue is 1 mg/kg bolus followed by 0.5 mg/kg/h. 12 h infusion [4]. Other dosing schedules also exist.

Other agents used in the treatment of carcinoid crisis include ketanserin (antagonist of 5-hydroxytryptamine receptor 2, alpha 1 adrenoreceptor, H1-histamine receptor), and chlorpheniramine (H1 and H2 Histamine receptor blockers) [3, 18, 29, 30].

Diarrhoea generally responds to standard antidiarrheal medications; however serotonin antagonists can also control diarrhoea and malabsorption.

23.8 Key Points

1. Carcinoid crisis is defined as a severe manifestation of carcinoid syndrome characterized by fluctuations in blood pressure, flushing, dyspnoea, pruritus and confusion.
2. Carcinoid crisis can be life threatening.
3. The most common triggers of carcinoid crisis are anaesthesia and surgery.
4. Suspect and anticipate carcinoid crisis in any mid-gut NET posted for a surgery, biopsy.
5. Pre-anaesthetic check-up should include 5-HIAA.
6. Care should be taken in those with a documented carcinoid syndrome.
7. The signs and symptoms of carcinoid crisis closely mimic anaphylactic reaction.
8. The predominant symptom is wide blood pressure fluctuations with a predominance of hypotension.
9. Prevent carcinoid crisis by preoperative intravenous short acting octreotide.
10. There are varying doses of octreotide between 150 and 500 μg. UK guidelines support infusion of 50 μg/h octreotide.
11. Start the infusion 2 h. preop and continue 48 h postop.
12. Hypotension is generally fluid non-responsive.
13. DO NOT USE catecholamines as first line to support blood pressure.
14. DO NOT USE iv calcium.
15. Titrate the infusion of octreotide.

16. Methylene blue may be used.
17. Octreotide should be readily available in the operation theatre and ICU.
18. Long-acting Octreotide depot preparation are useful for Carcinoid syndrome, not for CARCINOID CRISIS.

References

1. Kromas M, Passi Y, Kuzumi C, et al. Intraoperative carcinoid crisis: revised anaesthesia management. Ind J Anaesth. 2017;61(5):85–6.
2. Seymour N, Sawh SC. Mega-dose intravenous octreotide for the treatment of carcinoid crisis: a systematic review. Can J Anaesth. 2013;60(5):492–9.
3. Tapia Rico G, Li M, Pavlakis N, et al. Prevention and management of carcinoid crises in patients with high-risk neuroendocrine tumours undergoing peptide receptor radionuclide therapy (PRRT): literature review and case series from two Australian tertiary medical institutions. Cancer Treat Rev. 2018;66:1–6.
4. van Diepen S, Sobey A, Lewanczuk R, et al. A case of acute respiratory distress syndrome responsive to methylene blue during a carcinoid crisis. Can J Anaesth. 2013;60(11):1085–8.
5. Massimino K, Harrskog O, Pommier S, et al. Octreotide LAR and bolus octreotide are insufficient for preventing intraoperative complications in carcinoid patients. J Surg Oncol. 2013;107(8):842–6.
6. Condron ME, Pommier SJ, Pommier RF. Continuous infusion of octreotide combined with perioperative octreotide bolus does not prevent intraoperative carcinoid crisis. Surgery. 2016;159(1):358–65.
7. Gut P, Czarnywojtek A, Bączyk M, et al. Clinical features of gastroenteropancreatic tumours. Arch Med Sci. 2015;10:127–34.
8. Hellman P, et al. Effect of surgery on the outcome of midgut carcinoid disease with lymph node and liver metastases. World J Surg. 2002;26(8):991–7.
9. Petrik PK. Fatal small intestinal infarction due to occlusion by mesenteric carcinoid tumor. Am J Forensic Med Pathol. 1989;10(2):146–8.
10. Sakai D, et al. Ileal carcinoid tumor complicating carcinoid heart disease and secondary retroperitoneal fibrosis. Pathol Int. 2000;50(5):404–11.
11. Ratnavel RC, Burrows NP, Pye RJ. Scleroderma and the carcinoid syndrome. Clin Exp Dermatol. 1994;19(1):83–5.
12. Shah GM, et al. Biochemical assessment of niacin deficiency among carcinoid cancer patients. Am J Gastroenterol. 2005;100(10):2307–14.
13. Hegyi J, Schwartz RA, Hegyi V. Pellagra: dermatitis, dementia, and diarrhea. Int J Dermatol. 2004;43(1):1–5.
14. Chambers AJ, et al. Impairment of cognitive function reported by patients suffering from carcinoid syndrome. World J Surg. 2010;34(6):1356–60.
15. Berry EM, Maunder C, Wilson M. Carcinoid myopathy and treatment with cyproheptadine (Periactin). Gut. 1974;15(1):34–8.
16. Kinney MA, Warner ME, Nagorney DM, et al. Perianaesthetic risks and outcomes of abdominal surgery for metastatic carcinoid tumours. Br J Anaesth. 2001;87(3):447–52.
17. Woltering EA, Wright AE, Stevens MA, et al. Development of effective prophylaxis against intraoperative carcinoid crisis. J Clin Anaesth. 2016;32:189–93.
18. Koopmans KP, Brouwers AH, De Hooge MN, et al. Carcinoid crisis after injection of 6-18F-fluorodihy-droxyphenylalanine in a patient with metastatic carcinoid. J Nucl Med. 2005;46(7):1240–3.
19. Rubin de Celis Ferrari AC, Glasberg J, Riechelmann RP II. Carcinoid syndrome: update on the pathophysiology and treatment. Clinics (Sao Paulo). 2018;73:e490s.

20. Hannah-Shmouni F, Stratakis CA, Koch CA. Flushing in (neuro)endocrinology. Rev Endocr Metab Disord. 2016;17:373–80.
21. Maroun J, Kocha W, Kvols L, et al. Guidelines for the diagnosis and management of carcinoid tumours. Part 1: the gastrointestinal tract. A statement from a Canadian National Carcinoid Expert Group. Curr Oncol. 2006;13:67–76.
22. Corcuff JB, Chardon L, El Hajji RI, Brossaud J. Urinary sampling for 5HIAA and metanephrines determination: revisiting the recommendations. Endocr Connect. 2017;6:87–98.
23. Gkolfinopoulos S, Tsapakidis K, Papadimitriou K, Papamichael D, Kountourakis P. Chromogranin a as a valid marker in oncology: clinical application or false hopes? World J Methodol. 2017;7:9–15.
24. Gut P, Czarnywojtek A, Fischbach J, et al. Chromogranin a - unspecific neuroendocrine marker. Clinical utility and potential diagnostic pitfalls. Arch Med Sci. 2016;12:1–9.
25. Bodei L, Sundin A, Kidd M, et al. The status of neuroendocrine tumour imaging: from darkness to light? Neuroendocrinology. 2015;101:1–17.
26. Kunz PL, Reidy-Lagunes D, Anthony LB, et al. Consensus guidelines for the management and treatment of neuroendocrine tumors. Pancreas. 2013;42(4):557–77.
27. Phan AT, Oberg K, Choi J, et al. NANETS consensus guideline for the diagnosis and management of neuro-endocrine tumors: well-differentiated neuroendocrine tumors of the thorax (includes lung and thymus). Pancreas. 2010;39(6):784–98.
28. Soto Herrera M, Restrepo JA, Díaz JH, et al. Reversible right-sided heart failure secondary to carcinoid crisis. Case Rep Crit Care. 2013;2013:487801.
29. Janssen M, Salm EF, Breburda CS, et al. Carcinoid crisis during transedophageal echocardiography. Intensive Care Med. 2000;26(2):254.
30. Lyseng-Williamson KA. Telotristat ethyl: a review in carcinoid syndrome diarrhoea. Drugs. 2018;78(9):941–50.

Chronic Myeloid Leukemia Blast Crisis: An Emergency

24

Gaurav Prakash, Urmimala Bhattacharjee, and Chandan K. Das

24.1 Introduction

Chronic myeloid leukemia (CML) is a malignancy which heralded an era of targeted therapy with the advent of oral therapy with an oral drug Imatinib. Due to a slow indolent course and oral therapy, presently, the management of CML is largely an office based practice with survival of patients moving towards age matched general population. However, a small yet significant proportion of patients develop a catastrophic complication whereby CML transforms to an acute leukemia like illness with development of more than 20% blasts cells and this phase of CML is called as blast crisis (BC). Blast crisis is a state of medical emergency as it can lead to rapid deterioration of health of a patient over a few days. There is a high risk of involvement of non-hematopoietic vital organs, and it invariably leads to an early death if not treated properly.

In the next few sections we shall discuss specific issues related to diagnosis and management of a case with CML blast crisis.

24.1.1 Definition of Blast Crisis

The criteria for CML-BC include ≥20% blasts in the blood or bone marrow or the presence of any extramedullary proliferation of blasts (also known as myeloid sarcoma) [1]. Some of the researchers keep a cut-off of >30% blasts to diagnose CML-BC. The cut-off threshold may be different in various guidelines but presence of excess blast cells proliferation in a CML patient connotes poor prognosis [2].

G. Prakash (✉) · U. Bhattacharjee · C. K. Das
Department of Clinical Hematology and Medical Oncology, Postgraduate Institute of Medical Education and Research, Chandigarh, UT, India

V. Kumar et al. (eds.), *Onco-critical Care*,
https://doi.org/10.1007/978-981-16-9929-0_24

24.2 Evaluation of a Suspected Case of BC

24.2.1 Clinical Features Suggesting Development of Blast Crisis in a Known Case with CML

The clinical features of a patient with CML BC mimic a patient with acute leukemia which include pallor, easy fatiguability, loss of appetite, bleeding at various sites, and fever. In majority of patients, CML-BC occurs in a previously known case of CML following a chronic or an accelerated phase. However, according to European population based registry data, 2.2% patients of CML patients may present upfront with blast crisis phase [3]. In such cases, it is difficult to distinguish it from a de-novo case of acute leukemia on clinical parameters. A blood and marrow examination with PCR for bcr-abl transcript helps in differentiating these patients.

24.2.2 When to Suspect CML Blast Crisis in a Patient Presenting with a Myeloid Malignancy

A diagnosis of blast crisis needs high index of suspicion. If a known patient of CML presents with rapid decline in blood cell counts which cannot be attributed to anti CML treatment then it can be the first indicator of development of an accelerated phase or blast crisis. The second scenario to suspect development of blast crisis is rapid enlargement of spleen or lymph nodes in a known patient with CML. This organ enlargement may or may not be associated with other features like severe-bone pain, gum-bleeding, petechial hemorrhages, and fever.

In a patient who has blast crisis phase at the time of first presentation, a few simple pointers can help in differentiating it from acute leukemia. The features like presence of peripheral blood basophilia, presence of immature myeloid cells in the peripheral blood like myelocytes and metamyelocytes, and presentation with a massive splenomegaly point towards a possibility of CML-BC. In such cases, diagnostic workup should be initiated to confirm CML in blast phase and the same is discussed in the next section.

24.3 Diagnosis of CML BC

24.3.1 Investigation Specific to Diagnosis of CML-BC

The WHO definition of CML BC includes >20% blast cells in bone marrow or extramedullary blast proliferation apart from the spleen [1]. However the European Leukemia Net has set cutoff for BM blast count at >30% [4]. The crucial point to improve survival in CML-BC involves the prompt diagnosis and early treatment initiation depending on morphology and immunohistological features. A complete blood count to get percentage of blast cells and their immunophenotyping for correct lineage identification is essential.

The cornerstone of diagnosis of CML BC is identification of either t(9,22) via FISH probe or a bcr-abl fusion gene with help of PCR. In a new patient, these tests can be performed, both, from a peripheral blood sample or a bone marrow aspirate. Peripheral blood sample has advantage of ease of acquisition but a bone marrow examination also provides valuable additional information about haemato-morphology and status of other cell lines. A PCR can also identify the type of fusion transcript which can help to distinguish a patient of CML-BC with a case of Philadelphia positive ALL.

24.3.2 Investigation for Prognostication and Treatment Planning for CML-BC

The CNS infilteration rates of lymphoid BC match with that of a de novo ALL case and these patients may deteriorate rapidly due to CNS manifestations of the leukemia. CNS involvement in a patient with CML-BC is a very poor prognostic marker. Hence, CSF cytopathology assessment should be done in all patients. A CSF examination at the time of diagnosis also provides an opportunity to give prophylactic intra-thecal chemotherapy.

In CML-BC there is an array of nonrandom, chromosomal aberrations characteristic of clonal evolution similar to other hematologic malignancies. In addition to t(9,22), the major abnormalities like isochromosome 17q, trisomy 8 additional Ph chromosome significantly predicted shorter survival. Major additional cytogenetic abnosrmalities are seen in 90% of CML BC patients and they represent early events leading to hematopoiesis failure and blastic differentiation [5].

Another significant clinical marker of poor prognosis is a lack of achievement of significant cytogenetics response to the initial TKI therapy.

Unfavorable Prognosis [6]	Favorable Prognosis
1. Major clonal evolution 2. 50%blast cell 3. Short CML Chronic phase duration 4. Extramedullary disease 5. Age > 60 years 6. LDH high	1. Achievement of major hematologic response 2. Complete cytogenetic response to first-line treatment

24.4 Emergency Challenges Associated with CML BC

As the name "blast-crisis" suggests, it is a state of acute crisis which targets multiple organ systems simultaneously. From the perspective of hemato-oncology practice, CML-BC is a state of oncologic emergency and following conditions need immediate attention.

24.4.1 Hyperleukocytosis and Leukostasis

High WBC count is a common characteristic of a newly diagnosed patient with CML. In the state of blast crisis, the number of immature blasts increase exponentially. Hyperleukocytosis is usually defined as a state of WBC >1,00,000/microliter [7]. The immature cells are large in size and they also have a large size nucleus which makes them less flexible, therefore, these blast cells are unable to navigate through tight capillaries. As a result, these cells clog small capillaries of most vital organs and this leads to acute organ dysfunction. The main organs affected with leukocytosis are [1] pulmonary capillary bed- leading to hypoxia and type-1 respiratory failure and [2] the brain leading to headache, dizziness or seizures. The primary treatment of hyperleukocytosis with or without leukostasis is reduction of the white blood cell count. The cytoreduction can be achieved medically by using chemotherapeutic agent hyroxyurea but medical cytoreduction is a slower process and it may take 7–10 days to achieve clinically meaningful benefit. In cases where the dangers associated with leukostasis are imminent, a much faster reduction in cell count is needed and this is best achieved by doing leukapheresis. In patients with very high leukocyte counts multiple session of leukapheresis are required.

24.4.2 Tumor Lysis Syndrome

Tumor lysis syndrome (TLS) is a metabolic complication associated with aggressive malignancies and CML-BC is one of them. It results from rapid break down of malignant cells which have high levels of nucleic acid. Sudden catabolism of the nucleotides overwhelms the enzymes of nucleotide catabolism pathway and it leads to accumulation of uric acid and xanthine in patient's body. A rapid breakdown of cells also results into release of intracellular ions (mainly potassium and phosphate) into plasma leading to rapid and potentially fatal electrolyte imbalance.

TLS is characterized by hyperkalemia, hyperphosphatemia, hypocalcemia and hyperuricemia. Out of these metabolic alterations, hyperkalemia can lead to potentially fatal cardiac arrythmias. Therefore, 6-12 hourly monitoring of serum electrolytes is needed in patients with CML-BC who develop TLS.

24.4.3 Hypersplenism and Splenic Rupture

Splenomegaly is the commonest clinical examination finding in patients with CML and at the time of occurrence of blast crisis, there is further enlargement of the same. A massive spleen can lead to sequestration of a large number of cells of the peripheral blood and creates a condition of relative cytopenia. This condition is known as hypersplenism. Anemia and thrombocytopenia related to hypersplenism may lead to symptoms associated with them. Spontaneous splenic rupture is a very rare but well documented complication of massive splenomegaly. It is a catastrophic event which may produce massive hemoperitoneum and may lead to rapid exsanguination of a patient. An urgent laparotomy and splenectomy is the mainstay of its treatment.

24.4.4 Febrile Neutropenia

In patients with CML-BC there is leukocytosis due to large number of immature cells in the blood. However, it occurs at the expense of normal peripheral blood neutrophils. Moreover, in patients with leukemia the neutrophils also have functional defects [8]. Therefore, these patients are at a very high risk of neutropenic fever. High index of suspicion for infection and early utilization of a broad spectrum antibiotics is needed in these cases. Severe neutropenia is also an independent risk factor for development of invasive fungal infection. Hence, the patients with CML BC should receive antifungal prophylaxis which covers for filamentous fungi like aspergillus.

24.5 Management

The goal of treatment of CML blast crisis is to convert the blast phase into hematologic remission followed by allogeneic hematopoietic stem cell transplant, if possible.

Management of CML-BC depends on the following factors:

1. The nature of blast crises: lymphoid or myeloid
2. Blast crisis developing de-novo or in those previously treated with TKI
3. BCR-ABL1 kinase domain mutation

Tyrosine kinase inhibitors (TKI) are the frontline agents for treatment of CML, at present. In the Pre-TKI era, attempts were made to treat CML-BC with protocols designed to treat acute leukemia (AL). Lymphoid blast crisis generally has a better prognosis compared to myeloid blast crisis. The response rates to vincristine, and prednisolone and other drugs used for ALL such as 6-thioguanine, 6-mercaptopurine, cytosine arabinoside and methotrexate ranged from 15 to 50%. However the response duration is short (median duration is 14 months) and median overall survival only around 17 months. For myeloid blast crisis, AML-type induction therapies with combination chemotherapy agents like anthracyclines, cytosine arabinoside, 5-azacytidine, etoposide, fludarabine and decitabine achieved response rate of ~10%. Overall, treatment of CML-BC turned out to be less successful compared to de novo Acute leukemia.

Currently in the TKI era, the overall incidence and outcomes of blast crisis has improved with the better elimination of effect of BCR-ABL1 translocation. A TKI, as a single agent or in combination with chemotherapy regimen is the treatment of choice for CML blast crisis. For exmple, in cases with lymphoid blast crisis a TKI, dasatinib is clubbed together with vincristine, daunorubicin and prednisolone is the therapy of choice [9].

Choice of TKI: For de novo CML blast crisis, we can start with either imatinib 600–800 mg/day or dasatinib 140 mg once daily or nilotinib 400 mg, twice in a day based on kinase domain mutation profile.

If blast crisis evolves during imatinib therapy, treatment with a second-or third generation TKI either dasatinib 140 mg, nilotinib 2 × 400 mg, bosutinib 500 mg or ponatinib 30–45 mg (according to kinase domain mutation profile) with/without conventional chemotherapy drugs is the treatment of choice followed by allo-SCT [10]. In case of V299L, T315A, or F317L/V/I/C mutations, nilotinib is preferred over dasatinib. In case of Y253H, E255K/V, or F359V/C/I mutations, dasatinib is more effective than nilotinib. In case of T315I ponatinib is indicated.

24.6 Role of BMT

Allogeneic stem cell transplant (AlloSCT) gives the best chance of long-term remission or cure in CML-BC. Based on recent data, alloSCT is the treatment of choice once a second chronic phase (CP) is reached with single agent or combination TKI with chemotherapy [11]. Transplantation can be performed with HLA-identical related donor or matched unrelated donor, or a haplo-identical donor. Standard conditioning with busulfan and cyclophosphamide with or without total body irradiation is used. Post-transplantation maintenance with TKI appears reasonable. Maintenance with dasatinib is recommended in lymphoid blast crisis for prevention of CNS relapse of leukemia as dasatinib has ability to cross the blood brain barrier.

24.7 Conclusion

CML-BC is a medical emergency which needs immediate attention and multidisciplinary care. These patients need hospitalization and an early initiation of therapy in order to avoid complications which are imminent in these cases. A close monitoring of rapid hematologic, respiratory, neurologic, and renal dysfunction is required. The availability of various tyrosine kinase inhibitors has increased efficacy of treatment regimen for CML-BC. However, for young patients or for patients without comorbidities, an allogeneic bone marrow transplant is the treatment of choice to achieve a long disease free survival.

References

1. Arber DA, Orazi A, Hasserjian R, et al. The 2016 revision to the World Health Organization classification of myeloid neoplasms and acute leukemia. Blood. 2016 May 19;127(20):2391–405.
2. Hehlmann R. How I treat CML blast crisis. Blood. 2012 Jul 26;120(4):737–47.
3. Hoffmann VS, Baccarani M, Hasford J, et al. The EUTOS population-based registry: incidence and clinical characteristics of 2904 CML patients in 20 European countries. Leukemia. 2015 Jun;29(6):1336–43.

4. Hehlmann R. The new ELN recommendations for treating CML. J Clin Med. 2020 Nov 16;9(11):3671.
5. Ko TK, Javed A, Lee KL, et al. An integrative model of pathway convergence in genetically heterogeneous blast crisis chronic myeloid leukemia. Blood. 2020 Jun 25;135(26):2337–53.
6. Jain P, Kantarjian HM, Ghorab A, et al. Prognostic factors and survival outcomes in patients with chronic myeloid leukemia in blast phase in the tyrosine kinase inhibitor era: Cohort study of 477 patients. Cancer. 2017 Nov 15;123(22):4391–402.
7. Ganzel C, Becker J, Mintz PD, Lazarus HM, Rowe JM. Hyperleukocytosis, leukostasis and leukapheresis: practice management. Blood Rev. 2012 May;26(3):117–22.
8. Manukyan G, Papajik T, Gajdos P, et al. Neutrophils in chronic lymphocytic leukemia are permanently activated and have functional defects. Oncotarget. 2017 Oct 17;8(49):84889–901.
9. Alimena G, Breccia M, Latagliata R, et al. Dasatinib in the management of lymphoid blast crisis of Philadelphia-positive chronic myeloid leukemia with multiple extra-medullary and intracranial localizations. Leuk Res. 2009 Aug;33(8):e134–6.
10. Saussele S, Silver RT. Management of chronic myeloid leukemia in blast crisis. Ann Hematol. 2015 Apr;94(Suppl 2):S159–65.
11. Lubking A, Dreimane A, Sandin F, et al. Allogeneic stem cell transplantation for chronic myeloid leukemia in the TKI era: population-based data from the Swedish CML registry. Bone Marrow Transplant. 2019 Nov;54(11):1764–74.

Management of Complications and Toxicities Related to Chemotherapy in ICU

25

Raja Pramanik, Raghav Gupta, Praneeth Suvvari, and Seema Mishra

25.1 Introduction

As new treatments continue to evolve for cancer management, survival for patients has been increasing. Even metastatic cancers are getting converted to chronic diseases with life-prolonging newer therapies. As a result, we are seeing an upshoot in the number of cancer patients admitted to intensive care units (ICUs). Admission to the ICU may be due to acute toxicities of treatment or worsening of the cancer itself. The intensivist must be aware of the spectrum of chemotherapy-related toxicities and their management.

Most commonly, a cancer patient will be referred to the medical ICU when he or she becomes sick during curative or life-prolonging chemotherapy, and the goal is a possible salvage out of an immediate crisis. It is often helpful to discuss the case with the treating oncologists about the patient's disease's treatment trajectory, the drugs received, his anticipations, and immediate goals. For a patient on systemic chemotherapy, who presents with acute sickness in the ICU, the intensivist must consider in his bucket list of differentials chemotherapy-related toxicity, superadded infection (bacterial, fungal, or viral as per the setting), a manifestation of progression of cancer, worsening of pre-existing comorbidity. E.g., a patient on induction therapy of acute lymphoblastic leukemia presents with altered sensorium and shock.

R. Pramanik
Department of Medical Oncology, AIIMS Delhi, New Delhi, India

R. Gupta
Oncoanaesthesia & Palliative Medicine AIIMS Delhi, New Delhi, India

P. Suvvari
Basavatarakam Indo American Cancer Hospital & Cancer Research Center, Hydrabad, India

S. Mishra (✉)
Department of Onco-Anesthesia and Palliative Medicine,Dr. B.R.A. Institute Rotary Cancer Hospital, All India Institute of Medical Sciences, New Delhi, India

V. Kumar et al. (eds.), *Onco-critical Care*,
https://doi.org/10.1007/978-981-16-9929-0_25

The intensivist finds that his working diagnosis is high-risk febrile neutropenia, and he is prescribed intravenous antibiotics, fluids, and ionotropic support. A careful review, however, revealed that the patient has hyperglycemia (due to L-Asarginase and prednisolone received last week), ileus (due to vincristine) as well as fungal pneumonia. An MR-Venography revealed that the altered sensorium was due to cortical venous thrombosis (due to L-Asparaginase). The addition of antifungals, anti-coagulants, and hyperglycemia management made a huge difference, and the patient stepped out of the ICU in a week. Thus, working knowledge of chemotherapy drugs' possible toxicities comes in convenient and valuable for the intensivist.

Most chemotherapy-related toxicities cause a range of morbidities and involve different organ systems of the body depending on the drug. e.g., peripheral neuropathy, rash, hypertension, nausea, etc. Many of these toxicities are detected and managed in the OPD settings with supportive medications. Patients entering the ICU will generally be more seriously affected and sicker with either hemodynamic instability, altered sensorium, dyspnoea, renal dysfunction, or fever. The following chapter will broadly cover ICU management of these life-threatening chemotherapy-related complications and toxicities. Nevertheless, the intensivist should also be aware of other "less serious" toxicities as these may accompany the serious ones and confound the clinical manifestations of other toxicities.

Most commonly the hematopoietic system, dermatologic, gastrointestinal, pulmonary, cardiovascular, neurologic, are affected by chemotherapy.

With the advent of immunotherapy (Checkpoint inhibitors) and cellular therapies (CAR-T Cells), several newer "never-before-seen" toxicities are being increasingly being recognized by oncologists. Many of these cases will land up in intensive care units requiring specialized management and monitoring. Intensivists should keep themselves updated about these toxicity scenarios as well.

This chapter is designed to give an overview of these toxicities, arranged as per the organ systems affected and the drugs responsible.

25.2 Toxicities by Organ System

25.2.1 Myelosuppression

Myelosuppression is the most typical side effect of cytotoxic chemotherapy, manifesting as anemia, neutropenia, and thrombocytopenia due to dose-limiting suppression of bone marrow. Haemoglobin level less than 7 g/dL should be transfused according to guidelines published by the British Committee for Standards in Haematology in 2001; however, there is little available evidence to support ideal haemoglobin level [1, 2].

Current practice among hematologists uses a platelet count of 10,000/microlitre (without fever) and 20,000/μL (if fever present) as a threshold for prophylactic transfusion. As per the American Society of Clinical Oncology (ASCO) guidelines, in cases of actively bleeding thrombocytopenic patients, or those requiring invasive procedures such as bone marrow aspiration, biopsies, central venous insertions, and removals, a platelet count >20,000/μL is desired. A lumbar puncture can be performed if platelet counts >40,000–50,000/μL. More invasive surgical procedures with a high risk of bleeding or placement of an epidural catheter may require a platelet count greater than 80,000–100,000/μL in the absence of other coagulation abnormalities [3].

Neutropenia, defined as an absolute neutrophil count (ANC) ≤500 cells/mL, predisposes patients to febrile neutropenia and opportunistic infections and oncologic emergency requiring hospitalization or close Outpatient Department (OPD) monitoring. Around 10–50% of patients with solid cancers and more than 80% with haematological malignancies develop a fever with neutropenia during their chemotherapy regimen. Treatment should be done with empirical antibiotics primarily directed against gram-negative pathogens causing life-threatening sepsis. In only about a half of all febrile neutropoenias, an infectious aetiology is identified.

"Febrile neutropenia is defined as a one-time oral temperature of greater than 38.3°C or a sustained temperature of greater than 38°C for ≥1 h in a patient who has an Absolute Neutrophil Count(ANC) <500 cells/mL or ANC expected to decrease to <500 cells/mL within 48 h."

Patients with solid tumours who are receiving chemotherapy will generally have that will last less than 7 days. About 5–30% will have neutropenic fever, with maximum chances during the first cycle of treatment. On the other hand, patients receiving chemotherapy for hematologic malignancies or those post hematopoietic transplants have more prolonged neutropenia that may last 2 weeks or more. The most typical infection source is due to translocation of gut bacteria or catheter-related bloodstream infections. For patients presenting with febrile neutropenia, at least two blood cultures should be obtained, one each from a peripheral vein and a central venous catheter, if present. This is followed by empiric broad spectrum antibiotics with anti-pseudomonal coverage. The patient should undergo a detailed history and physical examination.

The Multinational Association for Supportive Care in Cancer (MASCC) risk index score can identify patients at low risk for mortality and other serious complications. Those with a MASCC score of 21 or more may be considered for outpatient antibiotic therapy [4].

Patients with fever and neutropenia having MASCC score less than 21 points are high risk for complications during neutropenia. They should be admitted to the hospital for evaluation and treatment of potential infection. Cefoperazone plus Sulbactam, Cefepime, piperacillin-tazobactam, ceftazidime, or an antipseudomonal carbapenem (imipenem or meropenem) are the agents widely used with proven efficacy. The choice of antibiotics should be guided by previous infections, institutional protocols, antibiograms and susceptibility patterns. Hypotension at presentation indicates the upfront addition of gram-positive coverage (Vancomycin/Teicoplanin/Linezolid). (Refer Table 25.1) [5].

Patients with neutropenic fever is monitored daily for fever and for new signs or symptoms. In an otherwise stable patient, we do not change or add antimicrobials for persisting fever but do additional work-up. Further, high-risk patients with hematologic malignancies where anticipated neutropenia is greater than 7 days should be evaluated for invasive fungal disease very closely, even requiring a CECT chest or paranasal sinuses. Empiric antifungal therapy is often started on day 4 of

Table 25.1 IDSA treatment guidelines for febrile neutropenia

Criteria	High risk (Any *One*)	Empiric treatment (Any *One*)	Specific additions to treatment
Fever ≥38.3 °C ANC ≤500 cells/mL	Anticipated neutropenia >7 days Clinically unstable Any medical comorbidities	Piperacillin/tazobactam Carbapenem Ceftazidime Cefepime	Vancomycin or linezolid for CRBSI, cellulitis, pneumonia, or hemodynamic instability Aminoglycoside + carbapenem for pneumonia or gram-negative bacteremia Metronidazole for abdominal symptoms or suspected *C difficile* infection Antifungal therapy (echinocandin, voriconazole, or amphotericin B) if hemodynamic instability or fever persists (>4 days)

Table 25.2 Cardiovascular manifestations of different classes of chemotherapy drugs

Chemotherapy agents	Cardiovascular manifestations
Anthracyclines	LVD, HF, arrhythmia
5-fluorouracil	Ischemia, HF, pericarditis, cardiogenic shock
Bevacizumab	Hypertension, thromboembolism
Tamoxifen	Thromboembolism
Cyclophosphamide	HF, mitral regurgitation, pericarditis
Trastuzumab	HF, LVD, arrhythmia
Cytarabine	Pericarditis

LVD left ventricular dysfunction, *HF* heart failure

persistent fever, especially in patients with acute leukaemia, those on high dose corticosteroids and post allogeneic hematopoietic stem-cell transplantation.

25.2.1.1 Role of Granulocyte Colony-Stimulating Factor (G-CSF)

GCSF use decreases both the nadir and the duration of neutropenia if administered prior to its development. Current recommendations for the use of GCSF are based on patient's risk factors for developing neutropenia (age ≥ 65; poor performance status; existing cytopenia due to marrow involvement of malignancy; severe comorbidities; concurrent radiation therapy; extensive prior chemotherapy; previous episode of febrile neutropenia; and planned dose intensity >80%) [6].

25.2.2 Cardiotoxic Side Effects of Chemotherapy Agents

Many conventional chemotherapeutic agents cause cardiotoxicity. 4 categories of cardiac toxicity may occur due to chemotherapy (Table 25.2): (1) direct cytotoxic effects and associated cardiac dysfunction (e.g., anthracyclines); (2) cardiac ischemia e.g., fluorouracil [5-FU]; (3) cardiac arrhythmias and (4) pericarditis (cyclophosphamide, cytarabine).

Other ways to classify cardiotoxicity include reversible versus irreversible, acute versus chronic, and late onset. Irreversible damage is also known as type 1 and reversible damage is termed type 2. While Type 1 (direct damage) is usually caused by a cumulative dose; type 2 damage is not due to cumulative toxicity.

25.2.2.1 Management of Cardiotoxicity

Anthracyclines: These drugs cause Type 1 cardiac damage leading to decreased ejection fraction and clinical heart failure. This is dose dependent and occurs above a cumulative threshold of dose which is specific for each anthracycline. Neither betablockers nor ACE inhibitors have any preventing a decline of EF. Dexrazoxane, is indicated in patients receiving more than 300 mg/m^2 of doxorubicin, but it has no role in the setting of acute heart failure due to anthracyclines.

5-FU: The incidence of cardiotoxicity with 5-FU is about 20%. The reasons include many factors including its pattern of administration. When 5-FU is administered as a bolus, there is less risk of cardiotoxicity than when 5FU is given as a continuous infusion. Typically, a patient on 5FU infusion may present with chest discomfort or acute onset hypotension, or dyspnoea. ECG will show signs of ischemia. The infusions should be immediately stopped, and the patient should be monitored and managed like an acute coronary syndrome.

Trastuzumab: Trastuzumab causes a reversible heart failure in around 5% when administered alone and up to 25% when combined with another agent. It is therefore not at all combined with anthracyclines but given with paclitaxel when needed. LVEF should be assessed before its initiation as well as at regular intervals during therapy. Trastuzumab administration should be withheld for at least 4 weeks if the LVEF is below institutional limits of normal, or there is more than 10% absolute decrease from pre-treatment values [7].

High dose Cyclophosphamide: Cardiotoxicity has been reported in 7–28% of patients receiving high dose cyclophosphamide, typically during the conditioning regimen of stem cell transplants, e.g., CyBU. Cyclophosphamide causes endothelial dysfunction and coronary artery vasospasms, which leads to LV dysfunction, progressing to pericarditis or haemorrhagic myocarditis.

TKIs: The Tyrosine kinase inhibitors, *Sunitinib* and sorafenib, work by inhibiting VEGF, PDGF and kit receptors. There have published reports of Sunitinib and sorafenib causing systolic LV dysfunction and heart failure in 3–10% patients. Hypertension, class effect of these drugs, has been reported in around half of patients on sunitinib. Sorafenib rarely causes cardiac ischemia in about 3% of patients and leads to hypertension in 20–40% [8].

Imatinib, Nilotinib, Dasatinib are TKIs used in patients with chronic myeloid leukaemia and Ph-positive acute lymphoblastic leukaemia. Nilotinib and Dasatinib cause QT prolongation. Imatinib is associated with oedema. Dasatinib has off target effects on the Src nonreceptor tyrosine kinases, causing pleural effusions, fluid retention and pericardial effusion.

Cardiac monitoring is recommended in all patients initiating a potentially cardiotoxic chemotherapy. Those on anthracyclines and trastuzumab therapy must have cardiac-function monitoring at baseline; and every 3–6 monthly during treatment.

Recognition of the above potential cardiotoxic manifestations is extremely important for the intensivist dealing with a patient on chemotherapy who presents with hypotension, shock, or respiratory distress, the cardinal manifestations of cardiac dysfunction. The drugs received, their temporal association with symptoms, and bedside echocardiography can help in detecting heart failure caused due to cardiotoxicity of chemotherapy.

25.2.3 Pulmonary Toxicity

Many chemotherapeutic agents may affect the lungs; a few, however, produce severe, potentially life-threatening toxicities causing such a patient to land up in the intensive care unit. It is also important to recognize other less severe and chronic side effects as these may be confounding and complicating such a patient's manifestations. It is also essential to recognize that a patient on chemotherapy who presents with respiratory distress may have several other complicating factors simultaneously, e.g., infection, involvement by underlying malignancy (e.g., lung metastases, lymphangitis, or leukemic infiltrates). Therefore, the intensivist must have a broad list of differentials.

Among the several mechanisms by which chemotherapies can cause pulmonary toxicity, most important ones are direct damage to pneumocytes or alveolar capillary endothelium, immunologic-mediated toxicity, and capillary leak. Depending on the severity of the clinical findings, a diagnosis of ALI/ARDS may be met.

Gemcitabine has been associated with NCPE, though rarely at approximately 0.1%. Radiographic findings include bilateral infiltrates and pleural effusions. Other chemotherapeutic agents rarely associated with NCPE and respiratory failure include intrathecal methotrexate, vinblastine, and mitomycin C [9].

Retinoic acid syndrome, or ATRA syndrome, is associated with a rapid differentiation of promyelocytes into neutrophils after the institution of therapy. It is characterized by a constellation of clinical findings, that include fever, weight gain, elevated WBC count, respiratory distress, interstitial infiltrates, effusions. It occurs at a median of 5 days. Radiographic findings suggest pulmonary oedema and can include peri bronchial cuffing, GGOs, consolidation, nodules, air bronchograms, and pleural effusion [10]. Some patients may have episodic hypotension, and acute renal failure. The syndrome is highly responsive to high-dose steroids and temporary cessation of ATRA.

Bleomycin is best known for causing late-onset, dose-dependent pulmonary fibrosis 1–6 months after administration in up to 10% of patients. Bleomycin exerts its cytotoxic effect in the lungs via the generation of reactive oxygen species and resultant oxidative injury to pneumocytes [11].

Acute pneumonitis is a known immune-related adverse event (irAE) following checkpoint inhibitors and is treated with systemic steroids (see later section on immunotherapy).

In most cases, the diagnosis of lung-related drug toxicity is a diagnosis of exclusion. Treatment typically involves discontinuing the offending agent, supportive care with bronchodilators and mechanical ventilation, taking care to avoid high inspired oxygen concentrations in cases of bleomycin and mitomycin C toxicity, and systemic steroids ranging 0.5–1.0 mg/kg/day depending on severity. In instances of noncardiogenic pulmonary oedema, diuretics should be utilized following cardiovascular assessment.

25.2.4 Neurologic Complications

Chemotherapy-induced peripheral neuropathy can be a debilitating side effect of cancer therapy. Agents commonly associated with peripheral neuropathy include vincristine, methotrexate, paclitaxel, cisplatin, oxaliplatin, thalidomide, and bortezomib. However, these patients are usually managed in the outpatient setting and would not require ICU admissions. Nevertheless, working knowledge of these side effects might help the intensivist manage these patients' symptoms.

More serious life-threatening situations include the following situations, which may present to the ICU.

In about 10% of patients receiving high-dose therapy, Busulfan can precipitate seizures within 24 hours of administration. Ifosfamide can precipitate encephalopathy in 10–25%, manifesting as decreased attention and agitation within hours of administration lasting 1–4 days. High-dose Ara-C can also cause painful corneal toxicity associated with blurred vision, photophobia, and conjunctival injection, which can be prevented and treated with glucocorticoid eye drops. The cerebellar syndrome has also been described with high dose cytarabine and includes dysarthria, ataxia, and nystagmus.

Intrathecal methotrexate administration can cause aseptic meningitis in 10% of patients and manifests as headache, lethargy, and nuchal rigidity. Subacute central neurologic toxicity associated with moderate to high doses of MTX can occur weeks to months after administration and may present with aphasia, dysarthria, hemiparesis, seizures, and behavioral abnormalities. Chronic neurotoxicity occurring greater than 6 months after therapy combined with whole-brain radiation can present as dementia, ataxia, and incontinence [12, 13].

All-trans-retinoic acid commonly causes headache and, in some cases, can be associated with increased intracranial pressure due to idiopathic intracranial hypertension, as evidenced by papilledema.

Cortical venous thrombosis (CVT) can be a disabling complication associated with coagulopathy caused by L-Asparaginase or following diarrhea and dehydration associated with 5Fluorouracil or capecitabine.

While approaching a patient on chemotherapy with CNS symptoms, the intensivist should also consider septic encephalopathy, CNS involvement by disease (e.g., CNS metastases or leptomeningeal involvement by the tumor), drug effect, dyselectrolytemia, etc. in his bucket list of differentials.

25.2.5 Renal and Bladder Toxicities

The bladder and kidneys are at risk of toxicity due to anticancer therapies because they are the route of elimination for many of these agents. Comorbid diseases such as hypertension, diabetes, hypovolemia, concomitant nephrotoxic drug use such as nonsteroidal anti-inflammatory agents, and advanced age may increase the risk of developing chemotherapeutic-induced kidney injury.

Cisplatin causes proximal renal tubular impairment in reabsorption of water and sodium and increased renal vascular resistance leading to a decrease in creatinine clearance on an average of 15%. Renal tubular damage also leads to electrolyte abnormalities such as hyponatremia, hypocalcemia, and hypomagnesemia in up to 10% of patients due to impaired resorption and excess renal losses. Renal salt wasting syndrome (RSWS) due to cisplatin can occur as early as 12 h after administration and may be difficult to distinguish from SIADH. RSWS is characterized by hyponatremia, polyuria, hypovolemia, and high urinary sodium concentration with high fractional excretion of sodium despite volume depletion. Treatment for RSWS is the restoration of volume and serum sodium via saline infusion (isotonic or hypertonic based on the severity of hyponatremia) or salt tablets. Free water restriction will not be effective since urinary losses include salt and water [14].

Ifosfamide and cyclophosphamide result in the renally cleared metabolite acrolein production, which is toxic to the bladder epithelium resulting in hemorrhagic cystitis. Prevention of hemorrhagic cystitis is accomplished by vigorous IV hydration and mesna, which binds to acrolein. In the event bleeding does occur, bladder irrigation to evacuate clots is necessary.

High-dose methotrexate (1–12 g/m^2) causes nephrotoxicity by precipitation in the renal tubules where it is actively secreted as well as the collecting ducts resulting in renal failure due to ATN and renal obstruction, respectively. Its solubility is pH and volume-dependent, requiring urine alkalinization with sodium bicarbonate and intravenous fluids prior to administration. In severe cases of renal failure and methotrexate toxicity (MTX serum level > 1 μmol/L), carboxypeptidase has been shown to rapidly decrease serum levels of methotrexate by hydrolyzing MTX to an inactive metabolite [15].

25.2.6 Thrombotic Complications

Venous thromboembolism (VTE) has been reported in >50% of cancer patients on autopsy. Some anticancer therapies have been shown to increase the risk of VTE further. In a large population-based study with 10 years of follow-up, in patients receiving tamoxifen, there was a relative risk of 2.4 for the development of deep vein thrombosis (DVT)/pulmonary embolism (PE). Cisplatin-based chemotherapies are associated with an increase in the risk of vascular events, including cerebrovascular events, arterial thromboses, superficial phlebitis, angina pectoris, as well as DVT/PE [16].

Thrombotic thrombocytopenic purpura has been most associated with gemcitabine, cisplatin and mitomycin. This occurs due to direct endothelial cell dysfunction due to the chemotherapeutic agent and resultant generation of small immune complexes and platelet aggregates. Compared to classic TTP-HUS, chemotherapy-related TTP is typically more insidious in onset, neurologic symptoms are less common, and it does not respond well to plasma exchange. The incidence ranges from 8.5% to 15% for mitomycin-related disease cases, 2.6% secondary to cisplatin, and 0.015% to 1.4% due to gemcitabine. The risk of gemcitabine induced TTP appears to increase at cumulative doses >20,000 mg/m^2 and has a relatively later onset of 7 months compared to mitomycin. Renal failure in most cases is progressive and requires renal replacement therapy, while mortality ranges from 9% to 100% depending on the chemotherapeutic agent; however, these estimates are based on small case reviews [17]. Plasma exchange has been utilized in both mitomycin- and gemcitabine-induced TTP with mixed results (response rates only 30% compared to 80% in classical TTP), and its role remains controversial. The response rate to immunosuppressive agents such as glucocorticoids, Rituximab, and vincristine has been discouraging as well.

25.2.7 Gastrointestinal and Hepatic Toxicities

The incidence of clinically significant grade 3–4 oral mucositis is 1–10% when associated with anthracycline-based regimens, while 5-FU–related mucositis approaches rates of >15%. Taxane and platinum-based regimens also have an incidence of oral mucositis in the range of 3–13%; however, concomitant radiation increases the risk up to sevenfold. Stem cell transplant recipients (predominantly acute leukemia and lymphoma patients) have the highest mucositis rates because of high-dose chemotherapy regimens followed by head and neck patients.

The onset of mucositis typically occurs 5–7 days after treatment with chemotherapy or radiation and may resolve in 2–3 weeks in the absence of myelosuppression. Treatment is mainly supportive with adequate hydration, topical anesthetics such as lidocaine, and systemic analgesia with morphine via PCA. Present guidelines do not recommend chlorhexidine to treat established oral mucositis. Patients may require total parenteral nutrition (TPN) [18].

Mucositis involving the gastrointestinal tract can result in clinically significant diarrhea leading to hypovolemia and electrolyte abnormalities. Subcutaneous octreotide (100 μg) is recommended when first-line therapy with loperamide is unsuccessful. Radiation-induced proctitis accompanied by rectal bleeding can be treated with sucralfate enemas [19].

At least 70% of patients receiving cancer chemotherapy will experience nausea and vomiting, leading to dehydration, malnourishment, and electrolyte abnormalities. Some of the chemotherapeutics agents with the highest emetogenic potential

(>60%) include carmustine, cisplatin cyclophosphamide (especially at higher doses), dacarbazine, procarbazine (oral), dactinomycin, doxorubicin. The current focus of supportive care is to successfully prevent nausea and vomiting with adequate pre-medications like Aprepitant, Fosaprepitant, and post medication, e.g. ondansetron, olanzapine, etc. Treatment is largely supportive with IV hydration and/or nutrition as well as an aggressive electrolyte replacement.

Neutropenic enterocolitis, or typhlitis, is a necrotizing process involving the bowel due to neutropenia, most commonly resulting from the chemotherapeutic treatment of leukemia. Onset is within the first month of chemotherapy initiation and maybe occult as in most cases or present with diarrhea, abdominal pain, and fever.

Vinca alkaloids like Vincristine, Vinorelbine etc. may cause ileus presenting as constipation and abdominal distension. It commonly occurs in patients with low serum albumin, those on azole prophylaxis, or non-compliant prophylactic laxatives. This is important to recognize as these agents form an essential component of multiagent chemotherapy used for leukemias and lymphomas.

Various forms of hepatotoxicity may occur because of anticancer therapies. Venoocclusive or sinusoidal obstructive syndrome is a feared complication of bone-marrow transplant. Other manifestations of hepatotoxicity include cholestasis; elevations in transaminases due to hepatocellular injury; steatosis as seen with L-asparaginase treatment, hepatitis B reactivation, and increased hepatitis C viremia due to Rituximab.

25.2.8 Immune Related Adverse Effects that can Present to the ICU

Immune Checkpoint inhibitors (ICI have dramatically impacted the management of patients with advanced melanoma, lung cancer, urothelial cancers, Hodgkin's lymphoma and kidney cancers, etc.

Immune-related adverse events (irAEs) following ICIs are typically transient but occasionally can be severe or fatal. These side effects can affect almost any organ of the body, the common ones being dermatologic, diarrhoea/colitis, hepatotoxicity, pneumonitis, and endocrinopathies.

Quick identification of irAEs and rapid initiation of local or systemic immunosuppression as indicated by guidelines give best outcomes. irAES are more common with Ipilimumab than with Nivolumab or Pembrolizumab (anti- PD1) or other anti-PD-L1 agents. Nivolumab plus ipilimumab combination is associated with more toxicity than either agent given alone. Broadly, the treatment of moderate or severe irAEs requires interruption of the checkpoint inhibitor and the use of glucocorticoid immunosuppression depending on the severity of the observed toxicity.

For patients with most grade 2 (moderate) irAEs, ICIs should be stopped temporarily and should be resumed only when the toxicity is grade 1 or less. Glucocorticoids (prednisone 0.5 mg/kg/day or equivalent) are started if symptoms do not resolve within a week. Notably, for grade 2 endocrinopathies, immunotherapy may be withheld until hormone replacement is initiated and subsequently resumed once acute symptoms have resolved.

For patients experiencing grade 3 or 4 irAE, the checkpoint inhibitor should be permanently stopped. High doses of glucocorticoids (prednisone 1 to 2 mg/kg/day or equivalent) is given. If symptoms subside to grade 1 or less, steroids are tapered very slowly over at least one month. If glucocorticoids are not effective in treating immunotherapy-related diarrhea/colitis after approximately three days, infliximab (5 mg/kg) needs to be considered. Infliximab, however, is not indicated for patients with immune-mediated hepatitis [20].

As immunotherapy is coming to the forefront and more and more agents are getting approvals in the first and second line of therapy for many cancers, the intensivist is expected to be aware and versed with these unique toxicities.

25.2.9 Cytokine Release Syndrome (CRS) Following CAR-T Cell Therapy

Chimeric Antigen Receptors (CAR)-T Cells is the latest model of cellular therapy approved for the treatment of relapsed and refractory acute lymphoblastic leukemia and some lymphomas. Although it is not currently available widespread, its use is expected to increase with time. However, it is associated with a peculiar side-effect, called "Cytokine Release Syndrome, CRS" which is most commonly managed in the intensive care unit.

CRS associated with CAR-T cell therapy is an acute systemic inflammatory response syndrome (SIRS) manifesting as fever, with or without multiple organ dysfunction. The other clinical manifestations include fatigue, headache, rash, diarrhoea, arthralgia, and myalgia. Mild CRS can progress to a more severe syndrome, typically including hypotension, hypoxia. Uncontrolled SIRS can lead to vascular leakage, circulatory collapse, vascular leakage, peripheral and/or pulmonary oedema, renal and cardiac dysfunction.

CRS is a clinical diagnosis that develops hours to days after treatment with immune therapy. No specific laboratory studies are not required to diagnose CRS. Immune effector cell-associated neurotoxicity syndrome (ICANS) is a neuropsychiatric syndrome that can occur in some patients who are treated with immunotherapy. ICANS may or may not accompany CRS. For mild CRS, symptomatic treatment with antihistamines, antipyretics, and fluids is typically sufficient [21]. For severe CRS caused by CAR-T cell therapy, initial treatment with Tocilizumab plus a glucocorticoid is recommended because the combination is associated with more rapid response and complete control. For severe CRS caused by bispecific antibody therapy (e.g., Blinatumomab), the infusion should be interrupted, and corticosteroids should be started [22].

25.3 Key Points

- Most antineoplastic agents have toxic side effects. When a patient on chemotherapy presents to ICU, often the scenarios are complicated with a combination of chemo toxicity, infection, neutropenia, worsening comorbidities, and active or progressive cancer.
- The intensivist should have a high index of suspicion for drug related adverse effects in case a patient on chemotherapy arrives in the ICU.
- Bleomycin causes pulmonary fibrosis while gemcitabine and cytarabine have been associated with ARDS.
- Anthracyclines may cause cardiotoxicity that lead to refractory heart failure if not identified and managed early.
- In patients with underlying risk factors for coronary artery disease, treatment with 5FU can cause coronary vasospasm leading to acute coronary syndromes.
- Oral and GI mucositis may lead to dehydration and malnutrition.
- Renal salt wasting syndrome may be caused by cisplatin.
- Paralytic ileus is a known side-effect of vinca alkaloids, including Vincristine, Vinblastine and Vinorelbine. These agents are also known to cause peripheral neuropathies.
- Ifosphamide can cause acute metabolic encephalopathy. Haemorrhagic cystitis is typically associated with Ifosphamide treatment.
- Acute cerebellar dysfunction is associated with high dose cytarabine therapy.
- Thrombotic thrombocytopenic purpura (TTP) has been associated with therapy with mitomycin, cisplatin, and gemcitabine.
- Mostly the treatment of chemotherapy drug toxicity is supportive management.
- Immune related adverse effects (irAEs) after ICIs can affect any organ system at any time. Withholding the ICI and early use of steroids as per the grade of the event is crucial.

References

1. Spiess BD. Red cell transfusions and guidelines: a work in progress. Hematol Oncol Clin North Am. 2007 Feb;21(1):185–200.
2. Murphy MF, Wallington TB, Kelsey P, Boulton F, Bruce M, Cohen H, et al. Guidelines for the clinical use of red cell transfusions. Br J Haematol. 2001 Apr;113(1):24–31.
3. Schiffer CA, Bohlke K, Delaney M, Hume H, Magdalinski AJ, McCullough JJ, et al. Platelet transfusion for patients with cancer: American Society of Clinical Oncology clinical practice guideline update. J Clin Oncol Off J Am Soc Clin Oncol. 2018 Jan 20;36(3):283–99.
4. MASCC FN risk index score [Internet]. [cited 2021 Apr 1]. Available from: https://www.mascc.org/mascc-fn-risk-index-score
5. IDSA GUIDELINES Bundle (free trial) - Fever and Neutropenia [Internet]. [cited 2021 Apr 1]. Available from: http://eguideline.guidelinecentral.com/i/53994-fever-and-neutropenia/9?
6. Gh L, Jm K. Summary and comparison of myeloid growth factor guidelines in patients receiving cancer chemotherapy. Cancer Treat Res. 2011 Jan 1;157:145–65.

7. Mackey JR, Clemons M, Côté MA, Delgado D, Dent S, Paterson A, et al. Cardiac management during adjuvant trastuzumab therapy: recommendations of the Canadian Trastuzumab working group. Curr Oncol Tor Ont. 2008 Jan;15(1):24–35.
8. Schmidinger M, Zielinski CC, Vogl UM, Bojic A, Bojic M, Schukro C, et al. Cardiac toxicity of sunitinib and sorafenib in patients with metastatic renal cell carcinoma. J Clin Oncol Off J Am Soc Clin Oncol. 2008 Nov 10;26(32):5204–12.
9. Briasoulis E, Pavlidis N. Noncardiogenic pulmonary edema: an unusual and serious complication of anticancer therapy. Oncologist. 2001;6(2):153–61.
10. Patatanian E, Thompson DF. Retinoic acid syndrome: a review. J Clin Pharm Ther. 2008;33(4):331–8.
11. Sleijfer S. Bleomycin-induced pneumonitis. Chest. 2001 Aug;120(2):617–24.
12. Stone JB, DeAngelis LM. Cancer-treatment-induced neurotoxicity--focus on newer treatments. Nat Rev Clin Oncol. 2016 Feb;13(2):92–105.
13. Plotkin SR, Wen PY. Neurologic complications of cancer therapy. Neurol Clin 2003 Feb;21(1):279–318, x. https://doi.org/10.1016/s0733-8619(02)00034-8
14. Hamdi T, Latta S, Jallad B, Kheir F, Alhosaini MN, Patel A. Cisplatin-induced renal salt wasting syndrome. South Med J. 2010 Aug;103(8):793–9.
15. Kintzel PE. Anticancer drug-induced kidney disorders. Drug Saf. 2001 Jan;24(1):19–38.
16. Hernandez RK, Sørensen HT, Pedersen L, Jacobsen J, Lash TL. Tamoxifen treatment and risk of deep venous thrombosis and pulmonary embolism: a Danish population-based cohort study. Cancer. 2009 Oct 1;115(19):4442–9.
17. Müller S, Schütt P, Bojko P, Nowrousian MR, Hense J, Seeber S, et al. Hemolytic uremic syndrome following prolonged gemcitabine therapy: report of four cases from a single institution. Ann Hematol. 2005 Feb;84(2):110–4.
18. Peterson DE, Boers-Doets CB, Bensadoun RJ, Herrstedt J, ESMO Guidelines Committee. Management of oral and gastrointestinal mucosal injury: ESMO Clinical Practice Guidelines for diagnosis, treatment, and follow-up. Ann Oncol Off J Eur Soc Med Oncol. 2015 Sep;26(Suppl 5):v139–51.
19. Sonis ST, Elting LS, Keefe D, Peterson DE, Schubert M, Hauer-Jensen M, et al. Perspectives on cancer therapy-induced mucosal injury: pathogenesis, measurement, epidemiology, and consequences for patients. Cancer. 2004 May 1;100(9 Suppl):1995–2025.
20. Haanen JBAG, Carbonnel F, Robert C, Kerr KM, Peters S, Larkin J, et al. Management of toxicities from immunotherapy: ESMO Clinical Practice Guidelines for diagnosis, treatment and follow-up. Ann Oncol. 2017 Jul 1;28:iv119–42.
21. Neelapu SS. Managing the toxicities of CAR T-cell therapy. Hematol Oncol. 2019 Jun;37(Suppl 1):48–52.
22. Siegler EL, Kenderian SS. Neurotoxicity and cytokine release syndrome after chimeric antigen receptor T cell therapy: insights into mechanisms and novel therapies. Front Immunol [Internet]. 2020 [cited 2021 Apr 1];11. Available from: https://www.frontiersin.org/articles/10.3389/fimmu.2020.01973/full

Radiation Induced Toxicities Requiring ICU Admission

26

K. P. Haresh and Subhash Gupta

26.1 Chapter

Life threatening complications of radiation therapy has drastically decreased today with the use of highly precise modern techniques of radiation. Yet, certain toxicities still remain a serious concern, especially in those who are treated with curative intent, requiring timely detection and intervention, in the setting of critical care.

26.2 Radiation Induced Lung Toxicity

Incidence of radiation induced pneumonitis in those patients receiving any form of thoracic radiotherapy is around 10–30%, in whom there is an increased risk of radiation induced lung fibrosis [1–4].

26.2.1 Pathology

Radiation induced lung injury (RILI) is caused by both direct and indirect side effects of radiation by causing DNA damage in the normal cells of the lung tissue. The consequent fibrosis results from increase in cytokines like IL-6, TGF-beta, TNF-alpha.

Phase 1: This phase begins with a few hours to days after radiation exposure. Patient is usually asymptomatic. This is characterised by hyperaemic, congested mucosa with leukocytic infiltration and increased capillary permeability. This is followed by an exudative alveolitis, with tracheo-bronchial hyper-secretion. Type 1 alveolar epithelial cell are destroyed and there is an increase in surfactant production [5].

K. P. Haresh (✉) · S. Gupta
Department of Radiation Oncology, AIIMS Delhi, New Delhi, India

V. Kumar et al. (eds.), *Onco-critical Care*,
https://doi.org/10.1007/978-981-16-9929-0_26

Phase 2 (Latent phase): Accumulation of secretions due to increase in number of goblet cells.

Phase 3 (Acute exudative phase): This phase occurs 3–12 weeks after radiation exposure and referred to clinically as radiation pneumonitis. Type 2 pneumocytes become hyperplastic, with formation of hyaline membranes as a result of alveolar epithelial desquamation and fibrin rich exudate into alveoli.

Phase 4 (Resolution or Fibrosis): There may be resolution of hyaline membranes and exudates, or there may be deposition of myofibroblast within the interstitium along with increase in collagen, leading to decrease in lung volume. Fibrosis can develop as early as 6 months to years after the exposure to radiation [6, 7].

26.2.2 Risk Factors

1. Dose of radiation: Volume of normal lung receiving 20 Gy should be less than 35 percent of total volume, and mean lung dose should be less than 23 Gy to decrease the risk of pneumonitis to less than 20 percent, as per the QUANTEC guidelines [8, 9].
2. Volume of irradiation.
3. Technique of irradiation: IMRT decreases the risk of grade 3 pneumonitis, as compared to 3DCRT (RTOG0617) [10].
4. Concurrent Chemotherapy: Anthracycline, paclitaxel, gemcitabine, pemetrexed [11, 12].
5. Prior Thoracic radiation.
6. Underlying lung pathology: COPD (chronic obstructive pulmonary disease), ILD (Interstitial lung disease), Lung collapse or volume loss.

26.2.3 Symptoms

(a) Non-productive cough
(b) Dyspnoea [13]
(c) Fever- low grade, more pronounced when severe
(d) Chest Pain- Pleuritic or sub-sternal
(e) Malaise, weight loss

26.2.4 Signs

(a) Crackles or pleural rub
(b) Dullness on percussion if pleura effusion is present. Radiation induced effusions do not increase in size on observation.
(c) Severe cases can present with tachypnoea, cyanosis, pulmonary hypertension

26.2.5 Diagnostic Evaluation

The direction of evaluation is to assess the severity of respiratory impairment, correlate radiological imaging with radiation portal, and most importantly, to rule out other causes of symptoms like infection, thrombosis, drug or disease related pneumonitis, ILD, COPD or heart diseases.

There are no specific lab investigations that point to a doubt of radiation pneumonitis and is usually a diagnosis of exclusion.

Imaging: Computed tomography (CT) is more sensitive than chest radiograph. It plays a key role when the radiation CT with dosimetric information is correlated with the diagnostic CT, as the findings are usually confined to the radiotherapy portals. Chest radiograph in the early phase typically shows perivascular haziness which progress into patchy alveolar filling densities, while in more chronic setting chest radiograph shows coarse reticular opacities with volume loss [14].

Pulmonary function test: Pre-radiotherapy pulmonary function tests are compared with the PFT when the patient is symptomatic. Typically, PFT demonstrates reduction in total lung volumes-Total lung capacity, forced vital capacity, tidal volume and lung compliance, like any other interstitial lung disease [15].

Bronchoscopy: The main role of flexible fibre optic bronchoscopy is to look for infection, drug hyper-sensitivity or underlying malignancy. Broncho alveolar lavage (BAL) is non-specific and usually consists of lymphocytes.

26.2.6 Treatment

The major part of treatment is based on symptomatic management comprising of anti-tussive treatment, supplemental oxygen and treatment of underlying co-morbid conditions like COPD and cardiac conditions that aggravate the symptoms. The only drug that has been found to be useful is Prednisolone at a dose of 40–60 mg/day, given for 2–4 weeks, gradually tapering over 3–12 weeks. If there is relapse of symptoms, full dose of steroids will have to be re-started for 2 weeks, with slower tapering of the same. Prophylaxis against Pneumocystis jiroveci may be considered if steroid therapy continues for more than a month [16].

Other experimental drugs inculde Pentoxyphilline 400 mg TDS, which is a xanthine derivative that enhances microvascular blood flow and also inhibit TNF and IL, leading to anti-inflammatory and immunomodulatory properties. Angiotensin converting enzyme inhibitor Captopril has also been tried.

PROGNOSIS: Once fibrosis has been established, and patient has severe respiratory distress and requires ICU admission, the prognosis is very poor, with no effective treatment modalities to date.

26.3 Radiation Induced Cardiotoxicity

Radiation induced cardiac toxicity is manifested in the form of the following in the order of incidence

- Pericarditis
- Cardiomyopathy
- Coronary Artery Disease(CAD)
- Valvular heart disease
- Conduction abnormality

Incidence: Incidence varies with different thoracic malignancies ranging from 0.5 to 37% in breast cancer, and as high as 54% in lymphomas, depending on the survival associated with certain malignancies [17]. Longer the survival, higher the chance of detecting cardiac toxicity, with usual presentations between 10 and 20 years after completion of treatment. The incidence also varies in patients treated with cardio toxic chemotherapy, treatment of left sided versus right sided breast cancer with radiotherapy, technique of radiotherapy, dose of radiotherapy received, underlying co-morbidities, and addictions like smoking [18].

Dose of radiotherapy: Although there seems to be no minimal safe dose of radiotherapy to the heart, studies shows the risk of a coronary event progressively increases with increase in radiation dose, with a relative risk increase of 7.4% for each 1 Gy of radiation to the heart. A case- control study calculated the risk of a coronary event for a 50 year old female with no coronary risk factors, to die from an ischemic heart disease before 80 years of age, 1.9% to 2.4%, and risk of at least one major coronary event increased from 4.5 to 5.4% if the mean dose received was 3Gy. If the mean dose received was 10 Gy, the same increased from 1.9 to 3.4% and 4.5 to 7.7% respectively [19, 20].

26.3.1 Pathophysiology

The primary mode of injury to the heart is thought to be due to generation of reactive oxygen species that disrupt DNA strands, leading to secondary inflammatory changes and subsequent fibrosis. The deposition of myofibroblasts and platelet adhesion leads to narrowing of intima of coronary vessels leading to coronary artery disease, fibrosis of cusps of valves, myocardium and conduction fibres lead to valvular heart disease, cardiomyopathy and conduction abnormalities respectively [21].

26.3.2 Symptoms

Pericarditis may present as acute pericarditis within a few weeks of radiation therapy, which presents with chest pain(supine position and inspiration) and low-grade fever. These are usually self-limiting. Around 20% of those who developed acute pericarditis, may subsequently develop chronic and constrictive pericarditis, which presents with chest pain, dyspnoea and orthopnoea, and peri-cardiac effusions, and rarely develop cardiac tamponade which presents with hemodynamic abnormalities with hypotension, tachycardia and jugular venous distension [22].

26.3.3 Diagnosis

2D ECHO cardiogram is the most important investigation to diagnose as well as to follow up patients with pericarditis. ECG shows non-specific ST and T-wave changes or ST segment elevation in all leads. Chest X-ray and CT may show pericardial effusion and pericardial thickening in chronic pericarditis. Cardiac MRI helps in accurate assessment of pericardial thickness. Cardiomyopathy shows abnormalities in ECHO, as regional wall motion irregularities, usually inferior, LVH and diastolic dysfunction.

26.3.4 Management

Majority of acute pericarditis is self-limiting and respond well to aspirin and colchicine. Large pericardial effusion can be drained per-cutaneously or surgically. Recurrent effusions are managed by pericardiotomy or pericardial stripping. Pericardiectomy is recommended in those with constrictive pericarditis, although the mortality is higher as compared to constrictive pericarditis due to other causes. Cardiomyopathy and coronary artery disease, is usually managed on life-long medications, and would present to ICU only in case of cardiac failure.

26.4 Radiation Induced CNS Toxicity

Like other grade 4 radiation induced toxicity, this too depends on the dose of radiation, volume irradiated, and dose per fraction, and additionally, it also depends on the status of primary disease in the brain.

Most common causes for grade 4 toxicity after CNS radiation includes:

- Raised intra cranial pressure (due to radiation induced oedema, obstruction of ventricles)
- Radiation necrosis
- Progression of disease in the brain-(primary brain tumour or metastasis)

26.4.1 Symptoms

- Headache
- Vomiting

- Drowsiness
- Seizures
- Neurological deficit

26.4.2 Diagnosis

After routine laboratory investigations, and ruling our any electrolyte imbalance or any basic pathology in lab parameters, the first most useful investigation is a non-contrast CT of the head to look for gross dilatation of the ventricular system. A contrast enhanced MRI Brain is the imaging modality of choice, although this may still pose difficulties in differentiating between a progressing primary disease verus a radiation induced necrosis. Radiation induced necrosis is anticipated when the patient has received radiation 2–3 years prior, to a Dmax of 65 to 72 Gy, although doses lesser than this has also been reported to cause the same. The only definite way to confirm diagnosis includes biopsy, although patients are rarely fit for the same [23].

26.4.3 Management

Most important part of management includes medical decompression comprising of the following:

- Intravenous steroids (Dexamethasone 8 mg TDS) with monitoring of blood sugar levels
- Intravenous proton pump inhibitors (Pantoprazole 40 mg OD)
- Intravenous Mannitol (20%) 100 ml TDS for 3–5 days
- Carbonic Anhydrase inhibitor (Tab Acetazolamide 250 mg TDS)
- Syrup Glycerol for 2 weeks

It is important to diagnose hydrocephalus from other causes of cerebral edema as this is an emergency and requires urgent neuro-surgical intervention in the form of ventriculo-peritoneal shunt.

26.5 Others

(a) Occasionally, patients who are posted for head and neck interstitial brachytherapy may require unexpected ICU management- during the insertion or removal of the catheters, due to unexpected bleeding and aspiration. All these patients are usually curable in view of small disease, by virtue of which they are amenable to brachytherapy, and must be aggressively salvaged.

(b) Rarely, grade 4 radiation induced dermatitis, especially in pelvic radiotherapy for carcinoma anal canal, rectum and cervix, with super added infections and consequent septic shock, which may have to managed aggressively with systemic antibiotics as well as simultaneous wound care. Although newer techniques of radiotherapy and more vigilant patient review while on radiotherapy have decreased such occurrences significantly

References

1. Chun SG, Hu C, Choy H, Komaki RU, Timmerman RD, Schild SE, Bogart JA, Dobelbower MC, Bosch W, Galvin JM, Kavadi VS, Narayan S, Iyengar P, Robinson CG, Wynn RB, Raben A, Augspurger ME, MacRae RM, Paulus R, Bradley JD. Impact of intensity-modulated radiation therapy technique for locally advanced non-small-cell lung cancer: a secondary analysis of the NRG oncology RTOG 0617 randomized clinical trial. J Clin Oncol. 2017 Jan;35(1):56–62. https://doi.org/10.1200/JCO.2016.69.1378. Epub 2016 Oct 31. PMID: 28034064; PMCID: PMC5455690.
2. Nishioka A, Ogawa Y, Hamada N, Terashima M, Inomata T, Yoshida S. Analysis of radiation pneumonitis and radiation-induced lung fibrosis in breast cancer patients after breast conservation treatment. Oncol Rep. 1999 May–Jun;6(3):513–7. https://doi.org/10.3892/or.6.3.513.
3. Keffer S, Guy CL, Weiss E. Fatal radiation pneumonitis: literature review and case series. Adv Radiat Oncol 2019 Aug 31;5(2):238–249. https://doi.org/10.1016/j.adro.2019.08.010. PMID: 32280824; PMCID: PMC7136627.
4. Wennberg B, Gagliardi G, Sundbom L, Svane G, Lind P. Early response of lung in breast cancer irradiation: radiologic density changes measured by CT and symptomatic radiation pneumonitis. Int J Radiat Oncol Biol Phys. 2002 Apr 1;52(5):1196–206. https://doi.org/10.1016/s0360-3016(01)02770-5.
5. Kouloulias V, Zygogianni A, Efstathopoulos E, Victoria O, Christos A, Pantelis K, Koutoulidis V, Kouvaris J, Sandilos P, Varela M, Aytas I, Gouliamos A, Kelekis N. Suggestion for a new grading scale for radiation induced pneumonitis based on radiological findings of computerized tomography: correlation with clinical and radiotherapeutic parameters in lung cancer patients. Asian Pac J Cancer Prev. 2013;14(5):2717–22. https://doi.org/10.7314/apjcp.2013.14.5.2717.
6. Small W Jr, Woloschak G. Radiation toxicity: a practical guide. Introduction. Cancer Treat Res. 2006;128:3–5.
7. Larici AR, del Ciello A, Maggi F, Santoro SI, Meduri B, Valentini V, Giordano A, Bonomo L. Lung abnormalities at multimodality imaging after radiation therapy for non-small cell lung cancer. Radiographics. 2011 May-Jun;31(3):771–89. https://doi.org/10.1148/rg.313105096.
8. Tsujino K, Hashimoto T, Shimada T, Yoden E, Fujii O, Ota Y, Satouchi M, Negoro S, Adachi S, Soejima T. Combined analysis of V20, VS5, pulmonary fibrosis score on baseline computed tomography, and patient age improves prediction of severe radiation pneumonitis after concurrent chemoradiotherapy for locally advanced non-small-cell lung cancer. J Thorac Oncol. 2014 Jul;9(7):983–90. https://doi.org/10.1097/JTO.0000000000000187.
9. Matsuo Y, Shibuya K, Nakamura M, Narabayashi M, Sakanaka K, Ueki N, Miyagi K, Norihisa Y, Mizowaki T, Nagata Y, Hiraoka M. Dose--volume metrics associated with radiation pneumonitis after stereotactic body radiation therapy for lung cancer. Int J Radiat Oncol Biol Phys 2012 Jul 15;83(4):e545–e549. https://doi.org/10.1016/j.ijrobp.2012.01.018. Epub 2012 Mar 19.
10. van Sörnsen de Koste J, Voet P, Dirkx M, van Meerbeeck J, Senan S. Rotterdam oncological thoracic study group. An evaluation of two techniques for beam intensity modulation in patients irradiated for stage III non-small cell lung cancer. Lung Cancer. 2001 May;32(2):145–53. https://doi.org/10.1016/s0169-5002(00)00214-2.
11. Wang CJ, Chang HT, Chang CY. Docetaxel-related interstitial pneumonitis. Ther Clin Risk Manag 2015 Dec 9;11:1813–1816. https://doi.org/10.2147/TCRM.S90488. PMID: 26677333; PMCID: PMC4677769.

12. Bielopolski D, Evron E, Moreh-Rahav O, Landes M, Stemmer SM, Salamon F. Paclitaxel-induced pneumonitis in patients with breast cancer: case series and review of the literature. J Chemother (Florence). 2017;29(2):113–7.
13. Rodrigues G, Lock M, D'Souza D, Yu E, Van Dyk J. Prediction of radiation pneumonitis by dose - volume histogram parameters in lung cancer--a systematic review. Radiother Oncol 2004 May;71(2):127–138. https://doi.org/10.1016/j.radonc.2004.02.015.
14. Linda A, Trovo M, Bradley JD. Radiation injury of the lung after stereotactic body radiation therapy (SBRT) for lung cancer: a timeline and pattern of CT changes. Eur J Radiol 2011 Jul ;79(1):147–154. https://doi.org/10.1016/j.ejrad.2009.10.029. Epub 2009 Dec 1.
15. Torre-Bouscoulet L, Muñoz-Montaño WR, Martínez-Briseño D, Lozano-Ruiz FJ, Fernández-Plata R, Beck-Magaña JA, García-Sancho C, Guzmán-Barragán A, Vergara E, Blake-Cerda M, Gochicoa-Rangel L, Maldonado F, Arroyo-Hernández M, Arrieta O. Abnormal pulmonary function tests predict the development of radiation-induced pneumonitis in advanced non-small cell lung cancer. Respir Res 2018 Apr 24;19(1):72. https://doi.org/10.1186/s12931-018-0775-2. PMID: 29690880; PMCID: PMC5937833.
16. Baden LR, Swaminathan S, Angarone M, Blouin G, Camins BC, Casper C, Cooper B, Dubberke ER, Engemann AM, Freifeld AG, Greene JN, Ito JI, Kaul DR, Lustberg ME, Montoya JG, Rolston K, Satyanarayana G, Segal B, Seo SK, Shoham S, Taplitz R, Topal J, Wilson JW, Hoffmann KG, Smith C. Prevention and treatment of cancer-related infections, version 2.2016, NCCN clinical practice guidelines in oncology. J Natl Compr Cancer Netw. 2016 Jul;14(7):882–913. https://doi.org/10.6004/jnccn.2016.0093.
17. Lenneman CG, Sawyer DB. Cardio-oncology: an update on Cardiotoxicity of cancer-related treatment. Circ Res. 2016 Mar 18;118(6):1008–20. https://doi.org/10.1161/CIRCRESAHA.115.303633.
18. Menezes KM, Wang H, Hada M, Saganti PB. Radiation matters of the heart: a mini review. Front Cardiovasc Med. 2018;5:83. Published 2018 Jul 9. https://doi.org/10.3389/fcvm.2018.00083.
19. Yeboa DN, Evans SB. Contemporary breast radiotherapy and cardiac toxicity. Semin Radiat Oncol 2016 Jan;26(1):71–78. https://doi.org/10.1016/j.semradonc.2015.09.003. Epub 2015 Sep 4.
20. Menezes KM, Wang H, Hada M, Saganti PB. Radiation matters of the heart: a mini review. Front Cardiovasc Med 2018 Jul 9;5:83. https://doi.org/10.3389/fcvm.2018.00083. PMID: 30038908; PMCID: PMC6046516.
21. Taunk NK, Haffty BG, Kostis JB, Goyal S. Radiation-induced heart disease: pathologic abnormalities and putative mechanisms. Front Oncol 2015 Feb 18;5:39. https://doi.org/10.3389/fonc.2015.00039. PMID: 25741474; PMCID: PMC4332338.
22. Clare GC, Troughton RW. Management of constrictive pericarditis in the 21st century. Curr Treat Options Cardiovasc Med. 2007 Dec;9(6):436–42. https://doi.org/10.1007/s11936-007-0038-x.
23. Smart D. Radiation toxicity in the central nervous system: mechanisms and strategies for injury reduction. Semin Radiat Oncol. 2017;27(4):332–9. https://doi.org/10.1016/j.semradonc.2017.04.006.

Haematuria in Critically Ill Cancer Patients

27

Sridhar Panaiyadiyan, Prabhjot Singh, and Brusabhanu Nayak

27.1 Introduction

Haematuria is defined as the presence of red blood cells in the urine. It may be denoted as gross haematuria when there is visible blood in the urine. Microscopic haematuria denotes ≥3 red blood cells (RBC) per high power field detected in urinalysis [1]. Various classification of haematuria exists based on aetiology (glomerular/non-glomerular), clinical presentation (symptomatic/asymptomatic), duration of symptoms (transient, intermittent or persistent) and time in relation to void (initial, terminal, total) [2]. While published literature on approach to haematuria in general populations are available, there is only a limited material discussing the management of haematuria, particularly in critically ill cancer patients. In this chapter, we will discuss the potential causes, pathophysiology, clinical presentation and approach to haematuria in such vulnerable patient population.

27.2 Epidemiology

The exact prevalence of haematuria in critically ill cancer patients is unknown, possibly because of under reporting. However, haematuria is not uncommon with a reported prevalence of 4–20% requiring urology consultations and hospitalization [3]. The presence of haematuria should be considered a sign of malignancy until proven otherwise. It is estimated that up to 4% of patients with microscopic haematuria and 40% of patients with gross haematuria could have an underlying malignancy [4].

S. Panaiyadiyan · P. Singh (✉) · B. Nayak
Department of Urology, All India Institute of Medical Sciences, New Delhi, India

V. Kumar et al. (eds.), *Onco-critical Care*,
https://doi.org/10.1007/978-981-16-9929-0_27

27.3 Aetiology

Haematuria can occur anywhere in the urinary tract due to pathology in the kidney, ureter, bladder and prostate. Haematuria may be stratified based on the significance of bleed [5] or on the site of origin [6]. A better way of classifying the aetiology of haematuria is to divide as medical or surgical causes. Table 27.1 describes the common medical and surgical causes of haematuria in critically ill cancer patients.

Various medical conditions such as glomerular disease, infectious, inflammatory, bleeding diathesis and anticoagulant overdose can lead to haematuria. These conditions require disease specific medical management to control haematuria.

Non-glomerular causes of haematuria are mostly of urological origin. These include haematuria from the kidney, urothelium or prostate because of benign and malignant lesions. Other etiologies are urolithiasis, arteriovenous malformation, and trauma.

Table 27.1 Causes of haematuria in critically ill cancer patients

Medical causes	Surgical causes
Glomerular haematuria 1. IgA nephropathy 2. MPGN 3. FSGN 4. MGN	Renal causes 1. Renal cystic diseases 2. Tumour- benign or malignant
Infectious 1. UTI- pyelonephritis, uncomplicated cystitis, prostatitis 2. GUTB	Urothelial causes 1. Benign and malignant lesions
Inflammatory 1. Haemorrhagic cystitis (a) Chemotherapy induced (b) Radiation induced	Prostate diseases 1. BPH 2. Prostate cancer
Bleeding disorders 1. Haemophilia 2. Thrombocytopenia 3. DIC	Urolithiasis 1. Renal stone 2. Ureter stone 3. Bladder stone
Hypercoagulability 1. RVT	Traumatic 1. Catheter related injury 2. Post biopsy
Anticoagulants 1. Warfarin 2. Heparin	Vascular malformations 1. AVM

Abbreviations: *IgA* immunoglobulin A, *MPGN* membranoproliferative glomerulonephritis, *FSGN* focal segmental glomerulonephritis, *MGN* membranous glomerulonephritis, *RPN* renal papillary necrosis, *UTI* urinary tract infection, *GUTB* genitourinary tuberculosis, *BPH* benign prostatic hyperplasia, *DIC* disseminated intravascular coagulopathy, *RVT* renal vein thrombosis, *AVM* arteriovenous malformations

27.4 Pathophysiology

27.4.1 Glomerular Haematuria

A recent review showed an increasing incidence of glomerular haematuria in the United States among patients over 60 years of age [7]. Among glomerular haematuria, IgA nephropathy is the most common cause accounting for 30% cases [8]. Other causes include membranous nephropathy, postinfectious glomerulonephritis, lupus nephritis, and crescentic glomerulonephritis [2].

The pathologic findings in IgA nephropathy are limited to glomerulus. The proliferative changes usually confined to mesangial cells. Deposits of IgA, IgG, and β1microglobulin are noted in renal biopsy. These deposits induce inflammatory reactions in the glomerulus [9].

27.4.2 Urinary Tract Infections (UTI)

Infection can occur in any part of the genitourinary tract with most common being cystitis. Although most of them are asymptomatic, common symptoms include dysuria, haematuria, irritative lower urinary tract symptoms (LUTS) such as frequency, urgency with or without incontinence, foul-smelling urine, and suprapubic discomfort [1].

Hospital acquired UTI are the most common nosocomial infections, with an overall incidence density of 9.6–11.3 per 1000 ICU days [10]. The most frequent microbiological agents responsible are Escherichia coli, Pseudomonas, Staphylococcus, Klebsiella, Proteus, Enterobacter, Citrobacter, Enterococcus or candida species [11].

In men, bacterial prostatitis is mostly caused by infection by Enterobacteriaceae family. Acute bacterial prostatitis in such patients can cause significant morbidity. Majority of them are secondary to ascending infections from urethritis or epididymo-orchitis. Rarely, they can be caused by haematogenous seeding of sepsis in immunocompromised patients [12].

27.4.3 Haemorrhagic Cystitis

Haemorrhagic cystitis is rare, yet frequent cause of haematuria, particularly in patients received radiation therapy for pelvic organ malignancies or oxazophosphorine class of chemotherapeutic agents. In this, haematuria occurs due to diffuse ooze from the bladder mucosa caused by diffuse inflammation (Fig. 27.1) [13].

Radiation-induced haemorrhagic cystitis can occur anywhere from days to years after radiation therapy. Haematuria in such inflammatory cases is frequently associated with severe pain [14]. Although haemorrhagic cystitis is the usual differential diagnosis assumed in a cancer patient with a history of radiation therapy, one has to be cognizant about a new onset malignancy. Further, Leapman et al. showed 9.6%

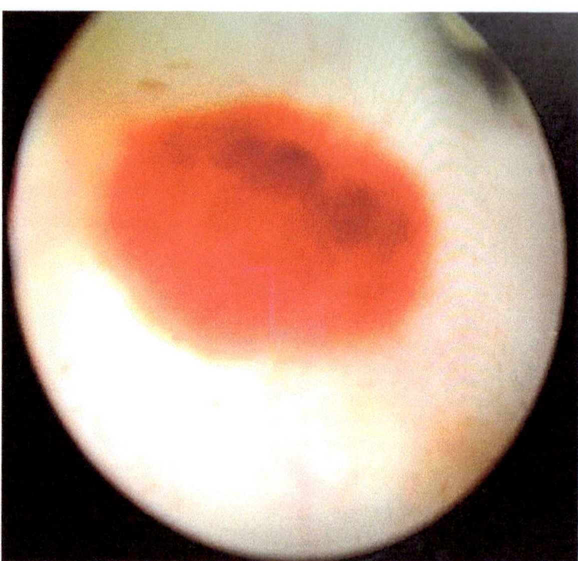

Fig. 27.1 Cystoscopic image showing diffusely affected bladder mucosa in a case of radiation-induced haemorrhagic cystitis

patients who received radiation therapy for prostate cancer presented with haematuria and revealed to have urinary bladder cancer [15]. The mechanism underlying radiation-induced cystitis is by progressive obliterative endarteritis. The vascular endothelium is damaged by the radiation exposure resulting in inflammation, ischemia, fibrosis, necrosis and mucosal sloughing [16]. Apart from the local vascular compromise, super-added infections further affect the tissue repair [17].

Chemical cystitis is a form of haemorrhagic cystitis, particularly caused by exposure to cyclophosphamide or ifosfamide chemotherapeutic agents. The estimated incidence is 2% to 40% following cyclophosphamide exposure [13]. Bladder mucosal inflammation is a result from the active metabolite acrolein produced by the liver. Acrolein causes inflammatory reactions, mucosal sloughing and subsequent fibrosis [18].

27.4.4 Renal Vein Thrombus

Renal vein thrombus (RVT) is a frequent cause of haematuria in newborn. However, it is rare in adults and results from the classical triad of endothelial injury, blood stasis and hypercoagulability. In contrast to children, RVT in adults is unilateral. The conditions associated with RVT include nephrotic syndrome, invasive tumours and trauma [19, 20].

27.4.5 Anticoagulants

Anticoagulants may cause drug-induced haematuria. However, studies have shown that at normal therapeutic levels, anticoagulant do not predispose to haematuria. Culclasure et al. in a prospective study, showed a comparable prevalence of haematuria between long-term anticoagulant users versus control group (3.2% vs 4.8%). Notably, 81% of patients had an underlying identifiable urological disease with more than one episode of microscopic haematuria [21]. Thus, unless overdosed anticoagulants do not cause haematuria.

27.4.6 Renal Mass

Pertaining to kidney, renal cell carcinoma (RCC) is the most common malignancy accounting for 90% of renal masses [22]. In recent years, RCC is frequently detected as an incidental finding on non-invasive images during evaluation of various non-specific symptoms [23]. In fact, haematuria in renal malignancy is a sign of advanced disease. In RCC, haematuria is caused by tumour infiltration into pelvicalyceal system or renal vein and/or inferior vena cava tumour thrombus extension [24].

27.4.7 Urothelial Diseases

Bladder carcinoma is the most frequent cause of painless gross haematuria in an adult. These hypervascular lesions rapidly grow and rupture, resulting in intermittent haematuria. Urothelial cancer can occur anywhere from calyx to urethra. Risk factors include tobacco use and occupational risk exposure to toxic agents such as aniline dye workers and painting industries [25]. Carcinoma-in situ may also present with irritative LUTS [26].

27.4.8 Prostatic Diseases

Common causes of prostate-related haematuria are benign prostatic hyperplasia (BPH), prostatitis and prostate cancer. In BPH, the underlying pathology causing haematuria is increased tissue vascularity due to increased micro-vessel density. At the molecular level, this has been related to a higher levels of local vascular endothelial growth factor in the hyperplastic prostate tissues [27]. In cases of advanced prostate cancer, haematuria results from tumour infiltrating bladder mucosa at the trigone [28].

27.4.9 Urolithiasis

In cases of urinary stones, haematuria is usually due to associated urothelial inflammation and infections. About 90% of cases have haematuria either, microscopic or gross [29].

27.4.10 Renal Arteriovenous Malformations

Renal arteriovenous malformations (AVMs) are abnormal vascular shunting between artery and vein. It may be congenital or acquired. Congenital lesions are tortuous and result from direct arteriovenous communication without an intervening vascular nidus. In contrast, acquired lesions are due to pseudoaneurysm or arteriovenous fistula in nature [30]. Renal biopsy, prior renal surgeries, trauma, malignancy are risk factors for acquired AVM [31].

27.4.11 Trauma-Related

Apart from causing UTI, an indwelling catheter can predispose to trauma-induce haematuria. Traumatic catheterization can results from underlying stricture urethra, prostate enlargement with large median lobe or attempt by an inexperienced person [32]. Occasionally, a confused, disoriented, restless patient in the ICU set-up can pull the urethral catheter in position leading to torrential bleeding.

27.5 Clinical Features

27.5.1 Presentation

Patients with gross haematuria may have varied clinical presentations. Table 27.2 describes clinical presentations based on different etiologies.

Table 27.2 Clinical presentations based on aetiology of haematuria

Aetiology	Haematuria	Associated symptoms
Glomerular	Gross and painless	Fever, rash, recent throat or skin infections
UTI	Microscopic or gross and with or without pain	Irritative LUTS, dysuria, cloudy urine, fever
Inflammatory cystitis	Persistent gross painful haematuria	Irritative LUTS
Urolithiasis	Microscopic or gross haematuria	Lithuria, lateralizing pain
Malignancy	Mostly gross and painless	Lateralizing pain, associated clots, constitutional symptoms, irritative LUTS, obstructive LUTS

Abbreviations: *UTI* urinary tract infection, *LUTS* lower urinary tract symptoms

27.5.2 History

The first step in evaluation is getting a detailed history from patients or primary caregivers in critically ill patients. Often, this provides the clue to diagnose the underlying cause. History should include about the severity, duration, frequency, time in relation to void.

Associated symptoms can be an additional diagnostic clue [1]. Presence of pain denotes acute condition. Pain in flank, back, lower abdomen, perineum or penis can help in localizing the site of haematuria. UTI, urine retention, clot retention may have suprapubic pain. Urothelial malignancy is usually painless; however, a clot colic can occur in upper tract urothelial cancer due to clots obstructing the ureter. Similarly, clots can cause urinary retention with pain in case of bladder cancer. Further, shape of clots suggests the site of origin. Amorphous clots signal bladder origin, whereas vermiform clots indicate bleeding from the upper tracts [20].

It is important to take a thorough personnel and family history. Chronic use of tobacco use suggests urothelial malignancy. Patients of diabetes, sickle cell trait of African American race, or chronic analgesic abuse can have renal papillary necrosis. A family history of bleeding diathesis, prostate cancer, renal cystic disease, urolithiasis should be obtained [33]. Finally, history of any anticoagulant intake with specific note on duration of the therapy and any recent change in the anticoagulant dose is obtained.

27.5.3 Physical Examination

The general examination is the first part of the physical examination including recording of patient haemodynamic status. Systemic examination should focus on abdomen and external genitalia. Renal angle tenderness may suggest an underlying renal pathology such as pyelonephritis, hydronephrosis due to urolithiasis or malignancy. The importance of genital examination should not be underestimated. An isolated varicosity on right side scrotum may be a sign of locally advanced right RCC due to blockade of the draining gonadal vein by venous thrombus. Finally, a digital rectal examination should be done to rule out prostatitis, or to look for a nodule concerning prostate cancer [1].

In addition, one must grossly examine the urine by naked eye for its colour and viscosity. A reddish-brown colour of the urine may signifies old blood, whereas a bright red colour denotes an active bleeding. Likewise, an increased viscosity of the haematuria denotes significant bleeding and risk of clot formation [1].

27.6 Diagnosis

27.6.1 Blood Investigations

Blood investigations include a complete blood count to evaluate baseline haemoglobin, total leucocyte and platelet counts. Moreover, it helps to rule out pancytopenia denoting bone marrow suppression especially in post chemotherapy patients. Renal function test is required to guide concomitant nephrology evaluation and to select appropriate radiological investigations. Liver function test may give information on transaminases. Coagulation profile tests including prothrombin time are not routinely required. However, it should be considered in patients suspected of bleeding diathesis and on anticoagulant therapy. A simultaneous blood typing and cross-matching are obtained in patients with significant haematuria requiring blood transfusion [20].

27.6.2 Urine Investigations

At first, a urine dipstick test is done, which has a sensitivity of over 90% for detecting RBCs. Presence of blood on the dipstick warrants a urine routine microscopic examination. Urinalysis is obtained to confirm haematuria and to look for dysmorphic RBC, cellular casts, or proteinuria. In suspected cases of UTI, a clean catch mid-stream urine is obtained for urine culture and sensitivity.

Urine cytology is highly specific (94.3%) for the detection of high-grade urothelial carcinoma. However, it requires multiple samples in view of low sensitivity (42.4%) [34]. In a relatively large study, the sensitivity and specificity of urine cytology for urothelial carcinoma were 45.5% and 89.5%, respectively [35].

27.6.3 Imaging Techniques

The most common initial investigation done for haematuria is ultrasonography (USG). In majority of cases, this helps in localising the site of bleeding. Further, it can detect clots in the bladder (Fig. 27.2) or pelvicalyceal system. Easy availability and portability enable bedside USG possible, which is an important concern in patients in critical care units. However, once the patient is stabilized, a multiphase contrast enhanced computed tomography (CECT) with urography is the gold

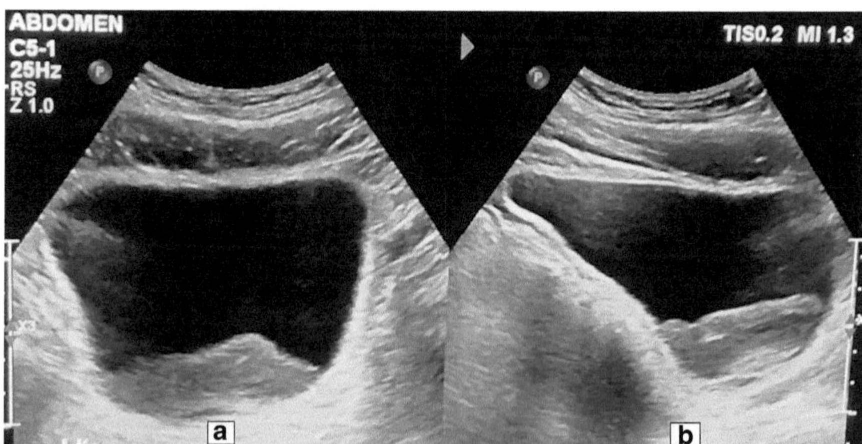

Fig. 27.2 Ultrasonography of urinary bladder showing clots inside the bladder

standard investigation for haematuria workup. The initial non-contrast phase helps in ruling out urolithiasis. Renal masses are better evaluated in the nephrogenic phase. Finally, an excretory phase is assessed for any filling defects which may suggest urothelial malignancies. In patients contraindicated for contrast study, magnetic resonance urography (MRU) is an alternative option. Occasionally, if CECT or MRU are not possible, USG of the kidney and bladder with retrograde pyelogram can give valuable information [1].

27.6.4 Cystoscopy

Cystoscopy is the most important investigation of haematuria evaluation, especially in cases suspicion of urothelial cancer. It is also the most reliable method to detect bladder cancer. One should perform cystoscopy for all patients with haematuria >35 years of age. In patients <35 years of age, cystoscopy is considered if there is concern for malignancy like history of smoking, irritative LUTS. It can be easily done in office set-up with minimal discomfort. In addition to the detection of bladder lesions, cystoscopy also helps in the evaluation of urethral lesions, urethral stricture, and lateralizing haematuria in cases of upper tract bleed [1].

27.7 Management

Management of haematuria in critically ill cancer patients should be in sequential steps with due concerns about their general conditions.

27.7.1 Initial Management

Irrespective of the causes, the initial step in the occurrence of gross haematuria is placement of a wide calibre (22 F) three-way catheter and continuous bladder irrigation (CBI) with normal saline. This washes out the clots from bladder and prevents clot retention. Meanwhile, other specific investigations are done to detect the cause of haematuria. Patients should be resuscitated with intravenous fluids and monitored continuously.

27.7.2 Medical Management

In cases of UTI, appropriate antibiotics are started as per the urine culture and sensitivity. Individual hospitals antibiogram should be adhered while considering treatment of UTI.

Glomerular haematuria warrants a concurrent nephrology consultation. It requires renal biopsy to know the exact pathology. Steroids and other immunosuppressants are the usual medical treatment. Antihypertensives, statin and other renal protective measures are advised to slow the disease progression. In cases of BPH-related haematuria, use of 5-alpha reductase inhibitor (finasteride) should be considered.

Haemorrhagic cystitis is one of the most troublesome case to manage in critically ill cancer patients. Often the specific cause is not found. However, a stepwise protocol is recommended to control the bleeding. Intravesical alum (1% alum solution) is considered the first-line therapy with a success rate of 66–100% [36, 37]. The 1% alum solution is made by dissolving 50 g alum in 5 litres sterile water, and CBI is started at a rate of 200–300 mL/hour. By its astringent action, alum causes protein precipitation on the urothelial at bleeding sites. It further causes vasoconstriction and decreased in capillary permeability [36]. If failed, other intravesical agents used sequentially are aminocaproic acid, formalin solution [37].

In cases of intractable haemorrhagic cystitis after failed intravesical therapy, hyperbaric oxygen (HBO_2) therapy can be considered. HBO_2 therapy is given in a specially designed pressure chamber. Inside the chamber, 100% oxygen is administered at 2–3 atmospheric pressure in multiple sessions [18]. Under such conditions, haemoglobin is fully saturated and dissolved oxygen is delivered to the local damaged tissues. Hyperoxygenation decreases oedema and promotes angiogenesis in the tissues affected by radiation-induced ischemia [38]. Response rates of 80% to 90% have been reported in the literature [18, 39]. Sandhu et al. studied the role of oral pentosan polysulfate, a synthetic glycosaminoglycan in post-radiation haemorrhagic cystitis. They showed a response rate of 58% with a durable response at median follow-up of 450 days [40]. Further, intractable cases may require endoscopic procedures like transurethral cauterization/fulguration of bleeding points. If unsuccessful, internal iliac artery embolization by interventional radiologist is considered. If haematuria is still uncontrolled, cystectomy and urinary diversion is the last resort [1].

27.7.3 Surgical Management

Patients with operable malignant conditions are subjected to standard surgical treatment only when the general conditions of the critically ill patients are improved and stabilized with initial medical management.

Refractory haematuria because of BPH requires transurethral resection of prostate (TURP). In advanced prostate cancer cases, androgen deprivation therapy (ADT) is considered as it decreases prostate tissue vascularity. If failed, they may require prostate artery embolization [1].

Radical nephrectomy is the standard surgical treatment for malignant renal mass. In cases of intractable haematuria in moribund, surgically unfit, or in patients with metastatic disease, a renal angioembolisation is initially considered. Once clinically stabilized, a renal mass biopsy is obtained. After pathological confirmation, targeted agents (tyrosine kinase inhibitors) are considered [41]. Bladder tumour is the most common urothelial malignancy and requires transurethral resection to confirm the pathological diagnosis [42]. Similarly, in a high-risk lesion radical nephroureterectomy is recommended. However, for low-risk and low-volume tumours an endoscopic resection and/or fulguration can be attempted [43]. Figure 27.3 shows the algorithm for the evaluation and management of haematuria in critically ill cancer patients.

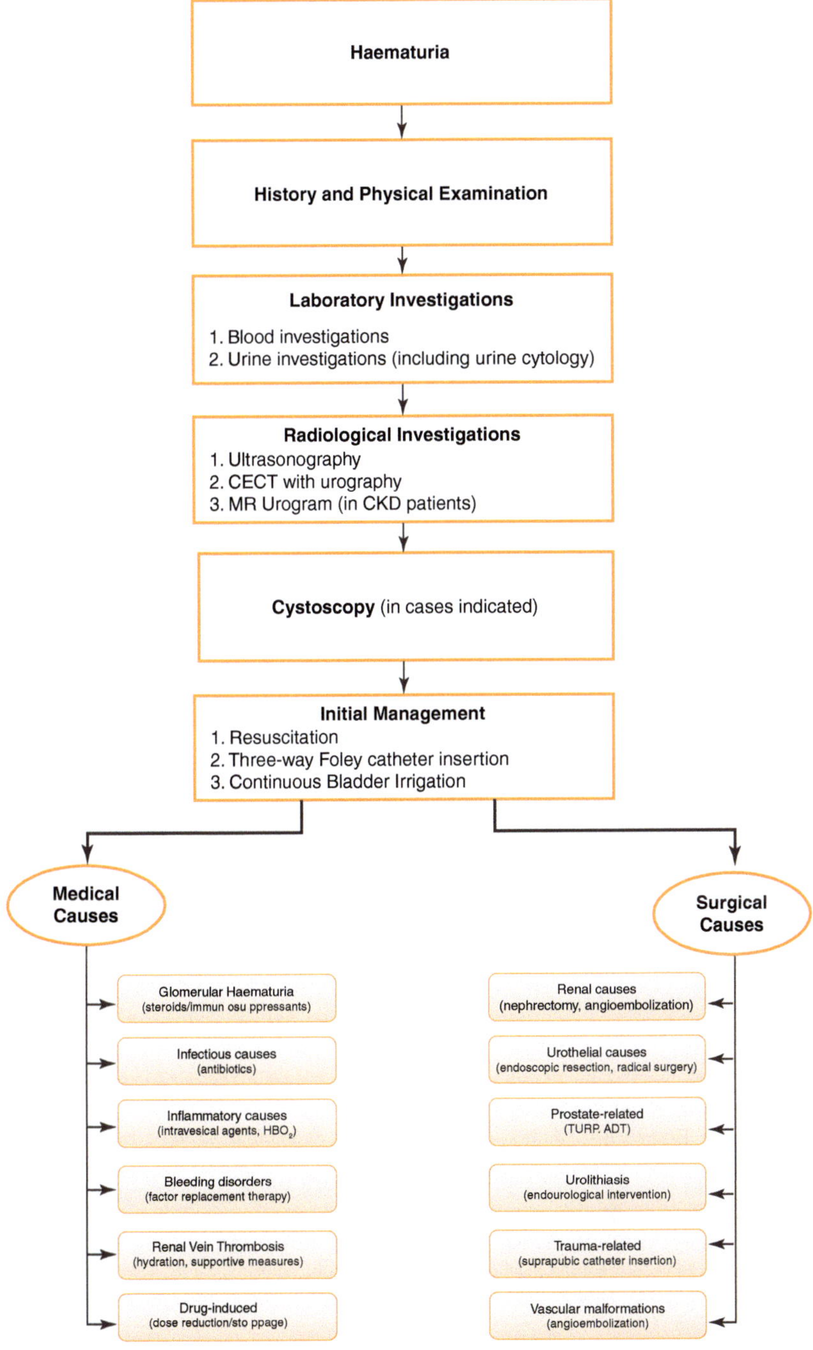

Fig. 27.3 Algorithm in the management of haematuria in critically ill cancer patients

27.8 Conclusion

Haematuria in critically ill cancer patients pose a varied clinical presentation with various underlying causes. While the initial treatment is usually the continuous bladder irrigation with normal saline, however, a multidisciplinary team is required for the thorough evaluation and management of such patients.

27.9 Key Learning Points

- Haematuria is not uncommon in critically ill cancer patients
- A variety of medical and surgical conditions can cause haematuria
- A systematic approach is to be done to reach the exact diagnosis
- A multidisciplinary team is required for the management

Acknowledgments None

Source of Funding None

References

1. Avellino GJ, Bose S, Wang DS. Diagnosis and management of hematuria. Surg Clin N Am. 2016;96:503–15.
2. Kalu CO, Abudayyeh A. Hematuria in the critically ill cancer patients. In: Nates JL, Price KJ, editors. Oncologic Critical Care. Cham: Springer International Publishing; 2020. p. 949–58.
3. Linder BJ, Boorjian SA. Management of emergency bleeding, recalcitrant clots, and hemorrhagic cystitis. AUA Update Series. 2015;34.
4. Grossfeld GD, Litwin MS, Wolf JS, Hricak H, Shuler CL, Agerter DC, Carroll PR. Evaluation of asymptomatic microscopic hematuria in adults: the American urological association best practice policy—part I: definition, detection, prevalence, and etiology. Urology. 2001;57:599–603.
5. Mariani AJ, Mariani MC, Macchioni C, Stams UK, Hariharan A, Moriera A. The significance of adult hematuria: 1,000 hematuria evaluations including a risk-benefit and cost-effectiveness analysis. J Urol. 1989;141:350–5.
6. Fogazzi GB, Ponticelli C. Microscopic hematuria diagnosis and management. Nephron. 1996;72:125–34.
7. Lin J, Cheng Z, Qian Q. Elderly patients with glomerular diseases and IgA nephropathy. Nephrology (Carlton). 2017;22(Suppl 4):20–6.
8. Fassett RG, Horgan BA, Mathew TH. Detection of glomerular bleeding by phase-contrast microscopy. Lancet. 1982;1:1432–4.
9. Suzuki H, Kiryluk K, Novak J, et al. The pathophysiology of IgA nephropathy. J Am Soc Nephrol. 2011;22:1795–803.
10. Mojtahedzadeh M, Panahi Y, Fazeli MR, Najafi A, Pazouki M, Navehsi BM, Bazzaz A, Naghizadeh MM, Beiraghdar F. Intensive care unit-acquired urinary tract infections in patients admitted with sepsis: etiology, risk factors, and patterns of antimicrobial resistance. Int J Infect Dis. 2008;12:312–8.
11. Laupland KB, Bagshaw SM, Gregson DB, Kirkpatrick AW, Ross T, Church DL. Intensive care unit-acquired urinary tract infections in a regional critical care system. Crit Care. 2005;9:R60–5.

12. Davis NG, Silberman M. Bacterial acute prostatitis. StatPearls; 2021.
13. Rastinehad A, Kavoussi L, Noble M. Hemorrhagic cystitis. AUA Update Series. 2007;26:65–76.
14. Haldar S, Dru C, Bhowmick NA. Mechanisms of hemorrhagic cystitis. Am J Clin Exp Urol. 2014;2:199.
15. Leapman MS, Stock RG, Stone NN, Hall SJ. Findings at cystoscopy performed for cause after prostate brachytherapy. Urology. 2014;83:1350–5.
16. Bevers RF, Bakker DJ, Kurth KH. Hyperbaric oxygen treatment for haemorrhagic radiation cystitis. Lancet. 1995;346:803–5.
17. Del Pizzo JJ, Chew BH, Jacobs SC, Sklar GN. Treatment of radiation induced hemorrhagic cystitis with hyperbaric oxygen: long-term followup. J Urol. 1998;160:731–3.
18. O'REILLY K. Hyperbaric oxygen in urology. AUA Update Series. 2002;21:26.
19. Zigman A, Yazbeck S, Emil S, Nguyen L. Renal vein thrombosis: a 10-year review. J Pediatr Surg. 2000;35:1540–2.
20. Willis GC, Tewelde SZ. The approach to the patient with hematuria. Emerg Med Clin North Am. 2019;37:755–69.
21. Culclasure TF, Bray VJ, Hasbargen JA. The significance of hematuria in the anticoagulated patient. Arch Intern Med. 1994;154:649–52.
22. Pantuck AJ, Zisman A, Belldegrun AS. The changing natural history of renal cell carcinoma. J Urol. 2001;166:1611–23.
23. Silverman SG, Israel GM, Herts BR, Richie JP. Management of the incidental renal mass. Radiology. 2008;249:16–31.
24. Psutka SP, Leibovich BC. Management of inferior vena cava tumor thrombus in locally advanced renal cell carcinoma. Ther Adv Urol. 2015;7:216–29.
25. Hicks D, Li C-Y. Management of macroscopic haematuria in the emergency department. Emerg Med J. 2007;24:385–90.
26. Lunney A, Haynes A, Sharma P. Moderate or severe LUTS is associated with increased recurrence of non - muscle - invasive urothelial carcinoma of the bladder. Int Braz J Urol. 2019;45:306–14.
27. Pareek G, Shevchuk M, Armenakas NA, Vasovic L, Hochberg DA, Basillote JB, Fracchia JA. The effect of finasteride on the expression of vascular endothelial growth factor and microvessel density: a possible mechanism for decreased prostatic bleeding in treated patients. J Urol. 2003;169:20–3.
28. Din OS, Thanvi N, Ferguson CJ, Kirkbride P. Palliative prostate radiotherapy for symptomatic advanced prostate cancer. Radiother Oncol. 2009;93:192–6.
29. Mayans L. Nephrolithiasis. Prim Care. 2019;46:203–12.
30. Cura M, Elmerhi F, Suri R, Bugnone A, Dalsaso T. Vascular malformations and arteriovenous fistulas of the kidney. Acta Radiol. 2010;51:144–9.
31. Crotty KL, Orihuela E, Warren MM. Recent advances in the diagnosis and treatment of renal arteriovenous malformations and fistulas. J Urol. 1993;150:1355–9.
32. Willette PA, Coffield S. Current trends in the management of difficult urinary catheterizations. West J Emerg Med. 2012;13:472–8.
33. Bolenz C, Schröppel B, Eisenhardt A, Schmitz-Dräger BJ, Grimm M-O. The investigation of hematuria. Dtsch Arztebl Int. 2018;115:801–7.
34. Chahal R, Gogoi NK, Sundaram SK. Is it necessary to perform urine cytology in screening patients with Haematuria? Eur Urol. 2001;39:283–6.
35. Mishriki SF, Aboumarzouk O, Vint R, Grimsley SJS, Lam T, Somani B. Routine urine cytology has no role in hematuria investigations. J Urol. 2013;189:1255–8.
36. Choong SK, Walkden M, Kirby R. The management of intractable haematuria. BJU Int. 2000;86:951–9.
37. Abt D, Bywater M, Engeler DS, Schmid H-P. Therapeutic options for intractable hematuria in advanced bladder cancer. Int J Urol. 2013;20:651–60.
38. Hader JE, Marzella L, Myers RA, Jacobs SC, Naslund MJ. Hyperbaric oxygen treatment for experimental cyclophosphamide-induced hemorrhagic cystitis. J Urol. 1993;149:1617–21.

39. Chong KT, Hampson NB, Corman JM. Early hyperbaric oxygen therapy improves outcome for radiation-induced hemorrhagic cystitis. Urology. 2005;65:649–53.
40. Sandhu SS, Goldstraw M, Woodhouse CRJ. The management of haemorrhagic cystitis with sodium pentosan polysulphate. BJU Int. 2004;94:845–7.
41. Ljungberg B, Albiges L, Bensalah K, et al (2020) EAU guidelines on renal cell carcinoma 2020. European Association of Urology guidelines. 2020 edition. Presented at the EAU annual congress Amsterdam 2020
42. Babjuk M, Burger M, Compérat E, et al (2020) EAU guidelines on non-muscle-invasive bladder cancer (TaT1 and CIS) 2020. European Association of Urology guidelines. 2020 edition presented at the EAU annual congress Amsterdam 2020
43. Rouprêt M, Babjuk M, Burger M, et al (2020) EAU guidelines on upper urinary tract urothelial carcinoma 2020. European Association of Urology Guidleines. 2020 edition. Presented at the EAU annual congress Amsterdam 2020

Acute Kidney Injury and Renal Replacement Therapy in Oncology ICU

28

Arunkumar Subbiah and Dipankar Bhowmik

28.1 Background

Acute Kidney Injury (AKI) is one of the most important determinants of outcomes in hospitalised patients, more so in critically ill patients admitted in the intensive care unit (ICU). Cancer patients are at a higher risk for developing AKI. In addition to the standard risk factors like increasing age, comorbid illnesses, nephrotoxic drugs and infections, patients with malignancy are more susceptible to develop renal dysfunction either as a direct complication of the cancer or due to the use of chemotherapeutic drugs. Acute and chronic kidney diseases are more prevalent in patients with cancer and with remarkable advancements in the field of chemotherapy, immunotherapy and targeted therapies, there are increasing reports of hitherto unknown renal complications. Recognising this link between cancer and kidney diseases and the increasing role of nephrologists in managing specific complications in cancer patients, a new subspecialty has been developed to provide the best nephrology care possible. This subspeciality, Onco-nephrology has been the subject of discussions in multiple conferences and is expected to develop further in the future [1].

Critically ill cancer patients in the ICU with acute kidney injury often require renal replacement therapy, have longer length of hospital stay and are at a high risk for mortality. A multi-disciplinary care team with coordinated efforts between the oncologist, nephrologist and intensivist is needed to improve outcomes for the patient. Apart from the immediate implications, patients with renal dysfunction require dose modifications in cancer chemotherapy and are more susceptible to adverse effects of drugs thereby limiting cancer care and possibility of cure. Moreover, persisting renal dysfunction and CKD tends to exclude many such

A. Subbiah · D. Bhowmik (✉)
Department of Nephrology, All India Institute of Medical Sciences Delhi, New Delhi, India
e-mail: dmbhowmik@aiims.edu

V. Kumar et al. (eds.), *Onco-critical Care*,
https://doi.org/10.1007/978-981-16-9929-0_28

patients from clinical trials of newer life-saving therapeutic options. In this chapter we will focus on the diagnosis and management of AKI in critically ill cancer patients.

28.2 Etiology of AKI

Patients with prior renal disease, CKD and comorbid-illnesses are more prone for developing AKI. In most of the patients there is often a combination of factors in play. There are some cancer-specific causes of AKI. In critically ill patients, the critical illness also adversely affects renal function [2].

In cancer patients, the various causes of AKI are as follows (Fig. 28.1) [3, 4].

1. Malignancy related causes
   (a) Paraneoplastic causes: Hypercalcaemia, tumour lysis syndrome
   (b) Obstructive uropathy especially in gynaecological, urological and retroperitoneal cancers
   (c) Infiltration into the kidney as in lymphoma
2. Treatment associated toxicity
   (a) Chemotherapeutics and related complications: Tumour lysis syndrome (TLS), thrombotic microangiopathy (TMA)
   (b) Radiation nephritis (following radiotherapy)
   (c) Post stem cell transplantation
   (d) Other drugs: NSAIDs (for cancer associated pain), contrast agents (in imaging studies), antibiotics (for infections)
3. Other related complications
   (a) Hypovolemia
   (b) Infections

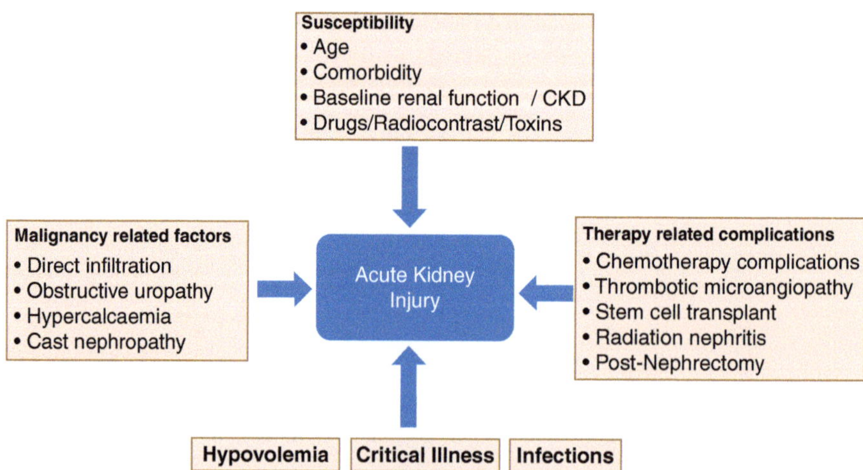

Fig. 28.1 Causes of acute Kidney Injury in cancer patients

Table 28.1 Cancer therapeutics and site of renal injury

Kidney compartment involved - Site of injury	Drugs
Glomeruli	VEGF inhibitors, sirolimus, interferon
Tubulo-interstitium	Cisplatin, methotrexate, immune checkpoint inhibitors, doxorubicin, Ifosfamide
Vessels	Gemcitabine, Mitomycin C, 5-fluorouracil

Cancer therapies, including the newer immune checkpoint inhibitors have multiple renal adverse effects. The various cancer therapeutic drugs affect different compartments of the kidney (Table 28.1).

28.3 Diagnosis of AKI in Cancer Patients

The definition of AKI and the diagnostic cut-offs used in different studies were different till a few decades back. The RIFLE (Risk, Injury, Failure, Loss of Kidney Function, and End-stage kidney disease) classification was proposed in 2004 for standardization of diagnosis of AKI and thereafter AKIN (Acute Kidney Injury Network) criteria in 2007 and KDIGO (Kidney Diseases Improving Global Outcomes) criteria in 2012 have come into practice [5].

The diagnosis of AKI relies on a combination of serum creatinine assessments and urine output. Patient is diagnosed with AKI if they fulfil either of the following broad criterion

- Increase in serum creatinine by 50% within 7 days
- Increase in serum creatinine by 0.3 mg/dL within 48 h
- Oliguria

Depending on the severity and duration of AKI, they are graded into successive stages. AKI stage 3 denotes dialysis requiring acute kidney injury. Early recognition of AKI has been the subject of investigation for the last 10 years. Even mild increase in serum creatinine by 0.3–0.5 mg% is associated with multifold increase in mortality in critically ill patients. This was the basis for including small changes in creatinine in the KDIGO (0.3 mg%) and AKIN (0.5 mg%) criteria. The staging of AKI according to KDIGO classification is as follows:

AKI Diagnosis: Abrupt increase in creatinine ≥0.3 mg/dL or 1.5-fold of baseline within 48 hrs.

- Stage 1: Increase in creatinine 1.5 to 1.9 times baseline.
- Stage 2: Increase in creatinine 2 to 2.9 times baseline.
- Stage 3: Increase in creatinine ≥3 times baseline or peak serum creatinine >4 mg/dL (with atleast 0.5 mg/dL increase) or need for RRT.

It is obvious from these definitions that serum creatinine is an integral part of diagnosis of AKI. However, cancer patients have loss of weight and muscle mass due to the chronic nature of disease, poor dietary pattern and loss of appetite, inflammation and chemotherapy. This affects creatinine production and hence serum creatinine may not be a suitable marker in cancer patients.

28.3.1 Cystatin C

Notwithstanding the inherent limitations of using serum creatinine to assess renal function, its role in diagnosing AKI in cancer patients is even more limited. Due to a reduced muscle mass and decreased production, serum creatinine increases late in cancer patients and hence may underdiagnose AKI. This has led to the search for alternate markers independent of patient's general condition.

Cystatin C (CysC), cysteine protease inhibitor synthesized by nucleated cells, is filtered by the glomeruli and is neither reabsorbed nor secreted making it an ideal marker to assess renal function. Also, it is unaffected by diet and change in muscle mass. This has made cystatin C a promising marker of renal function. Multiple studies have shown CysC to accurately predict AKI even in critically ill patients. Studies in cancer patients show similar result with no interference due to tumor burden while some show a elevated levels in patients with active malignancy. Hence, its value in oncologic AKI is still uncertain. The other limitations of using CysC include its prohibitive cost, availability (especially in smaller centres) and effect of inflammation on CysC levels.

28.3.2 Novel Biomarkers

The diagnosis of AKI depends on serum creatinine and urine output which have fallacies. Even cystatin C is not an ideal marker for AKI. This has propelled the search for a marker of renal function akin to troponin in myocardial injury. The ideal marker has to be easily measurable, rapid to increase following renal insult and should not be affected by other concomitant conditions. The various promising biomarkers are given in Table 28.2.

Neutrophil gelatinase associated lipocalin (NGAL) has shown promise in clinical studies and point-of-care testing methods are available for the same now. This allows rapid and early identification of AKI. One another biomarker kit measures TIMP2 and IGFBP7 and is available commercially. With regard to cancer patients, some of these markers have been studied in cisplatin associated nephrotoxicity [6]. Urinary markers like NGAL, beta-2-microglobulin, Calbindin and KIM-1

Table 28.2 Novel biomarkers in AKI

Category	Biomarkers
Inflammatory mediators	IL-6, IL-18
Cell injury biomarkers	Kidney injury molecule-1 (KIM-1), liver fatty acid binding protein (L-FABP), neutrophil gelatinase associated lipocalin (NGAL)
Cell cycle markers	Tissue inhibitor of metalloproteinases-2 (TIMP-2), insulin like growth factor-binding protein 7 (IGFBP-7)
Urinary low molecular weight protein	Cystatin C, retinol-binding protein, α1-microglobulin, β2-microglobulin

have shown promise in this scenario. However, they have not been validated and hence are limited only to research settings. Even with these biomarkers, the confounding role of inflammatory milieu seen in cancer has to be evaluated. Urinary microRNAs and exosomes also reveal kidney injury and may be of use in the future.

28.4 Epidemiology and Prognosis of Patients with Cancer and AKI

Data on the incidence of AKI is affected by the use of varied classification systems and diagnostic criteria. Though, the advent of the RIFLE scoring system standardised study definitions, many studies still used different criteria for diagnosis of AKI, the most common among that being requirement of RRT. This not only underestimates AKI but also makes it difficult to compare different studies. There has been some hope with routine use of AKIN and KDIGO classification systems for estimating the incidence of AKI.

In one of the largest studies on AKI in cancer patients from Denmark, 25.8% developed AKI among 37,267 patients on follow-up with a 5-year AKI risk of 27%. The incidence of AKI differs according to the type of malignancy, the stage and the general condition of the patient. In the Danish study, the highest risk was with kidney cancer (44%) followed by liver malignancy (33%) and multiple myeloma (31.8%) [7]. In a national survey from China with 1418 patients with malignancy associated AKI, Gastrointestinal cancer (50.1%) was most common followed by reproductive system malignancy (15.3%) and haematological malignancy (13.1%). Patients with hematological malignancy were significantly younger as compared to those with other causes of malignancy associated AKI. In a series of 1,63,071 cancer patients receiving chemotherapy, 9.3% developed AKI with highest risk for myeloma (26%) followed by bladder cancer (19%) and leukemia (15.4%) [8].

Patients having cancer have increased incidence of AKI compared to those without cancer and those in ICU have a higher risk of mortality. This risk is exponentially increased when the patient requires RRT. The length of ICU stay and hospital stay are significantly increased in oncology patients with AKI [2]. Moreover, AKI patients will require drug dose modifications especially of chemotherapeutic agents and cannot undergo contrast enhanced imaging studies unless strongly indicated (Fig. 28.2). This affects the standard of care in cancer patients and is probably the reason why cancer patients with AKI have a lower incidence of remission of malignancy. In the Belgian Renal Insufficiency and Anticancer Medications (BIRMA) study, 64% of cancer patients had a GFR < 90 mL/min/1.73 m^2 and over three-fourths of patients received at least one nephrotoxic chemotherapy drug [9]. Sensitisation of the treating team to the renal modifications of chemotherapeutic agents is therefore important.

Fig. 28.2 Vicious cycle of cancer and AKI

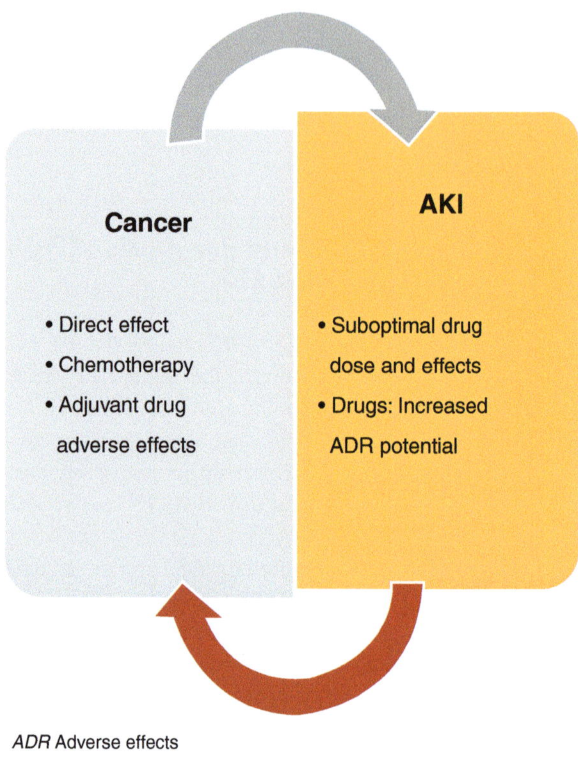

ADR Adverse effects

28.5 Prevention of AKI in Critically Ill Cancer Patients

There are no clinically proven drugs for prevention of AKI. The mainstay of prevention rests on general supportive measures [10]. In critically ill patients, hemodynamic instability and consequent impaired renal perfusion is the most important predisposing factor for AKI. The mean arterial pressure has to be maintained over 65 mm Hg by administering fluids to maintain the central venous pressure and/or inotropic support. Colloids are avoided as they increase the risk of renal injury. Among crystalloids, the advantages of balanced crystalloids over normal saline especially in the setting of hyperchloremic acidosis is often debated. Fluid overload is also common in patients in ICU and routine assessment of fluid status is quintessential. There is no specific inotrope which is renal protective and norepinephrine is at present the inotrope of choice. Vasopressin has shown promise in the Vasopressin vs Norepinephrine as Initial Therapy in Septic Shock (VANISH) trial and the Vasopressin versus Norepinephrine in Patients with Vasoplegic Shock after Cardiac Surgery (VANCS) trial. There are no specific recommendations for preferring vasopressin as the first choice yet and more studies will be required before this change can be made.

Diuretics are commonly used in patients with oliguria to improve urine output. This can be attempted if patient is overhydrated. In patients with eu/hypovolemia, use of diuretics increases the risk of AKI. Fenoldopam is a selective dopamine agonist believed to improve renal perfusion and prevent renal injury. Controlled trials have not shown a significant benefit for this therapeutic option. One of the most important components of patient management would be to avoid nephrotoxic drugs. Critically ill patients in the ICU usually have some component of sepsis and require broad spectrum antibiotics. Cancer patients are more severely immunosuppressed and most often have drug resistant sepsis necessitating use of higher antibiotics like vancomycin, aminoglycosides and/or colistin. These antibiotics increase the risk of AKI. Therapeutic drug monitoring based titrated dosing, use of appropriate antibiotics and newer modes of drug delivery like inhaled colistin are often tried to mitigate the nephrotoxicity. Antifungal drugs like amphotericin B are also used in these patients. The use of liposomal preparation offers scope to reduce the nephrotoxic potential of amphotericin B. Adequate hydration and correction of electrolyte disturbances has to be done.

In patients with obstructive causes of AKI due to malignancy, percutaneous nephrostomy tubes and internal ureteral stenting is effective. In cases of renal cancer, cytoreductive nephrectomy are performed which are nephron sparing and avoid complete loss of renal function. Most causes of chemotherapy related AKI can be prevented by hydration and renal function optimised dosing. In addition to hydration, in case of cisplatin, magnesium supplementation protects the patient from AKI. Forced alkaline diuresis, leucovorin rescue and glucarpidase are indicated for methrotrexate related nephrotoxicity. In case of haematological malignancies, there is a component of hypercalcaemia which needs to be managed appropriately to avoid AKI.

Tumor lysis syndrome (TLS) due to therapy related or spontaneous lysis of tumor cells causes severe electrolyte disturbances and AKI. Apart from hydration and frequent electrolyte monitoring, hypouricemic drugs namely allopurinol and febuxostat are the cornerstone of prevention. Recombinant urate oxidase, rasburicase was initially used only in the treatment of TLS but is now approved for prevention too. G6PD screening has to be done for patients at risk as rasburicase can cause haemolytic anemia in them.

28.5.1 Prevention of Post-Contrast Renal Injury

Patients with malignancy often undergo multiple imaging studies right from diagnosis to planning of therapy and then throughout the management course and on follow-up. This places them at a high risk of contrast-associated AKI. After onset, there is no treatment for contrast induced nephropathy (CIN). Hence, preventive strategies form the cornerstone of management [10]. Renal function has to be repeated 48–72 h after contrast administration for diagnosis of CIN and monitoring.

The standard precautions to prevent CIN include

- Identify risk factors for AKI—Comorbid illnesses like diabetes, heart failure; advanced age; use of nephrotoxic drugs—NSAIDS, diuretics, metformin, ACEi/ARB for hypertension, etc.

- Contrast related: Avoid high osmolar contrast dyes. When compared to low osmolar agents, iso-osmolar agents are associated with a lower risk of AKI and hence preferred in patients with eGFR<60 mL/min/1.73 m^2. Contrast volume to be limited to what is absolutely necessary.
- Periprocedural hydration is absolutely necessary—Normal saline should be given at 1 ml/kg/h for 3–6 h prior and after contrast administration. Oral hydration can be of benefit for outpatient imaging studies.
- N-acetyl cysteine (NAC) can be started 48 h prior to the procedure. Randomised trials have shown doubtful role for NAC but is still routinely used in most centers.

28.5.2 Role of Biomarkers

Serum creatinine is a late marker of acute kidney injury especially in cancer patients. The routine use of biomarkers in critically ill cancer patients may help us to diagnose AKI early and also constitute measures to prevent further renal dysfunction. The furosemide stress test and ultrasonographic measures like renal angina index have shown to be beneficial in some studies. Some markers like NGAL and KIM-1 have also been studied in cancer specific settings like cisplatin associated nephrotoxicity [6]. Biomarker guided management of use of nephrotoxic drugs and decision to initiate renosupportive strategies and renal replacement therapies needs to be determined in future studies.

28.6 RRT Modalities Used in a Cancer Patient with AKI

The indications for initiating renal replacement therapy (RRT) in critically ill cancer patients is similar to other groups of patients. Uncompensated metabolic acidosis, oligoanuria, treatment resistant hyperkalemia, volume overload and azotemia are common indications for RRT [5]. The common modes of RRT include

- Intermittent hemodialysis (IHD)
- Sustained low-efficiency dialysis (SLED)
- Continuous renal replacement therapy (CRRT)—Continuous venovenous hemodialysis (CVVHD)/hemofiltration (CVVHF)/hemodiafiltration (CVVHDF)
- Peritoneal dialysis

IHD is most often the modality of RRT in most centres. In IHD, 4 h sessions of dialysis are done on alternate days till renal recovery occurs. With intermittent RRT there is rapid correction of electrolyte disturbances, acid base balance and uremia. This can increase the risk of dialysis disequilibrium syndrome, cerebral edema and hypotension.

CRRT is a continuous therapy done 24 h a day. It offers the advantage of lesser hemodynamic instability and is preferred in critically ill ICU patients on inotropic support. The slower solute clearances and flow rates offer hemodynamic stability and a stable improvement in renal parameters. The high cost, need for anticoagulation, prolonged immobilisation are drawbacks of CRRT. Earlier studies have shown that either modalities can be used successfully in cancer patients based on the general condition of the patient and availability.

The various issues with these therapies resulted in the development of hybrid therapies (SLED) which combine the benefits of both continuous and intermittent therapies. SLED offers the benefit of longer duration of dialysis (6–8 h) with better hemodynamic stability compared to IHD and lesser costs compared to CRRT. The safety and efficacy of SLED in cancer patients has been shown in recent studies. Studies which compare SLED to CRRT have found it to be non-inferior to continuous therapies with regard to hemodynamic parameters and hard outcomes especially patient mortality.

Meta-analysis conducted by Tonelli et al., Ronco et al. and others have shown that intermittent therapies and continuous therapies have similar benefits in patient survival and AKI outcomes. The KDIGO AKI guidelines also suggests that continuous and intermittent RRT are to be used as complementary therapies. In those with hemodynamic instability and acute brain injury or cerebral edema, CRRT is to be preferred. Patients can be shifted between different modalities of RRT based on the clinical need. A comparison between the three modalities is given in Table 28.3 below.

The timing of initiation of dialysis in AKI has been the focus of randomised controlled trials in the last decade. Most of these trials compared outcomes in patients initiated on RRT early once AKI is diagnosed compared to those in whom RRT was withheld till clinically indicated. All these trials—ELAIN, AKIKI, IDEAL-ICU, STARRT-AKI not only failed to show benefit with early initiation of RRT but also revealed increased cost and dialysis complications in this group of patients. Only in patients in surgical ICU in ELAIN study, early dialysis initiation

Table 28.3 Different modalities of renal replacement therapy

	IHD	SLED	CRRT
Duration (in hours)	4	6–12	24
Mechanism	Diffusion	Diffusion	Diffusion (CVVHD) Convection (CVVH) Both (CVVHDF)
Blood flow (ml/min)	250–400	100–150	15–200
Dialysate flow (ml/min)	500–800	100–200	30–60
Solute removal	+++	+++	+++
Hemodynamic stability	Poor	Fair	Good
Vascular access	Vascular catheter or AV fistula		Vascular catheter
Anticoagulation	May not be needed	Low dose heparin sufficient	Always needed
Cost	+	++	+++
Complications	Hypotension Dialysis disequilibrium syndrome	Hypotension less common	Bleeding Dyselectrolemia Vascular access issues

had lower 90-day mortality. The differing criteria used for early initiation (KDIGO stage 2) and being restricted to surgical patients was the reason ELAIN trial had a different outcome compared to other trials. None of these trials were restricted to cancer patients but considering the common pathophysiology in all critically ill patients, the same criteria and concepts are followed in these patients.

TLS requires continuous correction of electrolyte abnormalities and CRRT may be beneficial in this scenario. If there is severe hyperkalemia, immediate reduction of potassium may be achieved with IHD. Acute peritoneal dialysis is performed in resource limited settings and is useful in most scenarios. There are concerns with uric acid removal in PD and hence may not be preferred in patients with TLS. Patients with myeloma especially cast nephropathy require removal of light chains which can be achieved with hemodialysis. However rapid removal of light chains requires specialized dialyzer like high cut-off dialyzers. Though HCO dialyzers showed promise in earlier clinical studies, randomised controlled studies on its utility—European Trial of Free Light Chain Removal (EULITE); and Studies in Patients with Multiple Myeloma and Renal Failure due to cast Nephropathy (MYRE) failed to show consistent benefit with regard to renal outcome and mortality. Till there is more evidence for its utility, routine hemodialysis is believed to stay as the standard of care for these patients.

28.7 Conclusions

Acute Kidney Injury is a common complication in cancer patients and is more common in those who are critically ill. Diagnosis rests on monitoring of renal function and urine output and is staged based on severity. Biomarkers have the potential to accurately diagnose AKI early thereby giving a scope for preventive strategies even before AKI sets in clinically. They have to be validated in cancer patients. Successful management of cancer associated AKI needs continued collaboration between the nephrologist, oncologist and intensivist. Advances in RRT modalities has helped improve outcomes in critical patients.

References

1. Rosner MH, Perazella MA. Acute kidney injury in the patient with cancer. Kidney Res Clin Pract. 2019 Sep;38(3):295–308.
2. Pickkers P, Darmon M, Hoste E, et al. Acute kidney injury in the critically ill: an updated review on pathophysiology and management. Intensive Care Med. 2021 Aug 1;47(8):835–50.
3. Lameire N, Vanholder R, Van Biesen W, Benoit D. Acute kidney injury in critically ill cancer patients: an update. Crit Care Lond Engl. 2016 Aug 2;20(1):209.
4. Campbell GA, Hu D, Okusa MD. Acute kidney injury in the cancer patient. Adv Chronic Kidney Dis. 2014 Jan;21(1):64–71.
5. Ostermann M, Bellomo R, Burdmann EA, et al. Controversies in acute kidney injury: conclusions from a kidney disease: improving global outcomes (KDIGO) conference. Kidney Int. 2020 Aug 1;98(2):294–309.

6. George B, Joy MS, Aleksunes LM. Urinary protein biomarkers of kidney injury in patients receiving cisplatin chemotherapy. Exp Biol Med Maywood NJ. 2018 Feb;243(3):272–82.
7. Christiansen CF, Johansen MB, Langeberg WJ, et al. Incidence of acute kidney injury in cancer patients: a Danish population-based cohort study. Eur J Intern Med. 2011 Aug;22(4):399–406.
8. Kitchlu A, McArthur E, Amir E, et al. Acute kidney injury in patients receiving systemic treatment for cancer: a population-based cohort study. J Natl Cancer Inst. 2019 Jul 1;111(7):727–36.
9. Janus N, Launay-vacher V, Byloos E, et al. Cancer and renal insufficiency results of the BIRMA study. Br J Cancer. 2010 Dec;103(12):1815–21.
10. Cosmai L, Porta C, Foramitti M, et al. Preventive strategies for acute kidney injury in cancer patients. Clin Kidney J. 2021 Jan 1;14(1):70–83.

Management of Oncologic Emergencies 29

Amol Kothekar, Mahima Gupta, and R. Natesh Prabu

29.1 Overview of Oncologic Emergencies

There is an increase in incidence of cancer cases globally due to increased life expectancy and growing exposure to risk factors. An oncologic emergency is an acute condition in a cancer patient, which is directly or indirectly related to either cancer itself or its treatment. Sometimes it may be the first sign of malignancy in patients with no previous history of cancer. Oncologic emergencies usually require urgent medical attention due to their potential life or limb threatening complications. It is highly desirable for an emergency physician and an intensivist to have knowledge of these emergencies for early diagnosis and treatment. In the present chapter, we will be discussing Syndrome of inappropriate antidiuretic hormone (SIADH), Hypercalcemia of Malignancy (HCM), Superior vena cava syndrome (SVCS) Hyperviscosity syndrome (HVS) and Malignant Spinal Cord Compression(MSCC). Conditions like febrile neutropenia, tumour lysis syndrome, and other toxicities due to Chemotherapy and radiotherapy are discussed elsewhere in the textbook.

A. Kothekar (✉) · M. Gupta
Department of Anaesthesia, Critical Care and Pain, Tata Memorial Center, Homi Bhabha National Institute, Mumbai, India

R. Natesh Prabu
Department of Critical Care Medicine St. John's Medical College, Bengaluru, India

V. Kumar et al. (eds.), *Onco-critical Care*,
https://doi.org/10.1007/978-981-16-9929-0_29

29.2 Syndrome of Inappropriate Antidiuretic Hormone (SIADH)

29.2.1 Introduction

Syndrome of inappropriate antidiuretic hormone (SIADH) is one of the commonest causes of hyponatremia in cancer patients [1]. It was first described by Schwartz et al. and demonstrated in two patients with bronchogenic carcinoma [2]. Further, it was demonstrated that the levels of Antidiuretic Hormone (ADH/arginine vasopressin-AVP) were 'inappropriately high' for the given serum osmolality, causing antidiuresis [2]. Later on, antidiuresis with normal or suppressed AVP was described due to mutation of vasopressin receptors or certain pharmacological factors [3]. The terminology-syndrome of inappropriate antidiuresis (SIAD) includes all the causes of antidiuresis without appropriate osmotic stimulus irrespective of AVP levels.

29.2.2 Pathophysiology of SIADH

SIADH is a disorder of water and sodium balance characterized by hypo-osomlar (true) hyponatremia with impaired urinary dilution capacity due to persistently high AVP levels despite hypo-osomlality [2]. Patients are either (mild) hypervolemic or euvolemic. Initially, there is a limitation of renal free water excretion causing dilutional hyponatremia (Phase of water retention). In the later phase, (6–8 days) there is additional sodium loss further contributing to low sodium levels (phase of solute loss and diuresis) [4] Fig. 29.1.

29.2.3 Diagnosis

It is reasonable to suspect SIADH in the presence of hyponatremia especially, if clinical signs of fluid depletion are absent. (euvolemic or hypervolemic hyponatremia).

The diagnostic criteria are mentioned below.

Diagnostic Criteria of SIADH

- The serum osmolality (Sr-osm) should be less than 280mosm/kg,
- Urine osmolality (Ur-osm) >100mosm/L during hyponatremia indicating inappropriate urine dilution for hypoosmolality
- Clinically there should be euvolemia and urine sodium > mmol/L (assuming normal salt intake)
- Rule out other causes of euvolemic hypotonic hyponatremia (glucocorticoid deficiency, hypothyroidism).
- Also, other supporting findings are correcting of hyponatremia with fluid restriction, failure to correct with volume expansion, plasma uric acid <4mgdL, fractional sodium excretion >1%; fractional urea excretion >55%, demonstrating elevated AVP levels during hypotonic state.

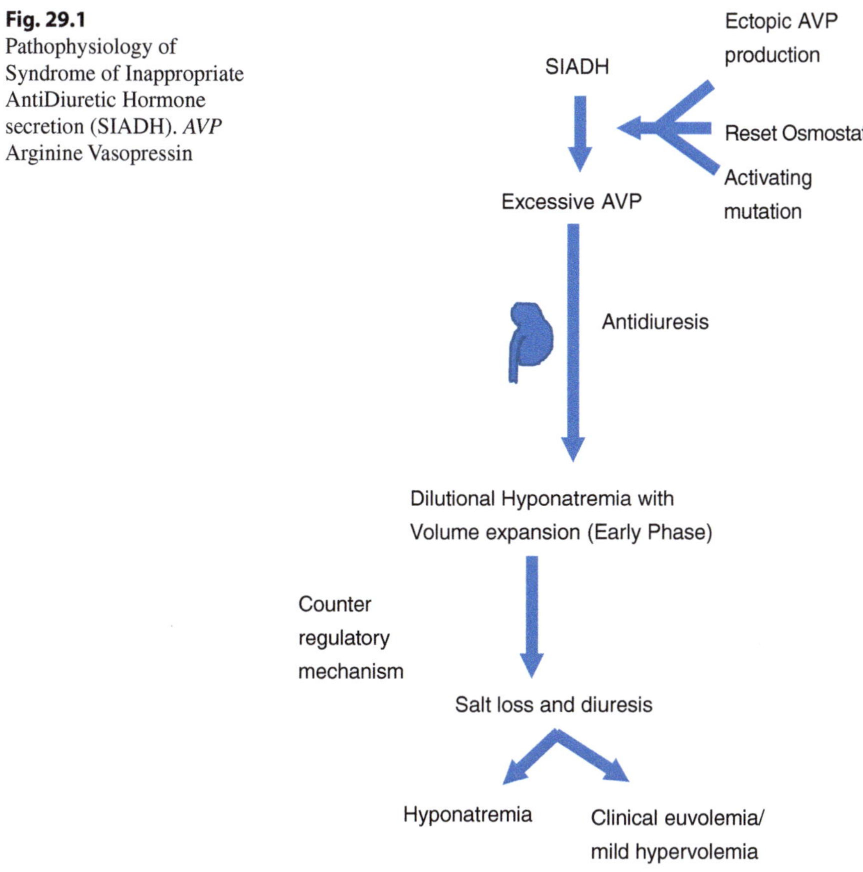

Fig. 29.1 Pathophysiology of Syndrome of Inappropriate AntiDiuretic Hormone secretion (SIADH). *AVP* Arginine Vasopressin

The SIADH is sometimes classified into four types based on the underlying pathology and levels of AVP (Table 29.1) [2, 5–7]. However, clinically it is not easy to identify the exact antidiuretic defect and response to AVP antagonists [8].

Similar clinical and laboratory picture can be seen in cerebral or renal salt wasting (CSW or RSW) especially in neurosurgical patients [9, 10]. Once sodium is corrected to normal, fractional excretion of urate (FEurate) drops to less than 11% in SIADH but it remain elevated (>11%) in CSW or RSW [11, 12].

29.2.4 Management

The main goals of treatment are to prevent (1) further worsening of symptoms/ sodium levels, (2) prevention of complications, (3) treatment of cause and (4) to avoid over correction. The grading of hyponatremia is described in Table 29.2.

Table 29.1 Syndrome of inappropriate antidiuretic hormone (SIADH) based on patterns of osmoregulatory defects [2, 5–7]

Type	Underlying pathology	Prevalance	Clinical Example
A	Very high AVP levels from ectopic source	30%	Malignancies e.g. Bronchogenic carcinoma
B	High AVP levels due to leak from neurohypophysis	30%	Injury to neurohypophysis or the inhibitory component of the osmoregulatory mechanism.
C	Ectopic secretion of AVP due to aberrant inputs. Threshold for AVP release/ suppression is altered. The entire osmoregulatory system is reset to lower levels. **(Reset osmostat).**	30%	Patients in long-term care facility, pregnancy, cleft lip and palate, corpus callosum agenesis, and hypothalamic cyst, tuberculosis, alcoholism, psychogenic polydipsia
D	Activating mutation of AVP V2receptor AVP levels is suppressed below normal	5–10%	Nephrogenic SIAD

AVP Arginine Vasopressin, *SIAD* Syndrome of Inappropriate Antidiuresis

Table 29.2 Grading of Hyponatremia based on severity

Grading	Serum sodium level	Clinical features
Mild hyponatremia,	130–135 meq/L	lethargy, inattention, restlessness, headache, nausea, vomiting.
Moderate hyponatremia	120–130 meq/L	confusion, altered sensorium, psychosis
Severe hyponatremia	<120 meq/L	severe life- threatening symptoms like seizures, coma.

The symptoms depend on the acuteness of hyponatremia. Patients with chronic hyponatremia may or may not show any symptoms

The priority in the treatment of acute severe hyponatremia in the first hour is to increase the serum sodium by 5 mmol/L with hypertonic saline, 100–150 mL of 3% saline over 20 min [13–15]. During acute phase, it is recommended to limit serum sodium rise to less than 10 mmol/L in 24 h, especially in patients at risk of developing osmotic demyelinating syndrome (malnutrition, alcohol consumption, liver failure, associated hypokalemia, severe hyponatremia). Once acute severe hyponatremia is appropriately treated, restrict fluid intake to either 800 mL/day (or previous day's urine output minus 500 mL). Fluid restriction alone may not be effective if urine osmolarity more than 500 mOsm/L and urine volume less than 1500 mL/day or combined value of urine sodium and potassium is more than serum sodium [16, 17]. In such cases, addition of oral salt (or urea) to increase osmotic load may help. Vaptans block the arginine vasopressin receptors (V2R) in principle cells of renal tubules causing pure water diuresis have shown beneficial effects [18, 19]. Tolvaptan is useful in SIADH in cancer patients especially with moderate to severe hyponatremia [20]. It is particularly useful when fluid restriction can't be followed or there is

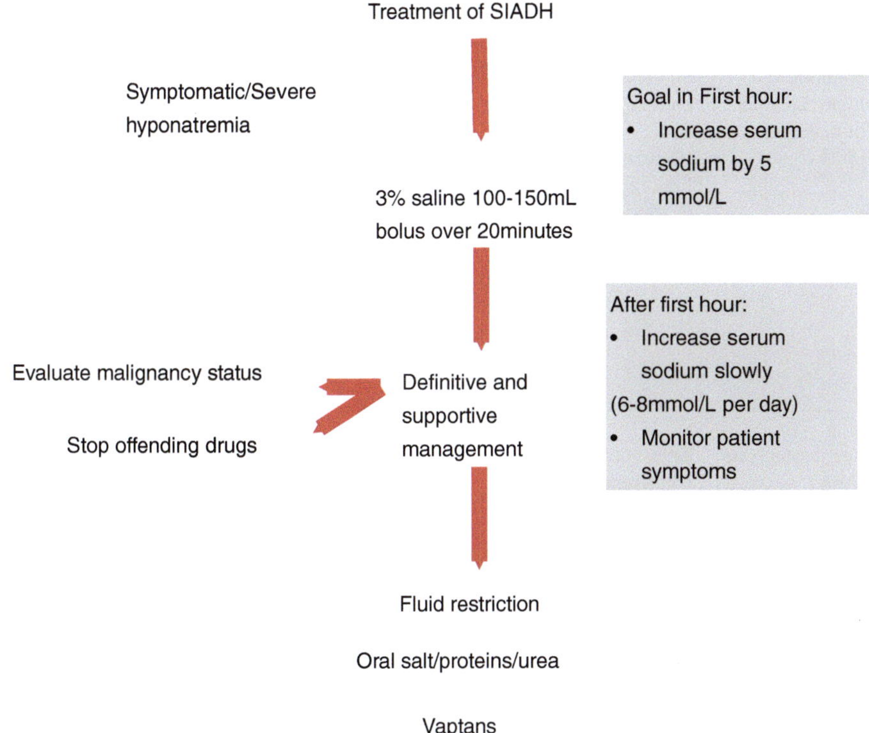

Fig. 29.2 Management of Syndrome of Inappropriate AntiDiuretic Hormone secretion (SIADH)

inadequate response to hypertonic saline. Attempts should be made to remove the stimulus that causes AVP secretion, e.g. pain, nausea, underlying infections, malignancy etc. Management of SIADH is summarized in Fig. 29.2.

29.3 Hypercalcemia of Malignancy (HCM)

Cancer patients, commonly with lung, kidney, gynecologic, head and neck cancers, and multiple myeloma can present with hypercalcemia of malignancy (HCM). HCM is more common during the later stages of these malignancies [21]. Due to the markedly elevated calcium levels, patients with HCM often have severe symptoms [22].

29.3.1 Pathophysiology of HCM

Pathophysiological mechanisms of HCM are described in Table 29.3. Humoral hypercalcemia of malignancy mediated by Parathyroid hormone-related peptide-PTHrP is the most common (80%) pathophysiological mechanism [22, 23].

Table 29.3 Pathophysiology of hypercalcemia of malignancy

Type	Malignancies	Mediator	Comments
Humoral hypercalcemia of malignancy (80%)	SCC(head and neck, esophagus, cervix, lung), RCC, Adenocarcinoma (Ovarian, prostate, Breast), Endometrial carcinoma, Human T-lymphotropic virus-associated lymphoma	Parathyroid hormone-related peptide (PTHrP)	• Naturally occurring hormone with close biochemical resemblance and functional overlap to parathyroid hormone (PTH). • Causes hypercalcemia by activation of osteoclasts and bone resorption and increased renal calcium reabsorption.
Local osteolysis (20%)	Breast cancer, Skeletal metastasis, Leukemia/ lymphoma Multiple myeloma	Local Chemokine (local PTHrP) Cytokines(IL-1,IL-6,IL-8,TNF-α, TGFα,β,MIP1α)	• Local factors from the tumour or metastasis causing osteolysis, • Local secretion of PTHrP in metastatic breast cancer
1,25 dihydroxy vitamin D related (<1%)	1,25(OH)2D Lymphomas, ovarian dysgerminoma	1,25(OH)2D	Increased calcium absorption form intestine and kidneys
Ectopic PTH (<1%)	Parathyroid carcinoma	Ectopic PTH	Parathyroid action

Table 29.4 Clinical features and severity of hypercalcemia

System	Clinical features
Neurology	Altered behaviour, lethargy, muscle weakness, coma
Renal	Polyuria, renal injury/failure, renal stones
Gastrointestinal	Nausea, vomiting, abdominal pain,
Cardiovascular	Heart block, short Qt interval.

29.3.2 Clinical Features

"Stones, bones, abdominal moans, and psychic groans," is known phrase to refer clinical symptoms of hypercalcemia [24]. The presentation is multisystemic (Table 29.4). The commonest symptoms that necessitate ICU admission are comatose state, seizures, renal failure, and cardiac complications. The clinical features depend on the severity and the rapidity of development of hypercalcemia. Hypercalcemia is traditionally defined as serum calcium levels more than 10.5 mg/dL. It is graded as per the severity, given below [24].

- Mild hypercalcemia: 10.5–11.9 mg/dL
- Moderate hypercalcemia: 12.0–13.9 mg/dL
- Hypercalcemic crisis: 14.0–16.0 mg/dL

29.3.3 Diagnosis

- The preferred method of diagnosis is by measuring the physiological 'free' ionized calcium. The reference range of ionized calcium in adults is 4.5–5.6 mg/dL or 1.05–1.3 mmol/L and any value higher than this, indicates hypercalcemia. Ionized calcium more than 7 mg/dL (1.75 mmol/L) is generally associated with coma. Unfortunately, measurement of ionized calcium is not universally available [25, 26]. hence total serum calcium concentration is used as surrogate.

Payne's formula is sometimes used to convert serum total calcium to ionized calcium.

Adjusted calcium (mmol/L) = Total calcium (mmol/L) + 0.02 [40—serum albumin (g/L)].

However, this formula is far from accurate especially in critically ill patients as changes in blood pH also affect protein-bound calcium [27]. In multiple myeloma, due to increased calcium binding to paraprotein serum total calcium may be falsely elevated despite normal ionized calcium [28].

29.3.4 Initial Management

1. Identify the presence of hypercalcemia and stratify the patients according to severity. At the same time, the evaluate disease status of the underlying malignancy. Realistic goals of the treatment can be planned, after discussion with the treating oncologist based on the intent of treatment, expected median survival etc. Patients who are either treatment naïve or have therapeutic options for disease cure or control should get priority over patients in terminal stage with no treatment options
2. Intravascular rehydration is the first line of management [29, 30]. Patients generally have extracellular volume depletion due to urinary sodium and water loss. This leads to reduced glomerular filtration rate perpetuating hypercalcemia. Rehydration with normal saline (NS), restores intravascular volume, breaks the perpetuating cycle and reduces any further risk of renal failure. NS is usually started at 200 ml/hr. Patients with cardiac failure or oliguria should be carefully monitored for fluid overload.
3. Diuretics may be added only when the intravascular volume is adequately restored to promote calcium excretion or if there are signs of fluid overload and should not be used routinely. Calcium excretion of diuretics is unpredictable and is associated with fluid and electrolyte imbalance [31].

4. In patients with renal failure or life-threatening hypercalcemia (severe hypercalcemia, cardiac and neurologic effects), hemodialysis with low calcium bath dialysate reduces serum calcium rapidly [32]. Hemodialysis may also be required in patients with heart failure if these patients may not tolerate large volumes of fluid loading.
5. Vitamin-D supplementation or thiazide diuretics can aggravate hypercalcemia and such medications should be stopped.

29.3.5 Definitive Management

Further management focuses on continuing measures to reduce the calcium levels by reducing the calcium production (bone resorption) along with enhanced calciuresis. The commonly used pharmacologic therapies for long term calcium level control are described below.

29.3.5.1 Calcitonin

Calcitonin acts by inhibiting osteoclastic bone resorption and renal calcium reabsorption. Calcitonin dose is 4 IU/kg every 12 h. It causes rapid (4–6 h) drop in serum calcium levels by 1–2 mg/dl [33, 34]. Usually tachyphylaxis develops by the third day hence bisphosphonates are added for sustained calcium lowering effect.

29.3.5.2 Bisphosphonates

Bisphosphonates act by blocking the osteoclastic bone resorption. It takes two to four days to show its effect which lasts for up to 3 weeks.

Doses: Zoledronic acid 4 mg intravenously giver over 15 min is (preferred) pamidronate 60–90 mg over two hours [35].

It has a well-established efficacy (up to 70%) and safety profile except for patients with severe acute kidney injury where it should be avoided [36].

Denosumab: It is a human monoclonal antibody to RANKL, which prevents the binding of the ligand to RANK receptors causing reduction in osteoclast activity by decreasing osteoclast maturation and hence bone resorption. It is effective in hypercalcemia refractory to bisphosphonates [37, 38]. Also, it can be used when the bisphosphonates are contraindicated like in renal failure as denosumab is not cleared by the kidneys.

Cinacalcet, a calcimimetic agent that activates the calcium-sensing receptor (CaSR) on the surface of parathyroid glands and non-parathyroid gland tissue (nephrons, intestine) helps reducing calcium levels by controlling PTH synthesis. It is recommended for patients with primary hyperparathyroidism in whom, surgery is contraindicated or not preferred. Recently it is tried with success in a patient with hypercalcemia associated with malignancy and it is emerging as a potential adjuvant [39–41].

29.3.5.3 Corticosteroid

Corticosteroids inhibit formation of 1,25-dihydroxyvitamin D (calcitriol) and hence are useful in calcitriol mediated hypercalcemia commonly seen with lymphomas

[42]. Additionally, they may also inhibit osteoclastic bone resorption by decreasing locally active cytokines.

29.3.6 Prognostication

HCM is associated with poor outcome even in patients who are on active treatment. Historically, median survival of 30 days has been reported in a retrospective study of 126 patients with cancer-associated hypercalcemia [43]. Current reported median survival in solid tumor with HCM is marginally improved to 40 days. The hospital mortality rate in hospitalized adult solid cancer patients with HCM (12.3%) is more than double the mortality rate in patients not having HCM (5.5%) [44].

29.4 Superior Vena Cava Syndrome (SVCS)

Superior vena cava syndrome (SVCS) is a condition caused due to the either intraluminal or extraluminal compression of Superior vena cava (SVC).

29.4.1 Etiology of SVCS

Common malignant and benign causes of SVCS are listed in (Table 29.5) [45–50].

Table 29.5 Etiology Superior vena cava syndrome (SVCS) (Ref. [25–28])

Malignant causes	Carcinoma of Lung (a) Non small cell Ca Lung (most common) (b) Small cell Ca Lung
	Lymphomas
	Metastases
	Thymomas
	Sarcomas
	Other adenocarcinomas
	Mesothelioma
Benign causes	Port-a-cath (most common)
	Dialysis catheter
	Fibrosing mediastinitis
	Pacemakers
	Radiation fibrosis
	Behchet's syndrome
	Retrosternal goiter
	Giant bulla
	Congential vascular defect
	Granulomas

29.4.2 Anatomy and Pathophysiology

Superior vena cava (SVC) is a thin walled compressible vessel, which drains blood from the head, upper libs and torso. It lacks strong architecture, similar to trachea or high internal pressure like aorta hence, is vulnerable to compression and obstruction. Any mass in the anterior and middle mediastinum can easily compress SVC. In cases of SVCS, pressure in SCV up to 20–40 mmHg has been reported in contrast to normal central venous pressure of 2–8 mm Hg [45]. This increase in venous pressure leads to development of collateral vessels, if the obstruction occurs gradually. The azygous vein, (Fig. 29.3) connects SVC with the Inferior vena cava (IVC) and thus provides the collateral pathway for obstruction. However, if the obstruction is distal to it, the occlusion is above (distal) the origin of azygous vein, the blood is diverted through small venous collaterals [51].

29.4.3 Diagnosis

29.4.3.1 Clinical Features

Diagnosis of SVC syndrome is primarily clinical and supported by imaging to demonstrate the obstruction. The signs and symptoms of SVCS are elaborated in Table 29.6 in order of their incidence [46]. The symptoms are usually exacerbated

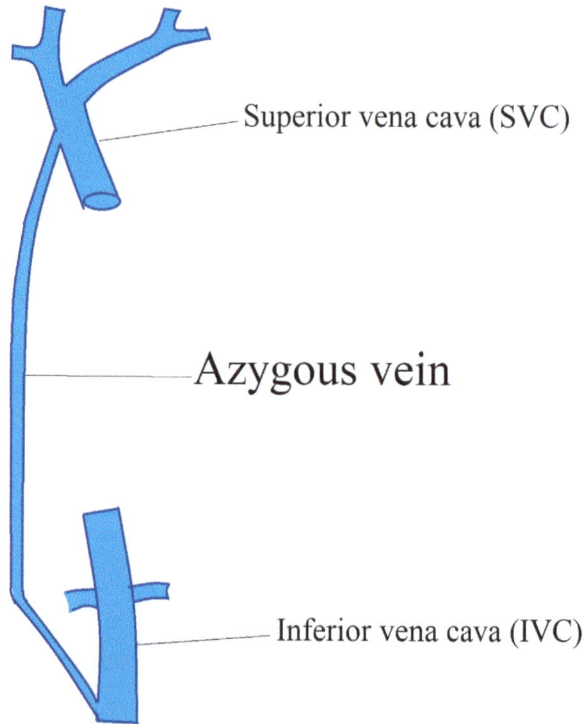

Fig. 29.3 Anatomy of Superior vena cava (SVC), Azygous vein and Inferior vena cava (IVC)

Table 29.6 Signs and symptoms OF Superior vena cava syndrome (SVCS)

Symptom/signs	Incidence (%)
Facial edema	60–100
Dsypnoea	38–70
Dilated chest vein collaterals	38–67
Distension of neck veins	27–86
Cough	22–58
Hoarseness of voice	15–20
Edema of upper extremities	14–75
Plethora	13–23
Syncope	8–13
Dizziness	2–10
Confusion	0–5
Stridor	0–5
Mental obtundation	0–3%

References [25, 29, 30, 33]

by maneuvers that increase supra-cardiac venous pressure like performing valsalva maneuver, leaning forward and lying supine.

29.4.3.2 Imaging

Chest X-ray may reveal widening of superior mediastinum (in cases of mediastinal masses) in about 75% cases. Ultrasonography can rule out thrombosis of subclavian, axillary and brachiocephalic veins in patients presenting with upper limb edema. Contrast enhanced CT imaging (CECT) will reveal the extent of tumor, involvement of surrounding structures, brain metastases, while venography can detect the presence of any intravascular thrombus [51]. Magnetic resonance imaging (MRI) venography can be used in patients allergic to iodine contrast. Diagnostic bronchoscopy may be required to detect endoluminal tumor growth.

29.4.3.3 Tumor Histology

Tissue diagnosis of the tumor is essential for treatment. Sputum examination and pleural fluid cytology for cases of carcinoma lung, peripheral lymph node biopsy for suspected lymphoma can establish the histology of the tumor. At times, thoracoscopy and mediastinoscopy may be required.

29.4.3.4 Management

The management of SVCS depends upon the severity of symptoms, probability of response to treatment (oncological etiology) and patient's performance status. Often, a multidisciplinary approach involving intensivist, medical oncologist and radiation oncologist and interventional radiologist is needed.

Patients presenting with symptoms such as coma, cerebral edema, syncope, airway and hemodynamic compromise (hypotension) require immediate admission to intensive care unit (ICU) for stabilization and control of symptoms, while waiting for the results of other investigations to formulate the future treatment plan.

I. **General care**

Patients should be nursed in 45-degree head up position to reduce the hydrostatic pressure in the veins of the upper torso. Venous access should be obtained in lower limbs.

II. **Anticipated difficult airway**

Difficult ventilation should be anticipated, especially if there is orthopnea, stridor or bronchial compression on imaging. Diuretics and corticosteroids can help reduce airway edema, but steroids may be avoided if lymphoma is the provisional diagnosis and biopsy is pending. Esophageal varices with occasional variceal bleeding may be present in chronic SVCS.

Interventional Radiology (Stents)

Endovascular stenting **provides immediate relief from severe symptoms and** has proven to be effective even in cases of relapsed malignancies [46]. Stenting may be avoided if rapid response to chemotherapy (lymphoma, small-cell lung cancer, and germ cell tumors) is expected or tumor is potentially amenable to surgery preceded by chemotherapy (thymoma). Kishi Scoring system (Table 29.7) can guide decision to initiate stent therapy based on the severity of symptoms [46, 47]. Stenting is feasible, if the patient can lie supine under local anaesthesia. Headache resolves first, followed by facial and truncal edema. Short-term anticoagulation is often required after stent placement. SVCS of benign etiology is managed with endovascular therapy. In SVCS due to thrombosis, stenting, catheter- directed thrombolysis

Table 29.7 Kishi Scoring system for decision to initiate stent therapy

Clinical signs		Weighting
Neurological signs	Awareness disorders or coma	4
	Visual disorders, headache, vertigo or memory disorders	3
	Mental disorders	2
	Malaise	1
Thoracic or pharyngeal-laryngeal signs	Orthopnea or laryngeal edema	3
	Stridor, dysphagia or dyspnea	2
	Coughing or pleurisy	1
Facial signs	Lip edema, nasal obstruction or epistaxis	2
	Facial edema	1
Vessel dilation	Neck, face or arms	1

A score of 4 or higher indicates a need for percutaneous stent placement

Adopted from Straka et al. Springer Plus (2016) 5:229 under Creative Commons license

(CDT) or mechanical thrombectomy can be considered. An intravascular device like pacemaker wires or central venous catheters may be removed [49].

Radiotherapy (RT)

RT can be palliative or definitive. Palliative RT is recommended for radiosensitive tumors like non-small cell lung cancer (NSCLC) encroaching critical structures in the mediastinum to halt progression of cardiac and respiratory symptoms. Definitive RT is administered with curative intent in cases of low- grade lymphoma, stage II or III NSCLC or SCLC with limited- stage disease. Radiotherapy can sometimes cause local edema with exacerbation of the symptoms, during treatment or SVCS due to radiation fibrosis later.

Chemotherapy and Immunotherapy

Lymphomas, germ cell tumors and small cell lung cancer (SCLC) respond well to chemotherapy generally within 24–48 h [47]. After the resolution of initial symptoms, definitive chemotherapy should be planned.

Surgery

After initial stabilization and chemotherapy, surgery is an option in resectable tumors like thymomas or Germ cell tumors.

29.5 Hyperviscosity Syndrome (HVS)

Hyperviscosity syndrome (HVS) is an oncologic emergency due to elevated blood viscosity either due to plasma or cellular components. They can produce life- threatening consequences due to hypoperfusion caused by sluggish blood flow and also due to impaired coagulation leading to bleeding.

29.5.1 Etiology

Aetiology of HVS in various diseases is discussed in (Table 29.8). Waldenstrom macroglobulinemia (WM) is one of the most common etiologies of HVS. Hyperleukocytosis and Leukocytosis are discussed separately.

29.5.2 Pathophysiology

An increase in blood viscosity either due to circulating cells or proteins cause sluggishness of blood flow leading to decreased microvascular circulation, and organ hypoperfusion while coagulation is impaired due to interference to platelet aggregation by the circulating proteins [52–54].

Table 29.8 Etiology of HVS

I. Increase in plasma proteins • Multiple myeloma (IgA, IgE, IgG3) • Waldenstrommacroglobulinemia • Cryoglobulinemia
IIa Increase in red cell mass • Neonates • Polycythemia rubra vera • Cyanotic heart disease **IIb Abnormal RBC** • Sickle cell anaemia
III. Leukocytosis • Leukemias (AML> ALL, CML. CLL) (Discussed under Hyperleukocytosis) **IV. Drugs** • Rituximab
VI. Miscellaneous • Rheumatoid arthritis • Systemic lupus erythematosus (SLE) • Sjogren's syndrome • HIV • Castleman's disease

Table 29.9 Clinical features of HVS

System	Symptoms and signs
Skin & musculoskeletal system	Mucosal bleeding, neuropathy[a]
Central nervous system (CNS)	Headache, dizziness, ischemic stroke, transient ischemic attack, ataxia, coma, seizure
Vascular system	Thromboembolism in arteries and veins Retinal venous congestion, blurring of vision Retinal ischemia, papilledema
Cardiovascular system (CVS)	Myocardial infarction, high output failure
Gastrointestinal system (GI)	Budd-chiari syndrome, mesenteric ischemia

[a]Neuropathy is due to paraprotein deposition in myelin sheath of the peripheral nerves

29.5.3 Clinical Features

Multiorgan involvement is frequently encountered, however, central nervous system and pulmonary vasculature are most commonly affected. The clinical features of HVS are summarized in (Table 29.9) [52–54].

29.5.4 Laboratory Parameters

Serum viscosity should be measured, if HVS is suspected. The reference range of serum viscosity is 1.4–1.8 centipoise(cp). Fundoscopy may reveal "string of sausages" appearance due to retinal venous engorgement, hemorrhages and retinal vein occlusion [52]. Peripheral smear can show "rouleaux formation" due to abnormal paraproteins cause aggregation of red blood cells.

29.5.5 Management of HVS

Intravascular hydration with crystalloid solution is the first step. Colloids and blood transfusion may be avoided due to risk of further increase in viscosity. In patients with WM, plasmapheresis can decrease serum viscosity and is done daily, till resolution of symptoms. In plasmapheresis, blood is centrifuged, and plasma is separated from the cellular components. The proteins are removed and replaced with albumin or fresh frozen plasma [52]. A single session reduces levels of serum proteins by 65% and reduces serum viscosity by 20% and removes large molecules such as IgA and IgM [52, 53].

29.6 Hyperleukocytosis and Leukostasis

Hyperleucocytosis is defined as total leucocyte count more than100,000 per microliter of blood (100×10^9/L) [55]. Leukostasis (symptomatic hyperleukocytosis) is tissue hypoperfusion due to extremely elevated leucocyte or blast cell count.

29.6.1 Etiology

Hyperleukocytosis is associated with specific subtypes of leukemia. In AML, hyperleukocytosis is associated with monocytic differentiation subtypes (M4, M5) while, in acute promyelocytic leukaemia (APML) and (ALL) an association with t (4:11) and t(9:22) is observed [56–58]. In chronic lymphocytic leukemia (CLL), symptomatic hyperleukocytosis occurs only if WBC is greater than 1,00,000 μ/ml [55].

29.6.2 Pathophysiology

Patients with hyperleukcocytosis are at risk for development of tumor lysis syndrome (TLS), disseminated intravascular coagulation (DIC) and leukostasis. There can be vascular obstruction and tissue hypoxia leading to a myriad of systemic manifestations. Two theories are being postulated for the pathophysiology of leukostasis. The rheological theory, where the viscosity of blood depends on the deforming capacity of the cells and the total volume of cells in the blood. In cases of high leukocrit, increased blood viscosity is due to increase in the volume of WBCs in the blood. As per this proposed theory, myeloblasts are bigger and less deformable than lymphoblasts and lymphocytes, so leukostasis is more commonly observed in AML than ALL and CLL where it occurs at much higher counts of WBC. While the other theory, focuses on the interaction of endothelium with the blast cells. It was proposed that the endothelium when activated by blast cells secretes cytokines and the adhesion molecules (VCAM and selectins) promote adhesion of blasts to the endothelium. Generally, leukostasis occurs at lower cell counts in myelomonocytic and monocytic AML (>50 × 109/L) compared to other AML and CML (>100 × 109/L). Leukostasis is rare in ALL and is seen at very high counts (>400 × 109/L) [59].

29.6.3 Clinical Features

Table 29.10 summarizes the clinical picture of Hyperleukocytosis [55, 60].

29.6.4 Management

Hyperleukocytosis management is aimed at reducing the WBCs and supporting circulation. In acute phase, patient should be admitted to ICU for monitoring and stabilization. Aggressive hydration is the initial step, measures for monitoring and treatment of TLS and DIC if suspected, should be in place. Once the patient stabilizes, further therapy in the form of induction chemotherapy (CT) and leucopheresis should be planned. Supportive management also includes cranial irradiation for leukostasis and neurological symptoms. Dexamethasone has been shown to prevent adhesion of the WBCs to the endothelium and hyperleukocytosis associated with arsenic trioxide treatment in APML [60].

Table 29.10 Clinical features of Hyperleukocytosis

System	Signs and symptoms
Central nervous system	Stroke, altered mental state, headache, focal neurological deficits, confusion, coma, blurred vision, tinnitus
Cardiovascular system	Congestive heart failure
Respiratory system	Pulmonary infarcts, pulmonary hemorrhage, Pseudo hypoxemia (leucocyte lacerny), tachypnea, dyspnea, Rhales
Genitourinary	Renal infarcts, stones (TLS), priapism
Gastrointestinal system	Bowel ischemia, splenic infarcts, Budd chiari syndrome
Hematological system	DIC, thrombosis, lab abnormalities—low fibrinogen, increased fibrin degradation products, and D-dimer.

29.6.4.1 Induction Chemotherapy (CT)

Induction CT reduces the cell burden in 24–72 h. If induction CT is not feasible, a low dose CT (hydroxyurea, cytarabine in cases of AML) can be considered [59]. These patients are at high risk for development of TLS.

29.6.4.2 Leukocytapheresis

The aim of leukocytapheresis is to improve tissue perfusion and to control or prevent the acute symptoms of leukostasis. In this procedure, WBCs or the blasts are removed from the patient's body and rest of the components are infused back. It is mostly performed in patients with AML and occasionally in ALL, CLL and CML. The improvement in symptoms gives an idea of the adequacy of leukocytapheresis. A single cycle reduces peripheral WBCs by 30–60% and maybe considered once or twice in a day [55]. Replacement fluid should provide a net positive fluid balance of 15%. Platelets, cryoprecipitate or plasma transfusion can be considered if indicated. In asymptomatic patients, Leukocytapheresis is discontinued when resolution of symptoms with WBC count $<50–100\times10^9$/L in AML and $< 400\times10^9$/L in ALL. In prophylactic apheresis, it is discontinued when the WBC count $<100\times10^9$/L and $< 400\times10^9$/L in AML and ALL respectively [59].

29.7 Malignant Spinal Cord Compression (MSCC)

It is the condition in which tumor (primary or metastasis) of spine jeopardizes the blood circulation or the function of spinal cord and can cause devastating impairment in quality of life, if left untreated.

29.7.1 Incidence and Risk Factors

MSCC can be due to primary spinal cord tumor or due to spinal metastases. Malignancies commonly presenting with spinal metastases are carcinomas of lung, prostrate and breast. It is estimated that up to 3–5% of cancer patients can have vertebral metastases on their first visit to the hospital [61]. Compression at thoracic level is far more common than lumbar level, while compression at cervical level is infrequent [62].

29.7.2 Clinical Features

The most common presenting symptom of MSSC is progressive back pain exacerbated by maneuvers that increase intraabdominal pressure like coughing, sneezing or bending forward. Localized pain is due to inflammation and periosteal stretching of the vertebral marrow. Movement associated pain, may indicate impeding fracture or unstable spine. Whereas, radicular pain presenting as pins and needle or burning sensation is due to nerve root compression by the tumor or the resultant vertebral collapse. The vertebral collapse can lead to paresis due to cord compression.

Often, patients present with weakness or heaviness in legs with loss of motor functions. Motor tracts are more sensitive to compression hence the loss of motor functions occur first followed by sensory loss and bladder bowel dysfunction [63]. In the initial stage, neurological symptoms may be reversible, but later on, vascular damage sets in and the neurological deficit is almost permanent.

29.7.3 Diagnosis

29.7.3.1 History and Physical Examination

A comprehensive history about the onset of symptoms, previous oncological diagnosis, and comorbidities should be taken. Thorough neurological examination should be done at baseline and repeated frequently for neurological deficit.

29.7.3.2 Imaging

Whenever MSCC is suspected, the patient should undergo neuroimaging at the earliest after initial stabilization. The whole spine should be imaged as multiple sites of metastases might exist in the same patient. MRI is the gold standard for the definitive diagnosis of MSCC with sensitivity of 93% and specificity of 98% [63] (Table 29.11). CT scan has a sensitivity of 66% and specificity of 99% respectively. If tissue diagnosis is needed, CT guided percutaneous biopsy of the most superficial and accessible lesion in the spine can be performed along with scan of chest, abdomen and pelvis for primary site, staging and prognostication.

Table 29.11 MRI grading of Malignant Spinal cord compression (MSCC)

Grades	Location of the tumor in spine
Grade 0	Tumor confined to bone
Grade 1	Tumor with epidural extension without contact with the SC or just SC abutment without displacement.
Ia	Epidural tumor without thecal sac compression
Ib	Epidural tumor with thecal sac compression but no cord contact
Ic	Epidural tumor with thecal sac compression and cord contact without compression
Grade 2	Tumor displaces or compresses the SC, without circumferential tumor extension or obliteration of the cerebrospinal fluid (CSF) space.
Grade 3	Tumor with circumferential epidural extension and/or that causes severe SCC with obliteration of the CSF space

29.7.4 Management

Early diagnosis and treatment can reduce the extent of neurological morbidity. Bed rest and steroids are the mainstay of initial management. If spine stability is a concern, patient should be nursed in flat position, with neutral spine including log rolling. Venous thromboembolism prophylaxis and ulcer prophylaxis should be given [64]. Glucocorticoids provide analgesia and decrease the production of prostaglandins and vascular endothelial growth factor, reducing the cord edema and preserve neurological function. A meta-analysis conducted by Kumar et al. concluded that steroids are most effective when given immediately or within 12 h of onset of symptoms. A bolus of 10 mg IV bolus followed by 16 mg of dexamethasone divided in four doses of 4 mg IV or orally [65]. Rapid resolution of tumor in a suspected steroid- responsive disease like lymphoma should be kept in mind especially if biopsy is pending. Once the diagnosis is confirmed, definitive treatment should be initiated. The management choices are radiotherapy, surgery or both.

29.7.4.1 Surgery

The indications of decompressive surgery are fractured or unstable spine, bony retropulsion and need for excision biopsy of the spinal lesion, or for tissue diagnosis in cases of unknown malignancy [66]. Surgery is also considered in in patients with radioresistant tumors like renal cell, melanoma, sarcoma, non-small cell lung, and gastrointestinal malignancies or radiosensitive tumor with previous radiation (relapse or recurrence).

The decision for surgery depends on the patient's general condition, stage of malignancy and prognosis [66].

Patient's prognosis can be determined by the Tokuhashi score as given in Table 29.12.

The spinal instability Neoplastic score (SINS) was developed to assess the level of spine instability and help identify patients at risk before the onset of neurological deficit. It has a sensitivity of 95.7% and specificity of 79.5% [66].

29.7.4.2 Radiotherapy (RT)

It is considered in radiosensitive tumour like, lymphoma, myeloma, germ cell tumors, breast, ovary, prostate and small cell lung cancer if there is no indication for urgent surgical decompression. Stereotactic RT has the advantage of local tumor destruction with minimal damage to the spinal cord. RT is less effective in radioresistant tumors like sarcoma, renal cell or melanoma but may be considered for palliation.

29.7.4.3 Pain Management and Rehabilitation

Opioids, paracetamol and NSAIDs along with stool softeners are the mainstay of pain management in these patients. Rehabilitation includes management of neurogenic bladder and bowel, prevention of decubitus ulcers, and rehabilitative care during acute hospitalization [67]. The patient should be mobilized with caution once

Table 29.12 Tokuhashi score

Predictive factor		Score (points)
General condition Karnofsky's performance status. (KPS)		
	Poor (KPS 10–40%)	0
	Moderate (KPS 50–70%)	1
	Good (KPS 80–100%)	2
Number of extraspinal bone metastases foci		
	≥3	0
	1–2	1
	0	2
Number of metastases in the vertebral body		
	≥3	0
	2	1
	1	2
Metastases to the major internal organs		
	Unremovable	0
	Removable	1
	No metastases	2
Primary site of the cancer		
	Lung, osteosarcoma, stomach, bladder, esophagus, pancreas	0
	Liver, gallbladder, unidentified	1
	Others	2
	Kidney, uterus	3
	Rectum	4
	Thyroid, prostate, breast, carcinoid tumor	5
Spinal cord palsy		
	Complete (Frankel A, B)	0
	Incomplete (Frankel C, D)	1
	None (Frankel E)	2

spine stability is ensured. Use of walkers and spinal braces should be encouraged. The presentation of neurogenic bladder and bowel depends upon the site of lesion. Upper motor neuron presents as urinary and fecal retention where the patients, self catheterize and use osmotic and motility agents for preventing constipation. Lower motor neuron lesions present with urinary and bowel incontinence and the patients maintain bladder voiding and bowel evacuation schedules. Decubitus ulcers should be prevented by regularly changing the bed position every two hours with log rolling to prevent areas of pressure necrosis and air mattress should be used. Occupational therapy during hospitalization should include fine motor dexterity and targeted task sequencing [67].

References

1. Berghmans T, Paesmans M, Body JJ. A prospective study on hyponatraemia in medical cancer patients: epidemiology, aetiology and differential diagnosis. Support Care Cancer. 2000;8(3):192–7. https://doi.org/10.1007/s005200050284.
2. Schwartz WB, Bennett W, Curelop S, Bartter FC. Syndrome of renal sodium loss and hyponatremia probably resulting from inappropriate secretion of antidiuretic hormone. Am J Med. 1957;23(4):529–42. https://doi.org/10.1016/0002-9343(57)90224-3.
3. Feldman BJ, Rosenthal SM, Vargas GA, Fenwick RG, Matsuda-Abedini M, Lustig RH, et al. Nephrogenic syndrome of inappropriate antidiuresis. N Engl J Med. 2005;352(18):1884–90. https://doi.org/10.1056/NEJMoa042743.
4. Leaf A, Bartter FC, Santos RF, Wrong O. Evidence in man that urinary electrolyte loss induced by pitressin is a function of water retention. J Clin Invest. 1953;32(9):868–78. https://doi.org/10.1172/JCI102805.
5. Robertson GL, Antidiuretic hormone. Normal and disordered function. Endocrinol Metab Clin N Am. 2001;30(3):671–94. https://doi.org/10.1016/s0889-8529(05)70207-3.
6. Janicic N, Verbalis JG. Evaluation and management of hypo-osmolality in hospitalized patients. Endocrinol Metab Clin North Am. 2003;32:459–81. https://doi.org/10.1016/s0889-8529(03)00004-5.
7. Feder J, Gomez JM, Serra-Aguirre F, Musso CG. Reset Osmostat: facts and controversies. Indian J Nephrol. 2019;29(4):232–4. https://doi.org/10.4103/ijn.IJN_307_17.
8. Robertson LG. Regulation of arginine vasopressin in the syndrome of inappropriate Antidiuresis. Am J Med. 2006;119(7 Suppl 1):S36–42. https://doi.org/10.1016/j.amjmed.2006.05.006.
9. Nelson PB, Seif SM, Maroon JC, Robinson AG. Hyponatremia in intracranial disease: perhaps not the syndrome of inappropriate secretion of antidiuretic hormone (SIADH). J Neurosurg. 1981;55(6):938–41. https://doi.org/10.3171/jns.1981.55.6.0938.
10. Wijdicks EF, Vermeulen M, Haaf JA, Hijdra A, Bakker WH, van Gijn J. Volume depletion and natriuresis in patients with a ruptured intracranial aneurysm. Ann Neurol. 1985;18(2):211–6. https://doi.org/10.1002/ana.410180208.
11. Sivakumar V, Rajshekhar V, Chandy MJ. Management of neurosurgical patients with hyponatremia and natriuresis. Neurosurgery. 1994;34(2):269–74. https://doi.org/10.1227/00006123-199402000-00010.
12. Maesaka JK, Imbriano L, Mattana J, Gallagher D, Bade N, Sharif S. Differentiating SIADH from cerebral/renal salt wasting: failure of the volume approach and need for a new approach to hyponatremia. J Clin Med. 2014;3(4):1373–85. https://doi.org/10.3390/jcm3041373.
13. Sterns RH, Nigwekar SU, Hix JK. The treatment of hyponatremia. Semin Nephrol. 2009;29(3):282–99. https://doi.org/10.1016/j.semnephrol.2009.03.002.
14. Spasovski G, Vanholder R, Allolio B, Annane D, Ball S, Bichet D, et al. Clinical practice guideline on diagnosis and treatment of hyponatraemia. Nephrol Dial Transplant. 2014 Apr;29(Suppl 2):i1–i39. https://doi.org/10.1093/ndt/gfu040.
15. Verbalis JG, Goldsmith SR, Greenberg A, Korzelius C, Schrier RW, Sterns RH, et al. Diagnosis, evaluation, and treatment of hyponatremia: expert panel recommendations. Am J Med. 2013;126(10 Suppl 1):S1–42. https://doi.org/10.1016/j.amjmed.2013.07.006.
16. Cuesta M, Ortolá A, Garrahy A, Calle Pascual AL, Runkle I, Thompson CJ. Predictors of failure to respond to fluid restriction in SIAD in clinical practice; time to re-evaluate clinical guidelines? QJM. 2017 Aug 1;110(8):489–92. https://doi.org/10.1093/qjmed/hcx036.
17. Furst H, Hallows KR, Post J, Chen S, Kotzker W, Goldfarb S, et al. The urine/plasma electrolyte ratio: a predictive guide to water restriction. Am J Med Sci. 2000;319(4):240–4. https://doi.org/10.1097/00000441-200004000-00007.
18. Schrier RW, Gross P, Gheorghiade M, Berl T, Verbalis JG, Czerwiec FS et al. SALT Investigators. Tolvaptan, a selective oral vasopressinV2-receptor antagonist, for hyponatremia. N Engl J Med. 2006 Nov 16;355(20):2099–112. https://doi.org/10.1056/NEJMoa065181. Epub 2006 Nov 14.

19. Verbalis JG, Adler S, Schrier RW, Berl T, Zhao Q, Czerwiec FS. SALT Investigators. Efficacy and safety of oral tolvaptan therapy in patients with the syndrome of inappropriate antidiuretic hormone secretion. Eur J Endocrinol 2011 May;164(5):725–732. https://doi.org/10.1530/EJE-10-1078. Epub 2011 Feb 11.
20. De las Peñas R, Escobar Y, Henao F, Blasco A, Rodríguez CA, Spanish Society for Medical Oncology. SEOM guidelines on hydroelectrolytic disorders. Clin Transl Oncol 2014 Dec;16(12):1051–1059. https://doi.org/10.1007/s12094-014-1234-2. Epub 2014 Oct 11.
21. Jick S, Li L, Gastanaga VM, Liede A. Prevalence of hypercalcemia of malignancy among cancer patients in the UK: analysis of the Clinical Practice Research Datalink database. Cancer Epidemiol. 2015; 39:901–7. https://doi.org/10.1016/j.canep.2015.10.012. Epub 2015 Nov 9.
22. Mirrakhimov AE. Hypercalcemia of malignancy: an update on pathogenesis and management. N Am J Med Sci. 2015 Nov;7(11):483–93. https://doi.org/10.4103/1947-2714.170600.
23. Clines GA, Guise TA. Hypercalcaemia of malignancy and basic research on mechanisms responsible for osteolytic and osteoblastic metastasis to bone. Endocr Relat Cancer. 2005 Sep;12(3):549–83. https://doi.org/10.1677/erc.1.00543.
24. Carroll MF, Schade DS. A practical approach to hypercalcemia. Am Fam Physician. 2003 May 1;67(9):1959–66.
25. Takano S, Kaji H, Hayashi F, Higashiguchi K, Joukei S, Kido Y, et al. A calculation model for serum ionized calcium based on an equilibrium equation for complexation. Anal Chem Insights. 2012;7:23–30. https://doi.org/10.4137/ACI.S9681.
26. Pfitzenmeyer P, Martin I, d'Athis P, Grumbach Y, Delmestre MC, Blondé-Cynober F et al. A new formula for correction of total calcium level into ionized serum calcium values in very elderly hospitalized patients. Arch Gerontol Geriatr. 2007 Sep–Oct;45(2):151–7. https://doi.org/10.1016/j.archger.2006.10.006. Epub 2006.
27. Nates LJ, Price JK. Oncologic critical care [e-book], 1st edition. Cham Switzerland: Springer International Publishing; 2020 [Cited 2021 April 12], pp. 1017–28. Available from http://93.174.95.29/main/4206DCE99287433B8AB4C9ECC4B4D3.
28. Pearce CJ, Hine TJ, Peek K. Hypercalcaemia due to calcium binding by a polymeric IgA kappa-paraprotein. Ann Clin Biochem. 1991;28(Pt 3):229–34. https://doi.org/10.1177/000456329102800305.
29. Hosking DJ, Cowley A, Bucknall CA. Rehydration in the treatment of severe hypercalcaemia. Q J Med. 1981 Autumn;50(200):473–81.
30. Stewart AF. Clinical practice. Hypercalcemia associated with cancer. N Engl J Med. 2005;352(4):373–9. https://doi.org/10.1056/NEJMcp042806.
31. LeGrand SB, Leskuski D, Zama I. Narrative review: furosemide for hypercalcemia: an unproven yet common practice. Ann Intern Med. 2008 Aug 19;149(4):259–63. https://doi.org/10.7326/0003-4819-149-4-200808190-00007.
32. Koo WS, Jeon DS, Ahn SJ, Kim YS, Yoon YS, Bang BS, et al. Calcium- free hemodialysis for the management of hypercalcemia. Nephron. 1996;72(3):424–8. https://doi.org/10.1159/000188907.
33. Silva OL, Becker KL. Salmon calcitonin in the treatment of hypercalcemia. Arch Intern Med. 1973;132(3):337–9.
34. McCurdy MT, Shanholtz CB. Oncologic emergencies. Crit Care Med. 2012 Jul;40(7):2212–22. https://doi.org/10.1097/CCM.0b013e31824e1865.
35. Major P, Lortholary A, Hon J, Abdi E, Mills G, Menssen HD, et al. Zoledronic acid is superior to pamidronate in the treatment of hypercalcemia of malignancy: a pooled analysis of two randomized, controlled clinical trials. J Clin Oncol. 2001 Jan 15;19(2):558–67. https://doi.org/10.1200/JCO.2001.19.2.558.
36. Saunders Y, Ross JR, Broadley KE, Edmonds PM, Patel S, Steering Group. Systematic review of bisphosphonates for hypercalcaemia of malignancy. Palliat Med. 2004;18(5):418–31. https://doi.org/10.1191/0269216304pm914ra.
37. Salahudeen AA, Gupta A, Jones JC, Cowan RW, Vusirikala M, Kwong C, et al. PTHrP-induced refractory malignant hypercalcemia in a patient with chronic lymphocytic leukemia

responding to denosumab. Clin Lymphoma Myeloma Leuk. 2015:15(9):e137–e140. https://doi.org/10.1016/j.clml.2015.06.007. Epub 2015 Jun 19.
38. Hu MI, Glezerman IG, Leboulleux S, Insogna K, Gucalp R, Misiorowski W, et al. Denosumab for treatment of hypercalcemia of malignancy. J Clin Endocrinol Metab. 99(9):3144–52. https://doi.org/10.1210/jc.2014-1001.
39. Asonitis N, Kassi E, Kokkinos M, Giovanopoulos I, Petychaki F, Gogas H, et al. Hypercalcemia of malignancy treated with cinacalcet. Endocrinol Diabetes Metab Case Rep. 2017 Dec 15;(2017):17–0118. https://doi.org/10.1530/EDM-17-0118.
40. Takeuchi Y, Takahashi S, Miura D, Katagiri M, Nakashima N, Ohishi H, Shimazaki R, Tominga Y. Cinacalcet hydrochloride relieves hypercalcemia in Japanese patients with parathyroid cancer and intractable primary hyperparathyroidism. J Bone Miner Metab. 2017;35(6):616–22. https://doi.org/10.1007/s0074-016-0797-0.
41. Sheehan MT, Wermers RA, Jatoi A, Loprinzi CL, Onitilo AA. Oral cinacalcet responsiveness in non-parathyroid hormone mediated hypercalcemia of malignancy. Med Hypotheses 2020 Oct;143:110149. https://doi.org/10.1016/j.mehy.2020.110149. Epub 2020 Jul 30.
42. Sternlicht H, Glezerman IG. Hypercalcemia of malignancy and new treatment options. Ther Clin Risk Manag. 2015 Dec 4;(11):1779–88. https://doi.org/10.2147/TCRM.S83681.
43. Ralston SH, Gallacher SJ, Patel U, Campbell J, Boyle IT. Cancer-associated hypercalcemia: morbidity and mortality. Clinical experience in 126 treated patients. Ann Intern Med. 1990 Apr 1;112(7):499–504. https://doi.org/10.7326/0003-4819-112-7-499.
44. Ramos REO, Perez Mak M, Alves MFS, Piotto GHM, Takahashi TK, Gomes da Fonseca L, et al. Malignancy-related hypercalcemia in advanced solid tumors: survival outcomes. J Glob Oncol. 2017;3(6):728–33. https://doi.org/10.1200/JGO.2016.006890.
45. Wilson DL, Detterbeck FC, Yahalom J. Clinical practice. Superior vena cava sydrome with Malignant Causes. N Eng J Med 2007;356(18):1862–1869. https://doi.org/10.1056/NEJMcp067190. Erratum in: N Engl J Med.2008 Mar 6;358(10):1083.
46. Straka C, Ying J, Kong FM, Wiley DC, Kaminski J, Kim NDW. Review of evolving etiologies, implications and treatment strategies for the superior vena cava syndrome. Springer plus. 2016 Feb 29;5:229. https://doi.org/10.1186/s40064-016-1900-7.
47. Friedman T, Quencer KB, Kishore SA, Winokur RS, Madoff DC. Malignant venous obstruction: superior vena cava syndrome and beyond. Semin Intervent Radiol. 2017 Dec;34(4):398–408. https://doi.org/10.1055/s-0037-1608863.
48. Batihan G, Usluer O, Kaya SO. Rare cause of superior vena cava syndrome: a giant bulla. BMJ Case Rep. 2018;11:e226477. https://doi.org/10.1136/bcr-2018-226477.
49. Garcia CR. Non-malignant superior vena cava syndrome in a patient with incidental diagnosis of a congenital vascular defect. BMJ Case Rep. 2017; https://doi.org/10.1136/bcr-2016-218844.
50. Israel RA, VanderLaan PA, Chee A. Man with superior vena cava syndrome and granulomas. Ann Am Thorac Soc. 2020 Jan;17(1):107–11. https://doi.org/10.1513/AnnalsATS.201905-348CC.
51. Nates LJ, Price JK. Oncologic critical care [e-book], 1st edition. Cham Switzerland: Springer International Publishing; 2020 [Cited 2021 April 12], pp. 1253–64. Available from http://93.174.95.29/main/4206DCE99287433B8AB4C9ECC4B4D3.
52. Shenoy S, Shetty S, Lankala S, Anwer F, Yeager A, Adigopula S. Cardiovascular oncologic emergencies. Cardiology. 2017;138(3):147-158. https://doi.org/10.1159/000475491. Epub 2017 Jun 28.
53. Khan UA, Shanholtz CB, McCurdy MT. Oncologic mechanical emergencies. Hematol Oncol Clin North Am. 2017;31(6):927–40. https://doi.org/10.1016/j.hoc.2017.08.001.
54. Gertz AM. Acute hyperviscosity: syndromes and management. Blood 2018 Sep 27;132(13):1379–1385. https://doi.org/10.1182/blood-2018-06-846816. Epub 2018 Aug13.
55. Nates LJ, Price JK. Oncologic critical care [e-book], 1st edition. Cham Switzerland: Springer International Publishing; 2020 [Cited 2021 April 12]. pp. 1147–54. Available from http://93.174.95.29/main/4206DCE99287433B8AB4C9ECC4B4D3.
56. Cuttner J, Conjalika MS, Reilly M, Goldberg J, Reisman A, Meyer RJ, et al. Association of monocytic leukemia in patients with extreme leukocytosis. Am J Med. 1980 Oct;69(4):555–8. https://doi.org/10.1016/0002-9343(80)90467-2.

57. Goldstone AH, Richards SM, Lazarus HM, Tallman MS, Buck G, Fielding AK et al. In adults with standard-risk acute lymphoblastic leukemia, the greatest benefit is achieved from a matched sibling allogeneic transplantation in first complete remission, and an autologous transplantation is less effective than conventional consolidation/maintainence chemotherapy in all patients: final results of the international ALL trial (MRC UKALL XII/ECOG E2993). Blood 2008 Feb 15;111(4):1827–1833. https://doi.org/10.1182/blood-2007-10-116582. Epub 2007 Nov 29.
58. Johansson B, Moorman AV, Haas OA, Watmore AE, Cheung KL, Swanton S, et al. Hematologic malignancies with t(4;11)(q21;q23)-- a cytogenetic, morphologic, immunophenotypic and clinical study of 183 cases. European11q23 workshop participants. Leukemia. 1998 May;12(5):779–87. https://doi.org/10.1038/sj.leu.2401012.
59. Padmanabhan A, Smith CL, Aqui N, Balogen AR, Klingel R, Meyer E, et al. Guidelines on the use of therapeutic apheresis in clinical practice- evidence based approach from the writing Committee of the American Society for apheresis: the eight special issue. J Clin Apher. 2019 Jun;34(3):171–354. https://doi.org/10.1002/jca.21705.
60. Ganzel C, Becker J, Mintz PD, Lazarus HM, Rowe JM. Hyperleuckocytosis, leukostasis and leukapheresis: practice management. Blood Rev. 2012 May;26(3):117–22. https://doi.org/10.1016/j.blre.2012.01.003.
61. Al-Qurainy R, Collis E. Metastatic spinal cord compression: diagnosis and management. BMJ. 2016 May 19;353:i2539. https://doi.org/10.1136/bmj.i2539.
62. Byrne TN. Spinal cord compression from epidural metastases. N Engl J Med. 1992 Aug 27;327(9):614–9. https://doi.org/10.1056/NEJM199208273270907.
63. Boussios S, Cooke D, Hayward C, Kanellos FS, Tsiouris AK, Chatziantoniou AA, et al. Metastatic spinal cord compression: unravelling the diagnostic and therapeutic challenges. Anticancer Res. 2018 Sep;38(9):4987–97. https://doi.org/10.21873/anticanres.1817.
64. Metastatic spinal cord compression review – Nice guidelines http://pathways.nice.org.uk/pathways/metastatic-spinal-cord-compression. Last updated - 4 November 2020.
65. Kumar A, Weber MH, Gokaslan Z, Wolinsky JP, Schimdt M, Rhines L. Metastatic spinal cord compression and steroid treatment: a systemic review. Clin Spine Surg. 2017;30(4):156–63. https://doi.org/10.1097/BSD.0000000000000528.
66. Loblaw A, George KJ, Misra V. Surgical and radiotherapeutic management of malignant extradural spinal cord compression. Clin Oncol (R Coll Radiol) 2020 Nov;32(11):745–752. https://doi.org/10.1016/j.clon.2020.07.022. Epub 2020 Aug 19.
67. Lawton AJ, Lee KA, Cheville AL, Ferrone ML, Rades D, Balboni TA et al. Assessment and management of patients with metastatic spinal cord compression: a multidisciplinary review. J Clin Oncol 2019 Jan 1;37(1):61–71. https://doi.org/10.1200/JCO.2018.78.1211. Epub 2018.

Tumour Lysis Syndrome

30

Shalabh Arora and Ajay Gogia

30.1 Introduction

Tumor lysis syndrome (TLS) is one of the most common oncologic emergencies. It is caused by the inability of the body's homeostatic mechanisms to handle the massive release of intracellular contents (potassium, phosphate and nucleic acids) from disintegrating tumor cells into the blood stream. Catabolism of nucleic acids to uric acid leads to urate deposition in renal tubules, resulting in acute kidney injury (AKI) and its associated complications. These metabolic disturbances can lead to clinical toxic effects including cardiac arrhythmia, seizures, multi organ dysfunction and death. This chapter outlines the epidemiology, risk factors, clinical features and principles of preventing and managing TLS.

30.2 Epidemiology

While TLS typically develops after the initiation of cytotoxic chemotherapy in patients with high grade hematological malignancies like aggressive non-Hodgkin's lymphoma (e.g., Burkitt's lymphoma) and acute lymphoblastic or myeloid leukemias, it may occur with any tumor type with rapidly proliferating component, large tumor burden or high sensitivity to cytotoxic agents [1, 2].

S. Arora · A. Gogia (✉)
Department of Medical Oncology, AIIMS, Delhi, India

V. Kumar et al. (eds.), *Onco-critical Care*,
https://doi.org/10.1007/978-981-16-9929-0_30

30.3 Etiopathogenesis

When cytotoxic therapy is initiated for a chemotherapy sensitive malignancy, particularly one with a large disease burden or rapid proliferation, there is rapid cell lysis, with release of intracellular contents (nucleic acids, potassium and phosphate) into the bloodstream. The nucleic acids are catabolized into hypoxanthine, xanthine and then to uric acid by the enzyme xanthine oxidase (Fig. 30.1). Uric acid has a pKa of 5.4–5.7 and is poorly soluble in water. Under physiological conditions, approximately 500 mg of uric acid is excreted by the kidneys daily. With rapid tumor cell lysis, uric acid precipitates into crystals in the acidic environment of the distal renal tubules and collecting system of the kidney. Deposition of urate crystals in the renal tubules leads to acute uric acid nephropathy with AKI. When allopurinol is administered for TLS prophylaxis and/or management, it blocks the catabolism of hypoxanthine and xanthine, leading to an increase in the levels of these metabolites, with the latter being much less soluble than uric acid. Additionally, as opposed to uric acid, the solubility of xanthine is not enhanced significantly by urinary alkalinization due to a much higher pKa (7.4 versus 5.8). Thus, patients with rapid tumor lysis who are receiving allopurinol are at risk for xanthine precipitation in the tubules, resulting in xanthine nephropathy or xanthine stone formation. Rasburicase, on the other hand, has a different downstream mechanism of action from allopurinol, and does not increase xanthine levels in the blood.

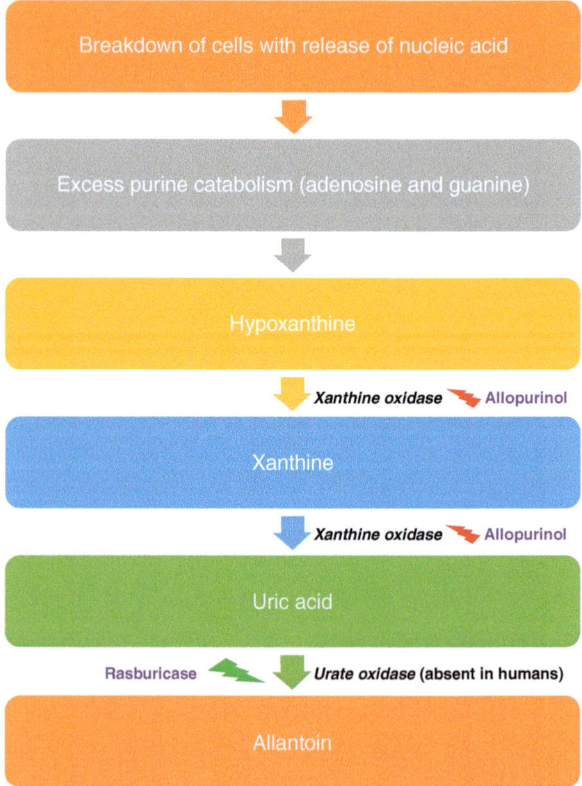

Fig. 30.1 Etiopathogenesis of tumour lysis syndrome

Rapid tumor cell lysis also leads to hyperphosphatemia since phosphorus concentration in malignant cells is significantly higher than in normal cells. Initially the kidneys respond by increased phosphate excretion and reduced tubular reabsorption of phosphorus but eventually the increased renal excretion is overwhelmed, and serum phosphorus levels rise. This hyperphosphatemia leads to calcium phosphate precipitation with secondary hypocalcemia. The risk of calcium phosphate deposition in renal tubules (nephrocalcinosis) with consequent AKI is particularly high when the calcium phosphate product (calcium concentration × phosphate concentration) is more than 60 mg^2/dL^2. Renal replacement therapy is often needed when calcium phosphate product is ≥70 mg^2/dL^2. Precipitation of calcium phosphate in the heart may lead to cardiac arrhythmias. Since the widespread use of hypouricemic agents, nephrocalcinosis has replaced hyperuricemia as the major mechanism of acute kidney injury in TLS.

Massive release of intracellular potassium may also exceed renal clearance capacity and lead to hyperkalemia, which is further accentuated by renal failure. This rapid rise in serum potassium leads to cardiac arrhythmias and may be life threatening.

30.4 Clinical Features

The clinical features associated with TLS stem from the associated metabolic abnormalities (hyperkalemia, hyperphosphatemia, and hypocalcemia). They include nausea, vomiting, anorexia, lethargy, hematuria, heart failure, edema, cardiac dysrhythmias, seizures, muscle cramps, tetany, syncope, and possible sudden death. Though uncommon, acute uric acid or calcium phosphate deposition with renal pelvic or ureteral stone formation can lead to flank pain. Urinalysis shows rectangular or rhomboid uric acid crystals.

Cairo and Bishop proposed a definition for TLS in 2004 along with a grading for clinical severity—these are the most widely used criteria to diagnose and classify TLS [3]. Laboratory TLS is defined by a 25% change from baseline or levels above or below normal for serum values of at least two parameters out of serum uric acid, potassium, phosphorus or calcium within 3 days prior and up to 7 days after initiating therapy (Table 30.1). Clinical TLS is defined by the presence of laboratory TLS in addition to one or more of the following that is not attributable to a therapeutic agent: increased serum creatinine, cardiac arrhythmia/sudden death or seizure (Table 30.2).

Table 30.1 Cairo-Bishop definition of laboratory tumor lysis syndrome

Uric acid	≥8 mg/dL or 25% increase from baseline
Potassium	≥6.0 mmol/L or 25% increase from baseline
Phosphorus	≥2.1 mmol/L (children), ≥1.45 mmol/L (adults) or 25% increase from baseline
Calcium	≤7.0 mg/dL or 25% decrease from baseline

Tumor lysis syndrome is defined by the presence of two or more of these criteria

Table 30.2 Cairo-Bishop definition and grading of clinical tumor lysis syndrome[a]

	Grade					
Complication	0	1	2	3	4	5
Creatinine	≤1.5 × ULN	1.5 × ULN	>1.5–3.0 × ULN	>3.0–6.0 × ULN	>6.0 × ULN	Death
Cardiac arrhythmia / sudden death	None	Intervention not indicated	Nonurgent medical intervention indicated	Symptomatic and incompletely controlled medically or controlled with device (e.g., defibrillator)	Life-threatening (e.g., arrhythmia associated with CHF, hypotension, syncope, shock)	Death
Seizure	None	–	One brief generalised seizure; seizure(s) well controlled by anti-convulsants or infrequent focal motor seizures not interfering with ADL	Seizure in which consciousness is altered; poorly controlled seizure disorder, with breakthrough generalized seizures despite medical intervention	Seizure of any kind which are prolonged, repetitive or difficult to control (e.g., status epilepticus, intractable epilepsy)	Death

[a]Clinical tumor lysis syndrome is defined by the presence of laboratory TLS plus at least one clinical complication

30.5 Risk Factors and Predictors of TLS

The most crucial aspect in management of TLS is identification of patients who are at high risk of developing it—so that prophylactic measures can be instituted before initiation of therapy and any abnormality may be promptly acted upon. Patients with one or more of the following factors are at relatively high risk of developing TLS and warrant some form of prophylaxis to mitigate the risk:

Patient Related Risk Factors

(a) Pretreatment hyperuricemia or hyperphosphatemia
(b) Pre-existing renal dysfunction
(c) Oliguria and/or acidic urine
(d) Dehydration or volume depletion

Tumor-Related Risk Factors

(a) Inherent chemotherapy sensitivity of the tumor
(b) High proliferation rate—lactate dehydrogenase is a surrogate for tumor proliferation
(c) Large tumor volume as evidenced by large tumor size (>10 cm), white cell count > 50,000 per cu mm, organ infiltration, extensive metastases or bone marrow involvement
(d) Renal infiltration or outflow tract obstruction

Patients with aggressive lymphomas and acute leukemias with high cell counts are also at risk of spontaneous TLS even without initiation of therapy—these patients should be recommended aggressive hydration and considered for TLS prophylactic agents even while full diagnostic work-up is underway.

Treatment-Related Risk Factors

(a) Intensity of anticancer therapy (multidrug regimens)
(b) Specific targeted agents e.g., venetoclax and obinutuzumab for chronic lymphocytic leukemia
(c) Exposure to nephrotoxins (e.g., concomitant vancomycin or aminoglycosides or contrast agents)
(d) Suboptimal fluid administration during therapy
(e) Exogenous potassium or phosphorus

Few highly effective targeted anticancer agents have recently entered the treatment landscape of certain malignancies, leading to an increase in frequency and severity of TLS in conditions that were previously only rarely associated with it. For example, venetoclax, a B-cell lymphoma 2 (BCL2) inhibitor initially used in CLL and with expanding indications, may lead to TLS in up to 13% of patients [4]. This high incidence of TLS in CLL patients with high tumor burden has led to a separate risk stratification and TLS prophylaxis system based on largest lymph node diameter and absolute lymphocyte count [5]. Similarly, high incidence of TLS has been observed with the use of anti-CD20 monoclonal antibody Obinutuzumab, cyclin-dependent kinase inhibitors dinaciclib and alvocidib, and chimeric antigen receptor T-cell therapy for lymphoid malignancies.

An expert panel on TLS was convened in 2008 to formulate evidence-based guidelines on TLS risk stratification and prophylaxis [6]. After an extensive review of all published literature on TLS (spanning almost half a century), the panel proposed a risk stratification system based on the type of tumor, tumor proliferation markers, burden of disease, expected response to treatment and renal/electrolyte impairment at the time of TLS diagnosis. It must be borne in mind that these criteria were arrived upon by expert consensus after review of literature and have not been prospectively validated.

30.6 Prevention of Tumor Lysis Syndrome

The management of established TLS is often difficult and resource intensive—hence all efforts must be made to identify patients at high risk of TLS early and institute preventive measures to prevent clinical TLS. There are two main strategies to prevent TLS—aggressive intravenous (IV) hydration and hypouricemic agents (allopurinol or recombinant urate oxidase). The specific type of prophylaxis depends on the risk category as ascertained using factors enumerated in Table 30.3.

(a) ***Laboratory monitoring***—Individuals at high risk of developing TLS should have their serum levels of uric acid, potassium, phosphate, calcium, creatinine and lactate dehydrogenase monitored every 4–6 h after initiation of therapy. Fluid intake and urine output should also be accurately recorded. Monitoring should be continued for approximately 24 h after the last dose of chemotherapy.

(b) ***IV hydration***—The goal of IV hydration is to improve renal perfusion and glomerular filtration to ensure high urine flow rate which in turn prevents uric acid or calcium phosphate precipitation in renal tubules. The recommended volume in adults and children is 2–3 L/m^2 body surface area per day with a target urine output of 80–100 mL/m^2/h [7]. For children weighing less than 10 kg, IV fluids should be administered at 200 mL/kg/day, with a target urine output of 4–6 mL/kg/h. Though guidelines recommend one quarter normal saline/5% dextrose solution as the fluid to be used, normal saline may be used interchangeably. Potassium, calcium and phosphate should be withheld from IV fluids initially due to the potential electrolyte disturbances in patients at risk for TLS. IV hydrations should be continued until tumor burden is resolved, there is no evidence of tumor lysis and the patient is able to maintain sufficient oral hydration. Patients with pre-existing renal or cardiac dysfunction are at risk of volume overload from hyperhydration and must be monitored closely for fluid status and urine output—diuretics may be used as required. In patients whose urine output remains low despite optimal hydration, a loop diuretic e.g., furosemide may be used to ensure a urine flow rate of at least 2 mL/kg/h. Loop diuretics are preferable to other diuretics as they also cause potassium excretion.

Table 30.3 Risk stratification for development of tumor lysis syndrome

Low risk (TLS incidence > 5%)	Intermediate risk (TLS incidence 1–5%)	High risk (TLS incidence <1%)
Most solid tumors	Highly chemotherapy-sensitive tumors e.g., neuroblastoma, germ cell tumor, small cell lung cancer, other cancers with bulky and advanced stage disease	N/A
Multiple myeloma	Plasma cell leukemia	N/A
Indolent NHL	N/A	N/A
Hodgkin lymphoma	N/A	N/A
CLL and WBC <50 × 10⁹/L treated only with alkylating agents	CLL treated with fludarabine, rituximab, or lenalidomide, or venetoclax and lymph node ≥5 cm *or* absolute lymphocyte count ≥25 × 10⁹/L, and/or those with high WBC ≥50 × 10⁹/L	CLL treated with venetoclax and lymph node ≥10 cm, *or* lymph node ≥5 cm *and* absolute lymphocyte count ≥25 × 10⁹/L and elevated baseline uric acid
AML and WBC <25 × 10⁹/L and LDH <2 × ULN	AML with WBC 25–100 × 10⁹/L or AML with WBC <25 × 10⁹/L and LDH ≥2 × ULN	AML and WBC ≥100 × 10⁹/L
Adult intermediate grade NHL and LDH within normal limits	Adult T cell leukemia/lymphoma, diffuse large B-cell, transformed, and mantle cell lymphomas with LDH > ULN, non-bulky	Adult T cell leukemia/lymphoma, diffuse large B-cell, transformed, and mantle cell lymphomas with bulky disease and LDH ≥2 × ULN
Adult ALCL	Childhood ALCL stage III/IV	N/A
N/A	Childhood intermediate grade NHL stage III/IV with LDH <2 × ULN	Stage III/IV childhood diffuse large B-cell lymphoma with LDH ≥2 × ULN
N/A	ALL and WBC <100 × 10⁹/L and LDH <2 × ULN	Burkitt's leukemia or Other ALL and WBC ≥100 × 10⁹/L and/or LDH ≥2 × ULN
N/A	Burkitt lymphoma and LDH <2 × ULN	Burkitt lymphoma stage III/IV and/or LDH ≥2 × ULN
N/A	Lymphoblastic lymphoma stage I/II and LDH <2 × ULN	Lymphoblastic lymphoma stage III/IV and/or LDH ≥2 × ULN
N/A	N/A	Intermediate risk disease with renal dysfunction and/or renal involvement or with renal dysfunction and/or renal involvement
Recommended prophylaxis		
Monitoring	Monitoring	Monitoring
Hydration	Hydration	Hydration
± Allopurinol	Allopurinol	Rasburicase

NHL Non-Hodgkin's lymphoma, *CLL* chronic lymphocytic leukemia, *WBC* white blood cells, *ALL* acute lymphoblastic leukemia, *AML* acute myeloid leukemia, *LDH* lactate dehydrogenase, *ULN* upper limit of normal, *ALCL* anaplastic large cell lymphoma

(c) ***Urine alkalinization*** to promote excretion of uric acid is not recommended as it is not backed by good quality evidence and may conversely increase the risk of calcium phosphate precipitation in the kidney and heart. Also, patients receiving rasburicase do not need urinary alkalinization. Sodium bicarbonate may, however, be used in cases of metabolic acidosis.

(d) ***Hypouricemic agents***—Allopurinol is a hypoxanthine analog that competitively inhibits xanthine oxidase, interfering with the metabolism of hypoxanthine and xanthine to uric acid (Fig. 30.1). A drawback of allopurinol is that inhibition of metabolism of these purine precursors may lead to xanthinuria with xanthine crystals being deposited in the renal tubules and worsening of AKI. However, it is widely used due to easily availability, low cost and ease of oral administration. One major limitation of allopurinol is that it only prevents new uric acid formation but has no effect on preexisting serum uric acid. For patients with pre-existing hyperuricemia (≥8 mg/dL), rasburicase is the preferred hypouricemic agent. The recommended dose is 100 mg/m^2 every 8 h (maximum 800 mg/day) in adults and 10 mg/kg/day in three divided doses for children. Treatment with allopurinol is usually started 24–48 h before cytotoxic therapy and continued until resolution of laboratory TLS. In cases of pre-existing AKI, the dose must be reduced by half for concerns of accumulation of allopurinol and purine metabolites.

Recombinant urate oxidase (rasburicase) is the preferred hypouricemic agent for children and adults at high risk for TLS. Urate oxidase is an enzyme present in most mammals but not in humans; it promotes the degradation of uric acid to the much more water-soluble compound allantoin (Fig. 30.1). Rasburicase is well tolerated and highly effective at rapid breakdown of pre-accumulated uric acid—in contrast to allopurinol, which only decreases new uric acid formation. When compared to allopurinol, rasburicase has demonstrated clear superiority in reduction of morbidity and laboratory TLS in both children and adults at high risk of TLS. The recommended dose of rasburicase is 0.2 mg/kg/day for high risk patients (serum uric acid ≥8 mg/dL) and 0.15 mg/kg/day for intermediate risk patients (serum uric acid <8 mg/dL), typically administered once daily for 5–7 days. However, a single dose of rasburicase 0.05–0.2 mg/kg was found to be as effective as prolonged dosing, with major economic benefit, and is practised at many institutions [8]. Importantly, rasburicase is contraindicated in patients with glucose-6-phosphatedehydrogenase (G6PD) deficiency as hydrogen peroxide, a breakdown product of uric acid, can cause methemoglobinemia and, in severe cases, hemolytic anemia.

30.7 Treatment of Established Tumor Lysis Syndrome

Patients who develop TLS despite prophylactic measures or spontaneously should undergo continuous cardiac monitoring and measurement of serum electrolytes, uric acid and creatinine every 4–6 h. Management of these cases includes intensive hydration with or without loop diuretics, treatment of specific electrolyte abnormalities per standard guidelines and the use of rasburicase if not already initiated.

(a) Hyperkalemia can cause cardiac dysrhythmias and sudden death. Glucose plus insulin or beta-mimetic agents can be used for transcellular potassium shift as a temporary measure. Calcium gluconate can be administered to reduce the risk of cardiac dysrhythmia. Oral potassium lowering agents e.g., sodium polystyrene sulfonate should be used, and renal replacement may be needed in refractory cases.
(b) Hyperphosphatemia can be managed with aggressive hydration and phosphate binders e.g., sevelamer hydrochloride or lanthanum carbonate.
(c) Hypocalcemia should be treated only if symptomatic (cardiac arrhythmia or tetany), and at the lowest dose needed to relieve symptoms in order to avoid calcium phosphate precipitation.

Renal replacement therapy may be needed in cases of electrolyte dysregulation that is refractory to medical management—the indications are generally similar to those in patients with other causes of AKI.

30.8 Key Points

Tumor lysis syndrome (TLS) is a rare but potentially life-threatening complication of highly proliferative or chemotherapy-sensitive cancers—most commonly hematological malignancies. Early identification of risk factors such as type of malignancy, chemotherapy regimen and age, followed by prompt institution of appropriate TLS prophylaxis can be life-saving. Vigorous hydration, fluid balance, electrolytes and hyperuricemia correction form the cornerstone of managing TLS.

References

1. Hande KR, Garrow GC. Acute tumor lysis syndrome in patients with high-grade non-Hodgkin's lymphoma. Am J Med. 1993;94(2):133–9.
2. Jeha S, Kantarjian H, Irwin D, Shen V, Shenoy S, Blaney S, et al. Efficacy and safety of rasburicase, a recombinant urate oxidase (Elitek), in the management of malignancy-associated hyperuricemia in pediatric and adult patients: final results of a multicenter compassionate use trial. Leukemia. 2005;19(1):34–8.
3. Cairo MS, Bishop M. Tumour lysis syndrome: new therapeutic strategies and classification. Br J Haematol. 2004;127(1):3–11.
4. Koehler AB, Leung N, Call TG, Rabe KG, Achenbach SJ, Ding W, et al. Incidence and risk of tumor lysis syndrome in patients with relapsed chronic lymphocytic leukemia (CLL) treated with venetoclax in routine clinical practice. Leuk Lymphoma. 2020;61(10):2383–8.
5. Seymour JF, Kipps TJ, Eichhorst B, Hillmen P, D'Rozario J, Assouline S, et al. Venetoclax–Rituximab in relapsed or refractory chronic lymphocytic leukemia. N Engl J Med. 2018;378(12):1107–20.

6. Cairo MS, Coiffier B, Reiter A, Younes A. Recommendations for the evaluation of risk and prophylaxis of tumour lysis syndrome (TLS) in adults and children with malignant diseases: an expert TLS panel consensus. Br J Haematol. 2010;149(4):578–86.
7. Coiffier B, Altman A, Pui C-H, Younes A, Cairo MS. Guidelines for the management of pediatric and adult tumor lysis syndrome: an evidence-based review. J Clin Oncol. 2008;26(16):2767–78.
8. Feng X, Dong K, Pham D, Pence S, Inciardi J, Bhutada NS. Efficacy and cost of single-dose rasburicase in prevention and treatment of adult tumour lysis syndrome: a meta-analysis. J Clin Pharm Ther. 2013;38(4):301–8.

Critical Care in Paediatric Tumours

31

Shuvadeep Ganguly and Deepam Pushpam

31.1 Overview

Pediatric oncology is a success story of modern medicine with long term survival of children with cancer currently exceeding 80% in most developed countries [1]. Much of this success is driven by advances in supportive care. One in three childhood cancer patients require critical care support during their treatment [2–4]. The outcome of pediatric cancer patients requiring intensive care have improved over the years but it still continues to remain modest [5]. There is also a survival gap between high income and low-middle income countries, part of which is due to lack of timely and proper critical care support. Hence, multi-disciplinary co-ordination is necessary to manage sick children with cancer [6].

Children with cancer require critical care either due disease related or due to treatment related complications. The common indications for intensive care admission include respiratory failure (26–58% cases), sepsis/septic shock (8–36%), neuro-oncological emergencies (10–31%), renal failure (5–15%) and tumor lysis syndrome (5–8%) [2, 6]. The etiological factors are summarized in Table 31.1. The management principles of most oncological emergencies remain same for children, however, the approach to etiology and certain aspects of management strategies differ from adults. In this chapter, the commonly encountered pediatric oncological scenarios requiring urgent critical care support are described i.e. hyperleukocytosis, tumor lysis syndrome (TLS), superior vena cava syndrome/superior mediastinal syndrome (SVCS/SMS), neuro-oncological emergency like malignant spinal cord compression with special focus on management issues specific to children.

S. Ganguly · D. Pushpam (✉)
Department of Medical Oncology, Dr. B.R.A. Institute Rotary Cancer Hospital, AIIMS, New Delhi, India

V. Kumar et al. (eds.), *Onco-critical Care*,
https://doi.org/10.1007/978-981-16-9929-0_31

Table 31.1 Common oncological emergencies in pediatric age group

Scenario	Common etiologies
A. **Malignancy related complications**	
1. Hyperleukocytosis	• Acute myeloid leukemia • Acute lymphoblastic leukemia • Chronic myeloid leukemia
2. Tumor lysis syndrome	• Burkitts lymphoma/leukemia • Acute lymphoblasicleukemia • Lymphoblastic lymphoma • High grade non Hodgkin lymphoma • Solid tumors (neuroblastoma, germ cell tumor)
3. Superior vena cava syndrome	• Non-Hodgkin lymphoma • Acute lymphoblastic lymphoma / leukemia • Neuroblastoma • Germ cell tumor
4. Malignant spinal cord compression	• Non Hodgkin lymphoma • Neuroblastoma • Rhabdomyosarcoma
5. Raised intracranial pressure	• Leukemic/lymphomatous infiltration of central nervous system • Intracranial extension of rhabdomyosarcoma, neuroblastoma • Medulloblastoma
B. **Treatment related complications**	
1. Infectious complications	• Febrile neutropenia
2. Cardiac complications	• Anthracyclines • High dose cyclophosphamide • Ifosfamide • Mediastinal radiation
3. Pulmonary toxicity	• Bleomycin • Thoracic radiation • Differentiation syndrome (ATRA) • Carmustine
4. Hemorrhagic cystitis	• Ifosafmide • Cyclophosphamide • Busulfan • Thiotepa
5. Hepatic dysfunction	• 6-Mercaptopurine • Methotrexate • Actinomycin-D • Cytarabine (high dose) • Busulfan
6. Renal dysfunction	• Platinum compounds • Methotrexate • Clofarabine • Cyclophosphamide/Ifosfamide
7. Neurological dysfunction	• Ifosfamide (encephalopathy) • Methotrexate (high dose) • ATRA (Pseudotumor cerebri) • Busulfan (seizure) • Central venous thrombosis (L-Asparaginase)
8. Pancreatitis	• L-Asparaginase

ATRA All-trans retinoic acid

31.2 Management of Common Pediatric Oncological Emergencies

31.2.1 Hyperleukocytosis

Hyperleukocytosis is defined as peripheral blood leukocyte count exceeding 1×10^5/μl, however, often symptomatic hyperleukocytosis may be observed even in lower counts. Hyperleukocytosis is observed in between 5 and 22% of childhood leukemias. It is more common in hypodiploid or infant/ MLL (mixed lineage leukemia) rearrangedacute lymphoblastic leukemia (ALL), and in French American British (FAB) subtype M4/5 or FLT3-ITD$^+$(Fms like tyrosine kinase 3-internal tandem duplication)acute myeloid leukemia (AML) [7, 8].

Clinical presentation: Hyperleukocytosis is often an incidental finding but symptomatic hyperleukocytosis may be observed in patients with counts >2×10^5/μl in AML and counts >3×10^5/μl in ALL. Lung and central nervous system (CNS) are commonly affected. Children may present with altered sensorium, irritability, blurred vision, seizures along with respiratory distress and hypoxia. Besides, bleeding manifestations including CNS bleeds, gastrointestinal bleeding, dactylitis, priapism may be observed. Concomitant metabolic derangement due to TLS with/ without renal failure may complicate the presentation [7, 9]. Incidence of symptomatic hyperleukocytosis is more common in AML than ALL [10].

The pathophysiology of clinical presentation in hyperleukocytosis is multifactorial. The most common aetiology is due to increase in blood viscosity, which contributes to leukostasis with thrombus formation and tissue hypoxia. Myeloblasts being larger in size, cause more symptomatic hyperleukocytosis. However, interaction of leukemic blasts with adhesion molecules expressed in endothelium also contributes to leukostasis [11]. Associated disseminated intravascular coagulation exacerbates the bleeding manifestations [7].

Management: The management of hyperleukocytosis is directed towards aggressive hydration to cause hemodilution along with supportive care to prevent TLS. With prompt establishment of diagnosis by immunophenotyping, it is also important to initiat chemotherapy if the child is stable.

(a) **Fluid management**: The recommended fluid remains potassium and calcium free N/2 5% dextrose at double the daily maintenance fluid requirement (3 l/m^2/day or 200 ml/kg/day for weight < 10 kg) with goal to maintain urine output ≥4 ml/kg/hr. for <1 year of age or ≥ 100 ml/m^2/hr. for older children. Aggressive hydration should be avoided in setting of severe anemia and/or congestive cardiac failure where 70–100% of daily maintenance may be attempted. Diuretics should be primarily avoided unless clinically indicated due to fluid overload/ congestive cardiac failure [7, 9].

(b) **Prevention of TLS**: Prevention of TLS is an important component of management of hyperleukocytosis and its management is discussed in detail separately. All patients should receive allopurinol, rasburicase is added in patients at high risk and established TLS along with regular monitoring and management of electrolyte abnormalities.

(c) **Blood product transfusion**: Platelet transfusion should be liberal as it does not increase blood viscosity. The target should be above 20,000/μl or above 50,000/μl in presence of coagulopathy to prevent CNS bleed. On the other hand, transfusion of packed red blood cells should be cautious and should be avoided as long as hemoglobin (Hb) is in 7–8 g/dl range and in any case, Hb > 10 g/dl should be avoided [7]. Monitoring of coagulation parameters are essential and correction of any coagulation abnormalities should be done with 10–15 ml/kg of fresh frozen plasma [9].

(d) **Definitive treatment***:* The definite therapy for hyperleukocytosis is to initiate chemotherapy as soon as possible. For ALL, after metabolic stabilization and hydration, initiation of steroids as per protocol is appropriate. In case of AML, as long as there are no contraindications for intensive treatment, it is important to promptly start induction therapy with standard/high dose cytarabine with/without anthracyclines [9, 12].

Hydroxyurea/low dose chemotherapy like cytarabine are commonly used to reduce tumor burden before initiation of definite therapy, however, there is lack of evidence of any benefit of this approach [13]. It may be restricted only in children not suitable for intensive treatment.

(e) **Role of leukapheresis/exchange transfusion***:* Leukapheresis is highly effective in reducing peripheral blood TLC burden by 20–50% in a single session. However, use of leukapheresis also failed to show any survival benefit and it may be restricted to those with symptomatic leukostasis [7, 9, 13, 14].

Exchange transfusion is an option for children with hyperleukocytosis with severe anemia. It is more suited for infants and younger children.It is carried out with packed red blood cells and plasma (2–3:1), with platelet supplementation and a recommended volume of 70–150 mL/kg, with an aim to reduce the blastsby at least 50% [9]. Similar to leukapheresis, while it has no demonstrated any survival benefit, but it may be considered in symptomatic and anemic younger children with leukostasis.

31.2.2 Tumor Lysis Syndrome

Tumor lysis syndrome (TLS) is a syndrome of metabolic derangements occurring due to lysis of malignant cells. TLS is often silent and reflected in laboratory values alone which is known as "Laboratory TLS". The exact incidence of laboratory TLS is anywhere between 42% in high grade NHL to 70% in acute leukemia, but clinically significant TLS occurs only in about 3% of cases [15].

TLS have been defined classically by Cairo and Bishop [16], which has been adopted for children as well [17]. The definition is summarized in Table 31.2. TLS is seen commonly after initiation of cytotoxic chemotherapy although spontaneous TLS is also seen especially in Burkitt's lymphoma and ALL [18].

Risk factors: TLS is more likely to occur in tumors with more bulk of disease and those with rapid proliferation rate and also in patients with already compromised renal function and deranged electrolytes. While TLS is observed in

Table 31.2 Definition of Tumor lysis syndrome (TLS) [16]

Laboratory TLS: Two or more of the following laboratory abnormalities within 3 days before to 7 days after initiation of chemotherapy		
Parameter	Value	Change from baseline
• Uric acid	>8 mg/dl or above the upper limit of normal Range for age in children	25% increase from baseline
• Potassium	>6.0 mEq/L	25% increase from baseline
• Phosphate	>6.5 mg/dl (for children)	25% increase from baseline
• Calcium	Corrected calcium <7.0 mg/dl or ionized calcium <1.12 mmol/l	25% decrease from baseline
Clinical tumor lysis syndrome: Laboratory TLS + any one of the below:		
• Kidney involvement: Increase in creatining by 0.3 mg/dl or value >1.5 times the upper limit of the age-appropriate normal range or oliguria (<0.5 ml/kg/hr. for 6 h) • Neurological: Seizure • Cardiac: Arrhythmia, death		

hematological malignancies, it is also observed in aggressive solid malignancies like germ cell tumor, neuroblastoma.

The following risk stratification is commonly used to identify children at higher risk of developing TLS [17, 19].

- **High risk:** Burkitt's lymphoma, Lymphoblastic lymphoma, ALL with TLC > 10^5/µl, AML monoblastic or TLC > 50,000/µl.
- **Intermediate risk:** ALL with count between 50,000/µl and 10^5/µl, AML with TLC between 20,000 and 50,000/µl
- **Low risk:** Other solid malignancies.

Pathophysiology and clinical features: Lysis of tumor cells causes release of intracellular contents in blood stream like potassium, phosphate as well as purines which metabolizes to uric acid [19]. In setting of hyperuricemia and hyperphosphatemia, there is increased chance of deposition of urate crystals and calcium phosphate crystals in renal tubules which may precipitate renal failure. On the other hand, hyperkalemia is itself life-threatening due to cardiac arrhythmias.

Clinically, TLS is often asymptomatic or may have non-specific symptoms like abdominal pain, anorexia, vomiting, irritability. Presence of electrocardiogram changes, tetany/seizure or oligo-anuria are ominous signs of established TLS [17, 20, 21].

Management: The management strategy of TLS is aimed towards in prevention of development of clinical TLS with appropriate prophylactic measure in high-risk cases. Definite chemotherapy needs to be delayed or withheld till stabilization to prevent exacerbation of the metabolic derangements.

(a) **Fluid management:** All patients deemed to be at intermediate/high risk for developing TLS should be started aggressive intravenous hydration with potassium and calcium free fluid at double the daily maintenance requirement as mentioned above in setting of hyperleukocytosis [17, 19]. Cautious use of diuretic may be considered to maintain adequate urine output >2 ml/kg/hr. Urine specific gravity should be <1.010. For established TLS, it is prudent to initially start with double hydration, however, renal replacement therapy should be considered at the earliest.

(b) **Urine alkalinization:** Urine alkalinization have been previously used in TLS to facilitate dissolution of uric acid, however, it leads to formation of xanthine and calcium phosphate crystals. It may further worsen nephropathy. Hence, urine alkalinization is not recommended in TLS [20].

(c) **Hyperuricemia:** For prophylactic purpose, children with intermediate and high risk for TLS should receive allopurinol at dose of 250–300 mg/m^2/day (in 2–3 divided doses). Allopurinol dose should be reduced to 50% in renal impairment [17, 19]. Children at high risk and established TLS should additionally receive recombinant urate oxidase (rasburicase) at recommended dose of 0.1 mg/kg/day for 5 days. Use of a single dose of rasburicase is also an equally effective option [22].

(d) **Hyperkalemia:** For potassium >6 mEq/l, children should be given regular insulin 0.1 IU/kg in 2 ml/kg of 25% dextrose. In presence of electrocardiogram changes, intravenous calcium gluconate (10%) 2 ml/kg should be infused over 20–30 min. Other options include use of potassium binding resins like Kayexalate (1 g/kg/dose q6-8h), use of sodium bicarbonate (1–2 mEq/kg intravenous infusion over 15–20 min) or salbutamol nebulization. Hyperkalemia refractory to above measures should be managed with hemodialysis [20, 21].

(e) **Hyperphosphatemia:** Serum phosphate >6.5 mEq/l is considered as hyperphosphatemia in children. It is important to ensure double maintenance hydration. Addition of oral phosphate binders (aluminium hydroxide or sevelamer) may be considered. Renal replacement therapy may be needed for refractory hyperphosphatemia [23].

(f) **Hypocalcemia:** TLS presents with hypocalcemia secondary to hypephosphatemia. For asymptomatic hypocalcemia, infusion of calcium is to be avoided to prevent calcium phosphate deposition. For symptomatic hypocalcemia or with electrocardiographic changes, intravenous infusion of 50–100 mg/kg of calcium gluconate should be done under cardiac monitoring [15].

(g) **Renal replacement therapy:** For established TLS and as well as refractory metabolic disturbances, renal replacement therapy should be sought at the earliest. Peritoneal dialysis is not effective, and it is preferable to do hemodialysis. For critically sick children, continuous hemofiltration is also an effective option [24].

31.2.3 Superior Vena Cava Syndrome and Superior Mediastinal Syndrome

Superior vena cava syndrome (SVCS) is a clinical syndrome caused by obstruction of superior vena cava; and the term superior mediastinal syndrome (SMS) is used when tracheal compression also co-exists [25]. SMS commonly co-exists in children with SVCS because of smaller chest volume and often these terms are thus used interchangeably.

SVCS is infrequently encountered in children; however, oncological cases remain one of the predominant etiologies [26]. In pediatric Non-Hodgkin lymphoma (NHL), it is seen in up to 6% of children [27]. The common etiologies are summarized in Table 31.3. It is also important to consider non-oncological etiologies in children with cancer because often multiple risk factors co-exist.

Clinical presentation: SVCS presents with predominantly with engorgement of veins of face and neck along with facial edema. Venous edema also causes airway edema which further exacerbates the airway compromise.

Children typically presents with cough/respiratory distress predominantly orthopnea along with lethargy/irritability and even confusion, headache due to cerebral edema [25].

Children with more aggressive disease like NHL/ALL are more likely to present with symptoms rather than disease like Hodgkin lymphoma where children may remain asymptomatic.

Management: SVCS/SMS in children differs from adults in terms of both etiology as well as management strategies. The broad aim of management is stabilization of the child along with prompt establishment of diagnosis.

(a) **Supportive care:** As soon as SVCS/SMS is suspected in a child, it is important to keep the child in head elevated position / sitting position to assist venous drainage with oxygen support and achieve intravenous access in lower limbs. The child must be started on maintenance intravenous fluids at least at 100% daily maintenance requirement (1.5 l/m^2/day) [25, 27, 28]. The fluid of choice is potassium and calcium free N/2 5% dextrose. Fluid rate may be increased to two-three times maintenance (3 l/m^2/day) in children in whom ALL/NHL is suspected along with prophylactic management/monitoring for TLS, as described above.
(b) **Avoidance of sedation:** Children with SVCS/SMS are at significantly high risk of sudden cardio-respiratory failure when administered any sedative/anesthetic agents. All such agents are to be avoided in any child suspected of SVCS/

Table 31.3 Common etiologies of superior vena cava syndrome in children

Oncological	Non oncological
• Non-Hodgkin lymphoma (T-lymphobastic lymphoma) • Acute lymphoblastic leukemia (T-acute lymphoblastic leukemia) • Neuroblastoma • Hodgkin lymphoma • Malignant germ cell tumor • Soft tissue sarcoma (Ewing's sarcoma) • Thymic tumors	• Infective or inflammatory (tubercular infection, fungal infection) • Congenital cardiac defects especially cyanotic heart diseases, post-operative • Central venous catheter related • Thrombophilia (inherited or acquired)

SMS [28]. Intubation is also to be avoided unless absolutely necessary as both intubation and weaning off ventilator is often difficult in such cases [29].

Investigations which need sedation/anesthesia in children (tissue biopsy, bone marrow aspiration/biopsy) should be deferred till symptomatic improvement.

(c) **Evaluation:** Beside history and general physical examination, it is important to obtain an urgent chest radiograph both postero-anterior and lateral view, which may demonstrate mediastinal widening along with tracheal compression. Complete blood count with peripheral smear, serum biochemistry including electrolytes and uric acid, serum lactate dehydrogenase (LDH), alpha fetoprotein (AFP), beta-human chorionic gonadotropin (βhCG) should be performed immediately. Pleural or pericardial fluid should be tapped for both diagnostic and therapeutic purposes. Fluid cytology may be diagnostic in case of NHL [28]. Bone marrow aspiration/biopsy may be carried out with local anesthesia in older children and may be diagnostic. If NHL is suspected and other investigations are non-contributory, fine needle aspiration from a peripheral lymph node may be carried out [25].

(d) **Steroid / cytoreductive therapy:** It is important to start steroid therapy as soon as SMS/SVCS is suspected [30]. Steroids decrease airway edema and also have rapid therapeutic effect on leukemia/lymphoma. Empirical steroid therapy is also reasonable. The dose of steroid is 6 mg/m^2/day of dexamethasone (divided q6-8h) or 5 mg/kg/dose of hydrocortisone q6h. Tissue biopsy should be obtained within 48 h of steroid therapy otherwise in a proportion of patients, histopathological diagnosis will be difficult to establish [31].

Other drugs which may be considered for empirical cytoreduction are cyclophosphamide (200 mg/m^2), vincristine (1–1.5 mg/m^2) or anthracyclines. These may be considered in life-threatening situations where rapid symptom improvement is essential [25, 32].

Definitive therapy should be started after confirmation of diagnosis. It is also important to monitor for tumor lysis after initiation of steroids/chemotherapy.

(e) **Radiation therapy:** Unlike adults, where radiation therapy plays a significant role in management of SVCS, there is no role of radiation therapy in management of SVCS/SMS of children [25].

31.2.4 Malignant Spinal Cord Compression

Malignant spinal cord compression is an uncommon neuro-oncological emergency in pediatric population occurring between 3 and 5% of children with cancer [33]. Often, the recognition is delayed but it is important to institute treatment at the earliest to preserve neurological outcome [34].

The common etiologies of malignant spinal cord compression in children is summarized in Table 31.4. Extradural tumors accounts for more than two-thirds of with neuroblastoma being the most common etiology [35].

Table 31.4 Common etiologies of malignant spinal cord compression in children:

Etiologies of malignant spinal cord compression in children		
Extradural	Intradural extramedullary	Intramedullary
• Neuroblastoma • Ewing's sarcoma • Soft tissue sarcoma • Lymphoma • Metastases	• Malignant peripheral nerve sheath tumor • Atypical teratoid/rhabdoid tumor • Medulloblastoma (drop metastases) • Rare (choroid plexus carcinoma, intracranial germ cell tumor)	• Ependymoma • Pilocytic astrocytoma • Glioma

Clinical presentation: Among children presenting with malignant spinal cord compression, it can be presenting feature for a newly diagnosed malignancy for about 75% of cases [35]. Motor deficit is the most common presenting feature followed by pain and sphincteric dysfunction. Infants and younger children may present late because signs are often missed by parents [36]. Contrast enhanced magnetic resonance imaging (MRI) of spine is diagnostic for all cases of spinal cord compression which should be done within 24 h of presentation.

Management: The management of the children presenting with cord compression should be aimed at instituting therapy immediately along with trying to establish etiology at the earliest.

While contrast enhanced MRI of spine can be diagnostic for intramedullary as well as extramedullary-intradural lesions with good enough certainty, for extradural lesions, it is appropriate to go ahead with an image guided biopsy at the earliest before instituting steroid therapy. Along with biopsy, investigations like complete blood count, peripheral smear, urinary metanephrines, serum LDH, AFP, βhCG and bone marrow aspiration/biopsy may be planned to establish diagnosis and for prognostic significance. Other imaging studies like MIBG (metaiodobenzylguanidine) scan, bone scan, contrast enhanced computed tomographic (CT) scan of chest should be planned as appropriate after stabilization [37].

(a) **Emergency steroid therapy***:* Steroid therapy should be initiated soon after biopsy or at the earliest if immediate biopsy is not feasible. There has been considerable variability regarding dose and schedule, although higher dose does not necessarily translate to better neurological recovery [38]. However, it is reasonable to start with a dose of 0.5–1 mg/kg of dexamethasone (maximum of 16 mg) intravenous followed by 0.15 mg/kg (maximum of 4 mg) every 6–8 hourly (maximum of 16 mg per day) to continue for 3 days and then rapid taper of over 2 weeks or as clinically indicated [37, 39].
(b) **Definitive therapy***:* Along with steroid therapy, it is also important to initiate definite therapy according to tumor type. For intramedullary as well as intradural extramedullary tumors, it is reasonable to go ahead with direct neurosurgical intervention with laminectomy for urgent cord decompression as well as obtaining gross tissue for histopathological examination.

For extramedullary tumors, which are chemotherapy sensitive like neuroblastoma/Ewing's sarcoma/germ cell tumor/lymphoma, instead of surgical intervention, it is reasonable to start with definite chemotherapy at the earliest [40, 41]. Radiation therapy may also be considered simultaneously if rapid resolution with chemotherapy is not anticipated. Surgical intervention should be considered in any case where diagnosis is uncertain, and biopsy is difficult and time-consuming.

(c) **Supportive care***:* In malignant spinal cord compression, it is also important to manage following aspects as well including spinal stabilization by keeping patient in neutral spine position, management of pain by opiates or gabapentin for neuropathic pain, management of constipation/urinary retention, monitoring for steroid toxicities, electrolyte abnormalities and also thromboprophylaxis for bed bound patients. It is also important to involve physical rehabilitation team soon after stabilization for facilitating neurological recovery [39].

31.3 Conclusion

Pediatric critical care support is challenging, and prompt identification and management of oncological emergencies is of paramount importance to provide excellence in care.

With recent advances in both field of pediatric oncology as well as critical care support, application of the evidence-based approach in management of childhood oncological emergencies is essential to achieve the best outcome.FundingNone

Conflicts of Interests None

Permissions to Use Copyrighted Materials Not applicable.

References

1. Cancer Statistics Review, 1975–2016 - SEER statistics. https://seer.cancer.gov/csr/1975_2016/. Accessed 2 Sep 2019.
2. Demaret P, Pettersen G, Hubert P, Teira P, Emeriaud G. The critically-illpediatrichemato-oncology patient: epidemiology, management, and strategy of transfer to the pediatric intensive care unit. Ann Intensive Care. 2012;2:14.
3. Haase R, et al. Die wachsendeBedeutung der pädiatrischenIntensivstation in der Behandlungo nkologischerPatienten - Erfahrungenüber 7 Jahre. KlinPädiatr. 2003;215:234–40.
4. Heying R, Schneider DT, Körholz D, Stannigel H, Lemburg P, Göbel U. Efficacy and outcome of intensive care in pediatric oncologic patients. Crit Care Med. 2001;29:2276–80.
5. Owens C, Mannion D, O'Marcaigh A, Waldron M, Butler K, O'Meara A. Indications for admission, treatment and improved outcome of paediatric haematology/oncology patients admitted to a tertiary paediatric ICU. Ir J Med Sci. 2011;180:85–9.
6. Sundaram M, Moussa AAH, Maaz AUR, Faqih N. The critically-IllPediatric oncology patients: what the intensivist needs to know? Pediatric critical care medicine. Indian J Crit Care Med. 2020;24:1256–63.

7. Ruggiero A, Rizzo D, Amato M, Riccardi R. Management of Hyperleukocytosis. Curr Treat Options in Oncol. 2016;17:7.
8. Sung L, Aplenc R, Alonzo TA, Gerbing RB, Gamis AS, AAML0531/PHIS Group. Predictors and short-term outcomes of hyperleukocytosis in children with acute myeloid leukemia: a report from the Children's oncology group. Haematologica. 2012;97:1770–3.
9. Jain R, Bansal D, Marwaha RK. Hyperleukocytosis: emergency management. Indian J Pediatr. 2013;80:144–8.
10. Bunin NJ, Pui CH. Differing complications of hyperleukocytosis in children with acute lymphoblastic or acute nonlymphoblasticleukemia. J Clin Oncol. 1985;3:1590–5.
11. Stucki A, Rivier A-S, Gikic M, Monai N, Schapira M, Spertini O. Endothelial cell activation by myeloblasts: molecular mechanisms of leukostasis and leukemic cell dissemination. Blood. 2001;97:2121–9.
12. Röllig C, Ehninger G. How I treat hyperleukocytosis in acute myeloid leukemia. Blood. 2015;125:3246–52.
13. Oberoi S, Lehrnbecher T, Phillips B, Hitzler J, Ethier M-C, Beyene J, Sung L. Leukapheresis and low-dose chemotherapy do not reduce early mortality in acute myeloid leukemia hyperleukocytosis: a systematic review and meta-analysis. Leuk Res. 2014;38:460–8.
14. Haase R, Merkel N, Diwan O, Elsner K, Kramm CM. Leukapheresis and exchange transfusion in children with acute leukemia and Hyperleukocytosis. A single center experience. Klin Pädiatr. 2009;221:374–8.
15. Russell TB. Tumor lysis syndrome. American Academy of Pediatrics. https://pedsinreview.aappublications.org/content/41/1/20#sec-4. Accessed 7 Apr 2021.
16. Cairo MS, Bishop M. Tumour lysis syndrome: new therapeutic strategies and classification: new therapeutic strategies and classification of TLS. Br J Haematol. 2004;127:3–11.
17. Rajendran A, Bansal D, Marwaha RK, Singhi SC. Tumor lysis syndrome. Indian J Pediatr. 2013;80:50–4.
18. Cheung WL, Hon KL, Fung CM, Leung AK. Tumor lysis syndrome in childhood malignancies. Drugs Context. 2020;9:1–14.
19. Coiffier B, Altman A, Pui C-H, Younes A, Cairo MS. Guidelines for the management of pediatric and adult tumor lysis syndrome: an evidence-based review. J Clin Oncol Off J Am Soc Clin Oncol. 2008;26:2767–78.
20. Howard SC, Jones DP, Pui C-H. The tumor lysis syndrome. N Engl J Med. 2011;364:1844–54.
21. Cheung WL, Hon KL, Fung CM, Leung AK. Tumor lysis syndrome in childhood malignancies. Drugs Context. 2020;9:1–14.
22. Syrimi E, Gunasekera S, Norton A, Velangi M, Motwani J, Hiwarkar P. Single dose Rasburicase is a clinically effective pharmacoeconomic approach for preventing tumour lysis syndrome in children with high tumour burden. Br J Haematol. 2018;181:696–8.
23. Tonelli M, Pannu N, Manns B. Oral phosphate binders in patients with kidney failure. N Engl J Med. 2010;362:1312–24.
24. Wilson FP, Berns JS. Onco-nephrology: tumor lysis syndrome. Clin J Am Soc Nephrol. 2012;7:1730–9.
25. Jain R, Bansal D, Marwaha RK, Singhi S. Superior mediastinal syndrome: emergency management. Indian J Pediatr. 2013;80:55–9.
26. Nossair F, Schoettler P, Starr J, Chan AKC, Kirov I, Paes B, Mahajerin A. Pediatric superior vena cava syndrome: an evidence-based systematic review of the literature. Pediatr Blood Cancer. 2018;65:e27225.
27. Arya LS, Narain S, Tomar S, Thavaraj V, Dawar R, Bhargawa M. Superior vena cava syndrome. Indian J Pediatr. 2002;69:293–7.
28. Rheingold SR, Meadows AT. Recognition and management of superior vena cava syndrome. In: Sills RH, editor. Practical algorithms in pediatric hematology and oncology. Basel: Karger; 2003. p. 96–7.
29. Ricketts RR. Clinical management of anterior mediastinal tumors in children. Semin PediatrSurg. 2001;10:161–8.

30. Wilson LD, Detterbeck FC, Yahalom J. Superior vena cava syndrome with malignant causes. N Engl J Med. 2007;356:1862–9.
31. Borenstein SH, Gerstle T, Malkin D, Thorner P, Filler RM. The effects of prebiopsy corticosteroid treatment on the diagnosis of mediastinal lymphoma. J Pediatr Surg. 2000;35:973–6.
32. Fischer MJ, Rheingold SR. Oncologic emergencies. In: Pizzo PA, Poplack DG, editors. Principles and practices of pediatric oncology. 6th ed. Philadelphia: Lippencott Williams and Wilkins; 2011. p. 1125–51.
33. Lewis DW, Packer RJ, Raney B, Rak IW, Belasco J, Lange B. Incidence, presentation, and outcome of spinal cord disease in children with systemic cancer. Pediatrics. 1986;78:438–43.
34. Tantawy AAG, Ebeid FSE, Mahmoud MA, Shepl OE. Spinal cord compression in childhood pediatric malignancies: multicenter Egyptian study. J Pediatr Hematol Oncol. 2013;35:232–6.
35. De Martino L, Spennato P, Vetrella S, Capasso M, Porfito C, Ruotolo S, Abate ME, Cinalli G, Quaglietta L. Symptomatic malignant spinal cord compression in children: a single-center experience. Ital J Pediatr. 2019;45:80.
36. Tokuc G. 1467 pediatric oncology patients presenting with spinal cord compression. Arch Dis Child. 2012;97:A416–7.
37. Bristol royal hospital for children clinical guideline Spinal Cord Compression (SCC) – Management in Haematology and Oncology Patients.
38. Skeoch GD, Tobin MK, Khan S, Linninger AA, Mehta AI. Corticosteroid treatment for metastatic spinal cord compression: a review. Glob Spine J. 2017;7:272–9.
39. Suspected spinal cord compression in children and young people with malignancy. http://www.lhp.leedsth.nhs.uk/detail.aspx?id=4114. Accessed 4 Apr 2021.
40. De Bernardi B, Quaglietta L, Haupt R, et al. Neuroblastoma with symptomatic epidural compression in the infant: the AIEOP experience: neuroblastoma and symptomatic epidural compression. Pediatr Blood Cancer. 2014;61:1369–75.
41. Mirzaei L, Kaal SEJ, Schreuder HWB, Bartels RHMA. The neurological compromised spine due to Ewing sarcoma. What first. Neurosurgery. 2015;77:718–25.

Neuro-Oncological Problems in the Intensive Care Unit

32

Barkha Bindu, Charu Mahajan, Indu Kapoor, and Hemanshu Prabhakar

32.1 Introduction

One of the main aspects of neurocritical care is to provide intensive monitoring to critically ill neurological patients. It requires specially trained personnel with skills to identify subtle neurologic changes and worsening status. The prognosis of oncology patients admitted to intensive care unit (ICU) is generally considered poor [1]. Mortality rate in solid tumour patients admitted to ICU is reportedly upto 50% [2]. Over the past few decades, the number of oncology patients admitted to ICU has significantly increased owing to improved outcomes. Therefore, identifying patients who will benefit from ICU admission and development of disease-specific approaches to ICU management is important.

Neuro-oncology patients are different from routine oncology patients in the absence of typical risk factors (like tobacco, alcohol etc.) and type of complications encountered (seizures, cerebral hemorrhage). They are often in a better general condition with fewer comorbidities compared to general oncological patients.

32.2 Reasons for ICU Admission

Most patients are admitted to ICU with the purpose of providing close neuromonitoring. A multidisciplinary team comprising of neurosurgeons, neurologists, neurointensivists and neuroradiologists can provide the best of care. A hybrid model of

B. Bindu
Department of Neuroanaesthesiology and Neurocritical Care, Paras Hospital, Gurugram, Haryana, India

C. Mahajan · I. Kapoor · H. Prabhakar (✉)
Department of Neuroanaesthesiology and Critical Care, All India Institute of Medical Sciences, New Delhi, India

V. Kumar et al. (eds.), *Onco-critical Care*,
https://doi.org/10.1007/978-981-16-9929-0_32

ICU suits this patient group best, where a neurointensivist provides continuous care with the assistance of neurosurgeons and neurologists.

Other reasons for ICU admission among neurological patients are seizures, septic shock, respiratory failure and hemodynamic instability [3]. The goals of neurocritical management are to optimise cardiovascular (maintain cerebral perfusion pressure), respiratory (oxygenation, ventilation), metabolic (glycemic control, fluid and electrolyte management), infectious (antibiotics) and nutritional status while also providing disease specific therapy.

32.3 Neuromonitoring

An important and common reason for admission to the neurocritical care unit is close neuromonitoring. It needs specially trained personnel who are well versed with various neuromonitoring devices. Multimodality neuromonitoring includes intracranial pressure (ICP) monitoring, continuous electroencephalography (EEG), jugular venous oximetry, near infrared spectroscopy, brain tissue oxygen tension, cerebral microdialysis etc. The challenge is to identify an ideal combination of global and regional monitors depending on the clinical situation. A detailed description of each of these techniques is beyond the scope of this chapter.

Depth of coma is assessed by either Glasgow Coma Score (GCS) or Full Outline of UnResponsiveness (FOUR) score. The total score in GCS ranges from 3 to 15 [4]. It has three components: eye opening (E), motor response (M), and verbal response (V). GCS does not account for brainstem reflexes, and it does not score verbal response in intubated patients. Hence, the FOUR score was developed which includes eye opening, motor responses, brainstem reflexes, and respiration [5]. The total score ranges from 0 to 16. Neurological examination must also include detailed pupillary assessment (size, symmetry, reactivity).

32.4 Systemic Care of Neuro-Oncological Patients

32.4.1 Intracranial Pressure and Cerebral Perfusion Pressure (CPP)

ICP is defined as the pressure exerted on the dura mater by contents within the cranial vault. With an intact skull, the sum of the volume of brain, CSF, and intracranial blood is constant. Increase in one component results in the displacement of the others (Monroe-Kellie hypothesis) [6]. Once compensatory mechanisms are exhausted, ICP rises exponentially. This inflection occurs at an ICP value of 20–25 mmHg. For treatment purposes, intracranial hypertension is defined as sustained (>5 min) rise in ICP above 22 mmHg [7]. Table 32.1 shows common causes of rise in ICP.

CPP is the difference between the mean arterial pressure (MAP) and the mean ICP [8].

Table 32.1 Causes of raised ICP

Mechanism	Cause
Focal brain edema	Neoplasms, contusion, abscess, ischemic and hemorrhagic stroke
Diffuse brain edema	Diffuse head injury, encephalitis, meningitis, metabolic encephalopathy, hypoxic ischemic injury
Obstruction of CSF circulation	Obstructive HCP, subarachnoid hemorrhage
Obstruction of major venous sinuses	Cerebral venous thrombosis
Vascular malformations	Arterio-venous malformations
Idiopathic	Benign intracranial hypertension

CSF cerebrospinal fluid, *HCP* hydrocephalus

$$\text{CPP} = \text{MAP} - \text{ICP}$$

Hence, when the ICP increases, CPP decreases. With intact cerebral autoregulation, CBF is maintained over a wide range of CPP. Below the lower limit of autoregulation (CPP < 40–60 mmHg) cerebral ischemia occurs, and above the upper limit of autoregulation, cerebral hyperaemia, vasogenic edema and hemorrhage might occur. CPP values higher than 70 mmHg are avoided because the measures used to maintain high arterial pressures like intravenous fluids or inotropes may cause cardiopulmonary complications [9].

A number of therapies are used to lower ICP, targeting one or more of the intracranial components. Figure 32.1 describes the step-wise management of intracranial hypertension [10, 11]. Table 32.2 discusses important aspects of various ICP lowering therapies. Management of raised ICP begins with general management. Hyperosmolar agents lower ICP by generating an osmolar gradient across the intact blood-brain barrier and promoting movement of water from normal brain parenchyma. Mannitol and hypertonic saline are the most commonly used agents [12]. Hyperventilation and hypocapnia effectively lower ICP by reducing cerebral blood volume through cerebral vasoconstriction [13]. Due to the associated risk of cerebral ischemia, hyperventilation must be used only in life-threatening intracranial hypertension and PaCO2 must be rapidly normalised once definitive therapy is administered [14]. Decompressive craniectomy may be an option in patients with cerebral contusions, subdural hematoma, and hemispheric acute ischemic stroke and intracranial hemorrhage [15].

32.4.2 Respiratory Care

Neuro-oncological patients often require tracheal intubation and mechanical ventilation due to depressed mental status and resulting inability to protect the airway. Bulbar weakness and impaired cough reflex are common. Hypoventilation and hypercarbia due to impaired consciousness can result in raised ICP. Thus, promptly securing the airway is essential to prevent secondary brain injury. Factors that

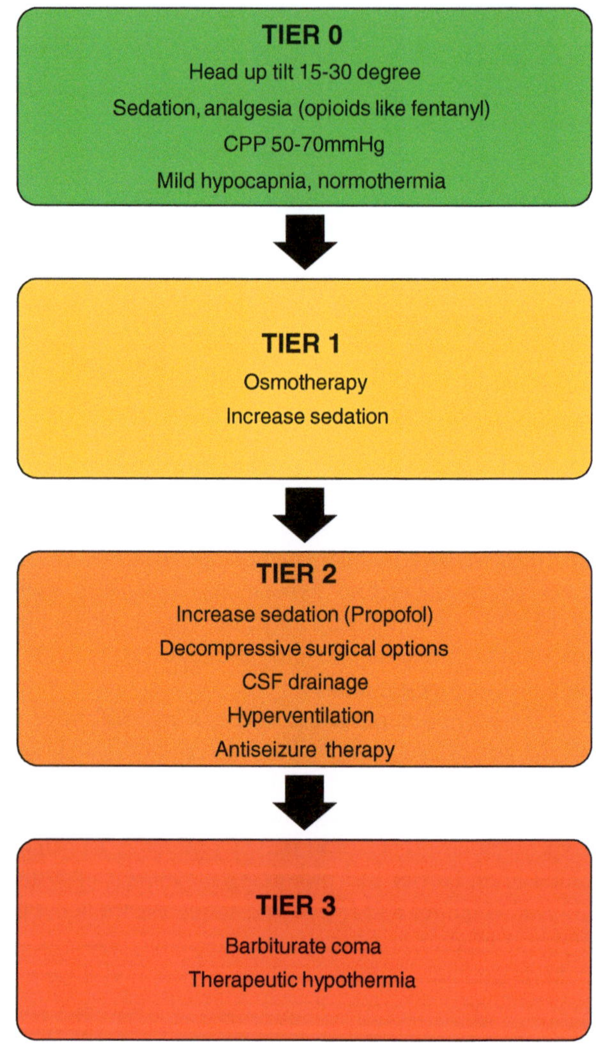

Fig. 32.1 Stepwise approach to intracranial hypertension

determine the need for intubation include level of consciousness, presence of gag and cough reflex, swallowing mechanisms, amount of secretions, and how long the patient is likely to be neurologically impaired [16]. However, in patients with concerns of futility of therapy, the decision to intubate must be taken cautiously.

Rapid sequence induction is the preferred method for securing the airway in patients at risk for elevated ICP. Induction should be performed using agents that are less likely to cause hypotension, maintaining MAP between 80 and 100 mmHg and preserving CPP >50 mmHg. Etomidate (hemodynamically stable), propofol (reduces CMRO2 and ICP, but can cause hypotension), fentanyl and non-depolarizing neuromuscular blockers such as rocuronium or vecuronium are commonly used agents for induction and intubation. Succinylcholine has rapid onset

Table 32.2 Salient points of various ICP lowering therapies

Tier 0 (General management)	Airway	Avoid hypoxia, hypercapnia
	Ventilation	Avoid hypoventilation Maintain normocapnia/mild hypocapnia
	Circulation	Avoid hypotension Maintain CPP of 50–70 mmHg
	Fluids	Avoid hypo-osmolar fluids and hyponatremia
	Sedation, analgesia	Avoid coughing, agitation
	Promote cerebral venous drainage	Head end elevation by 15–30°, neck in neutral position. Avoid tight tracheostomy and endotracheal tube ties, properly place cervical collar Avoid rise in intrathoracic and intra-abdominal pressures
	Fever	Antipyretics and hydrotherapy
	Glucocorticoids	Benefit in vasogenic edema Most effective in patients with brain tumors, abscesses, demyelinating diseases, and infections
Tier 1	Osmolar therapy	*Mannitol:* Dose: 0.25–1 g/kg body weight. Maintain serum osmolarity <320 mOsm/kg. An osmolar gap of 20 mmol/dL indicates inadequate clearance of mannitol and will increase the risk of rebound rise in ICP Reflection coefficient is 0.9, greater risk of accumulating inside brain Onset of action in 1–5 min, peak action in 40 min, duration of action is 90 min–6 h Adverse effects: Hypotension, rebound increase in ICP, volume overload, hypo/hypernatremia, hyperkalemia
		Hypertonic saline: Available in concentrations ranging from 3 to 23.4% Useful in hypovolemic patients since it remains intravascular longer Reflection coefficient is 1.0, crosses BBB less. Dose: Bolus of 3%: 2.5–5 mL/kg over 5–20 min, 5%: 2.5–5 mL/kg over 5–20 min, 7.5%: 1.5–2.5 mL/kg over 5–20 min, 23.4%: 30 mL over 10–20 min Given in continuous infusion Serum sodium beyond 160 mEq/dL is unlikely to provide any further benefit Preferably given via central line Needs frequent serum sodium level monitoring Duration of effect is 90 min–4 h Adverse effects: Thrombophlebitis, coagulation abnormality, hyperchloremic metabolic acidosis

(continued)

Table 32.2 (continued)

Tier 2 (Decompressive surgical options)	Resection of mass lesion	Abscess drainage, hematoma evacuation, resection of parenchymal contusion and lobar hemorrhage
	CSF drainage	Done using external ventricular drain (EVD) Reduces intracranial volume Useful when ICP elevation is due to ventricular obstruction Continuous drainage may be more beneficial than intermittent drainage
	Decompressive craniectomy	Involves removal of a portion of skull vault Reduces ICP and ICU stay Benefit in terms of functional outcome and mortality is not clear
	Hyperventilation	Recommended only as a temporizing measure in the setting of refractory hypertension and for brief periods (<2 h) in case of acute neurologic deterioration Effect is almost immediate but lasts for only 4–6 h after which pH of the CSF rapidly equilibrates to the new PaCO2 level PaCO2 of 30–35 mm Hg must be the target Prolonged prophylactic hyperventilation to a PaCO2 ≤25 mmHg is not recommended as there is a risk of cerebral ischemia Jugular venous oxygen or brain tissue oxygen measurements are recommended
	Antiseizure therapy	Seizure increases cerebral metabolic rate and cerebral blood flow with resulting increase in ICP There is insufficient evidence to recommend levetiracetam compared with phenytoin
Tier 3	Barbiturate coma	Cause coupled reduction in CBF and CMR, thus reducing ICP *Thiopentone:* Loading dose of 5 mg/kg over 30 min followed by infusion of 1–5 mg/kg hour until the electroencephalogram shows a burst suppression pattern. May cause hypotension *Pentobarbital* may result in hypotension needing vasopressor support Adverse effects: Hypotension, hypokalemia, respiratory depression, infections due to immune suppression, hepatic and renal dysfunction
	Therapeutic hypothermia	No definitive evidence Hypothermia reduces basal component of cellular metabolism along with suppression of electrical activity of brain Moderate hypothermia (target core temperature 32–34 °C) used Rewarming should be done slowly to avoid rebound severe intracranial hypertension Adverse effects: Shivering, cardiac arrhythmias, electrolyte disturbances, sepsis

CPP cerebral perfusion pressure, *ICP* intracranial pressure, *ICU* intensive care unit, *PaCO2* partial pressure of arterial carbon dioxide, *CBF* cerebral blood flow, *CMR* cerebral metabolic rate

and short duration of action, but, can cause transient rise in ICP, though clinically insignificant [17]. Ketamine causes ICP elevations in patients with hydrocephalus (HCP). But, in brain injury patients without HCP, it has no effect on cerebral perfusion and neurological outcomes [18]. In patients with raised ICP, care must be taken to minimize the duration the head end is lowered for intubation.

Normoxia and normocarbia must be maintained. Hypoxia must be avoided at all costs. Airway obstruction, hypoventilation, aspiration pneumonia, atelectasis etc. are usual causes of hypoxia. Use of hyperventilation and hypocapnia must be limited to acute ICP crisis situations only. Choice of ventilator mode is guided by PaCO2 values and patient-ventilator synchrony. There is no literature to guide the choice of mode of ventilation in these patients. Most commonly, mechanical ventilation is started with controlled modes and changed to assisted modes as neurological improvement occurs. Lung-protective ventilatory strategy using tidal volumes of 6–8 mL/kg body weight and plateau pressures below 30 cm H2O are advised [19]. Respiratory rate must be guided by the desired PaCO2 level. Fraction of inspired oxygen (FiO2) must be adjusted to maintain oxygen saturation of 95–100%. A PEEP of 5 cm H2O is commonly used. However, it might increase ICP and reduce CPP in patients with impaired cerebral autoregulation [16].

Sedation is often needed for patients on mechanical ventilation. Opioids, benzodiazepines and dexmedetomidine in continuous infusion are commonly used [20]. Propofol infusion is also commonly used. It has the advantage of decreasing ICP, but, may cause hypotension.

32.4.3 Planning Extubation in Post-neurosurgical Patients

Decision to extubate neuro-oncological patients in ICU is sometimes challenging. Generally, spontaneous breathing trial (SBT) is attempted in neurocritical patients while ensuring an FiO2 $< 40–50\%$, PEEP $< 5–8$ cmH2O, no neuromuscular blockade and absence of raised ICP, status epilepticus, cerebral vasospasm, or active neurologic ischemia [19]. It is also common practice in neurocritical care units to give prolonged CPAP trials before extubation, although there is no definitive evidence to this [21]. It is presumed that CPAP trials improve respiratory muscles strength and functional residual capacity [16]. Impaired consciousness and impaired cough reflex are common contributors to failed extubation. Level of consciousness, protective airway reflexes, amount of secretions and tolerability of SBT, all must be taken into consideration while deciding for or against extubation. Neuro-oncological patients often have impaired consciousness which alone must not preclude extubation trial, unlike in other oncological patients [22].

32.4.4 Infection

Common forms of infection in neuro-oncological patients include pneumonia, meningitis and ventriculitis, brain abscess, subdural or epidural empyema, and encephalitis. History of neurosurgery, cerebrospinal fluid (CSF) leakage, recent head injury, presence of cranial or extracranial infectious foci like otitis or sinusitis and immunocompromised state are the important risk factors for nosocomial intracranial infections [23]. Multidrug-resistant pathogens further complicate the management of these infections. Timely diagnosis and prompt initiation of appropriate antimicrobial therapy is important to improve the outcome.

Pneumonia can contribute to prolonged ICU stay and increased mortality. Good oral care, appropriate antibiotics, frequent position change, chest physiotherapy, early mobilization and swallowing rehabilitation can help in improving outcomes.

32.4.5 Fluid, Glycemic Control and Electrolytes

The choice of fluid in neurocritical patients remains controversial [24–26]. Crystalloids are commonly used in neurocritical patients. Balanced crystalloids may be used in patients not at risk of cerebral edema or raised ICP. Hyperchloremic metabolic acidosis is a common issue in neurocritical patients. It occurs due to extensive use of saline based solutions in these patients and is associated with acute kidney injury and increased mortality [27, 28].

After extensive research, it is now accepted that aggressive glycemic control is detrimental in these patients. A modest control of 140–180 mg/dL is considered appropriate [29].

Sodium is the single most important electrolyte in neurocritical patients. Fluctuations in serum sodium levels are both common and detrimental in them. While hyponatremia can cause cerebral edema, hypernatremia has been associated with acute kidney injury and increased mortality [30]. Brain tumours can cause sodium disturbances, more commonly Syndrome of Inappropriate Antidiuretic Hormone secretion (SIADH) and hyponatremia. Pituitary adenomas and craniopharyngiomas, especially after resection, can cause Diabetes Insipidus (DI) and hypernatremia.

Other common electrolyte disorders are of potassium, magnesium and calcium. Specifically, hypokalemia may precipitate arrhythmias, hypomagnesemia and hypocalcemia may cause seizures.

32.4.6 Gastrointestinal Care and Nutrition

Enteral nutrition must be initiated early, preferably within 48 h, in neurosurgical patients. Early nutrition can prevent hypercatabolism and infection. Early feeding has been found to be associated with a significant reduction in mortality rate, poor outcome and infectious complications [31]. A number of commercial feeds are available for use in neurocritical patients now-a-days. Glucose and electrolyte contents vary among these feeds. The choice of commercial feeds is influenced to some extent by patients' comorbidities and existing electrolyte abnormalities.

Majority of patients tolerate nasogastric or gastrostomy feeds well. Methods of calculating nutritional requirements of neurocritical patients are described in Table 32.3 [32]. Figure 32.2 shows one of the commonly used formulae, the Harris Benedict Equation, for calculating caloric requirements in critically ill patients [33]. Daily nutritional requirements of various electrolytes for adults are also described in Table 32.3 [34].

It must be remembered that oncological patients are at high risk of refeeding syndrome [35]. Refeeding syndrome is characterised by hypophosphatemia along with hypokalemia, hypomagnesemia, thiamine deficiency as well as abnormal sodium and fluid balance [36]. It can be prevented by identifying the high risk patients and starting feeds slowly along with replacement of electrolytes. Commercial multivitamin preparations that contain all vitamins may be added.

Stress ulcer prophylaxis using proton pump inhibitor or H2 receptor blocker is often indicated in neurocritical patients. Reasons include long term use of high dose steroids in brain tumour patients, mechanical ventilation, raised ICP etc. all of which can precipitate stress ulcers.

Table 32.3 Methods of calculating nutritional requirements in neurocritical care

Method	Description
Indirect calorimetry	• Considered the accepted standard • Based on the principle that energy expenditure can be calculated by measuring oxygen consumption & CO2 production • Must be done when steady state (stable acid base balance and CO2 production) is achieved • Costly, sensitive equipment required • High oxygen requirement, air leak around endotracheal tube cuff or through chest tube, fever, shivering, vasoactive drugs impair correct measurements
Harris-Benedict equation (Fig. 32.2)	• One of the most commonly used equations • It has an additional factor to compensate for elevated energy requirement due to injury or stress in hospitalised patients • Has 17–67% accuracy
Simplistic formulae	• Calories (Carbohydrates & fats): 25–30 kcal/kg/day • Protein: 0.8–1.2 g/kg actual body weight/day (patients without any additional stressors) 1.0–1.5 g/kg/day (in acute critical illness) 2–2.5 g/kg ideal body weight/day (in patients with BMI > 30 kg/m^2) • Potassium: 1–1.2 mEq/kg/day • Magnesium: 8–20 mEq/day • Calcium: 10–15 mEq/day • Phosphate: 20–30 mmol/day

CO2 carbon dioxide, *BMI* body mass index

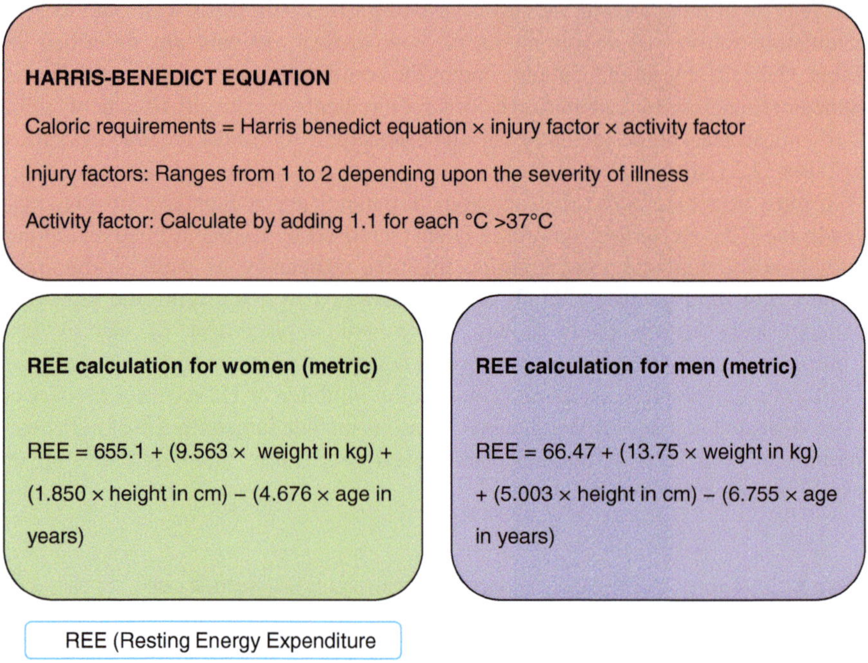

HARRIS-BENEDICT EQUATION

Caloric requirements = Harris benedict equation × injury factor × activity factor

Injury factors: Ranges from 1 to 2 depending upon the severity of illness

Activity factor: Calculate by adding 1.1 for each °C >37°C

REE calculation for women (metric)

REE = 655.1 + (9.563 × weight in kg) + (1.850 × height in cm) – (4.676 × age in years)

REE calculation for men (metric)

REE = 66.47 + (13.75 × weight in kg) + (5.003 × height in cm) – (6.755 × age in years)

REE (Resting Energy Expenditure

Fig. 32.2 Harris-Benedict equation

32.4.7 Venous Thrombosis Prophylaxis

The incidence of venous thromboembolism (VTE) in neuro-oncological patients is high. VTE prophylaxis is essential, but, must be weighed against the risk of bleeding. While mechanical prophylaxis using compression stockings must be applied to all neurocritical patients on admission to ICU, pharmacological prophylaxis with low molecular weight heparin must be initiated as early as possible. In postoperative patients of brain tumour excision, pharmacological prophylaxis is usually started within 24–48 h after surgery, if there is no contraindication.

32.5 End of Life Issues

Sometimes while managing neurocritical patients, a point may be reached when continuing treatment no longer offers any benefit, but its withdrawal is likely to lead to death. Determining this point of medical futility is extremely difficult and controversial [37]. Goals and treatment options must be clearly discussed with the family to ascertain whether or not a treatment holds any value for the patient and family. Once futility is established beyond doubt, the issue is of withdrawal or withholding of care [38]. In India, the legal provisions on this aspect are not clear, at present. Likewise, Do Not Resuscitate orders also are not a documented legal practice in India at present time.

32.6 Predictors of Survival and Prognosis

While mortality rate in cancer patients admitted to ICU is usually close to 50%, that in neuro-oncology patients is about 22%. Presence of multi-organ failure, respiratory, hemodynamic, hepatic, or renal dysfunction, mechanical ventilation or catecholamine infusion are associated with an increased risk of death in neurocritically ill patients. However, tumour type, GCS and disease control status reportedly do not influence ICU mortality rate [3]. In an Indian setting, age, diagnosis, GCS, pupillary status, serum albumin, and serum sodium were found to be independent predictors of survival in a neurosurgical ICU [39].

Several scoring systems have been developed to quantify outcomes of neurocritical care patients. GCS reportedly has less predictive power than simple acute physiology score II (SAPS II) scoring system in quantifying outcomes [40].

32.7 Key Points

1. One of the pivotal aspects of critical care management of neuro-oncological patients is to provide intensive neuromonitoring.
2. The goals of management are to maintain normoxia, normocapnia, normoglycemia, normothermia and avoid hypotension.
3. Early feeding is associated with significant reduction in mortality, poor outcome, and infectious complications.
4. End of life issues continue to be ambiguous to a large extent.

References

1. Kostakou E, Rovina N, Kyriakopoulou M, et al. Critically ill cancer patient in intensive care unit: issues that arise. J Crit Care. 2014;29:817–22.
2. Azoulay E, Moreau D, Alberti C, et al. Predictors of short-term mortality in critically ill patients with solid malignancies. Intensive Care Med. 2000;26:1817–23.
3. Tabouret E, Boucard C, Devillier R, et al. Neuro-oncological patients admitted in intensive-care unit: predictive factors and functional outcome. J Neurooncol. 2016;127:111–7.
4. Teasdale G, Jennett B. Assessment of coma and impaired consciousness. A practical scale. Lancet. 1974;2(7872):81–4.
5. Wijdicks EFM, Bamlet WR, Maramattom BV, et al. Validation of a new coma scale: the FOUR score. Ann Neurol. 2005;58(4):585–93.
6. Mokri B. The Monro-Kellie hypothesis: applications in CSF volume depletion. Neurology. 2001;56:1746–8.
7. Jantzen JP. Prevention and treatment of intracranial hypertension. Best Pract Res Clin Anaesthesiol. 2007;21:517–38.
8. Miller JD, Stanek A, Langfitt TW. Concepts of cerebral perfusion pressure and vascular compression during intracranial hypertension. Prog Brain Res. 1972;35:411–32.
9. Contant CF, Valadka AB, Gopinath SP, et al. Adult respiratory distress syndrome: a complication of induced hypertension after severe head injury. J Neurosurg. 2001;95:560–8.
10. Tripathy S, Ahmad SR. Raised intracranial pressure syndrome: a stepwise approach. Indian J Crit Care Med. 2019;23:S129–35.

11. Stevens RD, Shoykhet M, Cadena R. Emergency neurological life support: intracranial hypertension and herniation. Neurocrit Care. 2015;23:S76–82.
12. Gu J, Huang H, Huang Y, et al. Hypertonic saline or mannitol for treating elevated intracranial pressure in traumatic brain injury: a meta-analysis of randomized controlled trials. Neurosurg Rev. 2019;42:499–509.
13. Godoy DA, Seifi A, Garza D, et al. Hyperventilation therapy for control of posttraumatic intracranial hypertension. Front Neurol. 2017;8:250.
14. Curley G, Kavanagh BP, Laffey JG. Hypocapnia and the injured brain: more harm than benefit. Crit Care Med. 2010;38:1348–59.
15. Alexander P, Heels-Ansdell D, Siemieniuk R, et al. Hemicraniectomy versus medical treatment with large MCA infarct: a review and meta-analysis. BMJ Open. 2016;6(11):e014390.
16. Nyquist P, Stevens RD, Mirski MA. Neurologic injury and mechanical ventilation. Neurocrit Care. 2008;9:400–8.
17. Kovarik WD, Mayberg TS, Lam AM, et al. Succinylcholine does not change intracranial pressure, cerebral blood flow velocity, or the electroencephalogram in patients with neurologic injury. Anesth Analg. 1994;78:469–73.
18. Cohen L, Athaide V, Wickham ME, et al. The effect of ketamine on intracranial and cerebral perfusion pressure and health outcomes: a systematic review. Ann Emerg Med. 2015;65:43–51.e2.
19. Acute Respiratory Distress Syndrome Network. Ventilation with lower tidal volumes as compared with traditional tidal volumes for acute lung injury and the acute respiratory distress syndrome. N Engl J Med. 2000;342:1301–8.
20. Aryan HE, Box KW, Ibrahim D, et al. Safety and efficacy of dexmedetomidine in neurosurgical patients. Brain Inj. 2006;20:791–8.
21. Shah V, Suarez JI. General principles of neurocritical care. In: Prabhakar H, Zulfiqar A, editors. Textbook of neuroanesthesia and neurocritical care. 1st ed. Singapore: Springer; 2019. p. 3–23.
22. Godet T, Chabanne R, Marin J, et al. Extubation failure in brain-injured patients: risk factors and development of a prediction score in a preliminary prospective cohort study. Anesthesiology. 2017;126:104–14.
23. Beer R, Pfausler B, Schmutzhard E. Infectious intracranial complications in the neuro-ICU patient population. Curr Opin Crit Care. 2010;16:117–22.
24. Ginsberg MD, Palesch YY, Hill MD, et al. High-dose albumin treatment for acute ischaemic stroke (ALIAS) part 2: a randomised, double-blind, phase 3, placebo-controlled trial. Lancet Neurol. 2013;12:1049–58.
25. SAFE Study Investigators. Saline or albumin for fluid resuscitation in patients with traumatic brain injury. N Engl J Med. 2007;357:874–84.
26. Suarez JI, Shannon L, Zaidat OO, et al. Effect of human albumin administration on clinical outcome and hospital cost in patients with subarachnoid hemorrhage. J Neurosurg. 2004;100:585–90.
27. Sadan O, Singbartl K, Kandiah PA, et al. Hyperchloremia is associated with acute kidney injury in patients with subarachnoid hemorrhage. Crit Care Med. 2017;45:1382–8.
28. Riha HM, Erdman MJ, Vandigo JE, et al. Impact of moderate hyperchloremia on clinical outcomes in intracerebral hemorrhage patients treated with continuous infusion hypertonic saline: a pilot study. Crit Care Med. 2017;45:e957–3.
29. Kramer AH, Roberts DJ, Zygun DA. Optimal glycemic control in neurocritical care patients: a systematic review and meta-analysis. Crit Care. 2012;16:R203.
30. Aiyagari V, Deibert E, Diringer MN. Hypernatremia in the neurologic intensive care unit: how high is too high? J Crit Care. 2006;21:163–72.
31. Wang X, Dong Y, Han X, et al. Nutritional support for patients sustaining traumatic brain injury: a systematic review and meta-analysis of prospective studies. PLoS One. 2013;8:e58838.
32. McClave SA, Martindale RG, Vanek VW, et al. A.S.P.E.N. Board of Directors; American College of Critical Care Medicine; Society of Critical Care Medicine. Guidelines for the provision and assessment of nutrition support therapy in the adult critically ill patient: Society of

Critical Care Medicine (SCCM) and American Society for Parenteral and Enteral Nutrition (A.S.P.E.N.). J Parenter Enteral Nutr. 2009;33:277–316.
33. Walker RN, Heuberger RA. Predictive equations for energy needs for the critically ill. Respir Care. 2009;54:509–21.
34. Rao GSU, Bansal S. Neurological critical care. In: Prabhakar H, editor. Essentials of neuroanesthesia. 1st ed. San Diego, CA: Academic, Elsevier; 2017. p. 595–611.
35. Azim A, Ahmed A. Nutrition in neurocritical care. Neurol India. 2016;64:105–14.
36. Mehanna HM, Moledina J, Travis J. Refeeding syndrome: what it is, and how to prevent and treat it. BMJ. 2008;336:1495–8.
37. Schneiderman LJ, Jecker NS, Jonsen AR. Medical futility: its meaning and ethical implications. Ann Intern Med. 1990;112:949–54.
38. Reynolds S, Cooper AB, McKneally M. Withdrawing life-sustaining treatment: ethical considerations. Thorac Surg Clin. 2005;15:469–80.
39. Ramesh VJ, Rao GSU, Kandavel T, et al. Predictive model for survival among neurosurgical intensive care patients. J Neurosurg Anesthesiol. 2011;23:183–7.
40. Zhao XX, Su YY, Wang M, et al. Evaluation of neuro-intensive care unit performance in China: predicting outcomes of Simplified Acute Physiology Score II or Glasgow Coma Scale. Chin Med J. 2013;126:1132–7.

Mental Status Dysfunction in ICU Postoperative Cognitive Impairment

33

Jayanta Kumar Mitra, Priyank Tapuria, and Dona Saha

33.1 Introduction

Post-operative mental state changes (ranging from emergence delirium to cognitive dysfunction) poses a special challenge to the intensivist. It interferes with both the assessment and management of post-surgical patients. Existing evidence suggests that post-operative cognitive dysfunction (POCD) primarily affects the elderly population and is inversely related to the patients' educational status. While individual contributions of surgical and anaesthesia-related factors towards the development of POCD is still being researched upon, the common understanding of the phenomena principally implicates a state of neuro-inflammation precipitated by the surgical stress. Also, pre-operative cognitive status is known to be a significant determinant of developing POCD. It has serious long-term consequences in the elderly population, including prolonged hospital length of stay (LOS), decreased functional independence, increased risk of dementia, caregiver burden, healthcare costs, morbidity and mortality [1]. In the context of oncological critical care patient subset, multiple co-existing factors increase the likelihood of POCD. Being diagnosed with cancer—its personal, economic and social implications, added to the stress of undergoing complex and protracted surgeries—is emotionally taxing. Moreover, though malignancies can affect any age group, the primary bulk of cancer patients are elderly. These, along with the concerns regarding lifestyle modifications secondary to post-surgical atomic alterations (like, facial disfigurement in head and neck

J. K. Mitra (✉)
Anaesthesia, AIIMS Bhubaneswar, Bhubaneswar, Odisha, India

P. Tapuria
Cardiac Anaesthesia, AIIMS Bhubaneswar, Bhubaneswar, Odisha, India

D. Saha
Neuro Anaesthesia, AIIMS Bhubaneswar, Bhubaneswar, Odisha, India

V. Kumar et al. (eds.), *Onco-critical Care*,
https://doi.org/10.1007/978-981-16-9929-0_33

cancer, feeding in gastro-oesophageal cancers, bowel diversions in colorectal cancers, effects of penectomy and mastectomy on conjugal life) impose immense emotional burden on this patient population. While advancements in medical practices have improved the lifespan in onco-surgical patients, the impact of the treatment modalities on the neuro-psychological aspects of the cancer survivors have been somewhat neglected until recently. With an enhanced focus on improving the quality of life in onco-surgical patients—pre-operative assessment, prevention, diagnosis and treatment of post-operative neuro-cognitive disorders is poised to become increasingly important to the practice of oncological critical care.

33.2 Postoperative Delirium in ICU Patients

Perioperative neurocognitive disorder (NCD) is the term used to describe cognitive impairment in the preoperative or postoperative period. Cognitive decline diagnosed before operation (is called as neurocognitive disorder). Postoperatively it is divided according to time frame again; Immediate (Emergence delirium), up to 1 week (postoperative delirium) and 1–4 weeks (delayed neurocognitive recovery) and 1–12 months (postoperative neurocognitive disorder) [2].

Preoperative cognitive impairment is the term used for patients having objectifiable cognitive decline before surgery and anesthesia detected in pre-anesthetic check-up before elective surgery. It may range from subtle decline as mild MCI (Mild Cognitive Impairment) to major (Dementia).

Delirium is the term used for patients having acute onset changes in mental status like altered awareness about the environment and decreased attention as described in DSM5 criteria for diagnosing delirium. Emergence delirium is a transient state of marked irritation and dissociation seen after discontinuation of general anesthesia. Postoperative delirium (POD) is the term used for patients fitting in DSM 5 criteria but occurring within 1 week of surgery or until discharge. But we need to exclude the following

1. Preoperative drug use, alcohol
2. Prior history of dementia and delirium
3. Persistent effect of drugs
4. Other physiological variables like hypoxia/acidosis/electrolyte imbalance/infection.

POD and emergence delirium (from anesthesia) are not synonymous. Most patients may have completely normal emergence from anesthesia post-procedure. They might develop acute fluctuation in mental status after a period of lucid interval i.e. in postoperative day 1–3 [3]

Postoperative cognitive dysfunction (POCD) is the term used for patients having objectifiable cognitive decline from the baseline starting 1 week post-surgery up to 1 year [4]. This cognitive decline is quantified using various neuropsychological tests usually administered as a test battery (Table 33.1).

Table 33.1 Nomenclature of perioperative neurocognitive disorder in different time period

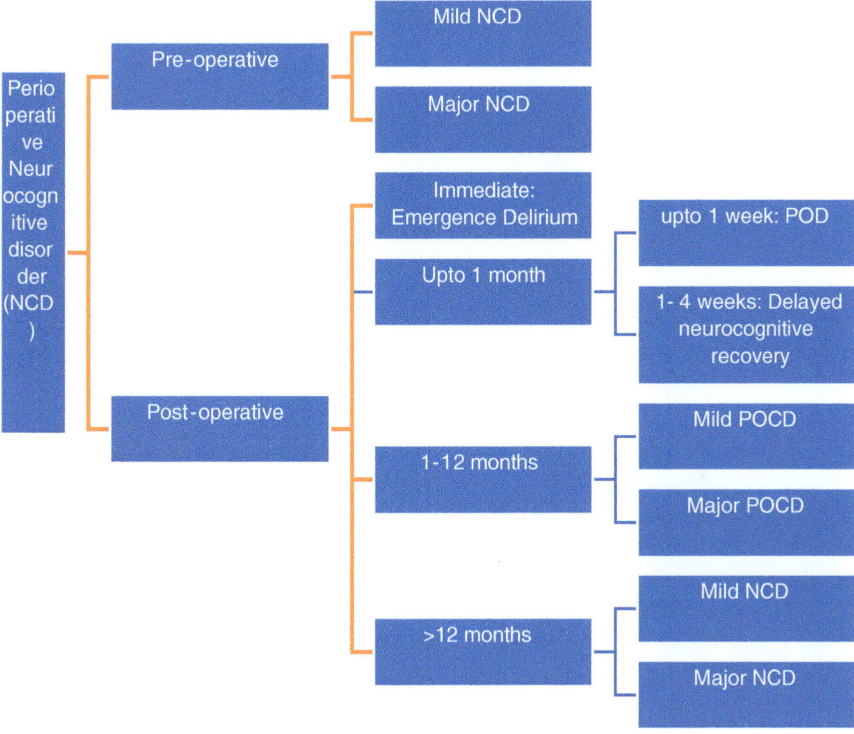

Modified from Evered et al. [2]

33.2.1 Pathogenesis of POCD in Cancer Patients

Numerous neurotransmitters like norepinephrine, lymphokines, melatonin have been implicated in the pathogenesis of POCD. Chemokines can disrupt blood-brain barrier *in vitro*, and suggested to be associated with pathogenesis of delirium. Its level has been found to be elevated in early postoperative period in patients who develop delirium after surgery. Cancer Surgery induced stress response leads to release of neuroendocrine factors and changes related to neuroinflammation, which may influence neuronal functioning, increased levels of glucocorticoids such as cortisol and cytokines lead to inflammatory response.

Anesthetic related central nervous system toxicity such as volatile anaesthetic induced apoptosis and B amyloid formation lead to cognitive impairment. The duration of cancer surgery and anaesthesia, intraoperative factors like hypoxia, hypercarbia, hypotension, and marked disturbance of homeostasis are risk factors resulting in POCD [5]. Many cancer surgeries are extensive and of long duration leading to major blood loss resulting in hypotension. In certain cancer surgeries, such as lobectomies and pneumonectomies there are increased chances of hypoxia and hypercarbia.

33.3 Cognitive Assessment Tools

A cognitive decline is defined as a decline from a previous level of performance in one or more cognitive domains (complex attention, executive function, learning, and memory, language, perceptual-motor, or social cognition [6]. The various tools for assessment of cognitive impairment in cancer surgical patients are as follows:

33.3.1 Mini Mental State Examination (MMSE)

MMSE [7] is a widely used tool for quantifying cognitive deficits. It includes orientation, attention, memory, language, and visual-spatial skills. It has been criticized as it takes a long time to complete an assessment.

33.3.2 Short Portable Mental Status Questionnaire (SPMSQ) [8]

It's a 10-point questionnaire. The questions are- what are the date, month and year; What is the day of the week; what is the name of this place; What is your phone number; How old are you; when were you born; who is the current president; who was the president before him; what was your mother's maiden name? can you count backwards from 20 by 3 s. The scoring is done by number of errors I the response 0–2 errors is normal mental function; 3–4 errors mild cognitive impairment; 5–7 errors moderate cognitive impairment; 8 or more errors severe cognitive impairment.

33.3.3 Montreal Cognitive Assessment (MoCA) [9]

It is a 30-point cognitive screening tool requires 10 min to finish. It can be done in pre-anesthetic check-up. It is available in 35 different languages. Can be done in visually impaired patients.

33.3.4 Clock Drawing Test [10]

It is a test in which the patient is asked to draw a clock and type of clock drawing errors are documented to differentiate between several cognitive and neuro psychiatric disorders especially dementia. It can demonstrate subtle cognitive deficits which are sometimes challenging to identify in routine bedside exams. It also has a great educational value for the patient and families.

33.3.5 Abbreviated Mental Test Score [11]

It is used to rapidly assess elderly patients for possibility of dementia. 10 point questionnaire. Each question correctly answered scores 1 point. A score of 6 or less suggests delirium or dementia. But further tests are required to conform the diagnosis.

33.3.6 Mini-Cog [12]

It is a 3-min cognitive screening tool which combines a clock drawing test with 3 item recall.

33.3.7 5 Item Recall and Fluency (5-IRF) [13]

It is a 2-min screening tool comprising a 5 item recall and a 1-min verbal fluency for animals where the patient is asked to name as many different animals.

Test	Description	Sensitivity/specificity
MMSE	Total of 30 points • 24–30 = Possible cognitive impairment • 18–23 = Mild to Moderate cognitive impairment • <17 = Severe cognitive impairment	In clinical setting: • Pooled sensitivity was 79.8% and • Specificity was 81.3% [14]
MoCA	Total of 30 points • Normal score > 26 • Requires 10 min to complete • Points are allocated as: visuospatial and executive functioning (5 points), animal naming (3 points), attention (6 points), language (3 points), abstraction (2 points), delayed recall (5 points), orientation (6 points), education level (1 point added if the individual has 12 years of formal education)	• Sensitivity is 90% in detecting MCI • Specificity of 87% in detecting MCI and Dementia [9]
Mini Cog	• 3-min screening test • Clock drawing task and 3 item recall • Dementia is correlated with a recall score of regardless of clock drawing task or recall score of 1–2 with an abnormal clock drawing score	• Sensitivity of 76% and specificity of 73% in detecting dementia [15] • Sensitivity of 99% and specificity of 93% in detecting dementia when compared to the MMSE with sensitivity of 91% and specificity of 92% [16]

Test	Description	Sensitivity/specificity
5-IRF	• Screening tool for dementia • Requires 2 min to complete • Comprises a 5-item address recall (e.g., John, Doe, 32, King Street, Louisiana) and a 1-min verbal fluency for animals • Dementia is correlated with 3 recall errors or < 8 animals named	• At a cut-off score of > 3 recall errors and < 8 animals name, the sensitivity is 79% and the specificity is 98% for detecting dementia [17]
Clock Drawing Test	• Most used cognitive screening tools for dementia	• Pooled sensitivity is 82% • Specificity is 75.7% using the Shulman system

33.4 Indications of Assessment

POD is a common complication following major surgeries and is often associated with adverse outcomes. Cancer surgeries are known to be of prolonged duration and most patients are elderly with multiple comorbidities, risking them for developing POD.

Recent studies have been able to identify certain risk factors in patients with different cancers. Incidence of POD is considerable in patients undergoing surgery for bone metastases. Risk factors identified were history of psychiatric disorders, preoperative serum albumin and CRP levels, and the dose of postoperative opioid analgesics [18].

In Head and neck cancer surgeries, age>70 years, Male gender, history of hypertension, long duration of surgery including neck dissection and flap reconstruction, need for blood transfusion, and ASA > 3 were all singled out as risk factors for POD [19].

Similarly POD was linked to Colorectal cancer group who are old age, with prior history of dementia, developing surgical site infection, operative approach open versus laparoscopic, poor nutritional status and encephalopathy [20].

The development of POCD is preventable in 30–40% of cases [21]. However after development of POCD, any intervention has not been so beneficial as they have been shown to be of little effect on severity, duration and recurrence [22]. This emphasizes the importance of primary prevention by risk factor assessment. Once the high risk groups are picked up, cognitive tools are applied to them for the following reasons: (1) screening for cognitive impairment; (2) differential diagnosis of cause; (3) rating of severity of disorder, or monitoring disease progression.

33.5 Interpreting Results

There are four areas of concern; these are how to analyse and interpret the results from the scales, timing when these scales are to be used, number of times the patient to be assessed and the whether to exclude patients with pre-existing mild cognitive impairment (MCI)

Among the different testing batteries available, how to analyse them, and determining how much dysfunction is clinically significant remains a matter of debate. There are three methods of analysing these results from the different assessment tools.

(a) Percentage change method:
Postoperative score – Preoperative score/Preoperative score
Averaging across groups should not be done because while some patients will decline, others improve over time and this difference can be masked.
(b) Standard deviation (SD) method: number of SD outside of which it is a decline. In patients who have low baseline score may give flawed result which is called as floor effect. Standard interpretation is ±2 SD from the preoperative values as either improvement or decline.
(c) Percent change method i.e., a decline of 20% from baseline. But patients with low scores to start with may require even smaller percentage change to be diagnosed with POCD.

The timing of test is important. Debate is still on over the optimal timing of perioperative cognitive testing [23]. Preoperative test scores can be affected at the morning of procedure due to preprocedural anxiety, therefore testing on the day of surgery should ideally be avoided and potential solutions when and where should the patient be tested preoperative includes:

- Memory Clinics: linked to surgical specialties concerned
- Primary Care Surgery Clinics: led by nurse
- Separate assessments when surgical decision is confirmed and patient is sent for a Pre anesthetic assessment

For postoperative scoring optimal postoperative cognitive testing has been suggested 1–3 months post procedure [24]. There are fallacies of both too early and late testing. Immediately after operation, patients who are tested can score worse than those who are tested weeks to months later possibly due to pain, residual drugs, and effect of acute medications. Similarly, long-term testing is confounded by loss to follow up, especially patients who experience the greatest decline are most likely to attrition. This may lead to significantly underestimation of the true incidence of POCD. The patients who have cancer have lower baseline assessment scores and post-surgery they tend to decline even further which may not be interpreted at first but with regular follow-ups its been seen that the incidence of POCD is even higher.

A patient assessed at a single point in time both preoperative and postoperative may give suboptimal result as he or she may be in many different cognitive trajectories. So, following the cognitive trend on a case-to-case basis is more reliable than a single point assessment. There is compelling evidence that patients who have declining trajectories before surgery, such as those who have mild cognitive impairment (MCI) or early dementia, are more likely to decline cognitively after surgery [25, 26]. While choosing patients for POCD assessment, care should be given not to exclude MCI patients like Alzheimer's disease, cerebral vascular disease and patients with dementia. All of these conditions are a significant risk factor of POCD by virtue of their pre-existing low cognitive reserve.

33.6 Management of Cognitive Dysfunction

To date, there are no specific treatments available for POCD, but the condition is of concern to elderly oncological patients, and it is important that anesthetists and surgeons consider ways to reduce its incidence and engage in a discussion of the risks with patients preoperatively.

33.6.1 Risk Factors

Preoperative	Intraoperative	Postoperative
Age > 70 years	Severe bleeding > 1000 ml	Severe pain
History of alcohol / illicit drug abuse	Intraoperative tight glucose control	Benzodiazepines, anticholinergics
Electrolyte imbalance	Bispectral index too low or too high	Delayed ambulation
Prior NCD	Intraoperative hypotension or hypocapnia	Malnutrition
Alzheimer's disease		

Special concerns in oncosurgical patients:

(a) Chronically malnourished
(b) Immunosuppressed
(c) Pre-existing comorbidities
(d) Low-level education
(e) Psychological factors—stress, anxiety after diagnosis
(f) Long operative duration with more blood loss and fluid shifts with consequent episodes of hypotension.
(g) Use of inotropes and vasopressors.
(h) Protracted ICU course
(i) Delay in initiating nutrition in surgeries involving gastrointestinal tract.
(j) Refeeding syndrome
(k) Chemotherapy, Radiotherapy and Hormone Therapy

At present a multidisciplinary care bundle approach to risk factor stratification and reduction is the most attractive management plan based on evidence of slight benefit from individual treatment.

33.6.1.1 Preoperative Management

1. Address psychological issues before taking up for surgery to reduce stress, anxiety, and depression on diagnosis of cancer.
2. To get a test battery including inventories commonly used to detect dementia and/or mild cognitive dysfunction prior to surgery. Which can be repeated at regular intervals post procedure as well.
3. Perioperative cognitive training.

33.6.1.2 Intraoperative Management

1. It is not clear whether maintenance with propofol-based total intravenous anesthesia (TIVA) or with inhalational agents affect incidences of postoperative delirium, mortality, or length of hospital stay. Low certainty evidence found that maintenance with propofol-based TIVA may reduce POCD [27].
2. No difference was found in the incidence of POCD with use of xenon or sevoflurane in elderly patients [28]. Although there are no studies done in oncosurgical patients so far.
3. Moderate-quality evidence suggest that optimized anesthesia guided by processed electroencephalographic (EEG) indices could reduce the risk of postoperative delirium in patients aged 60 years or over undergoing non-cardiac surgical and non-neurosurgical procedures. There are no data available for patients under 60 year [29].
4. Opioids and associated disturbances of calcium, sodium, and glucose homeostasis has been shown to cause post-operative cognitive dysfunction in elderly patients [30] so it is safe to assume that the same can be seen in onco-surgical patients as well although the evidence is scarce in this.
5. Multimodal interventions such as judicious use of regional anesthesia, use of antipsychotics, Bispectral index guided anesthesia and use of dexmedetomidine have shown to reduce the incidence of POCD [13].

33.6.1.3 Postoperative Management

1. Good postoperative pain management using multimodal analgesia.
2. Avoid postoperative benzodiazepine use.
3. There are no gold standard tests to measure cognitive function, but the combination of tests would help in diagnosis of cognitive impairment and to strategize for prevention of further impairment that would benefit in the overall outcome of patient.
4. Early recovery after surgery (ERAS) protocols are evidence based models that have been adopted in various surgical subspecialities. It has been shown to enhance recovery, shorten hospital stay, and reduce morbidity, and may be effective in preventing POCD [31].

33.7 Key Points

- POCD is a very well-known and disabling complication of cancer surgery. So it is beneficial to perform a serial cognitive assessment and categorize these patients according to correct nomenclature.
- Assessment of cognitive impairment in the preoperative setting includes a good detailed history and a formal evaluation using screening tools.
- The MMSE, MoCA, Mini-Cog, 5-IRF, clock drawing test, etc. are simple screening tools that can be utilized by all healthcare professionals at the bedside with acceptable sensitivity and specificity rates.
- Educating and training all levels of healthcare providers is of utmost importance as many patients' POD goes unrecognized by healthcare professionals.
- A multi-disciplinary approach with efforts to identify risk factors from preoperative setting is the key to management.
- Preventive measures against the development of POCD is the best strategy, followed by early recognition and management of perioperative symptoms.

References

1. Androsova G, Krause R, Winterer G, Schneider R. Biomarkers of postoperative delirium and cognitive dysfunction. Front Aging Neurosci. 2015;7:112. https://doi.org/10.3389/fnagi.2015.00112.
2. Evered L, Silbert B, Knopman DS, et al. Recommendations for the nomenclature of cognitive change associated with anaesthesia and surgery—2018. Br J Anaesth. 2018;121(5):1005–12. https://doi.org/10.1016/j.bja.2017.11.087.
3. Deiner S, Silverstein JH. Postoperative delirium and cognitive dysfunction. Br J Anaesth. 2009;103(Suppl.1):41–6. https://doi.org/10.1093/bja/aep291.
4. Inouye SK, Marcantonio ER, Kosar CM, et al. The short-term and long-term relationship between delirium and cognitive trajectory in older surgical patients. Alzheimers Dement. 2016;12(7):766–75. https://doi.org/10.1016/j.jalz.2016.03.005.
5. Rundshagen I. Postoperative kognitive dysfunktion. Dtsch Arztebl Int. 2014;111(8):119–25. https://doi.org/10.3238/arztebl.2014.0119.
6. Diagnostic and statistical manual of mental disorders (DSM-5®)—American Psychiatric Association. 5th ed. American Psychiatric Publishing; 2013.
7. Folstein MF, Folstein SE, McHugh PR. 'Mini-mental state'. A practical method for grading the cognitive state of patients for the clinician. J Psychiatr Res. 1975;12(3):189–98. https://doi.org/10.1016/0022-3956(75)90026-6.
8. Pfeiffer E. A short portable mental status questionnaire for the assessment of organic brain deficit in elderly patients. J Am Geriatr Soc. 1975;23(10):433–41. https://doi.org/10.1111/j.1532-5415.1975.tb00927.x.
9. Nasreddine ZS, Phillips NA, Bedirian V, et al. The montreal cognitive assessment, MoCA: a brief screening tool for mild cognitive impairment. J Am Geriatr Soc. 2005;53(4):695–9. https://doi.org/10.1111/j.1532-5415.2005.53221.x.
10. Park JK, Jeong EH, Seomun GA. The clock drawing test: A systematic review and meta-analysis of diagnostic accuracy. J Adv Nurs. 2018;74(12):2742–54. https://doi.org/10.1111/jan.13810.
11. Hodkinson HM. Evaluation of a mental test score for assessment of mental impairment in the elderly. Age Ageing. 1972;1(4):233–8. https://doi.org/10.1093/ageing/1.4.233.

12. Borson S, Scanlan JM, Chen P, Ganguli M. The mini-cog as a screen for dementia: validation in a population-based sample. J Am Geriatr Soc. 2003;51(10):1451–4. https://doi.org/10.1046/j.1532-5415.2003.51465.x.
13. Janssen TL, Alberts AR, Hooft L, Mattace-Raso FUS, Mosk CA, van der Laan L. Prevention of postoperative delirium in elderly patients planned for elective surgery: systematic review and meta-analysis. Clin Interv Aging. 2019;14:1095–117. https://doi.org/10.2147/CIA.S201323.
14. Mitchell AJ. A meta-analysis of the accuracy of the mini-mental state examination in the detection of dementia and mild cognitive impairment. J Psychiatr Res. 2009;43(4):411–31. https://doi.org/10.1016/j.jpsychires.2008.04.014.
15. Holsinger T, Plassman BL, Stechuchak KM, Burke JR, Coffman CJ, Williams JW. Screening for cognitive impairment: comparing the performance of four instruments in primary care. J Am Geriatr Soc. 2012;60(6):1027–36. https://doi.org/10.1111/j.1532-5415.2012.03967.x.
16. Borson S, Scanlan J, Brush M, Vitaliano P, Dokmak A. The Mini-Cog: a cognitive 'vital signs' measure for dementia screening in multi-lingual elderly. Int J Geriatr Psychiatry. 2000;15(11):1021–7. https://doi.org/10.1002/1099-1166(200011)15:11<1021::AID-GPS234>3.0.CO;2-6.
17. Stephen Long L, Shapiro WA, Leung JM. A brief review of practical preoperative cognitive screening tools. Can J Anesth. 2012;59(8):798–804. https://doi.org/10.1007/s12630-012-9737-1.
18. Hindiskere S, Kim HS, Han I. Postoperative delirium in patients undergoing surgery for bone metastases. Medicine (Baltimore). 2020;99(20). https://doi.org/10.1097/MD.0000000000020159.
19. Zhu Y, Wang G, Liu S, et al. Risk factors for postoperative delirium in patients undergoing major head and neck cancer surgery: A meta-analysis. Jpn J Clin Oncol. 2017;47(6):505–11. https://doi.org/10.1093/jjco/hyx029.
20. Yang Z, Wang XF, Yang LF, Fang C, Gu XK, Guo HW. Prevalence and risk factors for postoperative delirium in patients with colorectal carcinoma: a systematic review and meta-analysis. Int J Colorectal Dis. 2020;35(3):547–57. https://doi.org/10.1007/s00384-020-03505-1.
21. Inouye SK, Westendorp RGJ, Saczynski JS. Delirium in elderly people. Lancet. 2014;383(9920):911–22. https://doi.org/10.1016/S0140-6736(13)60688-1.
22. Burry L, Mehta S, Perreault MM, et al. Antipsychotics for treatment of delirium in hospitalised non-ICU patients. Cochrane Database Syst Rev. 2018;2018(6). https://doi.org/10.1002/14651858.CD005594.pub3.
23. Nadelson MR, Sanders RD, Avidan MS. Perioperative cognitive trajectory in adults. Br J Anaesth. 2014;112(3):440–51. https://doi.org/10.1093/bja/aet420.
24. Moller JT, Cluitmans P, Rasmussen LS, et al. Long-term postoperative cognitive dysfunction in the elderly: ISPOCD1 study. Lancet. 1998;351(9106):857–61. https://doi.org/10.1016/S0140-6736(97)07382-0.
25. Saczynski JS, Marcantonio ER, Quach L, et al. Cognitive trajectories after postoperative delirium. N Engl J Med. 2012;367(1):30–9. https://doi.org/10.1056/NEJMoa1112923.
26. Avidan MS, Searleman AC, Storandt M, et al. Long-term cognitive decline in older subjects was not attributable to noncardiac surgery or major illness. Anesthesiology. 2009;111(5):964–70. https://doi.org/10.1097/ALN.0b013e3181bc9719.
27. Miller D, Lewis SR, Pritchard MW, et al. Intravenous versus inhalational maintenance of anaesthesia for postoperative cognitive outcomes in elderly people undergoing non-cardiac surgery. Cochrane Database Syst Rev. 2018;2018(8). https://doi.org/10.1002/14651858.CD012317.pub2.
28. Cremer J, Stoppe C, Fahlenkamp AV, et al. Early cognitive function, recovery and well-being after sevoflurane and xenon anaesthesia in the elderly: A double-blinded randomized controlled trial. Med Gas Res. 2011;1(1):1–10. https://doi.org/10.1186/2045-9912-1-9.
29. Punjasawadwong Y, Chau-in W, Laopaiboon M, Punjasawadwong S, Pin-on P. Processed electroencephalogram and evoked potential techniques for amelioration of postoperative

delirium and cognitive dysfunction following non-cardiac and non-neurosurgical procedures in adults. Cochrane Database Syst Rev. 2018;2018(5). https://doi.org/10.1002/14651858.CD011283.pub2.
30. Fines DP, Severn AM. Anaesthesia and cognitive disturbance in the elderly. Contin Educ Anaesth Crit Care Pain. 2006;6(1):37–40. https://doi.org/10.1093/bjaceaccp/mki066.
31. Kotekar N, Shenkar A, Nagaraj R. Postoperative cognitive dysfunction—current preventive strategies. Clin Interv Aging. 2018;13:2267–73. https://doi.org/10.2147/CIA.S133896.

Critical Care Management in Patients Undergoing Brain Tumor Surgery

34

Kali Charan Das, Vanitha Rajagopalan, and Girija Prasad Rath

34.1 Introduction

Brain tumors are amongst the most dreaded of all forms of cancer. The duration and requirements of intensive care unit (ICU) management for neurosurgical patients after brain tumor resection are unclear. A general consensus is that all patients should be observed closely in an acute care setting for at least 12–24 hours after brain tumor resection surgery [1]. Postoperative intensive care aids prevent delay in detecting life-threatening complications, facilitation of early intervention, and reestablishment of homeostasis to hasten recovery. An uneventful and successful tumor surgery may have a bad outcome if the postoperative ICU management is inadequate. Even after the established importance of postoperative ICU management, certain sections of expertise have questioned the role of such a mandatory provision. Postoperative ICU stays after cardiac surgery have been challenged for years. Advanced intraoperative/anesthetic management led to early extubation and shifting of patients to step-down units; it helped reduce the burden in the conditions of limited resources and improve patient satisfaction [2]. Similar postoperative management has been applied in a certain group of neurosurgical patients, particularly for low-grade tumor surgeries with an uneventful intraoperative course, and it has shown some benefit.

Despite advancements in neurosurgery, neuroanesthesia, neuro-oncology, and neurointensive care, the morbidity and mortality due to intracranial neoplasms still remain high. Furthermore, clear-cut guidelines regarding postoperative management after brain tumor surgery is lacking [3]. This chapter discusses the common postoperative complications among neuro-oncological patients and their ICU management based on the current practices.

K. C. Das · V. Rajagopalan · G. P. Rath (✉)
Department of Neuroanaesthesiology and Critical Care, Neurosciences Centre, All India Institute of Medical Sciences (AIIMS), New Delhi, India

V. Kumar et al. (eds.), *Onco-critical Care*,
https://doi.org/10.1007/978-981-16-9929-0_34

34.2 Postoperative Neurointensive Care

Every patient undergoing neurosurgical intervention is admitted to the neuro-ICU (NICU) as part of our conventional practice [4]. A dedicated NICU is preferable as it is safer than the non-specialized ICU [5], and thence, a patient with indications for intensive care after brain tumor resection is usually admitted to the NICU.

The concept of whether or not every patient after elective neurosurgery required admission to the NICU started emerging due to the reduction in practices of prolonged postoperative mechanical ventilation and sedation. Following an uneventful intraoperative course and if extubated early, many patients may be transferred to the wards if they remain stable after several hours of observation. This idea of early patient discharge from the NICU also has economic benefits. Advanced age, high-risk anesthetic and surgery, prolonged surgery, extensive blood loss, and other major intraoperative complications are significant factors, which should be considered for patient admission to the NICU [6]. Patients with infratentorial tumor resection are preferably admitted and monitored in the NICU [6].

The importance of balancing between the advantages of a brief stay in the NICU and patient safety cannot be emphasized more. The concept of the creation of a recovery room became the reality to arbitrate between the two [7]. NICU admission is required if the patient does not become fully awake at the end of the surgery and cannot be extubated safely in the recovery room.

Neuro-oncology patients who are stable and without further postoperative deterioration can be safely managed in the recovery room. They may be transferred directly to the ward; their postoperative management is beyond the scope of this chapter. The management of patients with anticipated complications in the postoperative period requiring NICU admission is elaborated in this chapter.

34.3 Brain Tumor Types

There are more than 150 different types of documented brain tumors, but the two main groups are termed primary and metastatic. Tumors that originate from the tissues of the brain or its immediate surroundings are included in primary brain tumors. They are further classified as glial or non-glial (developed from blood vessels, nerves etc.) and benign or malignant. World Health Organization (WHO) classifies primary brain tumors based on histopathologic criteria and immunohistochemical data (Table 34.1). The incidence of tumors in CNS (both malignant and nonmalignant) is 28.57 per 100,000 population (Table 34.1). Metastatic brain tumors arise from sites other than the brain (such as the liver, lungs) and reach the brain, usually through the hematogenous route. Metastatic tumors are considered malignant tumors.

Postoperative neurosurgical care after tumor surgery aims to prevent or minimize complications related to anesthesia and surgery. Careful and serial neurological assessments by trained staff and management of systemic complications are the

Table 34.1 Brain tumors: types, incidence, diagnosis, and management [8]

Classification	Incidence (%)	Diagnosis	Management
Total: 28.57%			
Tumor of Meninges (7.88%)			
Meningioma	7.61 F:M 2:1	CT/MRI	Preoperative embolization followed by surgical excision with or without radiotherapy (RT)
Mesenchymal Tumors	0.08	Imaging with Histopathology	Surgical resection
Primary Melanocytomas	0.01	MRI with Histopathology	Surgical resection
Other Neoplasm	0.18	MRI / histopathology	Surgical or palliative
Tumors of Neuro-epithelium (6.61%)			
Glioblastoma	3.19 M > F	CT/MRI	Maximal surgical resection with chemoradiotherapy
Diffuse Astrocytoma	0.55 M:F 1:1	CT/MRI	surgical resection with adjuvant TMZ based CT (24 cycles) with RT
Glioma	0.46 M:F 1:1	CT/MRI	Surgical resection
Ependymal Tumors	0.42	Histopathology	Surgery with local RT
Anaplastic Astrocytoma	0.37 M:F 2:1	CT/MRI	Surgery followed by EBRT with adjuvant TMZ (42 cycles) or PCV
Pilocytic Astrocytoma	0.34 M:F 1.18:1	CT/MRI	Surgery alone or EBRT or conservative if surgery not possible
Neuoronal-Glial Tumor	0.28	MRI with Histopathology	Surgical resection
Embryonal Tumor (Medulloblastoma)	0.26 M:F 1.5:1	Histopathology and molecular analysis	Surgical resection with craniospinal irradiation and CT
Oligodendroglioma	0.2 M > F	Molecular analysis (IDH 1,2 mutation), OG NOS	Surgery or RT and adjuvant TMZ/PCV CT
Anaplastic Oligodendroma	0.11	MRI/MRS with OG NOS	Surgery with RT and adjuvant TMZ/PCV CT Anti VEGF (Bevacizumab)
Choroid Plexus Tumor	0.05, infants	MRI (frond-like lobulated IV mass)	Surgery/ stereotactic radiosurgery
Pineal Tumors	0.04 M < F	MRI (gold standard) Tumor markers (b-HCG, AFP)	Endoscopic third ventriculostomy (ETV) using ETV Score, Surgical resection, RT (Germinoma), RT-CT (all pineal tumor except pineocytoma)

(continued)

Table 34.1 (continued)

Classification	Incidence (%)	Diagnosis	Management
Tumor of Sellar Region (3.47%)			
Pituitary Tumor	3.29	Gad MRI with hormonal assay (TFT, GH, ACTH etc)	Transnasal transsphenoidal (TNTS) resection, with hormonal therapy
Craniopharyngioma	0.18 M = F	MRI	Surgery (TNTS or transcranial approach), EBRT, intra-cystic therapy (bleomycin, IFN α)
Tumor of Cranial Nerve and Spine (1.70%)			
Nerve Sheath Tumor (Schwannomma, Neurofibroma etc)	1.70	MRI, clinical signs, histopathology	Conservative (Neurofibromas), Surgery, Stereotactic Radiosurgery
Lymphomas (M/C Dlbcl)	0.46 M > F	MRI, PET, B cell, plasma cell markers	Whole-brain RT with high dose methotrexate (HD-MTX), myeloablative therapy etc
Germ Cell Tumors	0.10	MRI with tumor markers	Multimodal approach
Unclassified	0.19		Multimodal approach

CT Computed tomography, *MRI* magnetic resonance imaging, *M* male, *F* female, *PET* positron emission tomography

cornerstone of ICU care that can help minimize grave neurological sequel. Patients who are expected to require NICU care after elective or emergent tumor surgery include:

- Supra- and infratentorial craniotomy for tumor
- Craniofacial and transsphenoidal surgery
- Patients with serious medical comorbidities, elderly, or with unfavorable intraoperative course

The key elements for successful management of these patients are:

- Vigilance and early detection of surgical complications (stroke, seizures, and bleeding)
- Timely emergence and recovery from anesthesia
- Assessment of impaired consciousness
- Restoring and maintaining normal body temperature and prevention of shivering
- Pain management
- Management of postoperative nausea and vomiting (PONV)
- Prophylaxis for DVT and GI bleeding

34.4 Epidemiology

It is estimated that up to half of all post-neurosurgical patients will experience complications in their perioperative course. Ten percent (10%) of these complications are consequential and attract significant morbidity and mortality. The mortality rate for elective supratentorial tumor surgery and posterior fossa surgery are 1–7% and 2%, respectively. Transsphenoidal surgery has a perioperative mortality rate of 1%. However, most of the complications in neurosurgical patients are due to pain (80%), PONV (50%), and shivering (30%).

34.5 Complications

Intracranial hemorrhage (ICH) is one of the most serious complications and is seen in 1–3% of neurosurgical patients with mortality and morbidity of approximately 30% and 50%, respectively. ICH is independently linked with perioperative hypertension, coagulopathy, thrombocytopenia (<100,000/mm^3), high-grade vascular tumors, and emergent surgery. Tumors like high-grade astrocytoma, midline meningioma, and metastatic tumors may present with early postoperative seizures (10–20%). Prophylactic anticonvulsant administration is expected to reduce the incidence of early postoperative seizures by 30–50% but does not reduce the likelihood of developing late epilepsy.

CSF leaks occur in 2–5% of trans-sphenoidal surgeries; however, this is further lowered in procedures performed in the hands of experienced surgeons. Risk factors for leaks include preoperative radiation treatment, repeat procedures, large size tumors, and advanced age.

Complications following brain tumor surgery can be broadly distinguished according to the location of the tumor, which may be divided into three broad categories.

34.5.1 Intracerebral Hemispheric, and Convexity Tumors

Glioma, brain metastasis, and convexity meningioma are the most common types of brain tumors located in the cerebral hemispheres, although other types of primary or metastatic brain tumors may present in that location. The usual postoperative complications include new neurologic deficits (NNDs) and seizures [9].

34.5.1.1 Postoperative Neurologic Deficits

The NNDs in patients with intracerebral hemispheric and convexity tumors may include delayed awakening, hemiparesis, and aphasia. The diagnosis of NND should be made as early as possible. Hence, an awake patient at the end of the surgery is always preferred unless indicated otherwise, and prolonged postoperative sedation is contraindicated in patients with brain tumors. The occurrence of NND is an indication of an emergency computed tomography (CT) of the brain. Some of the common causes of NNDs are direct surgical damage of the brain tissue, ischemia (due to retraction, vessel handling, etc.), ICH, or peritumoral edema.

34.5.1.2 Direct Surgical Damage of the Brain Tissue

Direct surgical damage of the brain tissue that is functionally active and near eloquent areas lead to neuro deficits such as hemiparesis or aphasia. Emergency CT reveals a postoperative defect in the resected tumor bed which is almost indistinguishable from peritumoral edema. Magnetic resonance imaging (MRI) discriminates between the direct surgical damage of the neural tissue and ischemic changes due to microcirculation disturbance. Although postoperative ischemia most likely results in motor NNDs, both direct surgical injury of the brain tissue and microcirculation disturbances may also be present, and differentiation between them does not alter the critical care management of the condition. The patient can be safely extubated once the damage becomes irreversible and documented, and measures established to prevent associated secondary injuries and discharged to the neurosurgical ward. Active rehabilitation may lead to improved functional outcomes in these patients [10].

34.5.1.3 Brain Ischemia

Intraoperative damage of perforating arteries, arteries of the circle of Willis, deep veins, venous sinuses, and paradoxical air embolism (PAE) produce brain ischemia resulting in severe deficits like an acute ischemic stroke compared to impaired microcirculation alone. The presence of postoperative NND combined with the intraoperative information about surgical damage of the arteries helps to conclude the etiology of the ischemia even if the postoperative CT does not reveal any abnormality, thereby preventing any delay in the intensive care management may result in irreversible brain damage.

Immediately after the resection of brain tumors, specific implications are determined by the peculiar patients' characteristics. Blood pressure (BP) should be monitored continuously; mean BP (MBP) is the preferred monitoring endpoint as it is used for the calculation of cerebral perfusion pressure (CPP) which is the difference between MBP and intracranial pressure (ICP). The MBP should be maintained above 75 mmHg in adult patients during the first three postoperative days. During the first six postoperative hours, arterial hypertension must be prevented, as it may cause ICH [11]. A safe level for MBP seems to be 90–100 mmHg, considering other clinical conditions; however, there is no evidence to support this.

The administration of anticoagulants and antiplatelet agents is another area of concern, both being contraindicated up to 48 h after the intracranial surgery. Antiplatelet agents are avoided during the whole duration of the early postoperative period in neurosurgical patients [12]. LMWH may be initiated 48 h after the surgery in the prophylactic dose, as these patients with brain tumors are at high risk for development of venous thromboembolism [12].

In cases of severe ischemia with malignant cerebral edema, midline shift, and impending herniation, the step-wise protocol of basic principles of intracranial hypertension management should be followed.

34.5.1.4 Cerebral Venous Infarction

Cerebral venous infarction due to the perioperative obstruction of deep veins or venous sinuses is a less prevalent complication in patients with a brain tumor. CT reveals cerebral edema in the absence of secondary hemorrhage into the ischemic zone. The ensuing intracranial hypertension is resistant mainly to first-line therapy, and therapeutic hypothermia, decompressive craniotomy, or both may have to be instituted to control refractory intracranial hypertension.

34.5.1.5 Paradoxical Air Embolism (PAE)

Paradoxical air embolism (PAE) is an infrequent adverse event, and only a quick and meticulous therapeutic strategy can ameliorate the patient's outcome. Venous air embolism (VAE), an intraoperative complication, usually has a conducive outcome if the air does not pass into the systemic circulation through the pulmonary vasculature [8]. The two main sources of PAE are patent foramen ovale (PFO) which may occur in almost 25% of adults, and the trans-pulmonary air passage via bronchial arterial anastomoses when volume exceeds 50 ml per minute. Massive cerebral air embolism due to obstruction of cerebral arteries by the air bubbles leads to diffuse cerebral ischemia resulting in postoperative NND. The development of CT signs of ischemia is a time-dependent process; hence, an immediate postoperative CT may miss these changes. Only hyperbaric oxygenation and hypothermia are the two effective treatment modalities available and should be initiated as early as possible, failing which there may be irreversible ischemic brain damage, severe resistant NND, and poor outcomes result. Therefore, a high index of suspicion based on thorough analysis of the clinical picture, the surgical procedure, and the anaesthesiologist report may help in early diagnosis; and prompt treatment should follow.

34.5.1.6 Intracranial Hemorrhage

Epidural and subdural hematomas, hemorrhage into the operative cavity, or remote site intracerebral hemorrhage are diagnosed with an emergent CT as early as possible when suspected or in the routine postoperative imaging. The occurrence of the ICH is an indication for re-exploration and hematoma evacuation, except if the volume of the operative cavity hematoma is lesser than the resected tumor and peritumoral edema is not as large as compared to the preoperative state.

34.5.1.7 Peritumoral Brain Edema

Meningioma and malignant brain tumors (glioblastoma, metastasis) are notorious for developing severe post-resection edema [9]. Postoperative NND or intracranial hypertension usually does not occur with peritumoral edema due to the inner decompression due to tumor resection and the use of steroids (dexamethasone), which is effective in reducing the vasogenic edema associated with malignant tumors [13]. Use of proton pump inhibitors and blood glucose control is mandatory with dexamethasone.

Edema associated with brain tumors is vasogenic in nature due to a predominant disturbance at the level of the microvasculature. A pro-angiogenic peptide vascular endothelial growth factor (VEGF) is proposed to be partially responsible for the disruption of the BBB in brain tumors by stimulating the formation of endothelial gaps, which are associated with degeneration of the basement membrane leading to fluid leakage into brain parenchyma resulting in cerebral edema. It occurs especially in high VEGF-secreting tumors like gliomas, meningiomas, as well as metastatic tumors. They occur mostly in the region of low resistance (white matter).

They may present with features of raised ICP and seizures. They may often cause brain herniations (subfalcine, tonsillar, uncal, etc.) due to mass effects, which may lead to hemiplegia, pinpoint pupils, and cardiorespiratory dysfunction. Vomiting may be a prominent sign due to raised ICP. Various imaging views of MRI and contrast-enhanced CT are generally used for diagnosing vasogenic cerebral edema.

Treatment of Cerebral Edema

Although surgical management remains the mainstay of treatment for cerebral edema, critical care management has a significant role in acute settings. Therefore, the treatment measures for elevated ICP comprise general measures, medical interventions, and surgical interventions.

General Measures

- **Positioning goals:** The patient should be positioned with the head slightly elevated up to 30° with neck neutral to free jugular veins. It has been seen that head elevation decreases cerebrospinal fluid (CSF) pressure resulting in a decrease in ICP.
- **Hemodynamic goals:** Primary goal should be to maintain euvolemia, with careful monitoring of fluid balance and avoidance of hypotonic fluids. Cerebral perfusion pressure of more than 60 mmHg should be maintained. Vasopressors may be used in case of global autoregulatory failure to maintain CPP. Vasodilators should be avoided in case of hypertension.
- **Ventilatory goals**: Hypoxia and hypercarbia are potential vasodilators that can lead to raised ICP. Optimal normocapnia of 35–40 mmHg with a low threshold for intubation should always be considered. In intubated patients, proper ventilator management can enhance neurological recovery [14].
- **Temperature**: Fever can be detrimental in outcome following brain injury [15]. In general, normothermia should be the primary goal to achieve.

Medical Interventions

- **Anticonvulsants:** Seizures may threaten the airway and can cause hypercarbia leading to raised ICP with cerebral edema. Serial monitoring of electrolytes, blood sugar, and blood gas should be initiated in cases of seizures. The effectiveness of seizure prophylaxis following surgery is unclear [16]. Newer generation antiepileptic drugs such as levetiracetam may be used as prophylaxis following brain tumor surgery [17].

- **Osmotic therapy**: 20% mannitol at a dose of 0.5 to 1.5 g/kg is a commonly practiced osmotic diuretic to reduce ICP within 15 to 35 minutes after infusion. Diuresis following mannitol administration is significant [18], requiring close monitoring of electrolyte and fluid balance. Hypokalemia, alkalosis, as well as renal damage are potential toxic effects of its use. Alternatively, 3% to 23.4% hypertonic saline may be used. A central venous catheter should ideally be used in case of using osmotherapy for more than 24 hours. Weaning should always be gradual over 12–24 hours to prevent rebound raised ICP. Complications from hypertonic saline are mostly sodium and fluid overload [19].
- **Steroids:** The effect of steroids on peritumoral edema has been well documented, and it has been used widely throughout the world for the same purpose [20]. Due to its lack of mineralocorticoid activity as well as longer duration of action, dexamethasone has been the most popular steroid amongst all [21]. Administration of dexamethasone 4 mg 6 hourly 1 to 2 days prior to an elective surgical procedure demonstrated to reduce cerebral edema. They should always be started with minimal possible doses to reduce their side effects.
- **Future advances**: Given the role of VEGF in cerebral edema, VEGF inhibitors like semaxinib, AZD2171 have shown promise in animal trials. In animal models, selective COX-2 inhibitor like SC236 has shown efficacy in increasing survival benefit.

Surgical Intervention

- **Surgical interventions**: Cerebral edema due to brain tumor can never be fully managed by medical interventions hence the placement of an external ventricular drain, ventriculoperitoneal shunt (in cases of hydrocephalus), craniotomy with excision of any residual tumor and hematoma, or in many cases decompressive craniectomy are major options to treat raised ICP following postoperative cerebral edema.

34.5.1.8 Seizures

Patients with preoperative seizures should continue to receive their antiepileptic drugs (AEDs) postoperatively at adequate doses. Typical AEDs used are phenytoin, carbamazepine, valproate, or their combination [9]. AED therapy does not exclude the occurrence of postoperative seizures. Therefore, continuous EEG monitoring along with an emergent CT should be performed immediately whenever seizures or decreased level of consciousness occur postoperatively.

Postoperative seizures involving convulsive and nonconvulsive status epilepticus occur in 13–60% of patients with intracranial tumors [22]. Early seizure identification and initiation of treatment under the recent guidelines [23] enhances the results of treatment [9].

The role of prophylactic use of AEDs in patients without preoperative seizures is questionable. Data advocate both strategies [24]. High glutamate concentration in peritumoral edema fluid detected by cerebral microdialysis may trigger epileptogenesis and predispose to postoperative seizures. The patient needs prophylactic AED administration if the tumor has invaded the cortex and is located in areas of high epileptogenicity [9]. In practice, prophylactic AED is administered by the majority of neurosurgeons, especially due to the availability of AEDs with few side effects, such as levetiracetam. It is important to use an adequate dose of any AEDs, and this is best individualized based on the measurement of the plasma level of the drug. The duration of prophylactic AED therapy is another area of debate and is based on the experience in patients with severe subarachnoid hemorrhage (SAH) or traumatic brain injury (TBI). An acceptable proposition is that five or seven days of prophylactic AED treatment in patients with intracerebral hemispheric and convexity tumors. Early postoperative seizures are a notable risk factor for late postoperative seizures, which significantly worsen the quality of life and the outcome. Therefore, prophylactic treatment of early seizures improves the patient's safety during the early postoperative period and results in an improved quality of life during the late postoperative period.

34.5.1.9 Venous Thromboembolism

Patients with intracranial tumors are at risk for venous thromboembolism (VTE). The incidence may be as high as 30% for postoperative glioma cases. The risk factors for VTE include high-grade tumor and glioblastoma subtype, large tumor size of more than 5 cm, biopsy rather than subtotal or gross total resection, paraparesis, previous history of VTE, blood types A and AB, older age, obesity, and anti-Y vascular endothelial growth factor (VEGF) therapy [25, 26]. Mechanical prophylaxis with compression stockings, pneumatic devices, and pharmacological prophylaxis with enoxaparin administration may help to prevent VTE [27, 28].

Several options for anticoagulation exist (Table 34.2). Preferred drugs based on the CLOT study and, if financial considerations allow, is low molecular weight heparin (LMWH) such as enoxaparin, dalteparin, or tinzaparin, with warfarin as a backup choice if LMWHs are not feasible (Fig. 34.1) [29]. The use of bevacizumab, an anti-VEGF antibody for recurrent glioblastoma, may increase the relative risk of venous thromboembolism.

34.5.2 Posterior Fossa Tumors

Acoustic neuroma, meningioma, glioma, ependymoma, and medulloblastoma are the most frequent histological types of primary intracranial tumor localized in the posterior fossa. A tumor may grow from the cerebellum, cerebellopontine angle, or

Table 34.2 Management of venous thromboembolism

Immediate medical management	Chronic medical management
UFH: 80 U/kg IV loading dose f/b 18 U/kg/h according aPTT	Warfarin, according to INR
Enoxaparin: 1.5 mg/kg OD	Dalteparin: 150 U/kg OD
Dalteparin: 200 U/kg OD or 100 U/kg BD	Enoxaparin: 40 mg OD

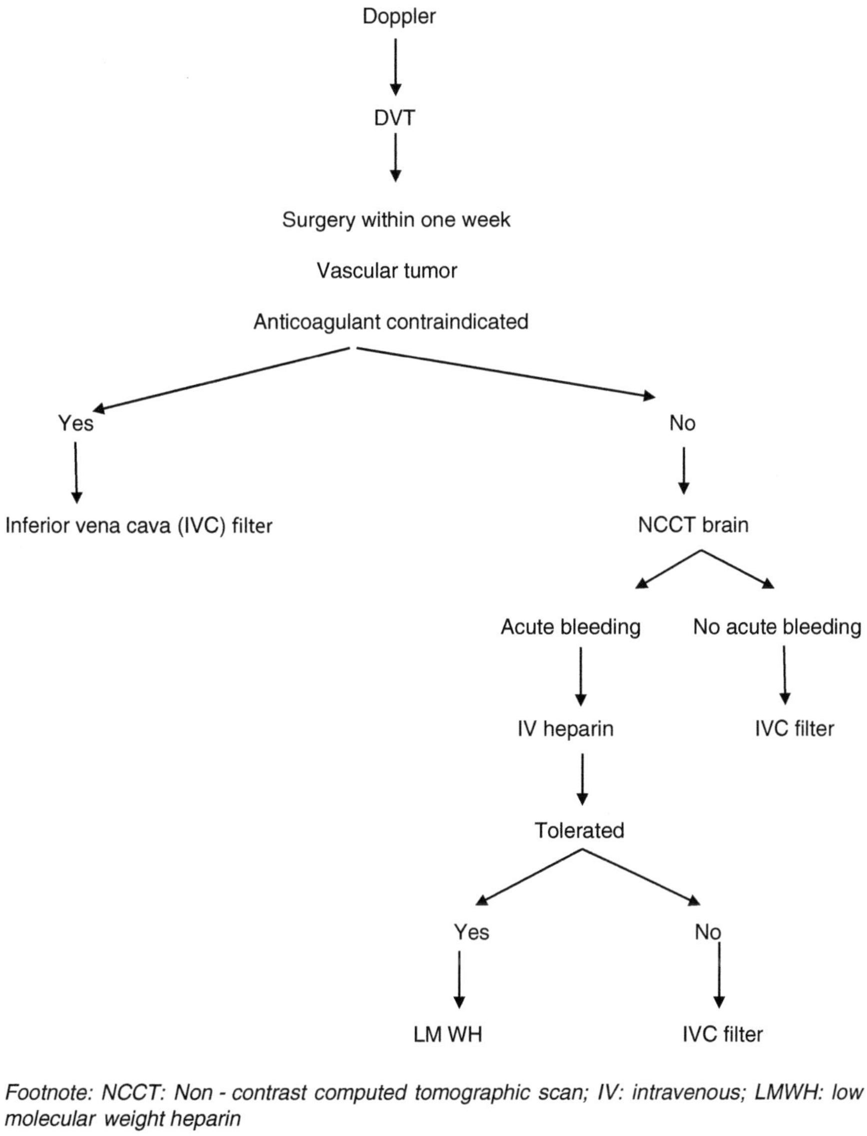

Doppler

DVT

Surgery within one week

Vascular tumor

Anticoagulant contraindicated

Yes

Inferior vena cava (IVC) filter

No

NCCT brain

Acute bleeding

IV heparin

Tolerated

Yes

LM WH

No

IVC filter

No acute bleeding

IVC filter

Footnote: NCCT: Non - contrast computed tomographic scan; IV: intravenous; LMWH: low molecular weight heparin

Fig. 34.1 Screening for deep vein thrombosis (DVT) and management of anticoagulation in neurosurgical patients. Footnote: *NCCT* Non-contrast computed tomographic scan, *IV* intravenous, *LMWH* low molecular weight heparin

from any layer of the brain stem, or may extend to the posterior fossa from the spinal cord, thalamus, pineal, or sellar region. Several anatomical factors peculiar to the posterior fossa may contribute to the development of postoperative complications. The posterior fossa contains the brain stem comprising of the ascending and descending sensorimotor pathways, nuclei of all the cranial nerves, the reticular activating system, the neural networks supporting extremely important reflexes as coughing, swallowing, and cardiorespiratory regulatory centers in a limited cavity surrounded by bones and the tentorium, housing the narrowest parts of the ventricular system—the fourth ventricle and the cerebral aqueduct. Knowledge regarding all these factors alerts the intensivists to impart utmost safety for patients with posterior fossa tumors during the postoperative period.

Infratentorial neurosurgery is an independent risk factor for respiratory insufficiency and mortality in patients undergoing tumor resection [30], and timely reintubation in patients with posterior fossa tumors in the postoperative period avoid complications. Direct surgical, ischemic, or hemorrhagic damage of the brainstem may lead to respiratory insufficiency. Respiratory insufficiency, dysphagia, or decreased level of consciousness in the postoperative period are indications for an emergent CT, which should be performed immediately after securing airway and breathing, as inadequate spontaneous breathing is a definitive sign of perioperative brainstem damage. Even small hematomas in the posterior fossa need to be surgically evacuated. No matter what is the cause of respiratory insufficiency is, incorrect airway management is an important factor leading to mortality and morbidity in patients with posterior fossa tumors [30]. Therefore, timely airway management would greatly increase patient safety and improve outcomes.

The causes of respiratory insufficiency are (a) bulbar palsy with disturbances in swallowing and coughing (damage of nuclei or IX-XII cranial nerve roots or corticobulbar tracts), (b) respiratory center damage, (c) injury to the reticular formation with the decline of consciousness, or (d) a combination of the above [31]. Assessment of the intubated patient for their preparedness for spontaneous breathing is impossible because [1] they are usually sedated, and the actual level of consciousness is unclear; [2] due to the pain and the discomfort they have impaired swallowing; [3] the cough reflex is impaired by the endotracheal tube due to the impedance of the glottic closure ("cough without glottic closure") [32, 33]. However, early extubation is preferred as soon as the criteria for extubation are fulfilled [34], else the duration of mechanical ventilation (MV) and the ICU stay might extend, with increased rates of pneumonia and worse outcome [35–37]. Reliable criteria or scales that predict the extubation success are lacking [38]. The high rate of extubation failures, especially in the neurocritical care population, emphasizes the incompetence of precise prediction of the extubation success or failure [39]. Therefore, the main focus regarding patient's safety is in the post-extubation period when the right decision should be made is a dilemma: to reintubate or not to reintubate. The Burdenko Respiratory Insufficiency Scale (BRIS) was developed for this reason [40]. It helps in the objectification of the patient's status to make a correct decision. BRIS consists of three parts: [1] assessment of the mental status with Richmond agitation sedation scale (RASS) [2] evaluation of the swallowing, cough, and airway patency [41] [3] measurement of PaO_2/FiO_2 ratio; with each part getting an independent score from 0 to 4, and then, the scores of each individual section are totaled. Obesity, due to its negative impact on respiratory function, increases the scoring by 1 point. The minimal total score is 0 (healthy person); the maximal total score is 12 in a patient with normal weight and 13 in an obese patient. The spectrum of BRIS parts extends from a normal criterion (normal consciousness, independent swallowing, effective cough, preserved airway patency, and normal PaO_2/FiO_2 ratio) to the criteria of the extreme degree of pathology (comatose state or deep sedation, severe lung injury with $PaO_2/FiO_2 < 200$, impaired airway patency with ineffective cough, and aspiration for two or more food consistencies). Each pathological condition is an indication for intubation and MV. Therefore, a score of 4 in any part of BRIS points towards immediate intubation and ventilation of the patient. A lot of intermediate clinical situations exist, where the patients have different combinations of the alteration of consciousness, swallowing disorders, cough impairment, loss of airway control, and lung injury. In such a situation, intubation decision is based on the individual demands of the patient and the experience of the intensivist.

BRIS has been developed for the uniformity of indications for intubation. A BRIS score of 3 or less means that the patient can breathe spontaneously with the need for enteral feeding via a nasogastric tube if cough and swallowing are impaired. A BRIS score of 4 as the sum points of all three parts of BRIS, but not as a single part, is still a grey zone. Some patients with a BRIS score of 4 require intubation and MV. Still, some patients will successfully keep adequate spontaneous breathing during their stay in intensive care and will be discharged to the ward, indicating that perhaps some additional factors determine the patient's ability to breathe spontaneously, which BRIS does not consider.

The posterior fossa is a small cavity with limited volume surrounded by bones and the tentorium. Even small hematomas or not very pronounced edema due to ischemia or intraoperative brain retraction may lead to intracranial hypertension. Routinely monitored supratentorial ICP may be normal, but a transtentorial ICP gradient will occur if the aqueduct or fourth ventricle is blocked [42]. Accordingly, the patients will develop neurological deficits such as consciousness decline and focal brainstem symptoms. The management based solely on normal supratentorial ICP is wrong and results in patient compromise.

Housing the narrowest parts of the ventricular system, even small additional volume in the posterior fossa leads to the rapid development of hydrocephalus due to ventricular system occlusion. The clinical picture includes signs of intracranial hypertension as severe headache, nausea, vomiting, decerebrate posturing, and declined consciousness. After immediate neuroimaging, emergent external ventricular drain (EVD) placement must be done. Rapid and excessive CSF diversion can cause severe and vitally dangerous complications such as brain dislocation and upward tentorial herniation (reverse herniation). Controlled CSF diversion is the only method for the mitigation of this complication.

34.5.3 Sellar/Suprasellar Region Tumors

Pituitary adenoma, craniopharyngioma, and para-sellar meningioma are the most frequent sellar region tumors, which are difficult to approach [43]. The evolution of endoscopic transsphenoidal surgery has considerably reduced the number of approach-related complications. Almost all histological types of sellar tumors, from the small-to-medium-size tumors with infra-sellar, latero-sellar, and antero-sellar extension can be successfully resected using the transsphenoidal approach. However, surgery of the large tumors with invasion of the suprasellar structures and the resection of craniopharyngiomas extending to the suprasellar region are still prone to the high risk of postoperative complications due to the diencephalon damage. Postoperative meningitis is another serious complication for patients with sellar tumors.

34.5.3.1 Damage of the Diencephalon

The diencephalon is a relatively small area with the highest agglomeration of vitally important centers of the entire brain. It comprises of the thalamus (primary precortical analysis of the sensory information except for olfaction), hypothalamus (highest center of the autonomic nervous system and the endocrine regulation), epithalamus (control of the autonomic functions, emotions, and the sleep-wake cycle), subthalamus (controls the extrapyramidal regulation of movements), and the pituitary gland (secretes all trophic hormones, contains vasopressin, oxytocin, and melatonin).

A direct surgical injury of diencephalon, ischemic or hemorrhagic lesions, or intraoperative traction and coagulation during the sellar-suprasellar region surgery results in local perioperative damage leading to diencephalic dysfunction. The diencephalon dysfunction syndrome (DDS), consisting of dysnatremia, alterations of consciousness, and at least one somatic organ dysfunction in patients with sellar tumors, is a recent concept [44].

34.5.3.2 Dysnatremia

Dysnatremia is the most common and widely discussed complication of sellar-suprasellar surgery. Most of these patients present with a complicated postoperative period with dysnatremia and require intensive care longer than 24 h [44]. The perioperative defacement of hypothalamus and pituitary gland function in patients with sellar tumors determines the rates of dysnatremia. Hypernatremia ($Na^+ > 145$ mmol/L) develops in up to 75–90% of patients postoperatively. Diabetes insipidus (DI) is the predominant cause of hypernatremia, leading to excessive fluid loss and hypovolemia [45]. The timely and adequate usage of desmopressin acetate (Minrin) and sodium-free fluid replacement according to their free water deficit in the patients with DI cannot be over-emphasized. Delay in recognition and treatment of hypovolemia leads to arterial hypotension and hypoperfusion of the peritumoral zone in the early postoperative period. Hyponatremia ($Na^+ < 135$ mmol/L) develops in up to 35% of postoperative patients [46]. It can be moderate ($Na^+ =$ 134–125 mmol/L) or severe (Na <125 mmol/L); acute, which develops within 72 h, or chronic, which develops more than 72 h postoperatively. Severe hyponatremia may result in coma, seizures, and adverse outcomes. The correction rates must be limited by 6–8 mmol/L per day of sodium for hyponatremia because a rapid increase in sodium level leads to a grave and possibly lethal complication - pontine or extra pontine myelinolysis [47]. The differential diagnosis of hyponatremia includes the syndrome of inappropriate secretion of antidiuretic hormone (SIADH), the cerebral salt wasting syndrome (CSWS), or adrenal insufficiency (AI), where the main pathophysiological difference is the volume status which determines the management. SIADH leads to hyper- or normovolemia, whereas both CSWS and AI are causes of hypovolemia. In SIADH, fluid restriction and vaptans are essential for treatment, while fluid replacement, glucocorticoids, and mineralocorticoids are needed for patients with CSWS and AI. Hypertonic saline solutions are indicated for CSWS and AI but should be avoided in SIADH except in severe hyponatremia cases causing coma or seizures.

Postoperative Glucocorticoid Therapy

Dexamethasone and hydrocortisone in combination are used in patients with sellar-suprasellar tumors [48]. Dexamethasone is tapered relatively fast, over 5–7 postoperative days [9, 49], to protect the patient from adrenal depression and development of primary AI. Hydrocortisone may be used for more extended periods in a dose of at least 150–200 mg per day [49]. Unstable patients may require higher doses of hydrocortisone up to 1200 mg per day. The correct dose of hydrocortisone should be individualized based on sodium, potassium, and glucose levels as well as BP, temperature, and several other clinical and laboratory parameters [48].

34.5.3.3 Consciousness Alterations

Consciousness alterations develop in patients with sellar tumors who have had a complicated postoperative period [44]. Coma is rare, but delirium is the most prevalent disorder of consciousness, hypoactive and mixed types of delirium being the most frequent types. The high rate of convulsive and nonconvulsive seizures is the most common complication of sellar tumor patients [44], requiring aggressive anticonvulsant therapy to improve consciousness and the outcome.

34.5.3.4 Organ Dysfunction

Since the hypothalamus is the highest center of the autonomic nervous system regulating the function of all the vital organs, perioperative damage to the diencephalon may lead to multi-organ dysfunction. However, studies with regards to this complication are scarce. Cardiovascular, respiratory insufficiency and paralytic ileus are the common types of organ dysfunction.

Postoperative Cardiovascular Insufficiency

Postoperative cardiovascular insufficiency in patients with sellar tumors is multifactorial. The common reasons are acute adrenal or thyroid insufficiency, hypopituitarism, hypovolemia in cases with the decompensated DI, or direct diencephalic injury [49]. The endocrine pathology that occurs in all cases of sellar-suprasellar tumors with a complicated postoperative period, despite normal endocrine function preoperatively, requires polyhormonal substitution (hydrocortisone, levothyroxine, and desmopressin) for successful management. Levothyroxine is administered intravenously in a dose of 2–3 μg/kg/day [48]. Desmopressin dose is based on the fluid balance and the plasma sodium level. Therefore, in adequate doses, postoperative polyhormonal substitutional therapy is paramount to prevent cardiovascular instability due to adrenal, thyroid insufficiency, hypopituitarism, and hypovolemia.

Direct perioperative diencephalic damage can cause arterial hypotension due to complete loss of vascular resistance leading to cardiovascular insufficiency

postoperatively [49]. The verification of the mechanism of the arterial hypotension led to the proposal of administration of alpha-adrenomimetics (norepinephrine, phenylephrine) as vasoactive agents of choice. A non-compensated thyroid insufficiency may cause bradycardia during the infusion of alpha- adrenomimetics [50], and its correction with a proper dose of thyroid hormones is needed [49].
The level of optimal BP in patients with sellar tumors having a complicated postoperative period should be maintained at the upper level of normal, which is mean BP between 95 and 110 mmHg [51].

Respiratory Insufficiency

Respiratory insufficiency is another frequent complication in patients with sellar-suprasellar tumors. Diencephalic injury can result in sudden sympathetic surge leading to neurogenic pulmonary edema, though a rare complication.

Intraabdominal Complications

Ileus is a serious clinical problem for neurocritical care patients and can also occur in patients with suprasellar tumors despite the fact that adequate thyroid replacement and is a significant risk factor for intraabdominal hypertension. Therefore, intraabdominal hypertension and abdominal compartment syndrome, when diagnosed, should be treated as an emergency.

Therefore, DDS is a severe condition requiring a multimodal approach for its successful management. The extent of organ dysfunction defines the severity of DDS and determines the outcome.

34.5.3.5 Postoperative Meningitis

Postoperative meningitis is another complication known to occur in patients with sellar tumors. Though a relatively sterile surgery, transsphenoidal surgery is associated with multiple risk factors for meningitis, including perioperative CSF leak, lumbar and external ventricular drainages, revision of the postoperative wound for defects of the disconnection of the CSF diversion system, and intraventricular injections of medications. There is no single effective prophylactic antibiotic regimen available to decrease meningitis rates. Of the several preventive measures employed, durable intraoperative skull-base plastics, prevention of postoperative CSF leaks, shorter duration of CSF drainage, and aseptic approach to the drainage management with decreased number of the system disconnection for obtaining CSF samples or injection of medications are the common ones. In patients with transcranial resection of suprasellar tumors, though postoperative meningitis is a rare phenomenon, CSF may collect under the cutaneous flap in the area of the surgical approach and pose a significant risk for meningitis.

Empirical Treatment

The recent guidelines recommend treatment with vancomycin for staphylococci and P. acnes coverage and either an antipseudomonal cephalosporin or an antipseudomonal carbapenem for coverage of aerobic gram-negative bacilli (GNB) [52]. The local prevalence of extended-spectrum beta-lactamase should be considered for choosing between cephalosporin and carbapenems. Despite its unfavorable pharmacokinetics, vancomycin at a dose of 15–20 mg/kg 2–3 times a day is the treatment of choice in methicillin-resistant staphylococcus aureus (MRSA) and methicillin-resistant enterococci (MRE). Due to its very low CSF penetration, teichoplanin is seldom used to treat post craniotomy meningitis (PCM). Linezolid has perfect CSF penetration; hence, it can be used for treatment with caution exercised on potential myelosuppression. Newer drugs such as telavancin, ceftaroline, and ceftobipirole have shown promise in treating gram-positive meningitis. For gram-negative bacteria, cephalosporins are generally preferred over carbapenems, as the latter is associated with seizures. For extended-spectrum beta-lactamase (ESBL), meropenem is the preferred choice. If the causative organism comes out to be A. baumanni or pseudomonas then colistin in high doses is an option. Carbapenem such as meropenem at higher doses can be combined with colistin if minimum inhibitory concentration (MIC) <8 mg/l. Colistin can be used intrathecally in addition to intravenous doses. The current IDSA guidelines recommend a daily dose of 10 mg colistimethate (125,000 IU colistimethate).

A 21 days course of directed antibiotic treatment in cases of GNB meningitis and 10–14 days for S. aureus meningitis is recommended.

34.6 Infections

Various neurosurgical procedures can lead to wound infections, barrier disruption leading to meningitis or encephalitis, while chemotherapy may lead to suppression of cell-mediated immunity as well as neutropenia. Poor nutritional status may also contribute to infections in patients with a brain tumor. Temazolamide, as well as corticosteroid use in these patients, makes them vulnerable to pneumocystis jiroveci pneumonia. Therefore, it is recommended to have serial lymphocyte count and initiate PCP prophylaxis (trimethoprim and sulfamethoxazole) whenever temazolamide based therapy or prolonged steroid therapy (one month) are used. Other rare infections associated with temazolomide and steroids include aspergillus, disseminated strongyloides, bronchopulmonary infections with Bordatella bronchiseptica, cryptococcal meningitis, disseminated tuberculosis.

Wound infections following craniotomy are more common in patients who have received bevacizumab. To date, only general recommendations for clean neurosurgery have been reported, and no consensus on the class of optimal antibiotic and the administration period has been established [53].

34.7 Special Issues in Postoperative Care

Pain, postoperative nausea, and vomiting (PONV), and residual neuromuscular blockade (RNMB) are important concerns during postoperative intensive care management of patients with an intracranial tumor, leading to arterial hypertension and result in the development of an early postoperative hematoma [54].

34.7.1 Post-craniotomy pain

Post-craniotomy pain is a very frequently encountered adverse effect following surgery. Understanding post craniotomy pain in these patients is of paramount importance as it may lead to delayed mobilization, prolonged hospital stays, increased morbidity, disability, and decreased quality of life. Many hypotheses are explaining the mechanism of pain, such as direct trauma to the skin, nerve injury, meningeal irritation due to debris, formation of neuromas, and central sensitization. Unfortunately, protocols for postoperative analgesia in neurosurgical practice are absent. Pain assessment is challenging in unconscious, aphasic, delirious, or disoriented patients [55], and can be precisely evaluated only in conscious patients. Local anesthetic agents' infiltration at the incision site helps in the control of postoperative pain [56]. This is a part of "pre-emptive analgesia," which can effectively prevent postoperative pain. The use of non-steroidal anti-inflammatory drugs (NSAID) and NMDA antagonists is also based on the same principle [57]. NSAIDs and paracetamol alone, and codeine-based analgesics are ineffective [50]. Systemic opioids, through effective analgesics, cannot be optimally used in patients with brain tumors due to several side effects like nausea, vomiting, cognitive impairment, respiratory depression, urinary retention, constipation, dependence, and tolerance. A continuous and titrated infusion of dexmedetomidine can modulate the pain perception and is suitable for postoperative analgesia and sedation in these patients.

34.7.2 PONV

PONV after craniotomy is present in about 70% of patients. In addition to discomfort to the patient, PONV causes arterial hypertension and increased risk of aspiration, intracranial hypertension, fluid-electrolytes disturbances, and acid-base imbalance. The combination of dexamethasone and 5HT-3 or Neurokinin (NK)-1 receptors antagonists reduces the Incidence of PONV. Administration of metoclopramide, droperidol, or gabapentin, in addition, is also found to be effective [58]. These strategies help to decrease the incidence of PONV but do not eliminate it. PONV plays a significant role in neurosurgical patients because it is a clinical sign of intracranial hypertension. The presence of PONV along with delayed arousal, with or without posturing, and focal neurologic symptoms such as anisocoria and pupillary dilatation warrant an emergent CT.

Neuromuscular blocking agents (NMBA) are part of the balanced anesthesia technique used during resection of brain tumors to ensure optimal surgical conditions. ***RNMB*** is one of the many causes of delayed awakening, and an emergent CT is desirable to rule out treatable intracranial causes without other reversible systemic causes. Unnecessary transportation to CT during the early postoperative period increases the risk of other complications in the neurosurgical patient [59]. Therefore, one should be aware of RNMB and train of four (TOF) monitoring applied in the perioperative period to assess the depth of neuromuscular blockade and adequately reverse it.

34.8 Nutrition

Nutritional support plays a significant factor in brain tumor patients achieving better outcomes. Any patient who undergoes surgery shows metabolic and hormonal changes mimicking a stress response. Cuthbertson in 1932. divided metabolic response into the early 'ebb' phase (12 hours) with reduced metabolic activity and oxygen consumption, followed by a 'flow' phase which is a catabolic state and requires nutritional support.

There is a 56% decrease in mortality in the ICU if nutritional support is started by Day 4 [60].

Overfeeding is as harmful as underfeeding as it may lead to hepatic dysfunction, hyperglycemia, and an increased risk of infections. There is always a risk of refeeding syndrome in a chronically ventilated cancer patient when feeding is initiated. Hence, it is better to gradually initiate feeding in these patients over a while and monitor serum potassium, magnesium, and phosphate levels in between.

Heyland et al. described the NUTRIC score, the first nutritional risk assessment tool developed and validated especially for critically ill patients to assess which patient will benefit from the provision of aggressive protein-energy nutrition. It depends on six variables, namely age, acute physiology, and chronic health evaluation (APACHE II) score, sequential organ failure assessment (SOFA), interleukin-6 levels, and the number of comorbidities and days from hospital to ICU admission.

34.9 Gastrointestinal Ulcer Prophylaxis

It is generally observed that neurological injury with prolonged mechanical ventilation (>48 h), major surgery (>4 h), coagulopathy, high doses of corticosteroids, and analgesics, especially NSAIDs, may contribute for the higher incidence of gastrointestinal (GI) ulcer in critically ill neurosurgical patients. Cushing ulcer in these patients is most likely because of stimulation of acetylcholine via the vagus nerve, which stimulates the M3 receptor of parietal cells, which ultimately leads to activation of hydrogen/potassium ATPase pump.

Routine use of GI ulcer prophylaxis such as proton pump inhibitors (PPI), H2 receptor antagonists (H2A), and antacids is not advised as they may lead to unwanted complications such as the emergence of resistant strains of bacteria and increased incidence of ventilator acquired pneumonia (VAP). Hence, it is always advised to observe the risk-benefit ratio to determine the aforementioned risk factors before starting any GI ulcer prophylaxis. In critically ill neurosurgical patients, PPIs have replaced H2A as H2A are associated with seizures, drug interactions, thrombocytopenia, etc. Early enteral feeding should be established as it helps in positive nitrogen balance, which alkalizes gastric pH and prevents further damage.

34.10 Multimodal Monitoring in Neurocritical Unit

The damage caused by secondary brain insult can be catastrophic and requires a point of care multimodal monitoring to prevent any such events. Although none of the devices can be 100% accurate in detecting impending ischemic events, the combination of various monitoring data can be extremely helpful in understanding brain function and preventing impending catastrophe. Invasive monitoring may be more accurate but is limited by the inherent risk of surgical implantation as well as its regional focus. With the advancement in neurocritical monitoring, noninvasive methods provide invaluable real-time information about cerebral blood flow (CBF), cerebral oxygenation, and intracranial pressure (ICP) but are limited by inaccuracy, lack of specificity, and high cost. Therefore, they are broadly categorized into three groups based on their monitoring parameters: ICP, CBF, and cerebral oxygenation.

34.10.1 ICP Monitoring

ICP is one of the most widely used parameters in a neurocritical care unit; its monitoring can be invasive or noninvasive (Table 34.3). Insertion of an external ventricular device (EVD) has many advantages in the form of an alternate drug delivery route as well as a measure to decrease ICP. However, the problem with EVD being invasive technique there is a higher risk of infection and bleeding especially during the insertion.

With respect to noninvasive methods to monitor ICP, a significant amount of studies have established a correlation between ONSD distension and an increase in ICP. It is generally considered that ONSD measurements below 5 mm correlate to normal ICP, while more than 6 mm diameter represents an elevated ICP (ICP >20 mmHg). Other methods such as infrared pupillometry can be used to quantitatively analyze changes in ICP by examining changes in pupil size in response to light stimuli. In normal ICP, the pupillary response to light should be a 34 to 36% decrease in size, whereas, in raised ICP, pupil response is decreased by 20% of normal constriction. Even an increased latency of N2 and P3 waveforms of the visual evoked potentials (VEP) can indicate changes in ICP.

34.10.2 Cerebral Oxygenation

There are different invasive as well as noninvasive modalities to determine cerebral oxygenation (Table 34.4).

34.10.3 Cerebral Blood Flow

Out of all parameters to assess brain perfusion, the most direct indicator of oxygenation and fuel delivery is cerebral blood flow (CBF); however, it is limited by the lack of a monitoring device that could monitor CBF continuously. Positron

Table 34.3 Intracranial pressure (ICP) monitors

Invasive	Noninvasive
Extra ventricular drains Intraparenchymal devices	Optic nerve sheath diameter (ONSD) Optic coherence tonometry Pupillometry Transcranial Doppler Visual evoked potential Distorted product otoacoustic emission

Table 34.4 Monitors of cerebral oxygenation

Invasive	Noninvasive
Jugular bulb oximetry	Electroencephalogram
Intraparenchymal oxygen monitor (Licox system, neurovent-PTO system)	
Cerebral microdialysis	

emission tomography (PET) scan remains the gold standard for determining CBF, which is limited by its inability to be used bedside. Q flow catheters using the thermal diffusion technique are the only device that can continuously monitor CBF and present real-time pictures of CBF. With respect to noninvasive devices, near-infrared spectroscopy (NIRS) measures regional cerebral oxygenation by indirectly measuring the metabolic state of the cerebral tissue.

34.11 End of Life Care

Palliative care of patients with brain tumors is a continuum starting with honest prognostication and amelioration of symptoms throughout the patient's illness. Symptoms at the end stage of glioma include progressive lethargy, inability to communicate, dysphagia, nausea, focal signs, incontinence, headache, and seizures. Hence, discontinuation of corticosteroids is not encouraged; AEDs are continued throughout life. Nausea and vomiting should be treated aggressively. The role of memantine in preventing cognitive impairment has been studied with a short follow-up trial, and the drug appeared to reduce the decline in memory, executive function, and processing speed.

34.12 Conclusion

Patients with a complicated postoperative period following intracranial tumor resection comprise a unique neurocritical care population. Most of the diagnostic, therapeutic, and prognostic practices can be adapted from the general guidelines and principles used in other neurocritical care patient populations. However, the patients belonging to distinct groups such as sellar-suprasellar tumors and posterior fossa tumors need specific guidelines for managing unique complications.

Conflict of Interest
None declared for each author.

References

1. Kelly D. Neurosurgical postoperative care. Neurosurg Clin N Am. 1994;5:789–810.
2. Sirio CA, Martich DG. Who goes to the ICU postoperatively? Chest. 1999;115:125S–9S.
3. Solheim O, Jakola AS, Gulati S, et al. Incidence and causes of perioperative mortality after primary surgery for intracranial tumors: a national, population-based study. J Neurosurg. 2012;116:825–34.
4. Rincon F, Mayer SA. Neurocritical care: a distinct discipline? Curr Opin Crit Care. 2007;13:115–21.
5. Diringer MN, Edwards DF. Admission to a neurologic/neurosurgical intensive care unit is associated with reduced mortality rate after intracerebral hemorrhage. Crit Care Med. 2001;29:635–40.
6. Bui JQH, Mendis RL, van Gelder JM, et al. Is postoperative intensive care unit admission a prerequisite for elective craniotomy? J Neurosurg. 2011;115:1236–41.
7. Herman MA, Gravenstein N, Gravenstein D. Postoperative neurosurgical care: recovery room misadventures and immediate concerns. In: Layon AJ, editor. Textbook of neurointensive care. London: Springer; 2013. p. 863–97.
8. Black S, Ockert DB, Oliver WC Jr, et al. Outcome following posterior fossa craniectomy in patients in the sitting or horizontal positions. Anesthesiology. 1988;69:49–56.
9. Wen PY, Schiff D, Kesari S, et al. Medical management of patients with brain tumors. J Neuro-Oncol. 2006;80:313–32.
10. Mukand JA, Blackinton DD, Crincoli MG, et al. incidence of neurologic deficits and rehabilitation of patients with brain tumors. Am J Phys Med Rehabil. 2001;80:346–50.
11. Taylor WA, Thomas NW, Wellings JA, et al. Timing of postoperative intracranial hematoma development and implications for the best use of neurosurgical intensive care. J Nerosurg. 1995;82:48–50.
12. Gerlach R, Krause M, Seifert V, et al. Hemostatic and hemorrhagic problems in neurosurgical patients. Acta Neurochir. 2009;151:873–900.
13. Raiten J, Thiele RH, Nemergut EC. Anesthesia and intensive care management of patients with brain tumors. In: Kaye AH, Laws ER, editors. Brain tumors. An encyclopedic approach. 3rd ed. Edinburgh/New York: Saunders, Elsevier; 2012. p. 249–81.
14. Nyquist P, Stevens RD, Mirski MA. Neurologic injury and mechanical ventilation. Neurocrit Care. 2008;9(3):400–8.
15. Hajat C, Hajat S, Sharma P. Effects of poststroke pyrexia on stroke outcome: a meta-analysis of studies in patients. Stroke. 2000;31(2):410–4.
16. Ansari SF, Bohnstedt BN, Perkins SM, Althouse SK, Miller JC. Efficacy of postoperative seizure prophylaxis in intra-axial brain tumor resections. J Neuro-Oncol. 2014;118(1):117–22.
17. Sayegh ET, Fakurnejad S, Oh T, Bloch O, Parsa AT. Anticonvulsant prophylaxis for brain tumor surgery: determining the current best available evidence: a review. J Neurosurg. 2014;121(5):1139–47.
18. Domaingue CM, Nye DH. Hypotensive effect of mannitol administered rapidly. Anaesth Intensive Care. 1985;13(2):134–6.
19. Fink ME. Osmotherapy for intracranial hypertension: mannitol versus hypertonic saline. Continuum: Lifelong Learn Neurol. 2012;18(3):640–54.
20. Miller JD, Leech P. Effects of mannitol and steroid therapy on intracranial volume-pressure relationships in patients. J Neurosurg. 1975;42(3):274–81.

21. Ryken TC, McDermott M, Robinson PD, et al. The role of steroids in the management of brain metastases: a systematic review and evidence-based clinical practice guideline. J Neuro-Oncol. 2010;96(1):103–14.
22. Cavaliere R, Schiff D. Clinical implications of status epilepticus on patients with cancer. Neuro-Oncology. 2003;5:331.
23. Brophy GM, Bell R, Claassen J, et al. Guidelines for the evaluation and management of status epilepticus. Neurocrit Care. 2012;17:3–23.
24. Wu A, Trinh V, Suki D, et al. A prospective randomized trial of perioperative seizure prophylaxis in patients with intraparenchymal brain tumors. J Neurosurg. 2013;118:873–83.
25. Perry JR. Thromboembolic disease in patients with high-grade glioma. Neuro-oncology. 2012 Sep;14(suppl_4):iv73–80.
26. Jenkins EO, Schiff D, Mackman N, Key NS. Venous thromboembolism in malignant gliomas. J Thromb Haemost. 2010;8(2):221Y227. https://doi.org/10.1111/j.1538-7836.2009.03690.x.
27. Agnelli G, Piovella F, Buoncristiani P, Severi P, Pini M, D'Angelo A, et al. Enoxaparin plus compression stockings compared with compression stockings alone in the prevention of venous thromboembolism after elective neurosurgery. New Engl J Med. 1998;339(2):80–5.
28. Goldhaber SZ, Dunn K, Gerhard-Herman M, Park JK, Black PM. Low rate of venous thromboembolism after craniotomy for brain tumor using multimodality prophylaxis. Chest. 2002;122(6):1933–7.
29. Jo JT, Schiff D, Perry JR. Thrombosis in brain tumors. Semin Thromb Hemost. 2014;40(3):325–31.
30. Flexman AM, Merriman B, Griesdale DE, et al. Infratentorial neurosurgery is an independent risk factor for respiratory failure and death in patients undergoing intracranial tumor resection. J Neurosurg Anesthesiol. 2014;26(3):198–294.
31. Mayer SA, Fink ME. Respiratory care: diagnosis and management. In: Rowland LP, editor. Merritt's neurology. Philadelphia: Lippincott Williams & Wilkins; 2001.
32. Salam A, Tilluckdharry L, Amoateng-Adjepong Y, et al. Neurologic status, cough, secretions and extubation outcomes. Intensive Care Med. 2004;30:1334–9.
33. Ko R, Ramos L, Chalela JA. Conventional weaning parameters do not predict extubation failure in neurocritical care patients. Neurocrit Care. 2009;10:269–73.
34. Coplin WM, Pierson DJ, Cooley KD, et al. Implications of extubation delay in brain-injured patients meeting standard weaning criteria. Am J Respir Crit Care Med. 2000;161:1530–6.
35. Hooda B, Chouhan RS, Rath GP, Lamsal R, Bithal PK. Incidence and predictors of postoperative pulmonary complications in patients undergoing craniotomy and excision of posterior fossa tumor. J Anaesthesiol Clin Pharmacol. 2019;35(2):254–60.
36. Bharati SJ, Pandia MP, Rath GP, Bithal PK, Dash HH. Respiratory complications in the early postoperative period following elective craniotomies. J Neuroanaesth Crit Care. 2015;2:114–20.
37. Guleria R, Madan K. Pulmonary complications in neurosurgical patients. Indian J Neurosurg. 2012;1:175–80.
38. Epstein SK. Decision to extubate. Intensive Care Med. 2002;28:535–46.
39. Navalesi P, Frigerio P, Moretti MP. Rate of reintubation in mechanically ventilated neurosurgical and neurologic patients: evaluation of a systemic approach to weaning and extubation. Crit Care Med. 2008;36:2986–92.
40. Popugaev KA, Savin IA, Goriachev AS, et al. A respiratory failure rating scale in neurosurgical patients. Anesteziol Reanimatol. 2010;4:42–50.
41. O'Neil KH, Purdy M, Falk J, et al. The dysphagia outcome and severity scale. Dysphagia. 1999;14:139–45.
42. Slavin KV, Misra M. Infratentorial intracranial pressure monitoring in neurosurgical intensive care unit. Neurol Res. 2003;25:880–4.
43. Kaltsas GA, Evanson J, Chrisoulidou A. The diagnosis and management of parasellar tumours of the pituitary. Endocr Relat Cancer. 2008;15:885–903.

44. Popugaev KA, Savin IA, Lubnin AU, et al. Structure and severity of acute diencephalon dysfunction syndrome. Neurocrit Care. 2012;17:S1.
45. Fenske W, Allolio B. Current state and future perspectives in the diagnosis of diabetes insipidus: a clinical review. J Clin Endocrinol Metab. 2012;97(10):3426–37.
46. Sata A, Hizuka N, Kawamata T, et al. hyponatremia after transsphenoidal surgery for hypothalamo-pituitary tumors. Neuroendocrinology. 2006;83:117–22.
47. Brown WD. Osmotic demyelination disorders: central pontine and extrapontinemyelinolysis. Curr Opin Neurol. 2000;13:691–7.
48. Gomes JA, Stevens RD, Lewin JJ 3rd, et al. Glucocorticoid therapy in neurologic critical care. Crit Care Med. 2005;33:1214–24.
49. Sakharova OV, Inzucchi SI. Endocrine assessment during critical illness. Crit Care Clin. 2007;23:467–90.
50. Gottschalk A, Ochroch EA. Is preemptive analgesia clinically effective? In: Fleisher L, editor. Evidence-based practice of anesthesia. Philadelphia: Saunders; 2008.
51. Popugaev KA, Savin IA, Goriachev AS, et al. Hypothalamic injury as a cause of refractory hypotension after sellar region tumor surgery. Neurocrit Care. 2008;8:366–73.
52. Popugaev KA, Savin IA, Goriachev AS, et al. Optimizing blood pressure in patients with sellar region tumors during complicated postoperative period. Zh Vopr Neirokhir Im N N Burdenko. 2012;76:20–7.
53. Tunkel AR, Hasbun R, Bhimraj A, Byers K, Kaplan SL, Scheld WM, van de Beek D, Bleck TP, Garton HJ, Zunt JR. 2017 Infectious Diseases Society of America's clinical practice guidelines for healthcare-associated ventriculitis and meningitis. Clin Infect Dis. 2017;64(6):e34–65.
54. Iacob G, Iacob S. Prophylactic antibiotherapy in Neurosurgery Romanian Neurosurgery. 2010;15:321–326.
55. Basali A, Mascha EJ, Kalfas I, et al. Relation between perioperative hypertension and intracranial haemorrhage after craniotomy. Anesthesiology. 2000;93:48–54.
56. Breivik H, Borchgrevink PC, Allen SM, et al. Assessment of pain. Br J Anaesth. 2008;101(1):17–24.
57. Nguyen A, Girard F, Boudreault D, et al. Scalp nerve blocks decrease the severity of pain after craniotomy. Anesth Analg. 2001;93(5):1272–6.
58. De Gray LC, Matta BF. Acute and chronic pain following craniotomy: a review. Anaesthesia. 2005;60:693–704.
59. Pugh SC, Jones NC, Barsoum LZ. A comparison of prophylactic ondansetron and metoclopramide administration in patients undergoing major neurosurgical procedures. Anaesthesia. 1996;51:1162–4.
60. Warren J, Fromm RE, Orr RA, et al. Guidelines for the inter- and intrahospital transport of critically ill patients. Crit Care Med. 2004;32:256–62.

Post-surgical Care in Head and Neck Cancer Patients

35

Nishkarsh Gupta and Rohini Dattari

35.1 Introduction

Head and neck cancer surgeries are complex surgeries requiring multi-disciplinary care that includes airway management, tracheostomy care, wound care, nutritional support to name a few. These surgeries predispose to wound infections together with poor wound healing due to exposure to radiotherapy, co-morbidities and proximity to soft-tissue planes and neurovascular structures further necessitating ICU management [1]. Admission to ICU by facilitating immobilization reduces mechanical disruption of microvascular anastomosis as well as allows more invasive hemodynamic monitoring [2]. Routine admission to ICU might be preferred by few surgeons for 24–72 h due to the availability of high level of nursing care in ICU [3]. This chapter gives an overview of critical care management following head and neck cancer surgeries.

35.2 Indications for ICU Admission and Care in Head and Neck Oncological Surgeries

Medical conditions of the patient as well as the complexity of the surgery requiring close monitoring of the patient in the immediate post-surgical period might be responsible for ICU admission. APACHE 2 score >10 and bilateral neck dissection have also been identified as risk factors for post-operative complications in oral cancer [4]. Various indices such as Kaplan-Feinstein score comorbidity index,

N. Gupta (✉)
Department of Onco-Anesthesia and Palliative Medicine, Dr. B.R.A. Institute Rotary Cancer Hospital, All India Institute of Medical Sciences, New Delhi, Delhi, India

R. Dattari
Department of Anaesthesia, Kasturba Medical College, Manipal, Karnataka, India

V. Kumar et al. (eds.), *Onco-critical Care*,
https://doi.org/10.1007/978-981-16-9929-0_35

Table 35.1 Indications for ICU admission in head and neck oncosurgeries

Medical indications	Surgeries
1. Respiratory failure requiring ventilatory support 2. Organ failure due to underlying co-morbidities requiring support 3. Reversible organ decompensation due to co-morbidities requiring critical care consultation 4. Hemodynamic instability 5. Need for diagnostic or therapeutic bronchoscopy due to pulmonary insufficiency or infection	1. Total thyroidectomy 2. Total laryngectomy with cervical emptying 3. Partial laryngectomy 4. Total/partial glossectomy plus cervical dissection 5. Transoral robotic surgery 6. Reconstructive flap surgery

Charlson Co-morbidity Index and Adult Comorbidity Evaluation have been used to predict complications in head and neck cancer patients. Abt et al. used Modified Frailty Index consisting of 15 variables to predict the need of critical care support following head and neck cancer resections specifically free flap reconstructions [5]. The authors noted that increasing scores were strongly associated with Clavien-Dindo 4 classification complications following head and neck resections. Varying rates of ICU admission has been reported in the literature following head and neck reconstruction. Retrospective analysis by To et al concluded 3 out of 47 patients (6.3%) undergoing free flap reconstruction required an elective ICU admission in the post-operative period [6]. The duration of ICU stay depends on the patient progression and could last from 24 to 72 h following elective surgeries [7]. In contrast, ICU stay in emergency interventions in the post-operative period or otherwise is determined by factors such as co-morbidities, intercurrent infections, type of intervention, underlying condition (Table 35.1).

35.3 Airway Patency

Maintenance of airway patency is the most important clinical goal in the immediate post-operative period. Post-operative hemorrhage and hematoma formation leading to airway compromise can occur in total laryngectomy with cervical dissection, radical parathyroidectomy, reconstructive flap surgery requiring close monitoring. In total laryngectomy with cervical emptying, any airway obstruction could be catastrophic as orotracheal intubation is impossible due to anatomical distortion of airway necessitating elective tracheostomy and ICU management for 24–72 h [8, 9]. Damage to bilateral recurrent laryngeal nerve, hypocalcemia, post-operative hemorrhage, post-operative airway edema following total thyroidectomy can compromise airway.

Elective tracheostomy in OR is preferred when prolonged intubation is anticipated along with monitoring and care in ICU. Accidental decannulation in such patients does not pose much problem unlike percutaneous technique as early recannulation without losing the trajectory is possible here. It has been reported that tracheostomy is done 'almost always' done in 39% and 'usually done' in 30% cases of uncomplicated free flap reconstruction in British maxillofacial units [10]. But tracheostomy can be associated with complications such as tube obstruction, lower respiratory tract infection, airway scarring, delayed oral intake, respiratory arrest [11, 12]. It is also a predictor of major post-operative complications and length of hospital stay [13]. Of late, many centers are avoiding elective tracheostomy in head and neck free flap reconstruction. In case of airway emergency in tracheostomized and laryngectomy patients, multidisciplinary guidelines for the management of such cases is available that can be followed [14] These guidelines advocate the presence of patent airway "green bed-head" sign at the bed head of tracheostomized patients and 'green algorithm' to be followed in the event of airway emergency. Similarly, "red bed-head" sign should be present at the bed head of laryngectomy patients and to follow 'red algorithm' for airway emergency.

In intubated patients shifted to ICU, the key issue is to determine the ideal time for extubation although there is paucity of literature suggesting the ideal time [15]. There are two schools of thought with one school preferring delayed extubation in maxillo-facial surgeries due to difficulty in determining the degree of post-operative inflammation and post-operative complications while the fast tract school preferring 'early extubation' by the use of multi-modal approach thereby avoiding prolonged intubation. But the latter technique is to be adopted only by highly competent specialized teams [16]. In head and neck reconstructive surgeries, planned postoperative intubation and mechanical ventilation has been followed routinely so as to allow the airway edema to subside and allow airway stabilization although it could lead to difficult weaning, ventilator associated pneumonia and respiratory insufficiency [17]. In addition, post-operative sedation can reduce the systemic blood pressure leading to reduction in flap perfusion pressure. It has been noted that immediate extubation after head and neck surgery can reduce the length of ICU stay without causing wound complications or affecting flap [18]. T. Singh et al. conducted a study to review the difference in outcomes in a group of 78 patients who had undergone tracheostomy(25 patients) or delayed extubation (53 patients with extubation 24–47 h after surgery) following microvascular free flap reconstruction for maxillofacial pathology [11]. The authors reported no difference in the duration of ICU stay between the groups but the length of overall hospital stay significantly prolonged in tracheostomy group (27.2 days) than in delayed extubation group (20.4 days, P = .03). 12% (3 patients) with tracheostomy developed serious complications related to the procedure that included cardiorespiratory arrest due to tracheostomy tube obstruction. In the delayed extubation group only one patient required a delayed (secondary) tracheostomy for persistent airway edema with failed delayed extubation (2%), and other two had a tracheostomy for other reasons (4%). 94% of patients in delayed extubation group did not require tracheostomy later. So, they reported that delayed extubation is safer in free flap reconstruction with unilateral neck dissection with good lung function and no obstructive sleep apnoea(OSA). Tracheostomy is to be preferred in oral resection or oropharyngeal resection with bilateral neck dissection or when additional access procedure is required. Presence of patient related risk factors such as OSA, obesity, poor lung function and difficult re-intubation may also require tracheostomy. This has been suggested in an algorithm by the authors.

So, immediate extubation or delayed extubation or tracheostomy should be individualized based on patient related factors, surgical factors, expertise of the anesthesiologist, available resources.

35.4 Analgesia and Sedation

Head and neck resections involve larger resections with prolonged operative times and many of these patients could be on pre-operative opioids for pain management which makes the pain management challenging in the post-operative period. In addition, the standard daily procedures such as mobilization, aspiration of secretions in tracheostomized patients, healing of wounds, etc. can also cause pain. Inadequately controlled pain can prolong the recovery and lead to pulmonary, cardiac complications, reduced mobility, persistent surgical pain, delayed wound healing. Hence, pain management is essential to reduce complications and promote recovery. If early extubation has not been planned, appropriate analgo-sedation is to be provided. Patient controlled analgesia (PCA) using morphine has been found to be beneficial [19]. Multi-modal analgesia using opioid sparing drugs such as paracetamol, NSAIDS, gabapentin, dexamethasone, α-2 agonists, iv lidocaine, acetaminophen, ketamine and using opioids as rescue analgesics helps to reduce the adverse effects of opioids and hasten the recovery [20].

Various pain scales can be used to monitor the level of analgesia based on the factors such as ability to communicate. In patients who can self-report the pain, Numeric rating scale (NRS) which has been visually enlarged has been determined to be the most valid scale for use in ICU patients [21]. Behavioral Pain Scale (BPS) and Critical Care Pain Observation Tool (CPOT) are the two validated pain behaviour scales used in patients unable to communicate [22–24]. Richmond Agitation Sedation Scale (RASS) can be used to determine the level of sedation in ICU patients.

35.5 Skin Graft Care

Securing the micro-vascular anastomosis is the main goal of free flap reconstruction. Intensive monitoring of the graft by serial assessment for 24–48 h is required as it has been noted that most complications occur in this period [25]. Early recognition of compromised flap perfusion would help in early intervention so as to maximise the chance of flap viability. Bed side clinical examination for capillary refill, temperature, flap colour and pin prick test can be performed usually hourly for the first 24 h can be performed to assess the graft patency and it can be complemented by using colour Doppler [26]. Other techniques such as microdialysis, fluorescence angiography, implantable Doppler, pO2 monitors, video-based application (Eulerian), Near Infrared Spectroscopy (NIRS), contrast enhanced duplex can also be used to monitor flap perfusion but they are expensive and require expertise.

Amongst these, implantable arterial Doppler has more data demonstrating efficacy, lower false positive rates with low flow variability [27]. Studies have demonstrated the beneficial effect of improved salvage rates and decreased flap losses as regional oxygen saturation drops earlier than change in flap colour which can be detected by these techniques [28, 29]. The head should be maintained in a neutral position in the frontal plane avoiding flexion or lateralization that can compress the graft.

35.6 Fluid Therapy

Optimal fluid therapy so as to maintain normovolemia and normotension should be the goal in post-surgical patients. Hypervolemia can lead to tissue edema while hypovolemia can cause flap thrombosis. ERAS programs advocate maintenance of near zero balance which is to maintain the preoperative weight in the immediate perioperative period, or goal directed fluid therapy [30]. Hence, tissue perfusion and efficient central hemodynamics should be the target avoiding positive net balance. Goal directed fluid therapy is based on fluid responsiveness which can be determined by cardiac output, stroke volume, or pulse pressure variation [31, 32]. This can be achieved by pushing the patient's blood toward the peak of the Frank Starling curve so that cardiac output and thereby oxygen delivery is maximized, both of which can be measured invasively with an arterial line, semi-invasively using Doppler, or noninvasively using bioreactance technology [33, 34]. If hypotension continues despite adequate fluid resuscitation, vasoactive support with vasopressors may be necessary to ensure adequate perfusion pressure especially in reconstructive flap surgeries as its success depends on continuous arterial and venous flow until neovascularization [35]. But the use of vasoconstrictors in flap surgery is controversial as animal studies have shown evidence of vasoconstriction in microcirculation [36] though it has been reported to not affect the flap outcome in head and neck [37] as well as microsurgeries [38]. An alternative to the use of vasoconstrictors is inotropes such as dobutamine can increase the mean and maximum blood flow through arterial anastomosis in head and neck surgery [39]. It is imperative to maintain a target mean arterial pressure of 70 mmHg particularly in flap surgeries.

The choice of fluid between crystalloids vs. colloids is still an ongoing debate. Theoretically, colloids are better than crystalloids as they have a longer plasma half-life and higher plasma expansion capacity but can prolong the clotting time and cause kidney injury. The ratio of the cumulative dose of colloids over the cumulative dose of crystalloids has been shown to be ranging roughly from 0.41 to 1 [40]. Although limited studies have compared the effects of crystalloids vs. colloids for volume therapy in major surgery, these studies have shown lower IV fluid volume requirement with colloid-based resuscitation (ratio around 1.6:1) without significant difference in clinical outcomes [41, 42]. Isotonic balanced crystalloids are preferred for maintenance therapy as 0.9% saline has been associated with hyperchloremic metabolic acidosis and acute renal injury [43]. Hence, fluid therapy has to be individualized and reassessed periodically.

35.7 Nutrition

The head and neck cancer patients might be nutritionally depleted prior to surgery increasing the risk of sepsis, poor wound healing, wound infections, muscle weakness, cardiac and pulmonary complications in the post-operative period [44]. Resumption of oral diet in the post-operative period might also be delayed due to the presence of swelling, swallowing impairment further affecting the nutrition. The extent of surgical resection and reconstruction after head and neck surgery has an impact on the degree of functional deficit which in-turn affects the nutrition in the post-operative period. Few patients might be able to resume oral intake while others might have to placed nil by mouth in whom enteral nutritional support is indicated. ESPEN guidelines recommend early initiation of nasogastric tube feeding (within 24 h) in such patients where oral feed cannot be resumed immediately and oral nutrition would be inadequate (<50%) for >7 days [45]. But the risk of wound dehiscence, fistula, aspiration should be carefully evaluated. There are studies that have compared early initiation (prior to post-operative day 6) of oral intake vs. late (postoperative day 6 or later) oral intake and have reported reduced duration of hospital stay without any increase in morbidity or adverse outcome in the early oral intake group [46, 47]. It has been seen that early resumption of oral feeding after primary total laryngectomy (from as early as 1 day post-surgery to 7 days) can reduce the length of stay with no difference in fistulae rates compared with delayed oral feeding of >7 days [48].

Standard polymeric enteral feed started slowly at a rate of 20 ml/h and increased gradually has been recommended [45]. Parenteral nutrition needs to be initiated only in the absence of normal gut function and/or enteral access is not possible and published guidelines can be followed to guide the practice [49].

35.8 DVT Prophylaxis

Recent studies have reported that head and neck surgical patients have considerably higher rates of venous thromboembolism (VTE) of nearly 20% in the highest-risk subgroups although historically it was believed that head and neck surgeries were low risk for VTE [50]. It has been noted that VTE in the post-operative period is associated with an increased length of hospital stay by more than 5 days and 6.56% excess mortality rate in patients undergoing oncological procedures [51]. The presence of risk factors such as malignancy, pulmonary co-morbidity, large and complex surgeries, advanced age, male sex, obesity (BMI > 25) contribute to increased risk in these group of patients. But a major concern in using antithrombotic agents in these patients is the risk of post-surgical hemorrhage can have profound consequences including loss of airway, cardiorespiratory arrest, compression of vascular anastomosis by hematoma following microvascular reconstruction. Hence the risk-benefit ratio for using anticoagulants is not so favourable in head and neck cancer surgery. Use of pharmacological prophylaxis has shown a significant reduction in VTE in patients undergoing head and neck cancer surgery with free flap reconstruction though an increase in bleeding complications has also been noted [50, 52]. Hence, anticoagulant use should be individualized based on the risk of both VTE and bleeding. Use of risk assessment models like the Caprini RAM may be useful to identify high risk patients who are likely to be benefitted from chemoprophylaxis. Chemoprophylaxis has been recommended in patients with Caprini score of 5–6 and dual prophylaxis (chemo and mechanical) in patients with Caprini score of 7 or more [53]. NICE guidelines recommend the use of pharmacological thromboprophylaxis for a minimum of 7 days in patients undergoing oral and maxillofacial surgery in patients in whom the VTE risk outweighs the bleeding risk. Mechanical thromboprophylaxis in the form of intermittent pneumatic compression, anti-embolism stockings can be used when the risk of bleeding is high [54]. ASCO guidelines also recommend pharmacological thromboprophylaxis in patients with malignancy undergoing major surgery with either LMWH or UFH in the preoperative period unless contraindicated and it should be continued for 7–10 days in the post-operative period. Mechanical prophylaxis can be added to pharmacological prophylaxis but should not be used as a monotherapy unless pharmacological prophylaxis is contra-indicated. Dual therapy may be used in high-risk patients [55].

35.9 Miscellaneous Care

1. Rehabilitation is an important component following head and neck surgeries. Early initiation of speech therapy (day 2 of surgery) as well as swallowing exercises (day 4 of surgery) has been recommended [56]. In order to improve swallowing, interventions that target specific physiological deficits and volitional control can be started so as to compensate for the changes to the anatomy and physiology and reduce the risk of aspiration, malnutrition as well as improve the quality of life. Few such intervention include postures such as chin tuck, head turn to reduce aspiration, maneuvres such as supraglottic swallow, Mendelsohn, therapeutic exercises such as thermal tactile stimulation, range of motion to name a few [57]. Post-operative pulmonary physical therapy helps to reduce the pulmonary complications, reduce the secretions and reduce the length of hospital stay. It includes incentive spirometry, intermittent positive pressure breathing, deep breathing exercises.
2. Perioperative antibiotic therapy
   The reported incidence of surgical site infection (SSI) in clean head and neck (H and N) surgical procedures without antimicrobial prophylaxis is <1% as compared to 24–48% infection rates in complicated H&N cancer surgical patients without antimicrobial prophylaxis [58–61]. Risk factors such as poor nutrition, advanced age, diabetes mellitus, anemia, peripheral vascular disease, preoperative chemotherapy and radiotherapy, long duration surgery, use of metal screws and plates predispose to higher risk of infection in head and neck cancer patients [62–65]. However, rational use should be encouraged due to the risk of development of antibiotic resistance by the bacteria by indiscriminate use of antibiotics.

YO-IFOS head and neck study group (Young Otolaryngologist Group of the International Federation of Otolaryngologic Societies) have provided a few recommendations for perioperative antibiotic prophylaxis in head and neck surgery [66]. In clean surgeries such as thyroidectomy, parotidectomy, parathyroidectomy antibiotic coverage is not recommended in the perioperative period although nutritional status, surgical safety, co-morbidities should be taken into consideration. Antibiotic use may be considered in neck dissection. In surgeries of oral cavity, oropharynx, nasopharynx, hypopharynx, larynx along with neck dissection (clean contaminated head and neck surgeries) where aero-digestive tract is entered antibiotics should be administered for at least 24 h. Clindamycin monotherapy as prophylaxis in patients with true allergy to beta lactam antibiotics should be avoided. Antibiotic prophylaxis including gram negative coverage for at least 24 h is recommended in major H&N reconstruction and microvascular free flap reconstruction. The antibiotic chosen should be based on the microbial flora and the resistance profile of the hospital.

A systematic review (39 studies) and meta-analyses (5 trials) by Vander Porten V reported the beneficial effects of cefazolin, ampicillin-sulbactum, amoxycillin-clavulanate administered for 24–48 h following clean contaminated head and neck surgery in preventing surgical site infection. Clindamycin and Benzylpenicillin were less effective. Antibiotic prophylaxis for >48 h did not further reduce the rate of wound infection [67].

35.10 Management of Post-surgical Complications

1. **Post-operative hemorrhage**

   Post-operative hemorrhage should be rapidly recognized and treated. The presence of cervicofacial vascularization and major cervical vessels can make homeostasis insufficient in head and neck region. Patients with previous history of surgery or irradiation to the neck are at a higher risk for bleeding due to fibrosis, vessel wall abnormalities and lack of plane of dissection. Antiplatelets and anticoagulants also increase the bleeding risk. Postoperative hemorrhage can be graded as minor, intermediate, major, or severe based on the quantity of blood loss, type of surgical management required, development of life-threatening complications or need for emergent life-saving intervention [68]. Minor hemorrhage is presence of bright red blood or blood clots that can be treated without operative management. Intermediate grade is presence of diffuse venous oozing or small arterial source bleeding resulting in operating room evaluation or intervention and managed with monopolar or bipolar cautery. Brisk or copious bleeding requiring operative intervention in the form of transoral or transcervical vessel ligation, or interventional radiology embolization is major bleeding. Severe bleeding results in life-threatening medical complications such as: Hypoxia/airway compromise requiring tracheostomy, Cardiopulmonary arrest and presents with hemodynamic instability requiring blood transfusion [68].

Airway, breathing and circulation must be carefully assessed. The hemogram, coagulation status, lactate level of the patient must be obtained. Hemodynamic status must be carefully monitored. Fluid resuscitation with crystalloids must be done. Transfusion of blood and blood products might be required in some patients.

2. **Post-operative hematoma**

Postoperative hematoma is a dreaded complication following head and neck surgery. The overall incidence of postoperative neck hematoma has been reported as 3.4% which can result in 540% increased odds of death (P < .001) , additional length of stay of 5.14 days (P < .001) and excess cost and $17,887.40 (P < .001) [69]. Pre-existing coagulopathy, male gender, black race, presence of ≥4 comorbidities (e.g., renal insufficiency, diabetes, coronary disease, hypertension) are some of the risk factors for post-operative hematoma [69]. Acute airway compromise can occur due to expanding post-operative hematoma necessitating evacuation of hematoma and either surgical or endotracheal airway management. It can also compromise the vitality of the microvascular flap.

Early symptoms and signs of hematoma include increased neck pain, asymmetry of the neck, increase in neck circumference, change in drain output, voice change, tightness and discoloration of the neck, hypertension. Late symptoms and signs include dysphagia, odynophagia, drooling of saliva, facial edema, tongue edema, tracheal deviation, breathlessness, stridor, agitation, tachycardia.

Supportive measures include head end elevation, 100% oxygen, iv steroids, nebulization with racemic epinephrine and administration of heliox. Surgical team should be informed for evaluation and management. An experienced personnel with airway expertise should attempt intubation. Difficult airway cart and Trach equipment should be available bed-side. Flexible fiberoptic nasopharyngo-video-laryngoscopy using a 6 mm scope (for adults) or 1.99 mm (pediatrics) can be helpful to identify displacement of the larynx, degree of laryngeal edema, location, and size of any mass although there could be a risk of complete airway collapse in these patients requiring caution. Immediate management by opening the suture line and evacuating the hematoma may be attempted in the absence of the surgeon to prevent and/or relieve total airway obstruction. Total airway collapse requires immediate surgical cricothyroidotomy to re-establish a patent airway due to completely swollen neck with distorted landmarks [70]. Once stable patient may be shifted to OR for definitive hemostasis.

Answering four questions—what is to be done? When? Where? And How? may help in the critical management of these patients [71].

(a) What is to be done ?—Opening the suture line, hematoma evacuation, intubation, awake fiberoptic evaluation of the airway are the options and the involved personnel must decide upon these options.
(b) When?—Act without delay or await the arrival of surgeon are the options
(c) Where?—Operating room, ICU, Emergency Department, bedside on the ward
(d) How?—Awake vs. under general anesthesia? If asleep: Intravenous vs. inhalational induction?

35.11 Conclusion

Head and neck cancer post-operative patients can pose unique challenges in the ICU requiring close monitoring for early recognition and prompt management so as to improve the surgical outcomes and reduce morbidity and mortality. Team effort by the anesthesiologists, surgical oncologists, physiotherapist, nutritionist, speech therapist can help to improve the outcome and reduce the complication rates.

References

1. Garantziotis S, Kyrmizakis DE, Liolios AD. Critical care of the head and neck patient. Crit Care Clin. 2003;19:73–90.
2. Arshad H, Ozer HG, Thatcher A, Old M, Ozer E, Agarwal A, et al. Intensive care unit versus non-intensive care unit postoperative management of head and neck free flaps: comparative effectiveness and cost comparisons. Head Neck. 2014;36:536–9.
3. Haddock NT, Gobble RM, Levine JP. More consistent postoperative care and monitoring can reduce costs following microvascular free flap reconstruction. J Reconstr Microsurg. 2010;26:435–9.
4. de Melo GM, Ribeiro KC, Kowalski LP, Deheinzelin D. Risk factors for postoperative complications in oral cancer and their prognostic implications. Arch Otolaryngol Head Neck Surg. 2001;127(7):828–33.
5. Abt NB, Xie Y, Puram SV, Richmon JD, Varvares MA. Frailty index: intensive care unit complications in head and neck oncologic regional and free flap reconstruction. Head Neck. 2017;39(8):1578–85.
6. To EWH, Tsang WM, Lai ECH, Chu MC. Retrospective study on the need of intensive care unit admission after major head and neck surgery. ANZ J Surg. 2002;72:11–4.
7. Kovatch KJ, Hanks JE, Stevens JR, Stucken CL. Current practices in microvascular reconstruction in otolaryngology-head and neck surgery. Laryngoscope. 2019;129:138–45.
8. Bannister M, Trotter P, Jawad A, Veitch D. Airway and head and neck high dependency unit: a single-centre experience. J Laryngol Otol. 2016;130:777–80.
9. Godden DRP, Patel M, Baldwin M, Woodwards RTM. Need for intensive care after operations for head and neck cancer surgery. Br J Oral Maxillofac Surg. 1999;37:502–5.
10. Marsh M, Elliott S, Anand R, Brennan PA. Early postoperative care for free-flap head & neck reconstructive surgery—a national survey of practice. Br J Oral Maxillofac Surg. 2009;47:182–52.
11. Singh T, Sankla P, Smith G. Tracheostomy or delayed extubation after maxillofacial free-flap reconstruction? Br J Oral Maxillofac Surg. 2016;54(8):878–82.
12. Castling B, Telfer M, Avery BS. Complications of tracheostomy in major head and neck cancer surgery; a retrospective study of 60 consecutive cases. Br J Oral Maxillofac Surg. 1994;32:3–5.
13. Patel RS, McCluskey SA, Goldstein DP, Minkovich L, Irish JC, Brown DH, et al. Clinicopathologic and therapeutic risk factors for perioperative complications and prolonged hospital stay in free flap reconstruction of the head and neck. Head Neck. 2010;32:1345–53.
14. McGrath BA, Bates L, Atkinson D, Moore JA. National Tracheostomy Safety Project. Multidisciplinary guidelines for the management of tracheostomy and laryngectomy airway emergencies. Anaesthesia. 2012;67(9):1025–41.
15. Zulian MA, Chisum JW, Mosby EL, Hiatt WR. Extubation criteria for oral and maxillofacial surgery patients. J Oral Maxillofac Surg. 1989;47:616–20.
16. Shackford SR, Virgilio RW, Peters RM. Early extubation versus prophylactic ventilation in the high-risk patient: a comparison of postoperative management in the prevention of respiratory complications. Anesth Analg. 1981;60:76–80.

17. Nkenke E, Vairaktaris E, Stelzle F, Neukam FW, St PM. No reduction in complication rate by stay in the intensive care unit for patients undergoing surgery for head and neck cancer and microvascular reconstruction. Head Neck [Internet]. 2009;31:1461–9.
18. Allak A, Nguyen TN, Shonka DC, Reibel JF, Levine PA, Jameson MJ. Immediate postoperative extubation in patients undergoing free tissue transfer. Laryngoscope [Internet]. 2011;121:763–8.
19. Jellish WS, Leonetti JP, Sawicki K, Anderson D, Origitano TC. Morphine/ondansetron PCA for postoperative pain, nausea, and vomiting after skull base surgery. Otolaryngol Head Neck Surg. 2006;135(2):175–81. https://doi.org/10.1016/j.otohns.2006.02.027. PMID: 16890064
20. Gupta P, Sharma H, Jethava DD, et al. Use of dexmedetomidine for multimodal analgesia in head and neck cancer surgeries: a prospective randomized double blind control study. IOSR J Dent Med Sci. 2015;14(4):8–13.
21. Chanques G, Viel E, Constantin JM, et al. The measurement of pain in intensive care unit: comparison of 5 self-report intensity scales. Pain. 2010;151(3):711–21.
22. Barr J, Fraser GL, Puntillo K, et al. Clinical practice guidelines for the management of pain, agitation, and delirium in adult patients in the intensive care unit. Crit Care Med. 2013;41(1):263–306.
23. Payen JF, Bru O, Bosson JL. Assessing pain in critically ill sedated patients by using a behavioral pain scale. Crit Care Med. 2001;29(12):2258–63.
24. Gélinas C, Fillion L, Puntillo KA, et al. Validation of the critical-care pain observation tool in adult patients. Am J Crit Care. 2006;15(4):420–7.
25. Pattani KM, Byrne P, Boahene K, Richmon J. What makes a good flap go bad? A critical analysis of the literature of intraoperative factors related to free flap failure. Laryngoscope. 2010;120(4):717–23.
26. Cornejo A, Ivatury S, Crane CN, Myers JG, Wang HT. Analysis of free flap complications and utilization of intensive care unit monitoring. J Reconstr Microsurg. 2013;29(7):473–79. https://doi.org/10.1055/s-0033-1345434. Epub 2013 May 9. PMID: 23661332.
27. Ho MW, Cassidy C, Brown JS, Shaw RJ, Bekiroglu F, et al. Rationale for the use of the implantable Doppler probe based on 7 years' experience. Br J Oral Maxillofac Surg. 2014;52:530–4.
28. Takasu H, Hashikawa K, Nomura T, Sakakibara S, Osaki T, et al. A novel method of noninvasive monitoring of free flaps with near-infrared spectroscopy. Eplasty. 2017;17:e37.
29. Koolen PG, Vargas CR, Ho OA, Ibrahim AM, Ricci JA, et al. Does increased experience with tissue oximetry monitoring in microsurgical breast reconstruction lead to decreased flap loss? The learning effect. Plast Reconstr Surg. 2016;37:1093–101.
30. Miller TE, Raghunathan K, Gan TJ. State-of-the-art fluid management in the operating room. Best Pract Res Clin Anaesthesiol. 2014;28(3):261–73.
31. Martina JR, Westerhof BE, van Goudoever J, et al. Noninvasive continuous arterial blood pressure monitoring with Nexfin®. Anesthesiology. 2012;116(5):1092–103.
32. Chen G, Meng L, Alexander B, Tran NP, Kain ZN, Cannesson M. Comparison of noninvasive cardiac output measurements using the Nexfin monitoring device and the esophageal Doppler. J Clin Anesth. 2012;24(4):275–83.
33. Martina Noble MI. The Frank–Starling curve. Clin Sci Mol Med. 1978;54(1):1–7.
34. Hofer CK, Cannesson M. Monitoring fluid responsiveness. Acta Anaesthesiol Taiwan. 2011;49(2):59–65.
35. Richard B, van Gijn D, D'Souza J, King W, Bater M. Free flap head and neck reconstruction with an emphasis on postoperative care. Facial Plast Surg. 2018;34:597–604.
36. Cordeiro PG, Santamaria E, Hu QY, Heerdt P. Effects of vasoactive medications on the blood flow of island musculocutaneous flaps in swine. Ann Plast Surg. 1997;39(5):524–31.
37. Kelly DA, Reynolds M, Crantford C, Pestana IA. Impact of intraoperative vasopressor use in free tissue transfer for head, neck, and extremity reconstruction. Ann Plast Surg. 2014;72(6):S135–8.
38. Chen C, Nguyen MD, Bar-Meir E, et al. Effects of vasopressor administration on the outcomes of microsurgical breast reconstruction. Ann Plast Surg. 2010;65(1):28–31.

39. Scholz A, Pugh S, Fardy M, Shafik M, Hall JE. The effect of dobutamine on blood flow of free tissue transfer flaps during head and neck reconstructive surgery. Anaesthesia. 2009;64(10):1089–93.
40. Rochwerg B, Alhazzani W, Sindi A, Heels-Ansdell D, Thabane L, Fox-Robichaud A, et al. Fluid resuscitation in sepsis: a systematic review and network meta-analysis. Ann Intern Med. 2014;161(5):347–55.
41. Yates DR, Davies SJ, Milner HE, Wilson RJ. Crystalloid or colloid for goal-directed fluid therapy in colorectal surgery. Br J Anaesth. 2014;112:281–9.
42. Feldheiser A, Pavlova V, Bonomo T, Jones A, Fotopoulou C, Sehouli J, Wernecke KD, Spies C. Balanced crystalloid compared with balanced colloid solution using a goal-directed haemodynamic algorithm. Br J Anaesth. 2013;110:231–40.
43. Semler MW, Self WH, Wanderer JP, Ehrenfeld JM, Wang L, Byrne DW, Stollings JL, Kumar AB, Hughes CG, Hernandez A, Guillamondegui OD, May AK, Weavind L, Casey JD, Siew ED, Shaw AD, Bernard GR, Rice TW, SMART Investigators and the Pragmatic Critical Care Research Group. Balanced crystalloids versus saline in critically ill adults. N Engl J Med. 2018;378:829–39.
44. van Bokhorst-de van der Schueren MA, van Leeuwen PA, Sauerwein HP, Kuik DJ, Snow GB, Quak JJ. Assessment of malnutrition parameters in head and neck cancer and their relation to postoperative complications. Head Neck. 1997;19:419e25.
45. Weimann A, Braga M, Carli F, Higashiguchi T, Hübner M, Klek S, Laviano A, Ljungqvist O, Lobo DN, Martindale R, Waitzberg DL, Bischoff SC, Singer P. ESPEN guideline: clinical nutrition in surgery. Clin Nutr. 2017;36(3):623–50. https://doi.org/10.1016/j.clnu.2017.02.013. Epub 2017 Mar 7. PMID: 28385477
46. Guidera AK, Kelly BN, Rigby P, MacKinnon CA, Tan ST. Early oral intake after reconstruction with a free flap for cancer of the oral cavity. Br J Oral Maxillofac Surg. 2013;51:224–7.
47. McAuley D, Barry T, McConnell K, Smith J, Stenhouse J. Early feeding after free flap reconstruction for oral cancer. Br J Oral Maxillofac Surg. 2015;53:618–20.
48. Seven H, Calis AB, Turgut S. A randomized controlled trial of early oral feeding in laryngectomized patients. Laryngoscope. 2003;113:1076e9.
49. Braga M, Ljungqvist O, Soeters P, Fearon K, Weimann A, Bozzetti F, ESPEN. ESPEN guidelines on parenteral nutrition: surgery. Clin Nutr. 2009;28(4):378–86.
50. Shuman AG, Hu HM, Pannucci CJ, Jackson CR, Bradford CR, Bahl V. Stratifying the risk of venous thromboembolism in otolaryngology. Otolaryngol Head Neck Surg. 2012;146(5):719–24.
51. Ahmad FI, Clayburgh DR. Venous thromboembolism in head and neck cancer surgery. Cancers. Head Neck. 2016;1(1) https://doi.org/10.1186/s41199-016-0014-9.
52. Bahl V, Shuman AG, Hu HM, et al. Chemoprophylaxis for venous thromboembolism in otolaryngology. JAMA Otolaryngol Head Neck Surg. 2014;140(11):999–1005.
53. Cramer JD, Shuman AG, Brenner MJ. Antithrombotic therapy for venous thromboembolism and prevention of thrombosis in otolaryngology–head and neck surgery: state of the art review. Otolaryngol Head Neck Surg. 2018;158(4):627–36.
54. No authors listed. Venous thromboembolism in over 16s: reducing the risk of hospital-acquired deep vein thrombosis or pulmonary embolism. London: National Institute for Health and Care Excellence (UK); 2019. PMID: 32924386.
55. Key NS, Khorana AA, Kuderer NM, Bohlke K, Lee AYY, Arcelus JI, Wong SL, Balaban EP, Flowers CR, Francis CW, Gates LE, Kakkar AK, Levine MN, Liebman HA, Tempero MA, Lyman GH, Falanga A. Venous thromboembolism prophylaxis and treatment in patients with cancer: ASCO clinical practice guideline update. J Clin Oncol. 2020;38(5):496–520. https://doi.org/10.1200/JCO.19.01461. Epub 2019 Aug 5. PMID: 31381464
56. Clarke P, Radford K, Coffey M, Stewart M. Speech and swallow rehabilitation in head and neck cancer: United Kingdom National Multidisciplinary Guidelines. J Laryngol Otol. 2016;130(S2):S176–S180.
57. Pauloski BR. Rehabilitation of dysphagia following head and neck cancer. Phys Med Rehabil Clin N Am. 2008;19:889–928.

58. Avenia N, Sanguinetti A, Cirocchi R, et al. Antibiotic prophylaxis in thyroid surgery: a preliminary multicentric Italian experience. Ann Surg Innov Res. 2009;3:10.
59. Johnson JT, Wagner RL. Infection following uncontaminated head and neck surgery. Arch Otolaryngol Head Neck Surg. 1987;113:368–9.
60. Saginur R, Odell PF, Poliquin JF. Antibiotic prophylaxis in head and neck cancer surgery. J Otolaryngol. 1988;17:78–80.
61. Mandell-Brown M, Johnson JT, Wagner RL. Cost-effectiveness of prophylactic antibiotics in head and neck surgery. Otolaryngol Head Neck Surg. 1984;92:520–3.
62. Callender DL. Antibiotic prophylaxis in head and neck oncologic surgery: the role of gram-negative coverage. Int J Antimicrob Agents. 1999;12(suppl 1):S21–7.
63. Simo R, French G. The use of prophylactic antibiotics in head and neck oncological surgery. Curr Opin Otolaryngol Head Neck Surg. 2006;14:55–61.
64. Lotfi CJ, Cavalcanti RDC, Costa e Silva AM, et al. Risk factors for surgical-site infections in head and neck cancer surgery. Otolaryngol Head Neck Surg. 2008;138:74–80.
65. Liu SA, Tung KC, Shiao JY, Chiu YT. Preliminary report of associated factors in surgical site infection after major head and neck neoplasm operations—does the duration of prophylactic antibiotic matter? J Laryngol Otol. 2008;122:403–8.
66. Chiesa-Estomba CM, Lechien JR, Fakhry N, Melkane A, Calvo-Henriquez C, de Siati D, Gonzalez-Garcia JA, Fagan JJ, Ayad T. Systematic review of international guidelines for perioperative antibiotic prophylaxis in Head & Neck Surgery. A YO-IFOS Head & Neck Study Group Position Paper. Head Neck. 2019;41(9):3434–56. https://doi.org/10.1002/hed.25856. Epub 2019 Jul 8. PMID: 3128206.
67. Vander Poorten V, Uyttebroek S, Robbins KT, Rodrigo JP, de Bree R, Laenen A, F Saba N, Suarez C, Mäkitie A, Rinaldo A, Ferlito A. Perioperative antibiotics in clean-contaminated head and neck surgery: a systematic review and meta-analysis. Adv Ther. 2020;37(4):1360–80. https://doi.org/10.1007/s12325-020-01269-2. Epub 2020 Mar 5. PMID: 32141017; PMCID: PMC7140756.
68. Pollei TR, Hinni ML, Moore EJ, et al. Analysis of postoperative bleeding and risk factors in transoral surgery of the oropharynx. JAMA Otolaryngol Head Neck Surg. 2013;139(11):1212–8. https://doi.org/10.1001/jamaoto.2013.5097.
69. Shah-Becker S, Greenleaf EK, Boltz MM, et al. Neck hematoma after major head and neck surgery: risk factors, costs, and resource utilization. Head Neck. 2018;40(6):1219–27.
70. Hung O, Murphy M. Airway management of the patient with a neck hematoma. In: Hung's difficult and failed airway management [online]. 3rd ed. New York: McGraw Hill; 2018.
71. Gerasimov M, Lee B, Bittner EA. Postoperative anterior neck hematoma (ANH): timely intervention is vital. APSF News Lett. 2021;36(1)

Critical Care of the Thoracic Surgical Patient

36

Virendra K. Arya and Ganesh Kumar

36.1 Introduction

The perioperative management of thoracic oncological surgical patients always poses a challenging task to the critical care physician. In addition to the primary pathology and the complications associated with it, most of these patients have additional factors, which play a crucial role in the surgical outcome. These patients are often smokers and elderly with co-morbidities like hypertension, diabetes mellitus, coronary arterial disease, renal insufficiency, and chronic obstructive pulmonary disease (COPD) [1]. Besides, patients with lesions in the lungs and oesophagus, have poor nutritional status and diminished respiratory reserve even in the preoperative period, which is further compromised in the post-surgical period affecting the outcome. With the advancement in surgical techniques like minimally invasive procedures and shift of anaesthetic technique towards fast track protocol, sicker patients are getting operated on recently [2]. Even though the postoperative complications associated with thoracic surgery is higher (1–37%) when compared to abdominal surgeries (5–15%) [3], with better risk stratification and modification in the preoperative period and excellent intraoperative and postoperative care in the intensive care unit (ICU), a better outcome can be achieved in these patients.

In this chapter, we will discuss the basic surgical concerns and post-operative care and monitoring of patients undergoing thoracic surgery along with immediate complications and their management.

V. K. Arya (✉)
Max Rady College of Medicine, University of Manitoba, Saint Boniface Hospital, Winnipeg, MB, Canada

Department of Cardiac Anaesthesia, PGIMER, Chandigarh, India

G. Kumar
Department of Cardiac Anaesthesia, PGIMER, Chandigarh, India

V. Kumar et al. (eds.), *Onco-critical Care*,
https://doi.org/10.1007/978-981-16-9929-0_36

36.2 General Concerns in Postoperative Management of Thoracic Surgical Patients

Thoracic surgeries are complex surgeries performed for various lesions involving lungs and other mediastinal structures like the trachea, bronchus, oesophagus, and various intrathoracic soft tissues. Neoplastic diseases forms the major bulk of surgeries involving these structures particularly the lungs. In addition to the routine postoperative complications like pain, nausea, vomiting, airway irritation associated with tracheal intubation, the necessity of one lung ventilation in these surgeries and preoperative compromise in the respiratory functions due to the primary pathology complicates the postoperative course in these patients. The increase in the number of video assisted thoracoscopy surgery (VATS) and mediastinoscopy procedures have increased the need for one lung ventilation even in patients who do not require the same in traditional thoracotomy surgeries [4].

As mentioned earlier, the introduction of minimally invasive thoracic surgeries and fast track anaesthesia protocol has reduced the surgical aggressiveness and facilitates early postoperative recovery in these patients [2]. Similarly the use of staplers and glues has brought down the incidence of air leaks and reduced the overall hospital and ICU stay [5]. Optimization of factors like smoking cessation [6], preoperative education and physiotherapy [7] has shown to reduce the morbidities mortalities associated with these surgeries.

Despite of all the advancements in patient care, the postoperative mortality of this group of patients remains high in the range of 2–5% with cardiopulmonary morbidity around 20–40% [8], indicating the importance of ICU care in these patients. The decision regarding the need of ICU care in these patients can be predicted based on preoperative patient risk factors like age, frailty score, American Society of Anaesthesiologist (ASA) physical status, thoracic revised cardiac risk index and intra-operative factors like the extent of lung resection, blood loss and injury to the adjacent structures [9].

36.3 Intensive Care Management

An intensive cardiorespiratory monitoring, adequate pain control, proper fluid and electrolyte management along with prevention, early detection and treatment of complications forms the basic elements in the ICU management of these patients. The prognosis of these patients mainly depends on the management of the acute physiological process, which leads to ICU admission rather than the primary pathology itself [10]. Hence an aggressive approach towards these patients in the ICU may lead to a better ICU discharge rate.

36.4 Monitoring in ICU

In addition to the standard ASA monitoring in the postoperative period which includes an electrocardiogram, heart rate, blood pressure and oxygen saturation using pulse oximetry, these patients require additional monitoring like continuous blood pressure monitoring using invasive methods particularly in patients who require inotropic or vasopressor support for hemodynamic stability. Serum electrolyte and respiratory gases status should be monitored frequently using arterial blood gas (ABG) analysis, chest X-ray for assessment of postoperative lung and pleural space status along with hourly urine output and overall balance needs to be monitored. This monitoring can be achieved by the placement of invasive arterial line, a central venous catheter (CVC) and Foley's catheter, most of which would have been placed already in the operating room.

The monitoring of airway pressures along with the inspiratory and expiratory volume from the pressure-volume loop in the ventilator are also necessary for early detection and treatment of any significant bronchospasms or air leaks.

36.5 Pain Management

Adequate pain relief is essential in the postoperative period for better chest physiotherapy and early patient mobilization, both of which play a crucial role in the prevention of alveolar atelectasis and superadded secondary infections. Regular monitoring of pain should be done using various validated scores and goals should be established for adequate pain management purposes. Nowadays multi modal analgesia has become the norm in pain management and it should be tailored to the individual patient characteristics. There is a huge shift in the last two decades where local analgesia and anesthesia techniques like thoracic epidural and paravertebral blocks using opioids and local anaesthetics respectively have replaced the traditional technique of high dose intravenous (IV) opioids, thereby reducing the complications associated with the IV opioids [11].

The segmental blocks achieved using local anaesthetic and opioid in the thoracic epidural technique has shown to be the only way in which adequate pain control can be achieved without affecting much of the motor and sympathetic functions thereby aiding in the preservation of good conscious level and cough reflex helping the fast recovery of respiratory function [12]. Paravertebral blocks can be achieved either in the preoperative period or in the postoperative period after the completion of surgery where the catheter is placed in the paravertebral space either by the anaesthesiologist or surgeon to achieve the same benefits as epidural blocks. The ability to achieve unilateral analgesia makes paravertebral block preferable in surgeries where the pain afferents originate predominately from one side of the thorax [13].

Despite known side effects like nausea, vomiting, pruritus, constipation, urinary retention and respiratory depression, systemic opioids still plays a major role in pain management of these patients due to its high efficacy. Mostly, systemic opioids are used in adjunct with other modalities or as patient controlled analgesia (PCA) techniques. Other techniques like intrathecal, intra pleural, intercostal and cryoanalgesia are used in less frequency due to the limitations associated with it like short duration of action or less efficacy in postoperative analgesia [4].

36.6 Care of Intercostal Catheters

The management of intercostal catheters is one unique knowledge a physician should know in the effective management of these patients [14]. The use of single drainage instead of multiple individual drains is favoured nowadays due to less pain in the former methods [15]. These catheters serve for two purposes, monitoring for bleeding and to assess for air leak [3]. Even though there is no consensus on the duration of keeping these drainage catheters most of the centers remove them within first 24 h. Despite various meta-analysis and randomized studies, there are no established guidelines concerning the optimal negative pressure attached to these drainage systems. Negative suction to the catheters plays a vital role in patients who underwent pleurodesis with talc as it helps in the approximation of parietal and visceral pleura. In case of persistent air leakage, a portable Heimleikh valve container can be used which helps in early ambulation and even discharge of the patient [3].

36.7 Fluid and Electrolyte Management

The liberal use of fluids in these patients, particularly in lung resection procedures, is associated with acute lung injury and pulmonary oedema. Fluid status should be monitored strictly in these patients, not to over or under hydrate along with special attention to diuresis and renal function [16]. The right atrial pressure measured from the CVC if present and fluid status assessed from Inferior vena cava (IVC), left ventricular (LV), right ventricular (RV) end diastolic volumes using transthoracic echocardiogram (TTE) may help in better fluid management. Simultaneously, the lung can be scanned for the presence of B lines before administrating any fluid bolus. In general, maintenance fluid at the rate of 1–2 ml/kg/h both in the intra- and postoperative period with a target balance of less than 1.5 l positive over the first 24 h is the norm in these patients particularly those undergoing lung resection surgery. Inotropes or vasopressors should be considered for maintaining blood pressure and tissue perfusion, if the volume threshold is reached and required hemodynamic is not achieved [17]. Monitoring of electrolyte should be done regularly to prevent arrhythmias and hypotension, particularly when patients are on diuretic therapy or vasoactive drugs. This can be achieved either by serum biochemistry from the laboratory or from the ABG analysis.

36.8 Physiotherapy and Early Mobilization

The role of physiotherapy cannot be ignored in prevention of pulmonary insufficiency caused by infections, accumulation of secretions and pulmonary oedema. In addition to physiotherapy, bronchodilators, fluid restriction and tracheal toileting help in faster recovery of pulmonary function. Deep breathing and coughing exercise along with incentive spirometry forms the major part of chest physiotherapy. Diuretics should be used if necessary and a low threshold to be kept for starting antibiotics, if infection is suspected even before the start of radiological deterioration [3].

Similarly, early mobilization reduces the incidence of infection, atelectasis and in addition it prevents the occurrence of deep vein thrombosis (DVT) in these patients.

36.9 Postoperative Ventilation, Weaning and Extubation

Unless there are known injury to the airway or lung parenchyma, most of these patients undergo uneventful weaning and extubation in ICU. Particular attention to be paid to those patients, who underwent thoracic surgery for removal of long standing intrathoracic mass, as there is possibility of tracheomalacia or bronchomalacia due to the prolonged mechanical effect of the benign mass and infiltrative nature of malignant masses [18]. Intubation in the intraoperative period also tricky in such patients. One should be ready with all the equipment needed for both the anticipated and unanticipated difficult mask ventilation and intubation [19]. In the authors institute, preoperative evaluation of the airway using flexible fiber-optic bronchoscope (FOB) and virtual or dynamic airway studies using multi detector CT scan [20] is done and intraoperatively the airway is secured using awake FOB guided intubation with flexometalic tracheal tube (TT). The main target is to place the TT tip distal to the point of maximal stenosis or compression in the airway. In cases where lung isolation is needed, the TT can be replaced with double lumen tube (DLT) using an airway exchange catheter (AEC). Occasionally, other methods of lung isolation techniques like bronchial blockers may be utilised [21]. Ideally, all the patients with intrathoracic masses which preclude securing the airway safely, should be operated in a setup where cardiopulmonary bypass (CPB) backup is available. In such cases, before inducing the patient, all the necessary steps like priming of bypass circuit, preparation of inguinal region for femoral cannulation should be ready to place the patient on CPB if the need arises either electively or in emergency basis.

In addition to the standard extubation criteria, these patients should be evaluated for laryngeal and diaphragmatic functions due to possibility of injury to the recurrent laryngeal nerve and phrenic nerve during the intraoperative course. This can be achieved using FOB and ultra-sonogram (USG) of the diaphragm respectively. In suspected cases of tracheomalacia, extubation can be done after placing an AEC in the trachea, so that in case of airway collapse, it can be secured by intubating with TT using the AEC as guidewire [22].

36.10 Immediate Complications and Its Management

36.10.1 Postoperative Bleeding

Postoperative bleeding in these patients is rare with an incidence of 1–3% in open and <2% in VATS [23–26]. It may be due to either surgical causes like injury to lung parenchyma, peri-bronchial veins, bronchial arteries, thoracic wall vessels and muscles or coagulopathy. Preoperative and immediate postoperative coagulation profile helps in anticipating and managing coagulopathy due to medical causes. Based on the coagulation profile and sonoclot values, medical bleeding can be managed with transfusion of fresh frozen plasmas, cryoprecipitate, platelet concentrates and factor VII. An intercostal drainage of more than 1000 ml in the first hour or more than 200 ml/h for more than 3–4 h, after ruling out the medical coagulopathy, need to be re-explored [3]. Measurement of haematocrit of the chest drainage may help to rule out bleeding from lymphatic or serous drainage in stable patients with high chest drainage. In case of unstable patients with minimal or no drain output, chest X-ray, central venous pressure (CVP) and sonographic examination should be done to rule out occult haemorrhage in the thoracic cavity, which may require evacuation [27].

36.10.2 Cardiac Arrhythmias

Arrhythmias forms the major known cardiac complications in these patients with atrial fibrillation (AF) forming the major bulk followed by other tachyarrhythmia's like supra ventricular tachycardia. The incidence of AF varies based on the surgical procedure from 10% in lobectomy to as high as 40% in pneumonectomy patients [28, 29]. It usually occurs in the 2nd and 3rd postoperative days [30] and various factors influence the occurrence of these arrhythmias which may be patiently related like age, pre-existing cardio respiratory illness, preoperative radiation history or surgical factors like type of pneumonectomy, anaesthetic agents used and bleeding severity [31, 32].

In hemodynamically unstable patients, new onset AF should be terminated using electrical cardioversion followed by chemical cardioversion. In the case of stable patients, chemical cardioversion will be sufficient [33]. During pharmacological treatment, the presence of patient co-morbidities and primary lung pathology should be considered, for example, amiodarone should be avoided in patients with severe lung parenchymal disease particularly in those who underwent right pneumonectomy and in such cases, flecainide can be preferred [34]. Similarly, for rate control, selective β1 blocker like metoprolol or calcium channel blocker like diltiazem should be preferred in patients with moderate to severe COPD and bronchospasm [35].

If the AF persists more than 48 h or if it recurs, based on the CHA_2DS_2-VASc score, patients with more than or equal to 2 should be started on anticoagulation therapy for the prevention of stroke [36].

36.10.3 Cardiac Ischemia

The incidence of cardiac ischemia and myocardial infarction in these patient ranges approximately 3% and 1.5% respectively [37]. Major thoracic surgeries are categorized as high risk surgery as per the American College of Cardiology and American Heart Association guidelines and recommends preoperative cardiac evaluation in the presence of associated cardiac symptoms like unstable angina, severe valvular disease, decompensated heart failure and arrhythmia [38]. Such high risk patients should be monitored continuously with electrocardiogram for ST segment changes and with TTE for cardiac functions and change in the valvular lesion severity or new regional wall motion abnormality. Preoperative medications should be started as soon as possible with particular attention to the fluid management to prevent pulmonary oedema [4].

36.10.4 Pulmonary Hypertension and Right Ventricular Failure

Pre-existing pulmonary pathology predisposes these patients for development of acute rise in pulmonary artery pressure particularly following right pneumonectomy. Abrupt increase in the blood volume following pulmonary resection and pre-existing pulmonary vascular changes leads to pulmonary hypertension and right ventricular failure causing hemodynamic instability [1]. Such patients develop low cardiac output, high CVP, hepatic congestion and fall in urine output. Point of care TTE examination will show dilated RV with reduced RV stroke volume, under filled LV, Tricuspid regurgitation that can be used to measure pulmonary artery pressure (PAP) [39]. Reduced LV stroke volume may manifest as low blood pressure, which in turn compromise the coronary perfusion leading to cardiac ischemia. In the presence of patent foramen ovale (PFO), right to left shunt can occur leading to hypoxemia and desaturation. This complication should be diagnosed and managed early to prevent the vicious cycle of deterioration. The initial step is to find an treat the correctable causes of increase in PAP like hypoxemia, hypercapnia, acidosis, pain and other factors which stimulate the sympathetic system. Volume management is critical in such situation as right ventricular volume overload may impair the left ventricular filling due to septal shifting and interventricular dependence. TTE and pulmonary artery catheter can help in such situations for effective preload management. Right ventricular output can be optimized by using inotropic agents like milrinone, dobutamine and epinephrine. Milrinone is preferred as it contributes to the reduction of PAP through its actions on phosphodiesterase (PDE)-3 enzymes. Systemic pressure should be maintained to prevent cardiac ischemia with the help of vasopressors like norepinephrine or vasopressin. Vasopressin is preferred over norepinephrine due to its lack of effect on pulmonary vasculature. Drugs like Sildenafil, inhaled epoprostenol and inhaled nitric oxide (NO) can be used to reduce the PVP until the pulmonary vasculature remodels to tolerate the increase in blood flow [40].

Some patients, may exhibit refractory hypoxemia even in the absence of raised PAP, particular those who underwent right pneumonectomy. They exhibit platypnea and orthodeoxia, which gets relieved in supine position. This occurs due to mediastinal shift causing changes in the relationship between left atrium and right atrium and distorting the inter-atrial septum causing diversion of IVC flow towards PFO [41].

36.10.5 Pulmonary Oedema

The incidence of respiratory complication ranges from 5 to 14% in this group of patients [42–44]. Numerous reports have been published mentioning about a specific syndrome called post-pneumonectomy pulmonary oedema (PPO), which typically develops within 48 h of surgery with diffuse infiltration in chest X-ray consistent with pulmonary oedema but without any evidence of cardiogenic causes like LV failure or raised pulmonary wedge pressure [45–47]. The incidence of PPO is 2.5–4% [45].

The proposed mechanism of PPO is ischemic reperfusion injury and the injury produced by reactive oxygen species to the pulmonary capillaries [48]. Measures to reduce its occurrences includes, restricting total fluid balance to less than 20 ml/kg in first 24 h, no replacement for third space fluid loss, not targeting a urine output of >0.5 ml/kg/h, use of invasive monitoring for better assessment, use of vasopressors for maintaining tissue perfusion and blood pressure when required, avoiding hyperinflation of the residual lung, avoiding posture with the residual lung in dependent side for prolong period and regular chest X-ray for monitoring [4, 48].

PPO has a higher mortality rate of 50% even with adequate treatment with diuretics, mechanical ventilation, nutritional support and adequate oxygenation. Inhaled NO and extra-corporeal membrane oxygenator support can be tried as last resort. NO at 10–20 parts per million has shown to reduce mortality to 30% in addition to other measures like early elective intubation, bronchoscopy and frequent postural changes [48].

36.10.6 Post-pneumonectomy Syndrome (PPS)

PPS is caused due to massive mediastinal shift leading to compression of the bronchus [49]. With the incidence of 1 in 640 [50], it occurs mostly in patients with right pneumonectomy [4]. In pneumonectomy patients, the mediastinum undergoes counter-clockwise rotation leading to stretching, distortion and compression of the ipsilateral bronchus between the pulmonary artery anteriorly and the vertebral body posteriorly [49, 50]. Females and children are more prone to PPS due to the more elastic nature of their mediastinal tissues and softer airway [51]. Usually PPS manifests as recurrent respiratory infections, stridor and exertional dyspnoea. Once diagnosed, it is managed with surgical repositioning of the mediastinum by placing saline filed silicone prosthesis in pneumonectomy space [52]. In inoperable conditions and for acute stabilization of patients, an airway stent can be placed [51].

36.10.7 Injury to Adjacent Structures

Injuries to the intrathoracic structures can occur in any intra thoracic procedures like pleuro-pulmonary procedures, oesophageal, mediastinal and intra-pericardial and even in minimally invasive procedures like subclavian puncture [53, 54]. Injury to the thoracic duct causes chylothorax, which leads to loss of proteins, calories and fluids leading to nutritional deficiency, immunological dysfunction and dehydration, even respiratory compromise if not drained [55].

Postoperative air leak is one of the most common complications in these patients due to injury to the airway or alveoli. The majority of air leaks are alveolar air leaks, which can be managed with watchful waiting with continuous drainage. In case of broncho-pleural fistula, immediate treatment with surgical repair is needed to reduce postoperative morbidities [56].

Injury to the phrenic nerve and recurrent laryngeal nerve is possible particularly in patients with extensive adhesions and in redo cases. Phrenic nerve injury may present with difficulty in weaning from ventilator and in post extubation patient it may presents with dyspnoea on exertion and exercise intolerance. It can be temporary or permanent. Permanent unilateral diaphragmatic palsy due to phrenic nerve injury is better managed with unilateral diaphragmatic plication [4, 57].

Patient with recurrent laryngeal nerve injury often have a weak and whispery voices and they have increased risk of aspiration and impaired ability to cough. Permanent damage should be managed with surgical procedures like medialization laryngoplasty [4, 57].

36.10.8 Infection

These patients are prone for developing surgical wound site infection and nosocomial pneumonia. Antibiotic coverage should be started even before the surgical incision and continued until 3rd postoperative day unless the patient develops infection during ICU stay. Physiotherapy, early mobilization, adequate pain control and bronchodilators aid in faster recovery of these patients in the postoperative period thereby reducing the possibility of acquiring infection [58].

Other complications include cardiac herniation and tamponade, lobar torsion and gangrene, deep vein thrombosis and pulmonary thromboembolism, renal failure, strokes, gastrointestinal bleeding, stress ulcers, pressure sores, malnutrition, delirium, and critical illness myopathy. These complications should be diagnosed early and managed aggressively for a better patient outcome.

References

1. McKenna SS. Critical care for the thoracic surgery patient. In: Sugarbaker's adult chest surgery. 3rd ed. New York: McGraw Hill; 2015, p. 70–9.
2. Varandhan KK, Neal KR, Dejong CH, Fearon KC, Ljungqvist O, Lobo DN. The enhanced recover after surgery (ERAS) pathway for patients undergoing major elective open colorectal surgery: a meta-analysis of randomized trials. Clin Nutr. 2010;29:434–40.
3. Iyer A, Yadav S. Postoperative care and complications after thoracic surgery. In: Firstenberg MS, editor. Principles and practice of cardiothoracic surgery. IntechOpen; 2013.
4. Muñoz de Cabo C, Hermoso Alarza F, Cossio Rodriguez AM, Martín Delgado MC. Perioperative management in thoracic surgery. Med Intensiva. 2020;44:185–91.
5. Temes RT, Willms CD, Endara SA, Wernly JA. Fissureless lobectomy. Ann Thorac Surg. 1998;65:282–4.
6. Vaporciyan AA, Merriman KW, Ece F, Roth JA, Smythe WR, Swisher SG, et al. Incidence of major pulmonary morbidity after pneumonectomy: association with timing of smoking cessation. Ann Thorac Surg. 2002;73:420–6.
7. Brasher PA, McClelland KH, Denehy L, Story I. Does removal of deep breathing exercises from a physiotherapy program including pre-operative education and early mobilisation after cardiac surgery alter patient outcomes? Aust J Physiother. 2003;49:165–73.
8. Brunelli A, Charloux A, Bolliger CT, Rocco G, Sculier JP, Varela G, et al. ERS/ESTS clinical guidelines on fitness for radical therapy in lung cancer patients (surgery and chemo-radiotherapy). Eur Respir J. 2009;34:17–41.
9. Meert A-P, Grigoriu B, Licker M, Van Schil PE, Berghmans T. Intensive care in thoracic oncology. Eur Respir J. 2017;49:1602189. https://doi.org/10.1183/13993003.02189-2016.
10. Berghmans T, Sculier JP. Is there any usefulness for a specific scoring system in assessing the prognosis of cancer patients admitted to the intensive care unit? Intensive Care Med. 2004;30:1849.
11. Joshi GP, Bonnet F, Shah R, Wilkinson RC, Camu F, Fischer B, et al. A systematic review of randomized trials evaluating regional techniques for post thoracotomy analgesia. Anesth Analg. 2008;107:1026–40.
12. Hughes R, Gao F. Pain control for thoracotomy. Continuing education in anaesthesia. Crit Care Pain. 2005;5(2):56–60.
13. Karmakar MK. Thoracic paravertebral block. Anesthesiology. 2001;95(3):771–80.
14. French DG, Dilena M, LaPlante S, Shamji F, Sundaresan S, Villeneuve J, et al. Optimizing postoperative care protocols in thoracic surgery: best evidence and new technology. J Thorac Dis. 2016;8(Suppl 1):S3–11.
15. Dawson AG, Hosmane S. Should you place one or two chest drains in patients undergoing lobectomy? Interact Cardiovasc Thorac Surg. 2010;11:178–81.
16. Algar FJ, Alvarez A, Salvatierra A, Baamonde C, Aranda JL, Lopez-Pujol FJ. Predicting pulmonary complications after pneumonectomy for lung cancer. Eur J Cardiothorac Surg. 2003;23:201–8.
17. Evans RG, Naidu B. Does a conservative fluid management strategy in the perioperative management of lung resection patients reduce the risk of acute lung injury? Interact Cardiovasc Thorac Surg. 2012;15(3):498–504.
18. Gaissert HA, Burns J. The compromised airway: tumors, strictures, and tracheomalacia. Surg Clin N Am. 2010;90(5):1065–89.
19. Frerk C, Mitchell VS, McNarry AF, Mendonca C, Bhagrath R, Patel A, et al. Difficult Airway Society intubation guidelines working group, Difficult Airway Society 2015 guidelines for management of unanticipated difficult intubation in adults. BJA. 2015;115(6):827–48.
20. Sams VG, Lawson CM, Shibli AB, Taylor DA, Branca PR. Severe Tracheobronchomalacia after prolonged intubation of multitrauma patient. Case Rep Surg. 2011;2011:Article ID 627012, 3 pages.

21. Campos JH. Lung isolation techniques for patients with difficult airway. Curr Opin Anaesthesiol. 2010;23(1):12–7.
22. Mitchell V, Dravid R, Patel A, Swampillai C, Higgs A. Difficult Airway Society Guidelines for the management of tracheal extubation. Anaesthesia. 2012;67:318–40.
23. Peterffy A, Henze A. Haemorrhagic complications during pulmonary resection: a retrospective review of 1428 resections with 113 haemorrhagic episodes. Scand J Thorac Cardiovasc Surg. 1983;17(3):283–7.
24. Sirbu H, Busch T, Aleksic I. Chest re-exploration for complications after lung surgery. Thorac Cardiovasc Surg. 1999;47(2):73–6.
25. Krasna MJ, Deshmukh S, McLaughlin JS. Complications of thoracoscopy. Ann Thorac Surg. 1996;61(4):1066–9.
26. Yim AP, Liu HP. Complications and failures of video-assisted thoracic surgery: experience from two centers in Asia. Ann Thorac Surg. 1996;61(2):538–41.
27. Litle VR, Swanson SJ. Postoperative bleeding: coagulopathy, bleeding, hemothorax. Thorac Surg Clin. 2006;16(3):203–7.
28. Asamura H, Naruke T, Tsuchiya R, Goya T, Kondo H, Suemasu K. What are the risk factors for arrhythmias after thoracic operations? J Thorac Cardiovasc Surg. 1993;106:1104–10.
29. Amar D. Cardiac arrhythmias. Chest Surg Clin North Am. 1998;8:479–93.
30. Vaporciyan AA, Correa AM, Rice DC, Roth JA, Smythe WR, Swisher SG. Risk factors associated with atrial fibrillation after noncardiac thoracic surgery: analysis of 2,588 patients. J Thorac Cardiovasc Surg. 2004;127:779–86.
31. Amar D, Zhang H, Roistacher N. The incidence and outcome of ventricular arrhythmias after non-cardiac thoracic surgery. Anesth Analg. 2002;95:537–43.
32. Asamura H. Early complications; cardiac complications. Chest Surg Clin North Am. 1999;9:527–41.
33. Rena O, Papalia E, Oliaro A. Supraventricular arrhythmias after resection surgery of the lung. Eur J Cardiothorac Surg. 2001;20:688–93.
34. Fernando HC, Jaklitsch MT, Walsh GL, Tisdale JE, Bridges CD, Mitchell JD, et al. The Society of Thoracic Surgeons Practice Guideline on the prophylaxis and management of atrial fibrillation associated with general thoracic surgery: executive summary. Ann Thorac Surg. 2011;92:1144–52.
35. Woude HJ, Zaagsma J, Postma DS, Winter TH, van Hulst M, Aalbers R. Detrimental effects of beta-blockers in COPD: a concern for nonselective beta-blockers. Chest. 2005;127:818–24.
36. Svendsen JH, Nielsen JC, Darkner S, Jensen GVH, Mortensen LS, Andersen HR, et al. CHADS2 and CHA2DS2-VASc score to assess risk of stroke and death in patients paced for sick sinus syndrome. Heart. 2013;99(12):843–8.
37. On Knorring J, Lepantalo M, Lindgren L, Lindfors O. Cardiac arrhythmias and myocardial ischemia after thoracotomy for lung cancer. Ann Thorac Surg. 1992;53:642–7.
38. Eagle KA, Berger PB, Calkins H, Chaitman BR, Ewy GA. ACC/AHA guideline update for perioperative cardiovascular evaluation for non-cardiac surgery. Circulation. 2002;105:1257–67.
39. Augustine DX, Coates-Bradshaw LD, Willis J, Harkness A, Ring L, Grapsa J, et al. Echocardiographic assessment of pulmonary hypertension: a guideline protocol from the British Society of Echocardiography. Echo Res Pract. 2018 Sep;5(3):G11–24.
40. Brunner N, Perez VA, Richter A, Haddad F, Denault A, Rojas V, et al. Perioperative pharmacological management of pulmonary hypertensive crisis during congenital heart surgery. Pulm Circ. 2014;4(1):10–24.
41. Bakris NC, Siddiqi AJ, Fraser CD Jr, Mehta AC. Right-to-left interatrial shunt after pneumonectomy. Ann Thorac Surg. 1997;63:198–210.
42. Nagasaki F, Flehinger BJ, Martini N. Complications of surgery in the treatment of carcinoma of the lung. Chest. 1982;82:25–9.
43. Deslauriers J, Ginsberg RJ, Dubois P, Beaulieu M, Goldberg M, Piraux M. Current operative morbidity associated with elective surgical resection for lung cancer. Can J Surg. 1989;32:335–9.

44. Tedder M, Anstadt MP, Tedder SD, Lowe JE. Current morbidity, mortality, and survival after bronchoplastic procedures for malignancy. Ann Thorac Surg. 1992;54:387–91.
45. Jordan S, Mitchell JA, Quinlan GJ, Goldstraw P, Evans TW. The pathogenesis of lung injury following pulmonary resection. Eur Respir J. 2000;15:790–9.
46. Bauer P. Postpneumonectomy pulmonary oedema revisited. Eur Respir J. 2000;15:629–30.
47. Zeldin RA, Normandin D, Landtwing D, Peters RM. Postpneumonectomy pulmonary edema. J Thorac Cardiovasc Surg. 1984;87:359–65.
48. De Decker K, Jorens PG, Van Schil P. Cardiac complications after non-cardiac thoracic surgery: an evidence-based current review. Ann Thorac Surg. 2003;75(4):1340–8.
49. Maurik AF, Stubenitsky BM, van Swieten HA, Duurkens VA, Laban E, Kon M. Use of tissue expanders in adult postpneumonectomy syndrome. J Thorac Cardiovasc Surg. 2007;134:608–12.
50. Jansen JP, Brutel de la Rivière A, Alting MP, Westermann CJ, Bergstein PG, Duurkens VA. Postpneumonectomy syndrome in adulthood. Surgical correction using an expandable prosthesis. Chest. 1992;101:1167–70.
51. Régnard JF, Pouliquen E, Magdeleinat P, Sohier L, Gourden P, Gharbi N, et al. Postpneumonectomy syndrome in adults: description and therapeutic propositions apropos of 8 cases. Rev Mal Respir. 1999;16:1113–9.
52. Rakovich G, Bussières J, Fréchette E. Postpneumonectomy syndrome. Multimed Man Cardiothorac Surg. https://doi.org/10.1510/mmcts.2008.003475.
53. Joyce LD, Lindsy WG, Nicolott DM. Chylothorax after median sternotomy for intrapericardial surgery. J Thorac Cardiovasc Surg. 1976;71:476–80.
54. Van Mulders A, Lacquet LM, Van Meghem W, Deneffe G. Chylothorax complicating pneumonectomy. Thorax. 1984;38:954–5.
55. Kutlu CA, Sayar A, Olgac G. Chylothorax: a complication following lung resection in patients with NSCLC: chylothorax following lung resection. Thorac Cardiovasc Surg. 2003;51:342–5.
56. Sunil S, Victor AF, Charles RB, Ellen RC, John DM, Hiran CF, et al. Management of alveolar air leaks after pulmonary resection. Ann Thorac Surg. 2010;89:1327–35.
57. Haithcock BE, Feins RH. Complications of pulmonary resection. In: Shields TW, LoCicero J, Reed CE, Feins RH, editors. General thoracic surgery. 7th ed. Philadelphia: Lippincott Williams & Wilkins; 2009, page 558.
58. Radu DM, Jauréguy F, Seguin A, Foulon C, Destable MD, Azorin J, et al. Postoperative pneumonia after major pulmonary resections: an unsolved problem in thoracic surgery. Ann Thorac Surg. 2007;84:1669–74.

Critical Care Management of Mediastinal Mass Surgery Patients

37

Minati Choudhury

Key Points

1. Operated mediastinal mass (MM) patients may develop major airway and cardiovascular compression.
2. Preoperative understanding of the relation of the MM to the surrounding structures, their degree of invasiveness and preparation for possible postoperative complications are key to successful management.
3. Availability of tube exchanger, fiberoptic intubation set, immediate availability of rigid bronchoscope, avoidance of muscle relaxant, positioning changes may avoid major respiratory catastrophes.
4. Though it is essential to know pre-operative lung function tests, their role inpostoperative period is doubtful.
5. Most of the treating team desires an analgesic technique that has acceptable safety profile, produces reasonable pain relief while supporting early rehabilitation and physical recovery. A multimodal analgesic strategy is much in practice rather than any individual technique as stand-alone.
6. These patients often prone for major bleeding, risk of superior-venacaval (SVC) syndrome, infection and cardiorespiratory disturbances.
7. The effect of pre and postoperative radiotherapy and chemotherapy makes the management more critical.
8. Antibiotic management and awareness about drug interaction is an important part of care.

M. Choudhury (✉)
Department of Cardiac Anaesthesia and Critical Care, Cardiothoracic and NeuroSciences Centre, AIIMS, New Delhi, India

V. Kumar et al. (eds.), *Onco-critical Care*,
https://doi.org/10.1007/978-981-16-9929-0_37

9. Nutritional supplement, maintainance of bronchial hyegine and timely physiotherapy is important for early recovery.
10. Reporting of critical incidents, prior clarification about which incident to be reported can prevent and treat most of the post operative adverse events after MM surgery, thereby provide best outcome.

37.1 Introduction

The mediastinum is considered to be the most worried region of human body because it contains the vital organs. The patients with MM often presents the anaesthesiologist and critical care physician with a formidable challenge not only during intraoperative period, but also during their post surgery critical care unit (CRCU) stay. Bleeding, severe respiratory as well as cardiovascular complications including inability to resuscitate can ensue during postoperative period leading to a big burden on the management team. This chapter narrates the management of these high-risk patients in CRCU during their post surgical period. Aortic aneurysms, esophageal masses, cardiac tumors, spinal masses and lung tumors are not the part of this chapter.

37.2 Mediastinal Mass: A General View

Knowledge regarding the type of MM is important because their heterogenous pathology that may give rise to compression of surrounding structure and their sequel [1]. The CRCU management mainly depends upon the size and pathophysiology of the mass (preoperative airway/cardiovascular compromise), surgical procedure involved, and extensiveness of surgery. Near fatal cardiac arrest also been reported in their post extubation period and CRCU stay inspite of a uneventful surgery [2–5].

Primary MM are named depending on their location into anterior, middle or posterior mediastinum (Table 37.1). Thymoma, benign cysts and neurogenic tumors accounts for 60% of the lesions, while germ cell tumors, lymphomas and granulomatous diseases comprises of 30% of the lesions and the rest 10% are t vascular origin [5]. Sixty five % of symptomatic patients have malignant lesions, while 75% of aymptomatic patients have benign lesion.

On the view of postoperative complication, the patients are categorized in to three groups depending upon their preoperative characteristics. The *low risk* patients are usually asymptomatic or with mild symptoms but without postural symptoms or any radiological evidence of airway compromise. The patients under *moderate risk* category have mild to moderate postural symptoms with a radiological evidence of airway compression <50%; and thosewith severe postural symptoms, stridor or cyanosis and radiological evidence of airway compression >50%, SVC syndrome or pericardial effusion considered to be in *severe risk* category [1].

Table 37.1 Classification/nomenclature of mediastinal mass

Position	Benign	Malignant
Superior mediastinum	Thymoma Retrosternal goiter Parathyroid adenoma	Malignant thyroid/ parathyroid mass
Anterior mediastinum	*Thymus* 1. Thymoma 2. Thymic cysts 3. Thymiclipoma 4. Thymic hyperplasia *Lymphnode* 1. Benign nodal hyperplasia 2. Angioblastic lymphoid adenopathy *Cystic hygroma* *Teratoid tumors* 1. Dermoid cyst *Cardiovascular* 1. Pericardial cyst 2. Aneurysm of ascending aorta 3. Benign cardiac tumors *Others* 1. Pancreatic pseudocyst 2. Paraganglioma 3. Hemangioma 4. Tumors of vagus and phrenic nerve	*Thymus* 1. Thymic carcinoid 2. Thymic carcinoma *Lymphnode* 1. Lymphoma *Teratoid tumors* 1. Teratoma 2. Embryonalcell carcinoma 3. Mixed Germ cell tumor 4. Seminoma *Cardiovascular* 1. Metastasis 2. Malignant cardiac tumors
Middle mediastinum	1. Benign bronchogenic cysts 2. Benign adenopathy 3. Hiatus hernia 4. Cardiac/vascular tumors 5. Benign mass of esophagus	*Metastasis* 1. Lymphoma 2. Malignant mass of esophagus
Posterior mediastinum	*Neoplasm* 1. Paraganglioma 2. Lymphoma 3. Thyroid tumors 4. Hemangioma 5. Mesenchymal tumor 6. Vertebral tumor *Vascular* 1. Descending thoracic aortic pseudoaneurysm 2. Pseudomeningocele Abdominal 1. Retroperitoneal mass 2. Hernia of foramen of Bochdalek Developmental 1. Neuroenteric cysts 2. Bronchogenic cysts 3. Extra lobar sequestration *Neurofibroma* *Schwannoma* *Chemodectoma* *Others* 1. Extramedullaryhematopoiesis 2. Lateral meningocele 3. Lymphoid hyperplasia 4. Paraspinus abscess	*Neuroblastoma* *Lymphoma*

Well-defined small mass usually have a smooth postoperative course and does not require admission in CRCU. However patients with large invasive mass, those with pressure symptoms, and systemic manifestations (e.g. myasthenia gravis-thymoma, carcinoid, hyrotoxicosis-benign/malignant thyroid tumors, paroxysmal hypertension-pheochromocytoma) behave differently and need additional care. Patients with a malignant mass often need prior chemotherapy (CT) and radiotherapy (RT) to reduce the tumor size as well as thrombectomy and resection of adhered cardiovascular structures under CPB, require strict postoperative monitoring.

The intensity of postoperative care and complications also greately related to the mode of surgical approach and structures resected. The usual surgical approaches are: median sternotomy, thoracotomy, median sternotomy+thoracotomy, bilateral subcostal thoracotomy, inverse T incision of upper mediastinum, anterior-cervico-thoracic trans clavicularapproach, trans-manubrialosteomuscular sparing approach and high posterior thoracotomy [6, 7]. Some patients may need concomitant anatomical resection of adjacent structures-including partial or complete removal of pericardium, wedge resection of lung, lobectomy, pneumonectomy, chest wall resection, diaphragm resection and oesophagectomy, SVC resection and reconstruction, brachiocephalic vein resection, arterial resection (carotid/brachiocephalic artery) need strict postoperative monitoring and additional care. There is a report in which tracheal necrosis occurred in CRCU after extensive surgery with prosthetic replacement of SVC after resection of thyroid tumor. This patient was successfully treated by tracheostomy and omentopexy. Patients with giant tumors who have severe pre-operative compression of lung and great vessels or heart may develop reperfusion pulmonary edema after surgical reestablishment of flow to the pulmonary parenchyma and myocardium.

37.3 Post-Operative Care and Management of Complication

The ideal approach is to start the care from preoperative period. Preoperative cessation of smoking 6 weeks preoperatively circumvents postoperative bronchorrhoea and promotes regeneration of cilia. Preoperative pulmonary rehabilitation, psychotherapy, physiotherapy, education regarding deep breathing, splinted coughing exercises; prophylactic exercises for deep vein thrombosis (DVT) as well as shoulder exercises have an important role in recovery [8].

It is important to ensure that the CRCU team is aware of the patient's procedure and possible time of arrival in the unit. It is always desirable to extubate the patient when he is fully awake. Patients who need cardiopulmonary bypass (CPB) for tumor resection require special attention in the post operative period due to add on problems secondary to CPB [9]. Box 37.1 depicts few of the post surgical complication.

Box 37.1 Complications of mediastinal mass resection

Respiratory • Aspiration • Atelectasis • Hemorrhage • Tracheomalasia • Laryngospasm/bronchospasm • Pneumonia • Airleak • Pulmonary embolism • Pneumothorax, hemothorax • Pleural effusion, emphysema, chylothorax *Cardiovascular* • Major vessel hemorrhage • Ischemia • Arrhythmia • Cardiac tamponade • Ventricular dysfunction and LCOS • Cardiac herniation • Heart failure • Right to left intracardiac shunt • Pulmonary edema • Pulmonary thromboembolism • Superior venacaval syndrome *Pain* • Wound infection • Vascular prosthesis thrombosis • Myocardial infarction • CVA	*Central nervous system* • Brain hemorrhage • Stroke *Bleeding and coagulopathy* *Gastro intestinal* • Hemorrhage • Nutrition • Esophageal perforation • Ileus *Nerve injury* • Phrenic nerve • Recurrent laryngeal nerve *Miscellaneous* • Multiorgan failure • Tumor seeding of neck incision • Sternal dehiscence • Mediastinal mass syndrome

The patients with huge symptomatic MM have complex physical and emotional needs which is best met by a multidisciplinary team approach involving nursing, nutrition, physiological support, physical rehabilitation team, critical care physician, concerned anaesthesiologist and surgeon.

Sudden clinical deterioration may occur in few cases due to sudden haemorrhage, mediastinal mass syndrome, exacerabration of associated disease symptoms (e.g. myasthenia gravis) or complication of antitumor therapies. Early identification (Early warning symptoms) of at risk individuals would prove beneficial to facilitate early and appropriate discussion of treatment goals and ceilings of care. The most common earning signs those need attention are hypotension, tachycardia, tachypnea, and sudden change in level of consciousness [10, 11]. According to most of the studies the early warning sign evidenced before 8 hrs in adults and 11 hrs in children.

37.3.1 Respiratory Problems and Care

Post surgery, patients in "low" risk category should be transferred to the postoperative care unit where aim should be rapid extubation and minimal hemodynamic monitoring e.g. ECG, blood pressure and oxygen saturation for the first 24 hr. Patients who are in "moderate risk" category/where risk is "severe" (e.g. extended sternotomy/major thoracotomy) in spite of complete removal of the mass need CRCU admission and more aggressive hemodynamic and respiratory monitoring. The patients who underwent a diagnostic excision may have sudden respiratory or cardiovascular collapse during postoperative period so all the measures for airway and circulation management should be kept ready. The extubated patients with satisfactory cardiorespiratory and normal neurological status can be moved from the recovery room [12].

Patients with prior chemo/radiotherapy required more strict monitoring because of more propensity for hemorrhage, airleak, surgical emphysema and pneumonia. The post operative respiratory complications are primarily related to tracheal compressionof >50% on preoperative CT scan and a mixed (restrictive+obstructive) picture of abnormal pulmonary function.

Those with diagnosed tracheal compression who underwent video-assisted diagnostic biopsy and have an appropriate tube in situ from operating room (OR), need strict vigilance, adequate sedation and muscle relaxation to prevent accidental extubation till a definite procedure is planned. A rigid bronchoscope set with appropriate size of endotracheal tube (ET) should be available in the emergency basis. If there is need for change of ET tube, it should be best done over a tube exchanger. The patient to be put in a "rescue" position (it is chosen on the basis of the anatomical relationship between the mass and compressive structure and improvement in symptoms of respiratory collapse in a particular position which may be upright sitted, prone or lateral decubitus) to prevent sudden respiratory collapse before securing the airway via the rigid bronchoscope with a single/double lumen endotracheal tube. Severe cardiovascular compromise and hypotension may occur during the time which may require rapid positional change/volume expansion/vasopressor or inotrope [13]. Some patients may be unresponsive and need emergency sternotomy to elevate the mass from compromised structures/CPB/ECMO to rescue.

Pneumonia, airway obstruction secondary to edema, and atelectasis are usually occurred within the first 48 hr. postoperatively. Patients with prior bleomycin therapy have some degree of pulmonary damage. As prolong postoperative ventilation with high inspired oxygen concentration is detrimental in these patients, it is wise to keep inspired oxygen concentration as low as possible but compactable with reasonable arterial saturation [14].

37.3.1.1 Airway Emergencies

Airway obstruction can occur at any part depending upon the extension of mass, postoperative edema or hemorrhage. Incidious development of hemorrhage can lead to unpredictable clinical deterioration. Sudden increase in airway pressure and blood in ET tube are the manifestation in a ventilated patient; and respiratory distress, stridor, facial swelling and desaturation in an extubated one. A decrease in airwy diamer to at least 50% develops these symptoms. Prevention of *aspiration* is important in extubated patients and urgent intubation is necessary in them if volume is more e.g. >200 cc/hr. Any hemodynamic instability need to be treated simultaneously with transfusion or vasopressures depending upon the necessity. Place the patient in the dependent position to preserve the non bleeding lung from blood spillage or pooling. Identification of the site of bleeding by clinical suspicion/bronchoscopy/CT followed by ballon tamponade/endobronchial ablation/surgical ligation of the bleeding vessel or emergent radiotherapy to the residual mass or embolization of pulmonary or bronchial vessels depending upon the cause. Do not forget that there is no optimal ventilator setting for massive hemoptysis. Keep the endoluminal ballon inflated for at least 24 hr. before assessing rebleeding. In case of non-availability of double lumen tube or bronchial blocker, bronchoscopy guided intubation of non-bleeding lung is done till further measures are taken. As it is often difficult to oxygenate them with a bag-valve mask, a small size endotracheal tube is amenable in these cases. A surgical airway e.g. tracheostomy or cricothyrotomy is done in difficult scenario. It is better to avoid long acting sedatives and muscle relaxants for further assessment. Neck hematomas can be decompressed by needle aspiration or surgical clamping of the arterial bleed [15, 16].

37.3.1.2 Tracheomalacia

Usually occur in long standing masses and cause central airway obstruction in the postoperative period. Cough, stridor, wheezing and respiratory distress in a extubated patient and low tidal volume delivery than set level in the ventilated patient are the manifestations. A larger diameter endotracheal tube overcome this problem. Paralyzing agents and heavy sedation can compromise the airway further and hence it is advisible to use paralytics as the last resort during intubation. Peroxygenation or addition of helium to oxygen may provide laminar flow thus act as a bridge to intubation [17].

37.3.1.3 Pneumothorax

The usual causes are: central venous catheter, a complication of mechanical ventilation or tumor pleural involvement. Elevation of plateu pressure, hypoxemia or desaturation gives the clinical clue to diagnosis. Tension pneumothorax is a medical emergency that immediate decompensation after clinical suspicion. Water-seal chest tube drainage with a low-pressure suction is done the till reexansion of lung [18–20].

37.3.1.4 Brochopleural Fistula

Though rare can be a possibility. Suspicion arises in a patient with perstent pneumothorax. Low tidal ventilation is the best preventive measure. Management includes low tidal ventilation (< 6 ml/kg) and close monitoring of auto-PEEP. In persistent cases, coiling, endobronchial stenting, injection of sclerosant or laser coagulation is applied [18–20].

37.3.1.5 Pleural Effusion (PE)

Occurs especially in patients operated for extensive malignant masses. Seconary infection is another possibility. Correlating pleural fluid transamylase and lactate dehydrogenase with that of serum can differentiate exudative vs transudative PE. One should not forget the alternative causes such as heart failure, thromboembolism, hypoalbuminemia and toxic effect of chemo or radiotherapy. The diagnosis confirmed by a X-ray chest or ultrasound. Chest tube drainage is the usual measure. Recurrent effusion and inadequately draining tubes may need pleurodesis or decortication.

37.3.1.6 Hemothorax

Intratoracic bleeding may occur in extensive mediastinal adhesion leading to increase chest tube drainage, respiratory distress and a convex pulmonary margin around the chest tube in chest radiography. Minimal bleeding is controlled by antififibrinolytis/transfusion of blood products. Massive hemothorax is managed by large bore chest tube drainage to overcome rapid clotting and blood transfusion at the same time. Bleeding>200 ml/hr/for 4 hrs/retained volume 500-ml/rapid-accumulation >1500 ml needs immediate re-exploration.

37.3.1.7 Mediastinal Emphysema

Though rare is a possibility in major resection. Subcutaneous emphysema is the usual manifestation in ventilated patients. Diagnosis is done with chest X-ray or computed tomography (CT). Most of the cases is managed with chest tube insertion.

37.3.1.8 Airleak

Airleak may occur in patients with co-existing emphysema or damage to lung during surgery or barotrauma due to prolong ventilator support. It is considered to be abnormal if persists for more than 5 days. Presence of bubbles in the water seal chamber of drainage system suggests its [21]. Continuous leak lead to progressive subcutaneous or mediastinal emphysema, presenting as swollen eyes and swollen face. Early extubation reduces this complication to a significant extent by reducing intrapulmonary pressure. Some authors inject autologous blood, talc or other sclerosing agents to stop the persistent parenchymal leak. Insertion of pigtail catheter with Heimlich valve or intrabronchial valves is helpful.

37.3.1.9 Bronchospasm

Bronchospasm is common and mainly due to histamine release from opioid or allergic response to other drugs as well as from tracheal secretion or suctioning. Inability to ventilate or decresed delivery of set tidal volume and hypoxemia or desaturation are the usual manifestations. Patients usually respond to inhaled bronchodilators or glucocorticoids.

37.3.1.10 Atelectasis

Atelectasis is common in patients who have prior chemo/radiotherapy and undergone extensive resection under CPB. Postoperative pain aggravate the situation in extubated patients by interfering with deep breathing and coughing. Chest physiotherapy, removal of secretion and continuous positive airway pressure (CPAP) or positive pressure ventilation improves the situation. Bronchoscopic guided removal of secretion is done in case of non-improvement.

37.3.1.11 Infectious Mediastinitis

Often fatal, observed after excision of a large adherent mass. Persuistent fever without any identifiable cause, mediastinal edema and increased mediastinal fat attenuation in MDCT is an important diagnostic clue. It should be treated with drainage of collections, debridement of necrotic tissue and antibiotic therapy.

37.3.1.12 Respiratory Failure

Most of the patients get extubated within first 6–8 hrs of surgery. Patients with atelectasis, airway obstruction, pneumonia or aspiration may need prolong support.

37.3.2 Cardiovascular Care

37.3.2.1 Myocardial Ischemia and Hemodynamic Instability

Prolong compression of heart by a large mass may lead to coronary flow compromise. It is also possibile in patients who underwent extensive resection and intervention of cardiac structures e.g. reconstruction of right ventricular outflow tract, opening of cardiac chambers for removal of tumor emboli, massive blood loss, anemia, hypothermia, pain or excessive use of inotropes. Though, there is no gold standard for bed side diagnosis; identification is usually based on ECG manifestations, hemodynamic instability, regional wall motion abnormality in echocardiography. Elevated creatinine kinase-MB or troponin-I are highly specific and diagnostic [22]. The key point in management is correction of underlying precipitating factors, adequate oxygenation and ventilation, treatment of arrhythmias if any. In hemodynamically stable patients, morphine, sublingual or intravenous infusion of nitroglycerine is helpful, hemodynamically unstable patients need an intraaortic ballon pump (IABP). Resistance cases need a cardiologist's consultation for thrombolysis and further management [23]. Invasion of cardiac chambers or pulmonary and brachiocephalic vessels may need reconstruction of these parts using a clamp or prolong CPB. These patients need continued inotropic/vasopressor support to manage postoperative hemodynamic instability.

Tumors involving aorta may need a stent insertion or a graft. These patients are prone for stroke, paraplegia, visceral ischemia, stent migration and infection in CRCU. Strict monitoring, timely diagnosis and intervention can decrease the morbidity and mortality. Anticoagulants should be started in the immediate postoperative period and continued till 3–6 months in case of SVC reconstruction by prosthesis. A dose titration is done under INR monitoring [24].

37.3.2.2 Cardiac Herniation

Cardiac herniation may occur early during post operative period in patient who undergoes extensive resection of pericardium. Sudden hypotension without much change in HR, features of SVC obstruction, increase in pulmonary artery pressure and (PAP) and pulmonary capillary wedge pressure (PCWP) in combination with respiratory signs like wheezing, increased end-expiratory airway pressure and decrease in expiratory tidal volume are the warning signs. There may be ST-T, T wave changes. The extra pericardial myocardium becomes ischemic and edematous; and if not reduced quickly can cause obstruction to ventricular flow leading to cardiac arrhythmia and cardiovascular collapse. A chest X-ray can confirm the herniation of the heart to the opposite hemithorax (spherical heart, displaced laterally, apex against the left chest wall and features of rotation of mediastinal structures. Immediate management includes: positioning of the patient (non-surgical site down), a reduction of tidal volume, and injection of air into surgical hemithorax (to reposition the heart temporarily. The patient may than shifted to the operating room in this position for an emergency thoracotomy and reposition of herniated heart into the pericardiac sac and repairing the defect of pericardium [25].

37.3.2.3 Arrhythmias

Arrhythmias, especially atrial fibrillation (AF), are the most common cardiac complications after mediastinal surgery. The important risk factors can be patient related (older age, limited pulmonary reserve, pre-existing cardiovascular problem), surgery related (anaesthetic agent, major bleeding, intrapericardial pneumonectomy), treatment related (previous thoracic radiation or ongoing chemotherapy), hypoxia, hypercarbia, acidosis or inadequate pain relief. AF with hemodynamic compromise is best managed with electrical cardioversion. In asymptomatic cases underlying causes need to be reversed first followed by pharmacotherapy. New onset AF are mostly transient and resolved by rate controlling agent. Selective beta blockers are the agent of choice in non-asmatics and diltiazem is reserved for those with active bronchospasm or COPD. Digoxin along with a betabloker acts well in some non-responsive cases. In case of continuous or paroxysmal recurrent AF amiodarone is the most reasonable drug. Amiodarone however is not given to the patient who have severe lung disease or pulmonary resection to some degree. Flecainide, disopyramide, ibutide and propafenone, labetolol and sotalol are some other drugs, which have specific indications, merits and demerits in such cases. Patients with documented magnesium deficiency need the supplementation in the form of intravenous (IV) magnesium sulphate. Immediately. Some of the AF patients need additional anticoagulation therapy if have risk factors like prior stroke/transient ischemic attack, hypertension, left ventricular dysfunction or postoperative AF that lasts for more than 48 hrs. Aspirin 325 mg daily or warfarin is the suitable agents with the monitoring of INR.

37.3.2.4 Right to Left Intra Cardiac Shunt

Some 1–2% patients with persistent patent foramen ovale can develop a right to left intracardiac shunt with persistent hypoxia during post operative period; if there is an associated decrease in RV compliance due to right lung intervention during the mass removal. Pulmonary thromboembolism (PTE), increased intrathoracic pressure, COPD and positive pressure ventilation may lead to shunt reversal. A bedside diagnosis can be made from a arterial blood gas analysis, echocardiographay or a combination of both. The patient can be managed by intravascular occlusion of the defect in the cardiac catheterization lab or a surgical closure.

37.3.2.5 Ventricular Dysfunction and Low Cardiac Output Syndrome (LSOS)

Ventricular dysfunction and low cardiac output syndrome (LSOS) may be evident in first 48 hr in case of prolong surgery, long CPB and manipulation of cardiac structures. Seriel hemodynamic monitoring in combination with echocardiography can give rise to a definite diagnosis. Raised CVP in the presence of hypotension with nonrespondent to volume therapy is an indirect indication of right ventricular (RV) dysfunction. A compromised cardiac output (CO) with gradual increase in lactate is the usual manifestation in LCOS. Volume therapy, maintainance of normal hematocrit are the initial step followed by supplementation of inotropes/vasopressors. An immediate decrease in HR or increase in venous oxygen saturation or blood pressure following volume administration indicate that preload reserve is present; whereas the lack of this response suggests that preload reserve is exhausted and the patient need an afterload reducing agent to improve CO. In brief dobutamine (5–10 μgm/kg/hr) and epinephrine (0.05–1 μgm/kg/hr) are commonly used agent to improve preload and decrease systemic afterload. Milrinone, dopamine or norepinephrine in combination with nitroglycerine or sodium nitroprusside can be tried to improve the condition. Severe vasomotor paresis may occur which is nonrespondent to routine inotropes and characterized by severe decreased in systemic vascular resistance and respond well to vasopressin. Mechanical circulatory support (ECMO) is considered in extreme cases [26].

37.3.2.6 Heart Failure

Though rare, may occur in patients with pre-existing ventricular dysfunction, COPD, PTE or cardiac herniation. The management is similar to that of any other heart failure case.

37.3.2.7 Pulmonary Edema

Lung damage during mass removal reduced lymphatic drainage 2^{nd}ry to extensive resection or accidental volume overload at any time post surgery and within 48 hr of pulmonary intervention are the contributory factors. Increase in peak airway pressure, acute respiratory insufficiency, pink forthy secretion in endotracheal tube, low PCWP and diffuse infiltrate in X-ray chest are the usual manifestations. The therapy includes restriction of fluid, administration of diuretics, bronchodilators, maintenance of adequate oxygenation and mechanical ventilation (in non-intubated patients) if necessary, high dose steroid and nutritional support. Extreme cases need inhaled nitric oxide and ECMO support.

37.3.2.8 Cardiac Tamponade

Cardiac tamponade though rare, is a possibility. Persistent hypotension and rising CVP with fluid therapy and muffled heart sound indicates it's presence. Echocardiography is diagnostic which shows impaired filling of RV because of increased pericardial pressure due to effusion. Treatment is urgent pericardiaocentesis followed by removal of fluid or blood by a median subxiphoid sternotomy or thoracotomy.

37.3.2.9 Chylothorax

Injury of thoracic duct may occur during the procedure giving rise to chylothorax and subsequent loss of calories, fluids, proteins, malnutrition and subsequent dehydration, immunologic dysfunction. Respiratory insufficiency may happen due to compressive effect. The management is mostly conservative and includes chest drain, replacement of nutrient loss by oral low fat medium chain triglycerides, use of somatostatin and octreotide to reduce flow of chyle in the thoracic duct and thereby providing time to heal. Total parenteral nutrition may further reduce the chyle flow. In uncontrolled cases, where more than 1.5 L/day in adult or 15 ml/kg / day in child for more than 2 weeks, thoracic duct ligation or embolization is done [27].

37.3.2.10 Thromboembolism

Thromboembolism, either deep vein thrombosis (DVT)/PTE is precipitated by a general postoperative hypercoagulable state or in presence of a malignant mass. Prevention of DVT includes LMWH, elastic stockings and early ambulation. If not contraindicated, heparin (5000 IU subcutaneously twice daily) can be started preoperatively and continued till discharge. If there are signs of DVT, treatment dose of heparin infusion is started after a Doppler confirmation and an IVC filter is put if necessary. Peumatic compression device is advocated in high riskpatients. Direct oral anticoagulants also have equal role in the management.

Subclinical PTE with a normal chest X-ray occurs in some high-risk patients. High index of suspicion, visualization of thrombus in echocardiography gives a clue to diagnosis in ventilated patients. Pulmonary angiography and CT angiogram are the most common diagnostic techniques. In established PTE severe RV dilation and strain pattern may be visible in Echocardiography. Systemic anticoagulation or thrombolytic administration are the initial step of management. Refractory cases are tackled with catheter embolectomy or surgical embolectomy [28].

37.3.3 Management of Bleeding and Coagulopathy

Chest tubes should be watched for drainage and air leak. Even in the presence of bubbling suction should not be applied if chest X-ray is normal. A balanced drainage system is applied in case of additional lobectomy or pneumonectomy [drainage system is filled with one cm of liquid] and the drains are removed within 24 hr. In case of intervention to heart or great vessels or in the presence of persistent minimal bubbling the drainage tubes to be kept for a longer time. In this case if the parenchyma is expanded without any suction a Heimlich valve container is attached for an early ambulation.

Bleeding and coagulopathy is mostly surgical. The main source of bleeding are: sternal wound, adhesions, peribronchial tissues, intercostal or other vessels e.g. SVC, aorta and pulmonaries, anastomotic sites and muscles. In some cases, bleeding is asymptomatic, slow and develops clotted hemothorax and empyema leading to respiratory compromise. Sometimes a patient bleed without any apparent cause e.g. surgical bleeding, medication and with a normal or near normal coagulation profile. These patients are treated symptomatically with replacement of blood, FFP, platelets or cryoprecipitate depending upon the coagulation profile until the bleeding stops. Patients with uncontrollable bleeding needs reoperations, which significantly increase the morbidity and mortality with septicemia, shock and prolong ventilation. Chest tube drainage of 1000 ml in one hr. or 200/hr. for 4 hrs. Warrants return to the operating room for surgical intervention to control the bleeding. A hemodynamically unstable patient with low hematocrit and radio-opaque surgical site implies blockade of chest tubes [29]. Medications like antiplatelet agents, aspirin in the post op period may also cause increase bleeding and corrected by FFP and vitamin K.

37.3.4 Nerve Injury

Phrenic nerve palsy in extubated patients manifested as shortness of breath and it became difficult to wean the intubated patient from ventilator. X-ray chest shows elevation of affected hemidiaphragm, which can further confirmed by fluoroscopy or ultrasound. Plication of hemidiaphragm improves the situation. Injury to recurrent laryngeal nerve 3.5(RLN) leads to ineffective cough and aspiration. This condition is diagnosed by laryngoscopy by observing the sluggish or absence motion of affected vocal cord. It is mostly temporary and pulmonary physiotherapy is advised to prevent aspiration. Medialisation laryngoplasty is done in extreme cases [30–32].

37.3.5 Pain Management

Acute pain following mediastinal surgery is multifactorial and usual contributory factors are: skin incision, damage to muscle group with extensive dissection, retraction of sternum or rib cage in thoracotomy, placement of chest drains, shoulder pain due to traction induced neural injury, sternal wire placement, acute intercostal neuritis, damage to costovertebral ligament, anxiety as well as the underlying neurohormonal changes due to the disease itself. The management is most often challenging and insufficient pain control increase the risk of post-operative adverse events like myocardial ischemia or infarction, arrhythmia, pulmonary dysfunction, poor sleep, slower rehabilitation, prolong wound healing, patient dissatisfaction, depression, increased morbidity, longer critical care unit stay and more cost involvement. Most desirable in these cases is an analgesic technique that has acceptable safety profile and produces adequate pain relief while promoting early mobilization. Patient education about few aspects of pain management (meaning of pain, risks of pain medications and how to overcome it) is important to overcome certain disbelief (addiction due to pain medication) about pain and thereby improve the quality of pain care. Preoperative detailed information and online instructional video regarding what they can expect from their surgical procedure and perioperative care support the pain management. Depending upon the site and extent of incision various ways adopted for pain management following MM removal and the main analgesic strategy by most of the practitioners is preemptive and multimodal [33, 34]. Table 37.2 describes pharmacokinetics and concern related to the commonly used analgesics and adjuvants.

Table 37.2 Commonly used analgesics for postoperative analgesia after mediastinal mass resection

Drugs	Onset of action	Elimination half life	Dose	Caution, Common SE
Non-opioids				
Paracetamol	O:30–35 min IV:8 min	1.9–2.5 hr	Same in all the routes. Adult: loading 2gm followed by 1 gm 4–6hrly.	4gm/day for 4 days with anticoagulant increase INR/ gastritis
Diclofenac sodium	Immediate	1.2–2 hr	O:50 mg 8hrly IV:37.5 mg 6hrly Maximum dose/ day: 150 mg	Allergy, acid-peptic disease, hypertension, cerebrovascular disease, peripheral vascular disease
Ibuprofen	1–2 hr	1.8–2 hr	O: Adult: 200 mg–400 mg, 4–6 hrly Children:20-40 mg/ kg/day	Hepato-renal toxicity, asthma
ketorolac	30 min	2.5 hr	O:20 mg STAT, then 10 mg q4–6 hrly, not to exceed 40 mg/day IM: 60 mg, single dose or 30 mg q 6 hr.; not to exceed 120 mg/day IV: 30 mg, single bolus or 30 mg q 6 hr.; not to exceed 120 mg/day	Renal impairment, >65 yr. old, duration of treatment should not be>5 days

Table 37.2 (continued)

Drugs	Onset of action	Elimination half life	Dose	Caution, Common SE
Opioids				
Morphine	5–10 minutes	3–4 hr	B:0.1–0.2 mg/kg I:0.05–0.1 mg/kg/hr. PCA:1–3 mg bolus, Lockout:5–15 min, 4 hr. limit 30–70 mg E: 5–20 mg 4 hrly	N, V, Accumulation in hepatic and renal impairment, histamine release, delirium, hypotension, giddiness
Fentanyl	1–2 min	3–4 hr	B:0.1–0.2 μg/kg I:0.05–0.1 μg/kg/hr. PCA:10–25 μgm bolus, lockout 5–10 min,4 hr. limit TDP:25–100 μgm/hr	Accumulation in hepatic impairment leading to respiratory depression
Alfentanyl	1–2 min	1–6 hr	B:10–30 μgm/kg I:20–60 μgm/kg/hr	N, V, agitation, confusion, respiratory depression
Remifentanyl	1–3 min	3–10 min	B:1 μ/kg I:20–60 μgm/kg/hr	Respiratory depression, bradycardia, hypotension, tolerance, pruritus
Codeine	30–45 min	4–6 hr	O:30–60 mg 4hrly	Respiratory depression
Tramadol	30–45 min	4–6 hr	IV bolus/E:50–100 mg 4–6 hrly	CI in severe respiratory depression, acute bronchial asthma, paralytic ileus, hypersensitivity, Use of MAO-I within 15 days
Oxycodone	Immediate release:10–30 min Sustained release:60 min	4–6 hr	SC:2.5 mg 4 hrly O:5–10 mg 4 hrly	Withdrawl on sudden stopping of the drug
Diamorphine	60 min	3–4 hr	IV bolus:0.05–1 mg/kg SC:5–10 mg 4 hrly O:5–10 mg 4 hrly	Confusion, drowsiness, N, V

(continued)

Table 37.2 (continued)

Drugs	Onset of action	Elimination half life	Dose	Caution, Common SE
Adjuvant drugs				
Ketamine	IV:30 sec	2.3–3.5 hr	B:0.25-1 mg/kg I:0.125–6.5 μgm/kg/min IT:67 mg/day in divided doses	Hallucination, agitation, anxiety, euphoria if continued beyond 48 hr. Caution in patients with IHD, increased intracranial and intraocular pressure
Clonidine	O:30–60 min IV:10 min	5–13 hr	B:2–5 μgm/kg I:0.3 μgm/kg/hr. O:50–100 μgm	Hypotension in high dose
Dexmedeto-midine	IV:3–5 min	Dose dependent, 60–120 min	B:1 gm/kg I:0.2–1 gm/kg/hr	Bradycardia, hypotension
Magnesium	IV:10 min	Varies with the dose	B:30 mg/kg I:10 mg/kg/hr	Delayed tendon refex, hypotension
Gabapentin	O:2 hr	4–7 hr	O:300–1200 mg 8 hrly	Drowsiness, blurred vision, N, V
Pregabalin	O:25 min–3 hr	Not known	O:50–100 mg 8 hrly	Same as gabapentin

O Oral, *IV* intravenous, *IM* intramuscular, *B* bolus, *I* infusion, *PCA* patient control analgesia, *TDP* transdermal patch, *CI* contraindication, *MAO-I* monoamino-oxidase inhibitor, *IT* intrathecal

37.3.5.1 Epidural and Spinal Analgesia

Medications are delivered into the epidural/subarachnoid space as single injection or continuously via indwelling catheter inserted into the space can block pain sensation locally and centrally, decrease or eliminate the need for systemic opioids. If the incision is transverse sterno-thoracotomy or posterolateral thoracotomy, the tip of the catheter should be at dermatome along which the incision to be made. In case of median sternotomy and muscle sparing incisions, catheter placement at T6 interspace is effective. Intraoperative use of epidural analgesia as an adjunct to general anaesthesia promote a smooth transition to immediate postoperative period. Initial doses with a combination of a local anesthetic (LA) and a relatively lipophilic opioid bolus or by continuous infusion is desirable. In patients with poor cardiac or pulmonary reserve judicious fluid and vasopressor administration avoids large fluid shift. Patient controlled epidural analgesia in the postoperative period should continue till the removal of drainage tubes. Typically, the epidural infusate combines a low concentration of long acting LA (0.5–1 mg/ml of bupivacaine or 1–2 mg/ml ropivacaine) and 5 μg/ml of fentanyl) or 5–20 μ gm/kg of morphine with or without

2 μg/ml of epinephrine [35]. One should not forget that epidural catheters placed several dermatomes from the surgical site require large volume of analgesics.

Several other drugs e.g. ketamine, clonidine, dextromethorphan and neostigmine can be used as an adjunct. A continuous infusion of 4–6 ml/hr. with demand bolus of 2–4 ml in every 10–15 minutes can provide optimal analgesia. Patients with refractory pain should be given intravenous non-steroidal anti-inflammatory drugs (NSAIDS) as an adjuvant. During transition to oral opioid, the first dose should be given immediately after discontinuation of patient controlled epidural [PCEA] but the epidural catheter is still in situ. Prompt identification and removal of dysfunctional epidural catheter as well as rapid initiation of another alternative prevent severe pain. Identifying that motor blockade should not occur with dilute local anaesthetic solutions, and postoperative motor weakness should warn immediate imaging studies and neurosurgical consultation best prevents the most catastrophic complication of epidural placement e.g. epidural hematoma.

Continuous fentanyl infusion PCEA or both provide excellent analgesia and overcome the limitations to the duration of associated with epidural bolus. Though analgesia is excellent, pain score increases with coughing and movement unlike morphine and these patients need adjuvant analgesics. The most common side effect of epidural fentanyl is pruritus whch can respond well to naloxone. Prolong infusion or simultaneous addition of sedative or opioids via other route may give rise to respiratory depression.

The main concern of EA opioids is that it can reduce coughing especially in patients with low FEV1 and it is not applied if there is local or systemic sepsis. Spinal/epidural hematoma is a concern in the patients if CPB required for tumor resection. Hign spinal anaesthesia (block till the level of T1) before anaesthetic induction can also reduce post sternotomy pain to a greater extent [36].

37.3.5.2 Paravertebral Blocks

Paravertebral blocks as a single injection of continuously via a catheter is more suitable in patients in whom coagulopathy is a concern. Plane LAs solution (e.g. bupivacaine 0.25–0.5 5) or equivalent are generally used at a rate of 10–15 ml/hr. [37]

37.3.5.3 Intercostal Nerve Blocks (ICNB)

Intercostal nerve blocks (ICNB) are quick and simple, have the advantage of localized analgesia without any sympathetic blockade. Can be given by the surgeon under direct visualization or percutaneously by the anaesthesiologist as single injections at least two dermatomes above and below the incision. Liposomal bupivacaine is used by many, have an extended duration of action up to 72 hrs. Inadequate posterior analgesia may happen and large amount of LA are needed if multiple injections are performed. It is important to calculate the total dose of LAs because ICNB are notable for high systemic blood levels and toxicity, mainly neurologic and cardiovascular. Apart from this, block failure, pneumothorax and significant bleeding from trauma to intercostal artery may happen [38].

37.3.5.4 Intrapleural Analgesia

0.25–0.5%bupivacaine is injected between the visceral and parietal pleura either as a single bolus /as an infusion via an indwelling catheter. The main concern of this technique is that LAs tends to pool in the dependent areas and lost through chest drains, thus limiting effectiveness.

37.3.5.5 Interscalene Block

This mainly covers the referred shoulder pain related to chest tube placement after thoracotomy, involving irritation of diaphragm. This pain involves phrenic nerve distribution and is not covered by an appropriately placed working thoracic epidural catheter also. Dilute Ropivacaine (0.1–0.2%) is efficacious without producing any motor block [39].

37.3.5.6 Erector Spine Block

Done under ultrasound guidance by injecting LA as bolus or continuous infusion deep into erector spine fascia and superficial to the transverse process under ultrasound guidance. There is spread of LA from C7 to T10 unilaterally. Lack of significant sympathetic blockade, risk of epidural related hematoma in patients with or without anticoagulant, and providing the analgesic cover of the entire chest wall making this technique more popular [40].

37.3.5.7 Serratus Anterior Plane Block and Pectoralis Block

Ultrasound guided injection of LA deep to the serratus anterior muscle, in the region of midaxillary line at the T4–T5 level provide pain relief in the distribution of cutaneous branch of intercostal nerves from T2 to T9. It decreases pain both after median sternotomy and thoracotomy with better hemodynamic stability compared to TEA and reduce opioid use [41].

37.3.5.8 Cryoanalgesia

Destruction of individual intercostal nerve by cryoprobe (−20 °C) during surgery provides postoperative analgesia which can last for 6 months. However, because of long-term neuralgia and paresthesia, this technique is rarely used [42].

37.3.5.9 Transcutaneous Electrical Nerve Stimulation (TENS)

Transcutaneous electrical nerve stimulation (TENS): may be useful in mild to moderate pain but is ineffective when pain is severe.

37.3.5.10 Systemic Analgesia

The use of multimodal regimen is important to decrease the deleterious effects of any one of the analgesics because of the variable sedative and respiratory depressant effect of different analgesics. Regimens that are commonly used include opioids, NSAIDs, tramadol, ketorolac and paracetamol [34].

Opioids, though have a narrows therapeutic window are usually the initial analgesic therapy following mediastinal surgery. Administration of opioids with or without PCA needs to be limited in opioid-naïve patients because of the increased risk of side effects [Table 37.2]. Respiratory depression is a potential concern; and at the same time one should appreciate that some patients hypoventilate because of inadequate analgesia. Morphine, fentanyl, hydromorphone, sufentanyl and remifentanyl are the various opioids used for patient controlled analgesia (PCA). Whether one is better than other is still a question. Morphine and fentanyl are the most common one used during patients hospital stay. For morphine, the recommended dose is 30–40 mg intravenously (IV)/90–120 mg per orally (O) over 24 hrs and that of fentanyl for an adult weighing >50 kg to provide tolerable postoperative pain score of less than 3. Intramuscular (IM) morphine 0.2 to 0.3 mg/kg; gabapentin 300 mg or tramadol sustained release 300 mg PO 45 minutes before anaesthesia induction is in practice by several authors to produce pre-emptive analgesia. Fentanyl repeated single bolus 10–15 μgm maximum up to 5 μgm/kg/day or infusion 0.5–2.5 μgm/kg/hr. when patient is intubated. In the post extubation period 0.1–0.5 μg/kg/hr. can be given [43]. Hydromorphone, a direct derivative of morphine, with a similar onset and duration of action like morphine can be given at a dose of 1–2 mg orally every 6 hrly. Though there are few reports, some authors demonstrated that both remifentanyl and sufentanyl PCA can produce acceptable analgesia during post sternotomy period [44, 45]. There is limited data on transmucosal (buccal) or transdermal fentanyl for postoperative pain relief in MM surgery patients.

Tramadol at a dose of 50–100 mg IV/PO every 6hrly as needed, has an improved side effect profile and equivalent analgesia as thoracic epidural morphine. The sustained released release tablets can be given 100 mg PO once daily, increased by 100 mg/day every 5 days, with a maximum dose up to 400 mg/day [46].

37.3.5.11 Non-opioid Analgesia

IV ketorolac and acetaminophen are two popular analgesics those can be used during first 24 hr. postoperatively to reduce opioid consumption and improve patient satisfaction. Acetaminophen at a dose of 1 gm every 6 hrly is acceptable for adults; have a concern of liver toxicity.

Naproxen is used by some practitioners in the absence of specific contraindications. Parenteral or oral oxycodone and paracetmol with codeine also used for treating post sternotomy pain. Use of magnesium sulphate limits postoperative pain and the dose of PCA morphine requested. Preoperative administration of 600 mg gabapentin reduces postoperative opioid consumption. This is used in elderly with caution because of it's possible side effect like sedation, dizziness and visual disturbances. Carbamazepine (200 mg orally) or along with amitriptyline (10 mg) can be given as an adjunct to overcome the psychological aspect of pain [47]. Figure 37.1 depicts the overview of pain management following MM surgery.

Usual pain management strategies for mediastinal mass surgery across the globe is: preoperative oral gabapentin, 600 mg or morphine 0.2–0.3 mg/kg im, intraoperatively: a regional technique along with morpine/fentanyl infusion till extubation followed by postoperatively: tramadol or paracetamol+codeine or morphine/fentanyl infusion till extubation and subsequently PCA.

If high intensity pain persists after 2–3 days the following protocol may be adopted depending upon the visual analogue score (VAS) for pain assessment.

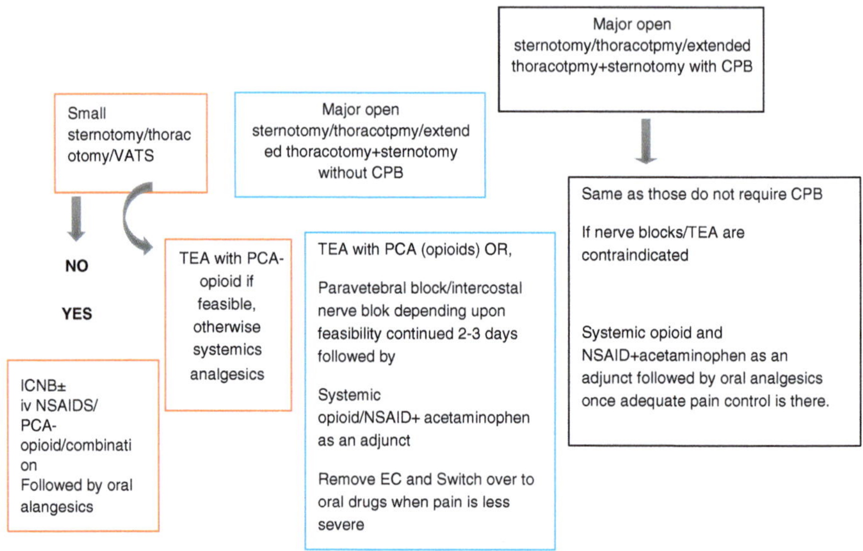

Fig. 37.1 Overview of pain management after mediastinal surgery

1. VAS > 50 mm: IV PCA with morphine/fentanyl+COX-2NSAID + paracetamol
2. VAS:>30 mm < 50 mm: paracetamol+ COX-2 NSAID+ tramadol
3. VAS:< 30 mm: IV paracetamol+ COX-2 NSAID

37.3.6 Acute Kidney Injury

Remains as a common complication during postoperative period especially in patients who need prolong CPB for mass resection, massive blood loss perioperatively, pre-existing renal dysfunction, diabetes mellitus, female gender, old age, or have chemotherapy induced complications (tumor lysis syndrome), chronic exposure to nephrotoxic agents are more prone. Renal replacement therapy benefits these patientsgreately. However, one should balance the benefits of RRT with the overall prognosis of the patient [48, 49].

37.3.7 Specific Post Operative Problems

37.3.7.1 Management of Immediate Complications After Tracheal Reconstruction

The invasive MM who require tracheal reconstruction and anastomosis in the same setting may develop anastomotic separation, glottis edema, recurrent laryngeal nerve injury, swallowing dysfunction, formation of trachea-innominate or tracheo-esophageal fistula during the immediate postoperative period. Tracheostomy before tracheal reconstruction increases the risk of postoperative anastomotic leak.

Granulation tissue around anastomotic site can lead to some grade of airway obstruction. Patient may develop some grade of stridor and relieved with debridement of granulation tissue with the help of rigid bronchoscopy and local injection of triamcinolone.

Anastomotic separation, a devastating complication, occurs within days to first two weeks of surgery [50]. Patient develop sudden stridor, cough, increased secretion, wound infection or subcutaneous emphysema. There may be sudden loss of airway which is highly fatal. Urgent stabilization of airway is important in these patients. As orotracheal intubation is difficult due to presence of laryngeal edema, bedside distal airway cannulation from the anastomotic site is a wise decision to save the patient. In case of stable patient, CT neck and chest can give a clue to diagnosis. In case of suspected separation, patient must be taken to the operating room immediately to establish the airway. In larger separation (>1 cm), neck is explored and management to be done with an airway appliance. A T-tube can be placed if upper airway is patent and in case of significant laryngeal edema a tracheostomy should be placed through the defect a repair is done once edema get subsided. Antibiotic therapy, voice rest, neck flexion and hyperbaric oxygen are used to promote early healing.

Tracheo-innominate fistulas are extremely rare during critical care unit stay and invariably carry a poor prognosis. Infection and inflammation causing anterior separation and erosion to the innominate artery is the cause. The typical manifestation is massive hemoptysis and severe cardiorespiratory compromise leading to death. Sentinel bleed may be an early sign in case of small tear. Emergent cough inflation or placement of a cuffed endotracheal tube can seal the bleeding site temporarily before shifting the patient to the operating room [51].

Glottic edema is common in case of extensive resection or manipulation of larynx. These patients are managed with steroid, diuretics, head elevation, voice rest and nebulized epinephrine. Tracheostomy is considered in case of persistent edema.

Transient recurrent laryngeal nerve palsy can occur in CRCU secondary to inflammation or traction. A weak cough indicates a diagnosis. Bedside laryngoscopy can visualize the vocal cord movement to make a diagnosis. Most of the cases improves over time. In extreme cases with bilateral RLNP palsy, tracheostomy is needed.

Swallowing dysfunction is common in the immediate postoperative period. The patient needs to kept nil per orally to avoid catastrophic aspiration. Improvement occurs in most of the cases over time. Consultation with a speech therapist is essential before allowing per orally.

37.3.7.2 Uncommon Masses

Almost 40% of patients with thymic mass have myasthenia gravis and need elective postoperative mechanical ventilation. Thymic carcinoids are another set of lesions usually associated with endocrine abnormalities, most commonly Cushing's syndrome or multiple endocrine neoplasia and are usually huge and calcified leading to difficult excision and chance of massive postoperative bleeding; thus, need additional care.

The patients who received bleomycin or radiotherapy preoperatively need to be taken seriously for preexisting pulmonary artery injury or adhesion of mediastinal structures' is important to keep the inspired concentration of oxygen as low as possible but compactable with best possible arterial oxygen saturation to prevent further pulmonary injury.

37.3.8 Fluid and Electrolytes

Post mediastinal surgery, intravenous fluids are given in reduced amount to prevent overhydration problem. Oral feeding is encouraged as soon as possible. The usual dose of maintenance fluid is 1–2 ml/kg/hr. to avoid a positive fluid balance of >1.5 L and to attenuate the risk of multifactorial postoperative acute lung injury. At the same time one should not forget about silent hypovolemia, acute kidney injury as well as impaired oxygen delivery. Inspite of adequate fluid therapy and in the absence of bleeding if there is sign of hypoperfusion inotrope/vasopressor support should be considered.

37.3.9 Nutrition

After major resection, metabolic alterations leads elevated energy expenditure, lean tissue catabolism, decrease synthesis of serum albumin and transferrin as well as fluid shift to the extracellular compartment.

Subsequently there is decrease in respiratory muscle strength poor wound healing, impaired immunity, increased risk of nosocomial infection and organ dysfunction. Patients, who are on mechanical ventilation, develop a decline in respiratory muscle strength after a few days of suboptimal nutrition. Indirect calorimetry is one of the best predictive model and considered to be the gold standard for measuring resting metabolic rate (RMR) and resting energy expenditure (REE) in these population.

It is important to remember that over feeding can increase in oxygen consumption and carbon dioxide production, which also have a deleterious consequence [52]. Nutritional management of a patient with a malignant mass are trickier because the metabolic demand of the patient is affected by the extensiveness of the mass, it's cell type, prior or ongoing radiotherapy and chemotherapy.

37.3.10 Infection and Antimicrobial Therapy

Benign and small masses are need routine antibiotic prophylaxis for 48 or 72 hrs. Depending upon the institutional protocols. However, those need extensive surgery or have huge malignant masses, prior chemo or radiotherapy, malnutrition, are prone for impaired neutrophil function-cell, T-cell or NK-cell defects and subsequent infection. Ventilator associated pneumonia, delayed wound healing and sepsis are not uncommon in these patients [53]. Patient receiving chemotherapy during perioperative period are more benefited with fluroquinolone prophylaxis which significantly lower the incidence of gram negative infection by 80% according to many authors. However, quinolones do not alter the incidence of gram positive bacterial and fungal infection [54].

One should not forget the hypersensitivity reaction, prolong Q-T interval, peripheral neuropathy and seizures associated with fluroquinolone use. Antibacterial and antifungal prophylaxis hardly have any role in these patients.

The ideal treatment for different infections that post MM resection patients encounter, should always be optimized with respect to the pharmacokinetics and pharmacodynamics of antimicrobials considered for therapy. One should not forget that immune compromised patients need more aggressive therapy and in that case side effects and toxicities of all agents need to be weighed against efficacy and safety.

37.3.11 Anticoagulation Prophylaxis and Therapeutics

Extensive malignant masses are at risk of postoperative thromboembolism which mostly occur during the initial six months of therapy. Apart from mechanical prophylaxis, unfractionated heparin at a dose of 5000 units can be given 8 hrly postoperatively for a minimum period of 7–10 days if no prosthetic agents are used. Alternatively, they can receive enoxaparin 20 mg subcutaneously every 2–4 hr. preoperatively and 40 gm daily thereafter; or fondaparinux 2.5 gm subcutaneously daily beginning 6–8 hr. postoperatively. Dose adjustment based on APTT is also recommended [55].

37.3.12 Postoperative Physiotherapy

Chest physiotherapy, coughing exercises, incentive spirometry and bronchodilators and endotracheal toilet improve postoperative pulmonary insufficiency. Patients with extensive resection and low FEV1 may need tracheostomy for prolong support of ventilation and clearing of secretion. Prevention of aspiration is important as it may result in multiorgan dysfunction and sepsis. If the patient has a tendency to aspirate, he should be kept nil or oral and nasogastric feeding initiated as required. Eating should only be allowed when he is fully alert and sitting up. Diuretics may need at times to reduce body fluid, lead to early mobilization and reduces complications like pulmonary atelectasis and DVT. If there is damage to the vocal cords then a speech pathology is sought for.

37.3.13 Miscellaneous Care

The CRCU team should be aware of a brief detailing regarding different drug therapies the patient undergoing, drug-drug interactions, adverse drug events and their management. The patients who are on mechanical ventilation for more than 48 hrs., associated coagulopathy and multiorgan failure are prone for stress ulcer and gastrointestinal bleeding. Histamine-2 receptor antagonist and proton pump inhibitors are commonly prescribed drugs for prophylaxis. One has to aware of the fact that these drugs are also associated with clostridium difficile infection as well as pneumonia.

37.4 Conclusion

Patients with extensive surgery may suffer from sudden cardiovascular collapse in the CRCU due to several reasons. Implementation of early warning symptoms can lead to early identification to facilitate timely intervention and appropriate level of care. Intermittent quality assurance and improvement as well as safety initiatives can improve the outcome of these patients.

References

1. Béchard P, Létourneau L, Lacasse Y, et al. Perioperative cardiorespiratory complications in adults with mediastinal mass: incidence and risk factors. Anesthesiology. 2004;100:826–34.
2. Levin H, Bursztein S, Heifetz M. Cardiac arrest in a child with an anterior mediastinal mass. Anesth Analg. 1985;64:1129–30.
3. Northrip DR, Bohman BK, Tsueda K. Total airway occlusion and superior vena cava syndrome in a child with an anterior mediastinal tumor. Anesth Analg. 1986;65:1079–82.
4. Goh MH, Liu XY, Goh YS. Anterior mediastinal masses: an anaesthetic challenge. Anaesthesia. 1999;54:670–4.
5. Strollo DC, Rosado de Christenson ML, Jett JR. Primary mediastinal tumors. Part 1: tumors of the anterior mediastinum. Chest. 1997;112:511–22.
6. Aigner C, Hoda MA, Klepetko W. Combined cervicothoracic approaches for complex mediastinal mass. Thorac Surg Clin. 2009;19:107–12.
7. Okereke IC, Kesler KA, Rieger KM, Birdas TJ, Mi D, Turrentine MW, Brown JW. Reasults of superior vena cava reconstruction with externally stented polytetrayluroethylene vascular prosthesis. Ann Thorac Surg. 2010;90:283–7.
8. Brasher PA, McClelland KH, Denehy L, Story I. Does removal of deep breathing exercises-from a physiotherapy program including pre-operative education and earlymobilization after cardiac surgery alter patient outcomes? Aust J Physiother. 2003;49:165–73.
9. Vaporciym AA, Rice D, Correa AM, Walsh G, Putnam JB, Swisher S, Smythe R, Roth J. Resection of advanced thoracic malignancies requiring cardiopulmonary bypass. Eur J Cardio Thorac Surg. 2002;22:47–52.
10. Sun L, Joshi M, Khan SN, Ashrafian H, Darzi A. Clinical impact of multiparameter continues non invasive monitoring in hospital wards: a systemic review and metaanalysis. J R Soc Med. 2020;113:217–24.
11. Blackwell JN, Keim-Malpass J, Clark MT, Kowalski RL, Najjar SN, Bourque JM, Lake DE, Moorman JR. Early detection of In-Patient deterioration: one prediction model does not fit at all. Crit Care Explor. 2020;11:e011.
12. Erdos G, Tzanova I. Perioperative anaesthetic management of mediastinal mass in adults. Eur J Anaesthesiol. 2009;26:627–32.
13. Chowdhury MM, Dagash H, Pierro A. A systemic review of the impact of volume of surgery and specialization on patient's outcome. Br J Surg. 2007;94:145–61.

14. Licker M, Fauconnet P, Villiger Y, et al. Acute lung injury and outcomes after thoracic surgery. Curr Opin Anaesthesiol. 2009;22:61–7.
15. Raiten JM, Blank RS. Anesthetic management of post thoracotomy complications. In: Slinger P, editor. Principles and practice of anesthesia for thoracic surgery. New York: Springer; 2011. p. 603.
16. Batuwitage B, Charters P. Postoperative management of difficult airway. BJA. 2017;17:235–41.
17. Zhengcheng L, Yang R, Shao F, Pan Y. Controlled tracheal suspension for tracheomalcia after resection of large anterior mediastinal mass. Ann Thorac Surg. 2015;99:2225–7.
18. Lawrence VA, Cornell JE, Smetana GW, American College of Physicians. Strategies to reduce postoperative pulmonary complications after noncardiothoracic surgery: systematic review for the American College of Physicians. Ann Intern Med. 2006;144:596–608.
19. Fisher BW, Majumdar SR, McAlister FA. Predicting pulmonary complications after nonthoracic surgery: a systematic review of blinded studies. Am J Med. 2002;112:219–25.
20. Hota P, Dass C, Erkmen C, Donuru A, Kumaran M. Post sternotomy complications: a multimodal review of normal and abnormal postoperative imaging findings. Am J Roentgenology. 2018;211:1194–205.
21. Mueller MR, Marzluf BA. The anticipation and management of air leaks and residual spaces post lung resection. J Thorac Dis. 2014;6:271–84.
22. London MJ. What is the best method for diagnosing perioperative myocardial infarction? In: Evidence based practice of anesthesiology. Ed: Fleisher LA. Saunders 2004;344–349.
23. Al-Hawwas M, Tsitlakidou D, Gupta N, Iliescu C, Cilingiroglu M, Marmagkiolis K. Acute coronary syndrome management in cancer patients. Curr Oncol Rep. 2018;20:78.
24. Lanuti M, De Delva PE, Gaissert HA, Wright CD, Wain JC, Allan JS, et al. Review of superior vena cava resection in the management of benign disease and pulmonary or mediastinal malignancies. Ann Thorac Surg. 2009;88:392–7.
25. Schummer W. Cardiac herniation with torsion after right pneumonectomy. Ind J Crit Care Med. 2017;21:473–4.
26. Masse L, Antonacci M. Low cardiac output syndrome: identification and management. Crit Care Nurs Clin North Am. 2005;17:375–83.
27. Emmet EM, Zoe B, Paul BA. Chylothorax: aetiology, diagnosis and therapeutic options. Respir Med. 2010;104:1–8.
28. Brunelli A. Deep vein thrombosis/pulmonary embolism: prophylaxis, diagnosis, and management. Thorac Surg Clin. 2012;22:25–8.
29. Litle VR, Swanson SJ. Postoperative bleeding: coagulopathy, bleeding, hemothorax. Thorac Surg Clin. 2006;16:203–7.
30. Raiten JM, Blank RS. Anesthetic management of post thoracotomy complications. In: Slinger P, editor. Principles and practice of anesthesia for thoracic surgery. New York: Springer; 2011. p. 603.
31. Ramachandran SK, Nafiu OO, Ghaferi A, Tremper KK, Shanks A, Kheterpal S. Independent predictors and outcomes of unanticipated early postoperative tracheal intubation after nonemergent, noncardiac surgery. Anesthesiology. 2011;115:44–53.
32. Rebuck JA, Rasmussen JR, Olsen KM. Clinical aspiration-related practice patterns in the intensive care unit: a physician survey. Crit Care Med. 2001;29:2239–44.
33. Sentürk M, Özca PE, Talu GK, Kiyan E, Camci E, Özyalçin S, Dilege S, Pembeci K. The effects of three different analgesia techniques on long-term postthoracotomy pain. Anesth Analg. 2002;94:11–5.
34. Rizzi A, Raveglia F, Scarci M, Cioffi U, Baisi A. The best to control pain after thoracic surgery: multimodal strategy again pain. Video-assist Thorac Surg. 2019;4:26–8.
35. Tan CN, Guha A, Scawn ND, Pennefather SH, Russell GN. Optimal concentration of epidural fentanyl and bupivacaine 0.1% after thoracotomy. Br J Anaesth. 2004;92:670–4.
36. Lee TW, Kowalski S, Falk K, Maguire D, Freed DH, Hay Glass GT. High spinal anesthesia enhances anti-inflammatory responses in patients undergoing coronary artery bypass surgery and aortic valve replacement replacement. Randomized Pilot Study. PLoS One. 2016;11:e0149942.

37. Yeung JH, Gates S, Naidu BV, Wilson MJ, Smith FG. Paravertebral block versus thoracic epidural for patients undergoing thoracotomy. Cochrane Database Syst Rev. 2016.
38. Khalil KG, Boutrous ML, Irani AD, et al. Operative intercostal nerve blocks with long-acting bupivacaine liposome for pain control after thoracotomy. Ann Thorac Surg. 2015;100:2013–8.
39. Singh P, Borle A, Kaur M, Trikha A, Sinha A. Opioid-sparing effects of the thoracic interfascial plane blocks: a meta-analysis of randomized controlled trials. Saudi J Anaesth. 2018;12(1):103.
40. Thiruvenkatarajan V, Adhikary S, Pruett A, Forero M. Erector spinae plane block as an alternative to epidural analgesia for post-operative analgesia following video-assisted thoracoscopic surgery: a case study and a literature review on the spread of local anaesthetic in the erector spinae plane. Indian J Anaesth. 2018;62:75.
41. Ökmen K, Ökmen BM. The efficacy of serratus anterior plane block in analgesia for thoracotomy: a retrospective study. J Anesth. 2017;31:579–85.
42. Yang MK, Cho CH, Kim YC. The effects cryoanalgesia combined with thoracic epidural analgesia in patients undergoing thoracotomy. Anaesthesia. 2004;59:1073–7.
43. Pang PWH, Sandler AN. A review of the use of fentanyl analgesia in the management of acute pain in adult. Anesthesiology. 1999;90:576–99.
44. Bjarnnes AK, Rusteen T, Lie I, Watt-Watson J, Leegard M. Pain characteristics and analgesic intake before and following cardiac surgery. Eur J Cardiovasc Nurs. 2016;15:47–51.
45. Hughes R, Gao F. Pain control for thoracotomy. Contin Educ Anaesth Crit Care Pain. 2005;5:56–60.
46. Bloch MB, Dyer RA, Heijke SA, James MF. Tramadol infusion for postthoracotomy pain relief: a placebo-controlled comparison with epidural morphine. Anesth Analg. 2002;94:523–8.
47. Vilte B, Strike E, Rutka K, Leibuss R. Pain management in intensive care unit patients after cardiac surgery with sternotomy approach. Acta Medica lituanica. 2019;26:51–63.
48. Kemlin D, Biard L, Kerhuel L, et al. Acute kidney injury in critically ill patients with solid tumours. Nephrol Dial Transplant. 2018;33:1997–2005.
49. Uchino S, Bellomo R, Kellum JA, et al. Patient and kidney survival by dialysis modality in critically ill patients with acute kidney injury. Int J Artif Organs. 2007;30:281–92.
50. Stock C, Gukasyan N, Muniappan A, et al. Hyperbaric oxygen therapy for the treatment of anastomotic complications after tracheal resection and reconstruction. J Thorac Cardiovasc Surg. 2014;147:1030–5.
51. Allan JS, Wright CD. Tracheoinnominate fistula: diagnosis and management. Chest Surg Clin N Am. 2003;13:331–41.
52. Mc Clave SA, Lowen CC, Kleber MJ, Nicholson JF, Jimmerson SC, McConnel JW, et al. Are patients fed appropriately according to their caloric requirement? JPEN J Parenteral Enteral Nutr. 1998;22:375–61.
53. Preventing infection in cancer patients. Centers for diseasecontrol. Nov19, 2015. http://www.cdc.gov/cancer/dcpc/resources/features/prevention
54. Gupta-Gvili A, Fraser A, Paul M, et al. Antibiotic prophylaxis for bacterial infection in afebrile neutropenic patients following chemotherapy. Cochrane Database Syst Rev. 2012;1:CD004386.
55. Wetson H, Kecling D, Laffan M, Tait R, Makris M. Guideline on the aspects of cancer related venous thromboembolism. Br J Hematol. 2015;170:540–648.

Critical Care of Hepatopancreatobiliary Surgery Patient

38

Sachidanand Jee Bharati, Wasimul Hoda,
and Brajesh Kumar Ratre

38.1 Introduction

Hepatopancreatobiliary cancers such as hepatocellular carcinoma (HCC), pancreatic and biliary tract carcinomas (i.e., cholangiocarcinoma and gallbladder carcinoma) are common gastrointestinal tumors. In most of the cases, the primary mode of treatment is surgical resection. The perioperative management in such cases are associated with clinical and surgical challenges. Patients may require post-operative intensive care unit (ICU) admission in case of extensive surgeries or if a complication occurs during the intraoperative period. Major hepatic resections are extensive and may need admission to the critical care unit in the immediate post-operative period. Therefore, multidisciplinary teamwork is essential to provide the best outcome for such patients.

38.2 Etiology

38.2.1 Hepatic Resection

The liver is a vascular organ. In order to prevent excessive blood loss during surgical resection of the liver, selective or total inflow occlusion (Pringle maneuver) or total vascular isolation of liver is done [1]. After resection, liver function is altered as a result of prolonged clamping, reduction in functional liver mass and potential ischemia/reperfusion injury to the remaining liver.

S. J. Bharati (✉) · B. K. Ratre
Department of Onco-Anaesthesia & Palliative Medicine, DR BRAIRCH, AIIMS, New Delhi, India

W. Hoda
Department of Anaesthesiology, Rajendra Institute of Medical Sciences, Ranchi, Jharkhand, India

V. Kumar et al. (eds.), *Onco-critical Care*,
https://doi.org/10.1007/978-981-16-9929-0_38

Common liver resections performed that may require ICU admission after surgery are left or right hepatectomies (~50% of liver volume is removed) or extensive right or left trisectionectomy (up to 80% of the liver is removed). Reduction of functional liver volume below 25% in normal livers or less than 40% in cirrhotic or with bile duct obstruction has been related to an increased risk of both liver failure and mortality [2].

Preoperative chemotherapy, preexisting cirrhosis, bile duct obstruction and intraoperative maintenance of low central venous pressure (less than 5 mmHg) with hemodynamic instability exaggerate the amount of postoperative hepatic injury [3]. These clearly indicate the need for ICU admission and close observation in the postoperative period. Therefore, details of preoperative dysfunction, intraoperative events such as bleeding, clamp time, intraoperative hemodynamic instability, transfusions are to be shared in details with physicians looking after the patient in ICU.

38.2.2 Pancreatic and Bile Duct Surgery

Usually, patients undergoing pancreatobiliary surgeries do not require ICU admission due to less hemodynamic instability and alteration in physiology. However, in prolonged surgeries such as Whipple procedure (pancreaticoduodenectomy) and surgery related to pancreatic head tumor or bile duct involving portal vein or extensive fibrotic resection may result in immediate ICU admission. They are closely observed in ICU for hemodynamic instability, leak at anastomotic site, formation of fistula, and collections in abdomen. Preexisting medical comorbidities, geriatric patients, intraoperative portal vein injury or repair associated with massive transfusions, hypotension and pancreatic or bile leaks are the other common indications for ICU admission.

38.3 Early Post-operative Treatment

The initial few days after major hepatopancreatobiliary surgery is crucial and needs a multidisciplinary approach. The postoperative outcome depends upon close cooperation between the anesthesiologist and the surgeon. Elderly patients with compensated liver cirrhosis and eventful intraoperative period increases the perioperative risk as compared to patients with preoperative normal liver function and child A classification. However, most of the patients undergoing major hepatectomy are monitored in ICU for initial 24 h before shifting to the ward [4]. ICU care does not vary from standard intensive care and it includes invasive monitoring of hemodynamics, mechanical ventilation, antiseptic precautions, glycemic control, and nutritional support [4].

As the patient is shifted to ICU, an initial assessment of vitals is done. Monitoring of vital parameters like pulse, blood pressure (BP), respiratory rate (RR), electrocardiogram (ECG), oxygen saturation (SPo2), and urine output are done. Samples for electrolytes, blood sugar, liver function, renal function, and coagulation profile are sent and monitored. Other important postoperative care includes fluid management, monitoring of urine and drain output, care of surgical wound, optimal analgesia, evaluation of cardiac & neurological functions, initiation of good nutritional support, and care for bowel movement.

38.3.1 Fluid and Electrolyte Management

After major hepatobiliary surgery, postoperative fluid management is of prime importance. In major hepatic resections, the postoperative fluid shifts may pose a challenge in the early postoperative period. Optimal perioperative fluid management is essential to reduce postoperative morbidity and mortality. In the postoperative period, replacement and maintenance of fluids are done with crystalloids such as 0.9% of normal saline (NS) and ringer lactate (RL). Colloids are used as plasma expanders and are not be used in case of shock.

Low central venous pressure (low-CVP) is considered to be the standard fluid therapy in major hepatic surgery. It helps in minimizing intraoperative blood loss. Therefore, in the postoperative period, the patients may have features of hypovolemia with oliguria and hypotension. It needs gentle volume re-expansion where albumin and fresh frozen plasma are helpful. Aggressive resuscitation may lead to hypoalbuminemia, pulmonary edema, and ascites. Goal directed fluid therapy (GDFT) when compared to low CVP in major open liver resections, do not show any difference in terms of intraoperative bleeding, morbidity or quality of surgical field [5].

Patients with preoperative cirrhosis are at greater risk of fluid shifts, vasodilation, and hypotension. In such cases, colloids are preferred in place of crystalloids. In the first 48 h, 50% of patients develop significant but self-limiting ascites. Sodium restriction, diuretics, and paracentesis are helpful in such cases [6].

Hyponatremia, hyperlactemia, hypophosphatemia, and potassium deranged levels are common after liver resection surgery. Hyponatremia is common in patients above class Child A. It is frequently seen with ascites and cirrhosis. Asymptomatic are managed with normal saline and serial monitoring of sodium level. Rapid correction is avoided and gradual correction of sodium deficit is done [7]. Estimation of serial lactate levels are important in the management of the early post hepatic resection period. Increased levels may indicate hypovolemia, if not corrected affects tissue perfusion, cardiac output and can lead to further liver dysfunction [8]. Lactate-containing fluids are to be avoided [9]. As there is increased uptake of phosphate by regenerating hepatic cells, Hypophosphatemia is a common presentation in all the patients undergoing major liver resections [10]. Therefore, the standard protocol involves replenishment of phosphate with maintenance fluids in the early post-operative period. There may be a transient and initial rise in serum transaminase and alkaline phosphatase levels due to hepatocellular damage [11]. A persisting raised levels indicate ongoing hepatic ischemia and reasons are to be explored and corrected. Prevention of hypothermia, careful examination of color & content of drains, and administration of antibiotics according to the institutional protocol are other important aspects in the management of early postoperative period.

38.3.2 Glycemic Control

Glucose metabolism is altered as there is a reduction in functional liver mass and liver dysfunction due to ischemia-reperfusion injury. The resulting altered hepatic physiology may lead to hypoglycemia. As glycogen storage is depleted, glucose is produced by the process of gluconeogenesis. Therefore, a tight glycemic control is needed in order to prevent hypoglycemia. Strict control of blood sugar in ICU is associated with less morbidity and mortality [12]. Maintenance of normoglycemia helps in reduction of infection after major liver resection. According to institutional protocol, insulin is given to maintain the blood sugar level between 90 and 120 mg/dl. Hypoglycemia is not uncommon after insulin therapy. At times, compromised hepatic mobilization of glucose in major liver resections may also warrant intravenous glucose administration [13].

38.3.3 Correction of Coagulopathy

Coagulopathy is common in early second to fifth postoperative period. It is due to the decreased synthesis by the remnant liver and increased consumption of coagulation factors. The common derangements seen are increased prothrombin time/ international ratio (PT/INR), partial thromboplastin time (PTT), and decreased platelets and fibrinogen [14, 15]. The initial coagulation derangements are self-limiting with no need for fresh frozen plasma (FFP) in non-cirrhotic patients. However, due to reduced hepatic protein synthesis and impaired hepatic reserve in cirrhotic patients, there is a need of FFP administration to correct underlying coagulopathy.

In case of obstructive jaundice, vitamin K injections are given in the preoperative as well as the postoperative period. Thrombocytopenia with platelet count less than 10,000/μ with active bleeding should be treated with transfusion of platelets. Therefore, a combination of fresh frozen plasma (FFP), vitamin K, octreotide, and human r-FVIIa may be used to reverse coagulopathy and prevent post-operative bleeding [4].

38.3.4 Ascites and Encephalopathy

After the immediate postoperative period, patients are at risk to develop ascites. Excessive sodium supplementation should be minimized. If additional volume expansion is needed, albumin or fresh frozen plasma should be used. Diuretics can be reinstituted after the immediate postoperative period. A general rule is to use a combination of Lasix and spironolactone, with 100 mg of spironolactone for every 40 mg of Lasix.

Encephalopathy is rare in patients after liver resection unless they are in liver failure or have pre-existing liver disease. Encephalopathy is treated with lactulose, oral antibiotic, rifaximin, and dietary protein restriction, as in other patients with end-stage liver disease. Infection, dehydration, and bleeding, as well as narcotic use, must be evaluated, as they can trigger decompensation that leads to encephalopathy [16, 17].

Early mortality in the postoperative period is low to about 2–5%. The important causes along with hemorrhage are sepsis, pneumonia, and multiorgan dysfunction syndrome (MODS). Treatment includes imaging, IV antibiotics, blood transfusions, and close drainage. Antibiotics are administered for 48 h postoperatively to minimize infection from bacterial translocation. Prophylactic use of octreotide has no significant effect on postoperative fistula formation or in the prevention of complications post-surgery [18]. However, the perioperative use of pasireotide has been found beneficial in the prevention of complications such as fistula, leak, and abscess formation [19].

38.4 Aftercare of Asymptomatic Patients

Asymptomatic post hepatectomy patients are followed up for any sign of recurrence. Intrahepatic recurrence within 1 year and the occurrence of solitary tumors along the line of resection are common [20]. Therefore follow-up even in asymptomatic patients is mandatory.

In pancreatic resection patients, according to the S3 guideline "Pancreatic carcinoma" no care is started until there are symptoms like the sense of not feeling well, pain, or weight loss [21]. However, regular clinical monitoring every 3–6 months and laboratory tests including blood sugar level should be done for early detection and management of diabetes [22].

38.5 Malnutrition and Maldigestion

Early nutrition in the postoperative period is an important component of enhanced recovery after surgery (ERAS) [23]. Malnutrition is common in cancer patients and about 30–50% of admitted patients present with issues related to it [24]. Nutritional deficiency encourages a sequence of serious consequences, such as jaundice, hepatic ascites, and hepatic failure [25]. Therefore, proper nutritional assistance after major hepatopancreatobiliary surgery can help in improving patient's immunity, disease prognosis, reducing incidence of infection, postoperative complications and enhancing overall quality of life.

Preoperative biliary obstruction, malignancy, and cirrhosis are important risk factors for nutrition-related complications in major hepatobiliary surgery. Other preoperative nutritional risk factors such as weight loss (greater than 14% lean body mass) over 6 months, serum albumin less than 3 g/dl, hematocrit below 30%, total body potassium less than 85% of normal, less than 25th percentile for mid-arm circumference, and skin test anergy are associated with postoperative complications [26]. Therefore, preoperative bilirubin, albumin, prealbumin, prothrombin time, transferrin, as well as replacement of vitamins and trace mineral deficits are to be considered and optimized preoperatively.

Both enteral and parenteral nutrition are associated with improved outcomes in high-risk hepatobiliary surgery [26, 27]. Early enteral nutrition is considered to be better in such patients as it is associated with improved gut flora, prevention of gastrointestinal atrophy, and loss of immunocompetence. Whereas, parenteral nutrition has been found to be associated with a greater risk of infection in prospective randomized trials after hepatic resection [28, 29]. Early low volume enteral feeding can be started immediately after surgery in ICU in cases of hepatic resections. Some may present with clinical signs of intolerance such as increased gastric residual volume. However, in mechanically ventilated patients, there is no need to stop enteral feeds unless the gastric residual volume is more than 200 ml on more than two occasions in a day. In hepaticojejunostomies or pancreatic surgery, surgeons are often reluctant to start early enteral nutrition due to the risk of anastomotic leaks. In such cases nutrition through feeding jejunostomy or feeding tube placed distal to the anastomosis should be started. Pancreatic enzyme supplementation with enteral feeds is given in major pancreatic surgeries.

The postoperative metabolic complications in the majority of liver resection surgery can be prevented by improving the preoperative nutrition and providing adequate postoperative carbohydrate and albumin supplementation. Patients undergoing liver resection may develop a varying degree of hypoglycemia during the early phase of liver regeneration. Severe hypoglycemia should be avoided with blood glucose monitoring and continuous intravenous infusion of 10% glucose solution for at least the early few days or before starting enteral carbohydrate feedings. As albumin is synthesized in the liver, hypoalbuminemia is corrected by supplementation of albumin for a week or up to 3 weeks till the albumin level returns to normal. As liver disease alters the metabolism of amino acids. Supplementation of branched-chain amino acids (BCAA) such as leucine, isoleucine, and valine helps in immunomodulation and helps in improving quality of life in patients undergoing major hepatic resection [30]. A fat-rich diet containing medium-chain triglycerides and few other fatty acids has also been found to be beneficial. In various trials, the short-term supplementation of BCAA in patients undergoing hepatic resections increases erythropoietin levels which have been found to be protective from ischemic injury on hepatic cells [31].

Biliary tract surgery affects liver function. In the postoperative period, patients are given a sufficient amount of water to preserve acid-base balance. In the early postoperative period, fat is restricted. Initially, parenteral nutritional support rich in energy content is given. As the patient improves, the parenteral nutrition is gradually withdrawn after 2–3 weeks and finally discontinued. Bile salts help in the emulsification of fat and in the absorption of calcium, iron, and other micronutrients. Supplementation of bile salt preparation help in postoperative recovery in patients with preoperative biliary obstruction and fistula [32, 33].

Prognostic nutritional index (PNI) is closely associated with postoperative outcomes in patients undergoing major pancreatic surgeries [34–36]. In a study involving 268 pancreatic cancer patients who underwent pancreatectomy, lower preoperative PNI was associated with poor outcomes and lower survival rates [34]. There has been a close association between the lower level of preoperative albumin,

PNI, and postoperative complication. Lower postoperative PNI in pancreatic surgeries is related to a greater incidence of postoperative pancreatic fistula [35].

In cases of pancreatic cancer, management of postoperative nutrition is vital and is closely associated with the postoperative prognosis. It becomes more challenging as pancreatectomy in cancer patients are associated with increased postoperative complication. Oral feeding is considered to be the initial and least invasive means of nutritional supplementation. In patients who cannot tolerate it, total parenteral nutrition (TPN) is initiated. However, TPN is associated with increased complications such as hyperglycemia, metabolic acidosis, and fluid retention. In contrast, enteral nutrition is considered to be a more "physiological" solution where nutrients are directly introduced into the gastrointestinal tract. Enteral nutrition also helps in the release of pancreaticobiliary secretion, regulation of GI hormones, maintenance of GI contraction, and blood flow [37]. If enteral nutrition fails to provide adequate calories, a combination of enteral and parenteral nutrition can also be given. The ultimate nutritional goal is to increase weight and absorption of fat & protein and decrease steatorrhea. In few selected patients, a diet rich in carbohydrates and protein with a mild degree of fat restriction is needed. In post pancreatoduodenectomy, prompt use of commercially available pancreatic exocrine enzymes are recommended. Oral supplementation of n-3 polyunsaturated fatty acids and medium-chain triglycerides can also be used in postoperative pancreatic cancer patients [38]. The assessment of energy expenditure involves indirect calorimetry which cannot be anticipated by equations. Still, patients with hepatopancreatobiliary cancer may need a calorie intake of up to 35 kcal/kg/day and 2 g/kg protein.

Cachexia and loss of body weight after pancreatic carcinoma resection is not uncommon [39]. It is one of the important prognosticators of poor outcomes and short survival. Factors such as preoperative weight loss >5 kg body weight, insufficient intake of calories in the postoperative period, food intolerance, and pancreatic exocrine insufficiency are responsible for cachexia in pancreatic surgery [40].

38.6 Liver Function

Liver dysfunction is not uncommon after hepatopancreatobiliary surgery and anaesthesia. It may vary from mild elevation of liver enzymes to progressive and refractory hepatic failure called as Postoperative hepatic failure (POHF). POHF is defined as "prolonged hyperbilirubinemia unrelated to biliary obstruction or leak, clinically apparent ascites, prolonged coagulopathy requiring fresh frozen plasma (FFP), and/or hepatic encephalopathy [41]." Incidence is reported to be 1.2–32% of cases with a mortality of about 1.6–2.8% of hepatectomy cases [42–44]. "Various perioperative risk factors responsible for the development of Postoperative Hepatic Failure (POHF) are age >70 years, male sex, cirrhosis, fibrosis, viral or other hepatitis, blood loss during surgery, need for blood transfusion, increased operative time ischemia, obstructive jaundice, preoperative chemotherapy such as irinotecan, oxaliplatin and avastin, steatosis or steatohepatitis, extended hepatectomy, small future liver remnant and preoperative hypoalbuminemia [45]."

Preoperative functional status of the liver can estimate the maximum amount of hepatic resection that can be done while preserving adequate liver function. In a normal liver, up to 75–80% of total liver volume can be resected safely. CT volumetric analysis can help in predicting the volume of the liver to be resected with respect to the measured volume of the entire liver [46]. As the regenerating process is fast, a residual otherwise healthy liver is estimated to be double in size within the first week of the postoperative period. Still, growth in parenchymal size does not indicate the full restoration of functional capacity.

Various preoperative assessments tools are available to guide the hepatic reserve, the feasibility of resection, and to predict postoperative morbidity and mortality.

- The child-Pugh clinical scoring system is considered to be a reliable and validated prognostic tool for patients undergoing hepatobiliary surgery. Child-Pugh class A patients may undergo major hepatectomy with resection of ≥4 segments. Child-Pugh Class B patients devoid of portal hypertension may undergo minor resections such as wedge to single segment resection. Child-Pugh class C is a contraindication for any kind of resection.
- Other scoring includes Model of End-Stage Liver Disease (MELD). MELD score ≥11 predicts liver failure post HCC resection. However, the Child-Pugh score is more widely used and it is considered to be a better tool in predicting postoperative outcomes [47].
- Portal hypertension and thrombocytopenia with platelet counts <1 lakh/μl is associated with significant mortality post hepatic resection. Therefore, guidelines for major resection in patients with underlying liver disease (cirrhotics) include "(1) Child-Pugh class A, (2) Platelet count >100,000/μl, (3) No clinically significant portal hypertension, (4) Anticipated remnant >40–50% and (5) Indocyanine green retention <15% [45]."
- 50–50 criteria and Mullen criteria are other postoperative criteria that have been used in predicting postoperative hepatic failure and mortality. The 50–50 criteria is an amalgamation of prothrombin time (PT) and serum bilirubin level. In patients who are admitted to ICU following postoperative liver failure after hepatic resections, PT less than 50% (or PT-INR > 1.7) and serum bilirubin greater than 50 μmol/l (or >2.9 mg/dl) is considered to be an excellent predictor of mortality on days 3–5 [48]. The Mullen criteria (bilirubin peak >7 mg/dl on postoperative days 1–7) have been found to be more precise than the 50–50 criteria in predicting death from hepatic failure after liver resection [49].

Most of the cases of benign postoperative jaundice without any apparent reasons resolve unexpectedly with supportive treatment. However, POHF is a life-threatening condition which need special care. So, all the cases of POHF are to be managed in ICU where liver functions and coagulation profile are monitored daily. Patients may present with associated hepatic encephalopathy which increases mortality. Increased level of ammonia due to liver failure is a key pathogenesis in the development of encephalopathy. Hepatotoxic drugs are avoided; lactulose and stool softeners are used. Coagulopathy is corrected with blood transfusions and fresh frozen plasma (FFP) transfusion. Mild cases are managed with supportive treatment with fluid management, correction of tissue oxygenation, infection prophylaxis, and nutritional support. The goal is to promote recovery from immediate injury to hepatic tissue, promote regeneration, correction of electrolytes & hypophosphatemia, and infection control. Severe cases may present with severe acidosis, jaundice, and hemodynamic instability. The treatment includes prevention of multiorgan failure and sepsis. The use of *N*-acetylcysteine does not help in reducing mortality in the management of hepatic failure after liver resection [50]. Liver transplantation may be considered in refractory cases not responding to supportive treatment [51].

38.7 Exocrine Insufficiency

Pancreatic exocrine insufficiency (PEI) is a common and known complication after pancreaticoduodenectomy (PD) in pancreatic malignancy. The Spanish pancreatic association has defined PEI as the "inability of the pancreas to perform digestion with disturbed pancreatic function [52]."

PEI after pancreatic resection is associated with long hospital stay, increased morbidity-mortality, poor nutritional status, and low quality of life [53–56]. Common symptoms are abdominal pain, diarrhea, steatorrhea, a sense of heaviness in the abdomen, and weight loss. The degree of exocrine insufficiency depends upon the extent of surgical resection, remnant pancreatic mass, digestive asynchrony, and perioperative octreotide use [57–61].

Pancreatic enzyme replacement therapy (PERT) is the mainstay of treatment of PEI. However, there are no fixed guidelines as to when to start PERT in the postoperative period [62]. The United Kingdom National Institute of Clinical Excellence has recommended perioperative use of PERT in all patients of pancreatic malignancy undergoing pancreatic resection [63].

In the preoperative setting, the patients are counseled about the probable development of PEI in the postoperative period. Preoperative patient counselling and education are vital regarding the correct use of PERT. Enzymes are used with all the meals, snacks, and drinks. Usually, PERT is started with a dose of 50,000–75,000 units of lipase with a meal and 25,000–50,000 units with every snack [64, 65]. With time, a patient is able to adjust the dose of PERT according to his symptoms and diet. However, patients are followed up and managed accordingly with serial anthropometric measurements, change in pancreatic functions, blood sugar optimization, and supplementation of diet with vitamins and micronutrients [66–68].

38.8 Vitamin Deficiency

Hypophosphatemia is a common presentation in the early days of hepatic resection. It needs attention and prompt correction [69]. The exact mechanism of hypophosphatemia is unclear. However, increased utilization during liver regeneration and renal wasting mechanism has been suggested. Interestingly, failure to develop hypophosphatemia is an indicator of postoperative hepatic insufficiency and increased mortality [70].

The clinical features of hypophosphatemia include respiratory depression, diaphragmatic insufficiency, seizures, and cardiac instability. Hepatocellular regeneration is adenosine triphosphate (ATP) dependent and if phosphate is not replenished adequately, the regeneration process may be impaired significantly [71].

In a study involving 35 liver resections, 21% had significant postoperative hypophosphatemia (<2.5 mg/dl) which was associated with increased complications (80%) as compared to normophosphatemic patients (28%) [72]. Contradictory to it, lower phosphate levels in the early postoperative period in 2342 patients following both proximal and distal pancreatectomies were associated with a greater risk of morbidity and postoperative pancreatic fistula (POPF) [73]. Therefore, persistent lower phosphate levels should be taken seriously with suspicion of postoperative leak or fistula. It needs prompt radiological evaluation and treatment [74].

Deficiencies of micronutrients such as vitamin A, iron, zinc, and selenium can be seen after pancreaticoduodenectomy (PD). In long-term survivors of PD, patients are advised to have diets rich in micronutrients. They are screened for osteopenia and levels of trace elements and fat-soluble vitamins. Micronutrients like vitamin B6, B12, and 25-OH-vitamin D3 must be monitored in post-PD patients and supplemented as required [75]. Bowel function cannot be neglected and its optimization with the help of diet, enzyme supplementation, and antidiarrhoeal therapy helps in improving the overall quality of life.

38.9 Diabetes Mellitus

About 50% of the pancreatic mass is removed during pancreatoduodenectomy which results in endo as well as exocrine pancreatic insufficiency. American Diabetes Association has defined "New-onset diabetes mellitus" (NODM) after pancreatectomy as pancreatogenic or type 3c diabetes mellitus [76]. In a study, it was found that the incidence of NODM after PD was 22% and most of the patients had developed in the first postoperative period. It is difficult to predict the incidence of NODM, as patient's insulin sensitivity, environmental and genetic factors vary and play an important role [77]. However, Percentage pancreatic remnant volume (%RV) post PD which can be determined by computer tomography (CT) preoperatively was found to be an independent predictor of NODM. A %RV of <48.8% was found to be a predictor of NODM [78].

Postoperatively, glucose metabolism insufficiency is reflected as increased blood sugar and glycosylated hemoglobin and low levels of insulin and C-peptide. According to American Diabetes Association to prevent the development of NODM, it is recommended to have an annual follow-up, lifestyle changes, and use of oral hypoglycemic drugs if there is impaired glucose intolerance or HbA1c above 6.4% [79]. It is therefore prudent to inform the risk of postoperative NODM during preoperative counseling. Patients and their families should be made aware of its early detection and management in the postoperative period.

38.10 Pain Management

Patients experience significant pain in the early postoperative period. The reason being the large subcostal incision that is given for major hepatopancreatobiliary surgery. Effective pain management helps in early ambulation, better respiratory functions, hemodynamic stability, and smooth extubation in the postoperative period. Postoperative pain management becomes challenging in a post-hepatectomy patient as there is significant coagulopathy and alteration in pharmacokinetics of drugs used for pain management, such as narcotics and sedatives.

Opioids are the mainstay analgesics to be used. However, inappropriate use of narcotics and sedatives in ICU can lead to oversedation. Prolonged respiratory depression results in atelectasis, aspiration, and postoperative pneumonia. Therefore, narcotics and benzodiazepines should be used in minimal doses to achieve optimal analgesia. If available remifentanil is the choice of opioid because of its limited hepatic metabolism [80]. Fentanyl is easily available and are considered to be a better option in case of renal dysfunction [81].

For patients who require postoperative mechanical ventilation, propofol is considered to be a better choice. The reason being the level of sedation that can be easily titrated, reversed, and allows more reliable serial neurologic assessment in ICU [82]. Dexmedetomidine can be used as a probable substitute for propofol because of its rapid onset and metabolism [83].

Non-steroidal anti-inflammatory drugs (NSAIDs) are better avoided in post hepatectomy patients. The reasons are the risk of peptic ulceration, bleeding, the risk of hepatorenal syndrome, and renal failure [84]. However, intravenous paracetamol can be used in a dose not greater than 2 g/day in patients with liver impairment [85].

Epidural pain management may be considered as an optimal analgesic technique after hepatic resection. However, continuous epidural analgesia is frequently avoided due to the risk of coagulopathy, thrombocytopenia, and hematoma formation. In a review of eight patients with epidural catheters, good pain control was achieved, with only one case of oversedation requiring naloxone. Although postoperative coagulopathy did occur, it was not to the extent that factor transfusion was needed before catheter removal, and there were no cases of hemorrhage. Patient-controlled analgesia (PCA) has been also found to be safe and effective in achieving optimal analgesia after hepatic resection [86]. However, Patient-controlled analgesia with basal rate infusion of narcotics is to be avoided as the metabolism of narcotics is difficult to be predicted in post-hepatic resection patients. Intrathecal morphine in a dose of 0.3–0.5 mg can be used as an alternative in patients with coagulopathy. This reduces the systemic requirement of morphine in the early postoperative period. Intrathecal morphine with PCA has been found to be a better alternative to a thoracic epidural in a resource-limited setting. It is associated with lower morbidity and overall complications [87].

References

1. Man K, Fan ST, Ng IO, Lo CM, Liu CL, Wong J. Prospective evaluation of Pringle maneuver in hepatectomy for liver tumors by a randomized study. Ann Surg. 1997;226(6):704.
2. Khan AS, Garcia-Aroz S, Ansari MA, Atiq SM, Senter-Zapata M, Fowler K, Doyle MB, Chapman WC. Assessment and optimization of liver volume before major hepatic resection: current guidelines and a narrative review. Int J Surg. 2018;1(52):74–81.
3. Clavien PA, Selzner M, Rudiger HA, et al. A prospective randomized study in 100 consecutive patients undergoing major liver resection with versus without ischemic preconditioning. Ann Surg 2003;238(6):843–50. Discussion 851–2.
4. Thorat A, Lee WC. Critical care issues after major hepatic surgery. In: Hepatic surgery. InTech Open; 2013. p. 83–103.
5. Jongerius IM, Mungroop TH, Uz Z, Geerts BF, Immink RV, Rutten MV, Hollmann MW, van Gulik TM, Besselink MG, Veelo DP. Goal-directed fluid therapy vs. low central venous pressure during major open liver resections (GALILEO): a surgeon-and patient-blinded randomized controlled trial. HPB. 2021;23(10):1578–85.
6. Wrighton LJ, O'Bosky KR, Namm JP, Senthil M. Postoperative management after hepatic resection. J Gastrointest Oncol. 2012;3:41–7.
7. Sterns R, Cappuccino J, Silver S, et al. Neurologic sequelae after treatment of severe Hyponatremia: a multicenter prospective. J Am Soc Nephrol. 1994;4:1522.
8. Basaran M, Sever K, Ugurlucan M, et al. Serum lactate level has prognostic significance after pediatric cardiac surgery. J Cardiothorac Vasc Anesth. 2006;20(1):43–7.
9. Watanabe I, Mayumi T, Arishima T, Nakao A, et al. Hyperlactemia can predict the prognosis of liver resection. Shock. 2007;28:35–8.
10. Salem RR, Tray K. Hepatic resection-related hypophosphatemia is of renal origin as manifested by isolated hyperphosphaturia. Ann Surg. 2005;241(2):343–8.
11. Imamura H, Kokudo N, Sugawara Y, Sano K, Kaneko J, Takayama T. Pringle's manoeuvre and selective inflow occlusion in living donor liver hepatectomy. Liver Transpl. 2004;10(6):771–8.
12. Van den Berghe G, Wouters P, Weekers F, Verwaest C, Bruyninckx F, Schetz M, et al. Intensive insulin therapy in the critically ill patients. N Engl J Med. 2001;345:1359–67.
13. Huo TI, Lui WY, Huang YH, Chau GY, Wu JC, Lee PC, et al. Diabetes mellitus is a risk factor for hepatic decompensation in patients with hepatocellular carcinoma undergoing resection: a longitudinal study. Am J Gastroenterol. 2003;98:2293–8.
14. De Pietri L, Montalti R, Begliomini B, Scaglioni G, Marconi G, Reggiani A, Di Benedetto F, Aiello S, Pasetto A, Rompianesi G, Gerunda GE. Thromboelastographic changes in liver and pancreatic cancer surgery: hypercoagulability, hypocoagulability or normocoagulability?. Eur J Anaesthesiol EJA. 2010;27(7):608–16.
15. Shontz R, Karuparthy V, Temple R, Brennan TJ. Prevalence and risk factors predisposing to coagulopathy in patients receiving epidural analgesia for hepatic surgery. Reg Anesth Pain Med. 2009;34:308–11.
16. Wright G, Jalan R. Management of hepatic encephalopathy in patients with cirrhosis. Best Pract Res Clin Gastroenterol. 2007;21(1):95–110.
17. Al Sibae MR, McGuire BM. Current trends in the treatment of hepatic encephalopathy. Ther Clin Risk Manag. 2009;5:617.
18. Yeo CJ, Cameron JL, Lillemoe KD, Sauter PK, Coleman J, Sohn TA, Campbell KA, Choti MA. Does prophylactic octreotide decrease the rates of pancreatic fistula and other complications after pancreaticoduodenectomy?: Results of a prospective randomized placebo-controlled trial. Ann Surg. 2000;232(3):419.
19. Allen PJ, Gönen M, Brennan MF, Bucknor AA, Robinson LM, Pappas MM, Carlucci KE, D'Angelica MI, DeMatteo RP, Kingham TP, Fong Y. Pasireotide for postoperative pancreatic fistula. N Engl J Med. 2014;370(21):2014–22.
20. Chiappa A, Zbar AP, Audisio RA, Leone BE, Biella F, Staudacher C. Factors affecting survival and long-term outcome in the cirrhotic patient undergoing hepatic resection for hepatocellular carcinoma. Eur J Surg Oncol (EJSO). 2000;26(4):387–92.

21. Adler G, Seufferlein T, Bischoff SC, et al. S3-guidelines "exocrine pancreatic cancer" 2007. Z Gastroenterol. 2007;45:487–523.
22. Malka D, Hammel P, Sauvanet A, et al. Risk factors for diabetes mellitus in chronic pancreatitis. Gastroenterology. 2000;119:1324–32.
23. Wilmore DW, Kehlet H. Management of patients in fast track surgery. BMJ. 2001;322:473–6.
24. La Torre M, Ziparo V, Nigri G, et al. Malnutrition and pancreatic surgery: prevalence and outcomes. J Surg Oncol. 2013;107:702–8.
25. Masuda T, Shirabe K, Yoshiya S, et al. Nutrition support and infections associated with hepatic resection and liver transplantation in patients with chronic liver disease. JPEN J Parenter Enteral Nutr. 2013;37(3):318–26.
26. Fan ST, Lo CM, Lai EC, et al. Perioperative nutritional support in patients undergoing hepatectomy for hepatocellular carcinoma. N Engl J Med. 1994;331:1547–52.
27. Richter B, Schmandra TC, Golling M, et al. Nutritional support after open liver resection: a systematic review. Dig Surg. 2006;23:139–45.
28. Gramlich L, Kichian K, Pinilla J, et al. Does enteral nutrition compared to parenteral nutrition result in better outcomes in critically ill adult patients? A systematic review of the literature. Nutrition. 2004;20:843–8.
29. McCullough AJ, Tavill AS. Disordered energy and protein metabolism in liver disease. Semin Liver Dis. 1991;11:265–77.
30. Okabayashi T, Iyoki M, Sugimoto T, Kobayashi M, Hanazaki K. Oral supplementation with carbohydrate-and branched-chain amino acid-enriched nutrients improves postoperative quality of life in patients undergoing hepatic resection. Amino Acids. 2011;40(4):1213–20.
31. Ishikawa Y, Yoshida H, Mamada Y, Taniai N, Matsumoto S, Bando K, Mizuguchi Y, Kakinuma D, Kanda T, Tajiri T. Prospective randomized controlled study of short-term perioperative oral nutrition with branched chain amino acids in patients undergoing liver surgery. Hepatogastroenterology. 2010;57(99–100):583–90.
32. Wendel D, Mortensen M, Harmeson A, Shaffer ML, Hsu E, Horslen S. Resolving malnutrition with parenteral nutrition before liver transplant in biliary atresia. J Pediatr Gastroenterol Nutr. 2018;66(2):212–7.
33. Ravindranath A, Yachha SK. Bile acid synthetic defects: simplified approach in a nutshell. Hepatobiliary Pancreat Dis Int. 2019;19(1):80–4.
34. Kanda M, Fujii T, Kodera Y, Nagai S, Takeda S, Nakao A. Nutritional predictors of postoperative outcome in pancreatic cancer. J Br Surg. 2011;98(2):268–74.
35. Sato N, Mori Y, Minagawa N, Tamura T, Shibao K, Higure A, Yamaguchi K. Rapid postoperative reduction in prognostic nutrition index is associated with the development of pancreatic fistula following distal pancreatectomy. Pancreatology. 2014;14(3):216–20.
36. Mahendran R, Tewari M, Dixit VK, Shukla HS. Enhanced recovery after surgery protocol enhances early postoperative recovery after pancreaticoduodenectomy. Hepatobiliary Pancreat Dis Int. 2019;18(2):188–93.
37. Gianotti L, Besselink MG, Sandini M, Hackert T, Conlon K, Gerritsen A, Griffin O, Fingerhut A, Probst P, Hilal MA, Marchegiani G. Nutritional support and therapy in pancreatic surgery: a position paper of the International Study Group on Pancreatic Surgery (ISGPS). Surgery. 2018;164(5):1035–48.
38. Haji S, Ohyanagi H, Takeyama Y. Nutritional management in pancreatoduodenectomy patients. Nihon Geka Gakkai zasshi. 2010;111(1):27–30.
39. Maréchal R, Demols A, Gay F, et al. Prognostic factors and prognostic index for chemonaïve and gemcitabine-refractory patients with advanced pancreatic cancer. Oncology. 2007;73:41–51.
40. Bruno MJ, Haverkort EB, Tijssen GP, Tytgat GN, van Leeuwen DJ. Placebo controlled trial of enteric coated pancreatin microsphere treatment in patients with unresectable cancer of the pancreatic head region. Gut. 1998;42:92–6.
41. Jarnagin WR, Gonen M, Fong Y, DeMatteo RP, Ben-Porat L, Little S, Corvera C, Weber S, Blumgart LH. Improvement in perioperative outcome after hepatic resection: analysis of 1,803 consecutive cases over the past decade. Ann Surg. 2002;236(4):397.

42. Rahbari NN, Garden OJ, Padbury R, Brooke-Smith M, Crawford M, Adam R, Koch M, Makuuchi M, Dematteo RP, Christophi C, Banting S. Posthepatectomy liver failure: a definition and grading by the International Study Group of Liver Surgery (ISGLS). Surgery. 2011;149(5):713–24.
43. Hyder O, Pulitano C, Firoozmand A, Dodson R, Wolfgang CL, Choti MA, Aldrighetti L, Pawlik TM. A risk model to predict 90-day mortality among patients undergoing hepatic resection. J Am Coll Surg. 2013;216(6):1049–56.
44. Mullen JT, Ribero D, Reddy SK, Donadon M, Zorzi D, Gautam S, Abdalla EK, Curley SA, Capussotti L, Clary BM, Vauthey JN. Hepatic insufficiency and mortality in 1,059 noncirrhotic patients undergoing major hepatectomy. J Am Coll Surg. 2007;204(5):854–62.
45. Qadan M, Garden OJ, Corvera CU, Visser BC. Management of postoperative hepatic failure. J Am Coll Surg. 2016;222(2):195–208.
46. Shoup M, Gonen M, D'Angelica M, Farnagin WR, DeMatteo RP, Schwartz LH, Tuorto S, Blumgart LH, Fong Y. Volumetric analysis predicts hepatic dysfunction in patients undergoing major liver resection. J Gastrointest Surg. 2003;7(3):325–30.
47. Schroeder RA, Marroquin CE, Bute BP, Khuri S, Henderson WG, Kuo PC. Predictive indices of morbidity and mortality after liver resection. Ann Surg. 2006;243(3):373.
48. Paugam-Burtz C, Janny S, Delefosse D, Dahmani S, Dondero F, Mantz J, Belghiti J. Prospective validation of the "fifty-fifty" criteria as an early and accurate predictor of death after liver resection in intensive care unit patients. Ann Surg. 2009;249(1):124–8.
49. Filicori F, Keutgen XM, Zanello M, Ercolani G, Di Saverio S, Sacchetti F, Pinna AD, Grazi GL. Prognostic criteria for postoperative mortality in 170 patients undergoing major right hepatectomy. Hepatobiliary Pancreat Dis Int. 2012;11(5):507–12.
50. Squires RH, Dhawan A, Alonso E, Narkewicz MR, Shneider BL, Rodriguez-Baez N, Olio DD, Karpen S, Bucuvalas J, Lobritto S, Rand E. Intravenous N-acetylcysteine in pediatric patients with nonacetaminophen acute liver failure: a placebo-controlled clinical trial. Hepatology. 2013;57(4):1542–9.
51. Sgroi A, Serre-Beinier V, Morel P, Bühler L. What clinical alternatives to whole liver transplantation? Current status of artificial devices and hepatocyte transplantation. Transplantation. 2009;87(4):457–66.
52. Sabater L, Ausania F, Bakker OJ, Boadas J, Domínguez-Muñoz JE, Falconi M, Fernández-Cruz L, Frulloni L, González-Sánchez V, Lariño-Noia J, Lindkvist B. Evidence-based guidelines for the management of exocrine pancreatic insufficiency after pancreatic surgery. Ann Surg. 2016;264(6):949–58.
53. van Dijk SM, Heerkens HD, Tseng DSJ, Intven M, Molenaar IQ, van Santvoort HC. Systematic review on the impact of pancreatoduodenectomy on quality of life in patients with pancreatic cancer. HPB (Oxford). 2018;20:204–15.
54. Heerkens HD, van Berkel L, Tseng DSJ, Monninkhof EM, van Santvoort HC, Hagendoorn J, Borel Rinkes IHM, Lips IM, Intven M, Molenaar IQ. Long-term health-related quality of life after pancreatic resection for malignancy in patients with and without severe postoperative complications. HPB (Oxford). 2018;20:188–95.
55. Bartel MJ, Asbun H, Stauffer J, Raimondo M. Pancreatic exocrine insufficiency in pancreatic cancer: a review of the literature. Dig Liver Dis. 2015;47:1013–20.
56. Gianotti L, Besselink MG, Sandini M, Hackert T, Conlon K, Gerritsen A, Griffin O, Fingerhut A, Probst P, Abu Hilal M, Marchegiani G, Nappo G, Zerbi A, Amodio A, Perinel J, Adham M, Raimondo M, Asbun HJ, Sato A, Takaori K, Shrikhande SV, Del Chiaro M, Bockhorn M, Izbicki JR, Dervenis C, Charnley RM, Martignoni ME, Friess H, de Pretis N, Radenkovic D, Montorsi M, Sarr MG, Vollmer CM, Frulloni L, Büchler MW, Bassi C. Nutritional support and therapy in pancreatic surgery: a position paper of the International Study Group on Pancreatic Surgery (ISGPS). Surgery. 2018;164:1035–48.
57. Nakamura H, Murakami Y, Uemura K, Hayashidani Y, Sudo T, Ohge H, Sueda T. Predictive factors for exocrine pancreatic insufficiency after pancreatoduodenectomy with pancreaticogastrostomy. J Gastrointest Surg. 2009;13:1321–7.

58. Tran TC, van Lanschot JJ, Bruno MJ, van Eijck CH. Functional changes after pancreatoduodenectomy: diagnosis and treatment. Pancreatology. 2009;9:729–37.
59. Sikkens EC, Cahen DL, de Wit J, Looman CW, van Eijck C, Bruno MJ. A prospective assessment of the natural course of the exocrine pancreatic function in patients with a pancreatic head tumor. J Clin Gastroenterol. 2014;48:e43–6.
60. Bruno MJ, Haverkort EB, Tytgat GN, van Leeuwen DJ. Maldigestion associated with exocrine pancreatic insufficiency: implications of gastrointestinal physiology and properties of enzyme preparations for a cause-related and patient-tailored treatment. Am J Gastroenterol. 1995;90:1383–93.
61. Gullo L. Somatostatin analogues and exocrine pancreatic secretion. Digestion. 1996;57(Suppl 1):93.
62. Working Party of the Australasian Pancreatic Club, Smith RC, Smith SF, Wilson J, Pearce C, Wray N, Vo R, Chen J, Ooi CY, Oliver M, Katz T, Turner R, Nikfarjam M, Rayner C, Horowitz M, Holtmann G, Talley N, Windsor J, Pirola R, Neale R. Summary and recommendations from the Australasian guidelines for the management of pancreatic exocrine insufficiency. Pancreatology. 2016;16:164–80.
63. National Institute for Health and Care Excellence. Pancreatic cancer in adults: diagnosis and management. NICE guideline [NG85], Recommendations.
64. Imrie CW, Connett G, Hall RI, Charnley RM. Review article: enzyme supplementation in cystic fibrosis, chronic pancreatitis, pancreatic and periampullary cancer. Aliment Pharmacol Ther. 2010;32(Suppl 1):1–25.
65. Seiler CM, Izbicki J, Varga-Szabó L, Czakó L, Fiók J, Sperti C, Lerch MM, Pezzilli R, Vasileva G, Pap A, Varga M, Friess H. Randomised clinical trial: a 1-week, double-blind, placebo-controlled study of pancreatin 25 000 Ph. Eur. minimicrospheres (Creon 25000 MMS) for pancreatic exocrine insufficiency after pancreatic surgery, with a 1-year open-label extension. Aliment Pharmacol Ther. 2013;37:691–702.
66. Phillips ME. Pancreatic exocrine insufficiency following pancreatic resection. Pancreatology. 2015;15:449–55.
67. O'Keefe SJ, Cariem AK, Levy M. The exacerbation of pancreatic endocrine dysfunction by potent pancreatic exocrine supplements in patients with chronic pancreatitis. J Clin Gastroenterol. 2001;32:319–23.
68. Armstrong T, Strommer L, Ruiz-Jasbon F, Shek FW, Harris SF, Permert J, Johnson CD. Pancreaticoduodenectomy for peri-ampullary neoplasia leads to specific micronutrient deficiencies. Pancreatology. 2007;7:37–44.
69. Schmidt LE, Dalhoff K. Serum phosphate is an early predictor of outcome in severe acetaminophen-induced hepatotoxicity. Hepatology. 2002;36(3):659–65.
70. Sushrutha CS, Venugopal HG, Vinay BN, Balakrishna SN, Shilpa MC, Sathish O, Babu R, Ashok Kumar KV, Nagesh NS. Post hepatectomy hypophosphatemia and its association with initial liver insufficiency and morbidity. Int Surg J. 2018;5(7):2427–31.
71. Campbell KA, Wu YP, Chacko VP, et al. In vivo 31P NMR spectroscopic changes during liver regeneration. J Surg Res. 1990;49:244–7.
72. Buell JF, Berger AC, Plotkin JS, et al. The clinical implications of hypophosphatemia following major hepatic resection or cryosurgery. Arch Surg. 1998;133:757–61.
73. Mueller JL, Chang DC, Fernandez-del Castillo C, Ferrone CR, Warshaw AL, Lillemoe KD, Qadan M. Lower phosphate levels following pancreatectomy is associated with postoperative pancreatic fistula formation. HPB. 2019;21(7):834–40.
74. Sadot E, Zheng J, Srouji R, Strong VE, Gönen M, Balachandran VP, D'Angelica MI, Allen PJ, DeMatteo RP, Kingham TP, Fong Y. Hypophosphatemia as a predictor of organ-specific complications following gastrointestinal surgery: analysis of 8034 patients. World J Surg. 2019;43(2):385–94.
75. Keim V, Klar E, Poll M, Schoenberg MH. Postoperative care following pancreatic surgery: surveillance and treatment. Dtsch Arztebl Int. 2009;106(48):789.

76. Mellitus D. Diagnosis and classification of diabetes mellitus. Diabetes Care. 2005;28(S37): S5–10.
77. Reaven GM. Pathophysiology of insulin resistance in human disease. Physiol Rev. 1995;75(3):473–86.
78. Singh AN, Pal S, Kilambi R, Madhusudhan KS, Dash NR, Tandon N, Sahni P. Diabetes after pancreaticoduodenectomy: can we predict it? J Surg Res. 2018;227:211–9.
79. Timper K, Donath MY. Diabetes mellitus type 2-the new face of an old lady. Swiss Med Wkly. 2012;142(2930).
80. Uchida K, Yasunaga H, Miyata H, Sumitani M, Horiguchi H, Kuwajima K, Matsuda S, Yamada Y. Impact of remifentanil introduction on practice patterns in general anesthesia. J Anesth. 2011;25(6):864–71.
81. Chandok N, Watt KD. Pain management in the cirrhotic patient: the clinical challenge. In Mayo Clinic proceedings 1 May 2010 (vol. 85, no. 5). Elsevier. p. 451–8.
82. Khamaysi I, William N, Olga A, Alex I, Vladimir M, Kamal D, Nimer A. Sub-clinical hepatic encephalopathy in cirrhotic patients is not aggravated by sedation with propofol compared to midazolam: a randomized controlled study. J Hepatol. 2011;54(1):72–7.
83. Wang ZX, Huang CY, Hua YP, Huang WQ, Deng LH, Liu KX. Dexmedetomidine reduces intestinal and hepatic injury after hepatectomy with inflow occlusion under general anaesthesia: a randomized controlled trial. Br J Anaesth. 2014;112(6):1055–64.
84. Bosilkovska M, Walder B, Besson M, Daali Y, Desmeules J. Analgesics in patients with hepatic impairment. Drugs. 2012;72(12):1645–69.
85. Mimoz O, Incagnoli P, Josse C, Gillon MC, Kuhlman L, Mirand A, Soilleux H, Fletcher D. Analgesic efficacy and safety of nefopam vs. propacetamol following hepatic resection. Anaesthesia. 2001;56(6):520–5.
86. Roy JD, Massicotte L, Sassine MP, Seal RF, Roy A. A comparison of intrathecal morphine/fentanyl and patient-controlled analgesia with patient-controlled analgesia alone for analgesia after liver resection. Anesth Analg. 2006;103(4):990–4.
87. Sakowska M, Docherty E, Linscott D, Connor S. A change in practice from epidural to intrathecal morphine analgesia for hepato-pancreato-biliary surgery. World J Surg. 2009;33(9):1802–8.

Critical Care Management in a Patient of CRS and HIPEC

39

S. V. S. Deo, Babul Bansal, and Jyoutishman Saikia

39.1 Introduction

Cytoreductive surgery (CRS) along with Hyperthermic intraperitoneal chemotherapy (HIPEC) has been standard of care for a subset of patients with peritoneal surface malignancies (PSM) including primary peritoneal malignancies like mesothelioma and peritoneal involvement secondary to ovarian, colorectal, gastric and appendicular malignancies. As a first step, cytoreductive surgery (CRS) is performed after which chemotherapeutic agents heated to 41–43 °C are infused intraoperatively using a dedicated HIPEC machine. As chemotherapeutic drugs can penetrate the peritoneal membrane for a maximum of 3 mm, CRS is performed to increase the effect of these drugs [1]. CRS includes an amalgamation of multiple complex procedures like excision of the primary tumor, omentectomies, peritonectomies, bowel and other organ resections as considered necessary to achieve a macroscopically tumor free peritoneal cavity. Multiple factors decide the efficacy of HIPEC such as patient factors, clinical factors, treatment parameters, type of drug and techniques, drug concentration, carrier solution, perfusate volume, temperature and duration of treatment [2]. A high variability exists with regard to HIPEC treatment globally based on disease type and institutional protocols.

Blood loss and massive transfusions can frequently be a part of such major operations which can pose an added insult to the perioperative course. In general, this procedure involves prolonged duration of anesthesia, fluid and electrolyte shifts, thermal stress, along with toxic effects of chemotherapy and acid base disturbances. In a systematic review by Chua et al., including data from retrospective and prospective studies reporting CRS with HIPEC, authors reported a mean operative time ranging from 5 to 10 h and significant blood loss as high as 3.5 L [3].

S. V. S. Deo (✉) · B. Bansal · J. Saikia
Department of Surgical Oncology, AIIMS, BRA-IRCH & NCI, New Delhi, India

V. Kumar et al. (eds.), *Onco-critical Care*,
https://doi.org/10.1007/978-981-16-9929-0_39

Perioperative and critical care management plays a very important role for optimal outcomes following CRS and HIPEC. This chapter will focus on the critical care management issues related to CRS and HIPEC.

39.2 Basic Surgical Concerns and Need for Admission in ICU

Multiple factors decide shifting the patients to ICU intubated or following extubation in the operating room. Some of the important ones are: existing major comorbidities of cardiac or respiratory system, blood loss, transfusion requirements, hemodynamics, metabolic factors towards end of surgery. Most of the time patients are shifted to ICU immediately after surgery (46–74%). In approximately 50% of cases endotracheal tube (ETT) is removed in the operating theatre (OT) [4]. Centers without ICU facilities can gain from experiences of high-volume centres on case selection or situations (e.g. Low volume disease, less blood loss etc.) where an ICU can be avoided. The following factors are important for a favorable postoperative outcome [5]

(a) Immediate or early extubation
(b) Epidural analgesia,
(c) Postoperative monitoring in ICU
(d) Immediate initiation of parenteral nutrition in postoperative period
(e) Stringent fluid status monitoring

Stress response in the postoperative period involves all major organ systems like cardiovascular, respiratory, coagulation, renal and endocrine system [6, 7]. During postoperative course patients may experience hyperthermia-related coagulopathy, hyperglycaemia, low-grade fever and mild pain. Besides these, secretory diarrhoea may occur in the first week. Other biochemical changes can be observed like transient severe hypophosphatemia (due to renal tubulopathy) and altered liver function tests (transaminitis following extensive electrocautery use on the liver capsule). Inflammatory markers like C-reactive protein and interleukins usually return to normal within 12–24 h. Total leukocyte count and platelet counts also decreases within a couple of weeks. Recommendations were laid down for postoperative care and ICU admission by the Society of Onco-anaesthesia and perioperative care and are described in Table 39.1 [5].

39.3 Monitoring in ICU (Hemodynamics/Coagulation Profile/Temperature/Electrolytes)

39.3.1 Haemodynamic Monitoring

These patients need invasive blood pressure monitoring and frequently also may require central venous pressure monitoring besides standard monitoring practices

Table 39.1 Postoperative and ICU care recommendations [5]

Sl no	Recommendation		Evidence available (yes/no)/consensus only
1	Should not routinely extubate the trachea on operating table		Yes
2	Attempting extubation in the operating room should be done in low-volume (low PCI) cases		Yes
3	Haemodynamically unstable patients should be transferred to ICU with endotracheal tube in situ		Consensus
4	Those patients undergoing massive blood loss, high arterial lactate and diaphragmatic striping may be considered for transfer to ICU with endotracheal tube in situ		Consensus
5	The decision to transfer patient to ICU with endotracheal tube in situ or with after tracheal extubation in patients who have undergone prolonged (>10 h) surgery, presence of preoperative bad pulmonary functions and major cardiac or non-cardiac comorbidities should be individualised		No
6	Fluid therapy in postoperative period should be based on	Fluid therapy guided by mean arterial pressure, heart rate and urine output	Consensus
		Fluid therapy guided by arterial lactate concentration	Consensus
7	Starting early enteral nutrition or parenteral nutrition in patient who cannot tolerate enteral nutrition		Yes

such as electrocardiogram, noninvasive blood pressure, pulse oximetry, end-tidal CO2 monitoring and core-body temperature monitoring [8]. In patients with significant disease burden (PCI >15) cardiac output monitoring can additionally be used. Goal-directed therapy (GDT) in CRS-HIPEC had shown to decrease morbidity and thereby shorten postoperative hospital stay. Additionally, there was no difference in mortality.

Throughout the surgery at regular intervals arterial blood gas monitoring is often needed to assess gas exchange, electrolyte, glucose and lactate levels [8]. Serum magnesium level monitoring is preferred both before initiating HIPEC phase and also in the postoperative period. This is because hypomagnesaemia can occur after fluid infusion (dilution) and following platinum-based chemotherapy perfusion [9]. Ionized calcium should also be monitored and corrected if there is massive transfusion of blood and blood products.

39.3.2 Goal for Intraoperative Urine Output

Following CRS-HIPEC, acute kidney injury (AKI) can be witnessed in 21–48% of patients [10]. Some of the predictors of development of AKI are higher age, BMI, pregabalin use (preoperatively), platinum-based chemotherapy, massive blood loss, high blood pressure and low intraoperative diuresis. Factors associated with development of AKI were low intraoperative urine output, angiotensin II receptor antagonist use and raised blood pressure [9]. Urine output is used as a surrogate marker for intraoperative measurement of renal perfusion. The target urine output during various phases are 0.5 mL/kg/h during CRS phase, 2–4 mL/kg/h during the HIPEC and 1–2 mL/kg/h after HIPEC across various studies [11]. However fluid therapy should also be individualized from patient to patient.

There are also controversies about hydration and higher diuresis during HIPEC. Firstly, chemotherapy is administered intraperitoneally rather than usual intravenous route. Secondly, with variation in surface area the degree of absorption and serum concentration may vary. Thirdly, clearance of a drug depends on the renal blood flow rather than urine output. Finally, the etiology of renal failure can be often multifactorial instead of attributing only to platinum. Thus, maintaining euvolaemia by individualising fluid therapy seems essential.

39.3.3 Coagulation Monitoring

The etiology of coagulopathy is multifactorial and depends on various factors like the duration of surgery, PCI, resection extent, blood loss and hemodilution. This in turn depends on the volume of replacement fluids (crystalloids and colloids), packed red cells transfusion and temperature attained (hypothermia). Postoperatively, coagulopathy peaks at 24 h and can remain up to 72 h [12]. Intraoperative monitoring of coagulation parameters periodically is advisable. Most centres use prothrombin time (PT), activated partial thromboplastin time (aPTT) and international normalised ratio (INR) for monitoring in preoperative and postoperative period [13]. Thromboelastography (TEG or ROTEM) is used additionally in some centres [13, 14].

39.3.4 Fluid Management

An important aspect of haemodynamics in patients undergoing CRS-HIPEC is sustaining an optimal fluid balance. Intraoperative fluid loses may reach as high as 12 mL/kg during CRS phase [15]. To ensure optimal haemodynamic goals without causing volume overload adequate perioperative crystalloids and colloids are needed. Hydroxyethyl starch (HES) was found to have a adverse impact on the renal function in patients undergoing HIPEC. HES causes increased perioperative bleeding compared with crystalloids and albumin and increased reduction in maximum amplitude on TEG. Isotonic normal saline has high chloride content which can induce hyperchloremia and metabolic acidosis. Ringer's lactate and acetate-based solutions, have an electrolyte composition nearly similar to plasma and are generally preferred.

Increased fluid administration can be dangerous as it could lead to overload and tissue oedema thereby causing abdominal, cardiac or pulmonary complications. An increase in morbidity has been associated with fluid overload. Restrictive fluid regimens have demonstrated decreased perioperative mortality in other major surgical procedures. However, restricted fluid therapy can cause suboptimal tissue and renal perfusion in the face of extreme haemodynamic changes that occur during the phases of CRS-HIPEC. Secondary to surgical dissection, an extensive loss of protein in the ascitic fluid was observed. Hence, albumin replacement was found to be beneficial in patients requiring extensive debulking and large-volume ascitic fluid drainage.

39.3.5 Temperature Management

In the perioperative period among patients undergoing CRS-HIPEC, maintaining a normothermic status is a challenging goal. Wide variations in temperature can be caused by extensive CRS and HIPEC [16]. During the HIPEC phase hyperthermia raises metabolic rate, consequentially resulting in increased heart rate, demand for oxygen, end-tidal carbon dioxide, lactatemia and metabolic acidosis [16]. These peak of the hyperthermia usually reaches a peak level by 60 min after starting infusion. Once the temperature normalizes these hyperdynamic alterations reverse. Hyperthermia can lead to coagulopathies, renal and liver dysfunction, neuropathies and seizures. High body temperatures can be prevented by using forced air warmers at ambient temperature, using cold intravenous fluids (<6 °C), cooling mattress and ice packs placed in the axilla and head and neck area before initiating HIPEC. Cooling (active or passive) the patient before starting the HIPEC phase can also be done. During the CRS phase, a lower body temperature (hypothermia) can be associated with cardiac morbidity, decreased humoral and cell-mediated immunity and acid–base abnormalities [14]. Hence, body temperature should be kept at normothermic levels forced air warming with blankets and blood/fluid warmers.

39.4 ICU Management

39.4.1 Coagulation and Blood Products

Substantial blood loss may occur during cytoreductive surgery, and transfusion may be necessary. A hemoglobin transfusion threshold of 8 g/dL is considered by many centers.

Commonly used drugs include antifibrinolytic group i.e., tranexamic acid and epsilon aminocaproic acid. These are used routinely for high blood loss during various surgeries (e.g., cardiac surgery, orthopedic and spine surgery). Little literature exists for the use of tranexamic acid during CRS with HIPEC.

Abnormal coagulation can also be caused by hyperthermia but that in practical this is less likely at usual core body temperatures during HIPEC [16]. Most institutions consider sending blood studies for hemoglobin, platelets, fibrinogen, and coagulation parameters as necessary based on blood loss, and correct abnormalities. Thromboelastography can be useful tool to help diagnose coagulopathy.

The timing of removal of the epidural catheter can be affected by alteration in coagulation parameters and platelet counts following CRS and HIPEC. The reasons for coagulopathy can be multifactorial, including dilution related to blood loss, chemotherapy effects, and other factors. Most patients return to normal by postoperative day 6.

39.4.2 Fluid Therapy

39.4.2.1 Restrictive Fluid Therapy

Restrictive or goal directed fluid therapy is suggested rather than a liberal administration, to decrease complications related to fluid overload. Some of the useful points are highlighted below:

- A Crystalloid solution is used for maintenance IV fluid therapy at 4 mL/kg/h.
- Aim for urine output between 0.5 and 1 mL/kg/h during cytoreduction and 4 mL/kg/h during HIPEC.
- If the patient remains hypotensive and SVV and urine output thresholds have been reached, start a vasopressor.
- Ongoing bleeding as a source of hypotension should be investigated, and laboratory studies used to determine whether blood product transfusions are needed.
- Continue goal directed therapy in the postoperative period, adding vasopressors as necessary to maintain hemodynamic stability. Aim for urine output of >0.5 mL/h.

39.4.2.2 Restrictive Versus Goal Directed Versus Liberal Fluid Therapy

Early advocates for CRS with HIPEC included liberal fluid administration, particularly during HIPEC phase. But, practice has gradually shifted towards more restrictive fluid therapy for all major abdominal procedures, including CRS with HIPEC. Many institutional protocols now-a days include restrictive or goal directed fluid therapy. This practice change has resulted in low complication rates, morbidity and mortality [17]. Liberal fluid administration during CRS with HIPEC has also been associated with increased perioperative pulmonary and cardiac morbidity. For instance, in a randomized trial of goal directed versus standard fluid therapy for 80 patients (CRS with HIPEC), the incidence of major abdominal complications has decreased significantly (10.5 versus 38%). Additionally, the length of hospital stay also decreased (19 versus 29 days) in the group who received goal directed therapy (GDT). In a retrospective review of 169 CRS with HIPEC cases before and after an institutional change from liberal to restrictive fluid therapy, restrictive fluid therapy was associated with decreased 60-day complications and reduced hospital length of stay. Renal failure and peak creatinine rates were similar between groups [18].

39.4.3 Electrolytes

It is prudent to check blood gases and electrolytes every 30 min during HIPEC and during the two hours after infusion of HIPEC is complete. Abnormalities in electrolytes occur commonly as chemotherapy is infused during HIPEC [19]. The metabolic acidosis is multifactorial including:

(i) Massive fluids shifts and electrolyte disturbances due to hyperthermia generated in the peritoneal cavity.
(ii) Hyperthermia induced vasodilation and systemic hypotension lead to increased lactic acid production.
(iii) Lysis of tumor cells releasing organic acids.

As intra-abdominal pressure increases, respiratory acidosis occurs during the HIPEC phase, due to increased airway pressure and decreased functional residual capacity. Dextrose infusions containing carrier solutions can cause hyperglycemia and hyponatremia. Intravenous insulin infusion is usually required to correct hyperglycemia. Other electrolyte disturbances can also be encountered including hypomagnesemia, hypokalemia, and hypocalcemia .Postoperative electrolyte disturbances are very common as large intraoperative fluid shifts can occur following intravenous fluids administration and absorption of carrier solutions used during HIPEC.

39.4.4 Transfusion of Blood and Blood Products

CRS and HIPEC procedures are among the most extensive abdominal surgeries in terms of duration, multi-visceral resections and stripping of parietal peritoneum over large surface area resulting in significant blood loss. As per an Australian study 77% of patients undergoing CRS & HIPEC require intraoperative blood transfusion. High tumor burden (i.e. PCI > 15), extensive surgery (operative length more than 9 h or more than three peritonectomy procedures), preoperative anemia and impaired coagulation profile (INR > 1.2) are risk factors for massive blood transfusion (MBT) [20].

The deleterious effects of blood transfusion in colorectal surgeries are well known. It is associated with increased postoperative morbidity and inferior long-term outcomes [21, 22]. In patients undergoing CRS and HIPEC, a dose-dependent relationship between amount of packed red blood cell (PRBC) transfusion and oncological outcomes has been established [23]. Also, in a single centre experience of 936 patients, it was found that MBT (5 or more units) was associated with an increase in peri-operative grade III/IV morbidity and mortality. MBT was also associated with a significant compromise in long term survival among patients of colorectal carcinoma and pseudomyxoma peritonei. This is because allogenic blood transfusion aggravates systemic inflammation and transfusion-related immunomodulation [24].

Therefore, it is suggested that strategies to reduce incidence of MBT be implemented to achieve better perioperative and oncological outcomes. This can be achieved by increasing the threshold of blood transfusion, reduction of intraoperative blood losses and preoperative correction of anemia.

Restrictive approach (trigger of hemoglobin <7 g/dL in asymptomatic patients without significant cardiac comorbidity) and liberal approach ('10/30' approach: transfusion for hemoglobin <10 g/dL or hematocrit <30%) are the two approaches to blood transfusion. Upon meta-analysis, restrictive strategy was equivalent to liberal strategy in terms of peri-operative morbidity and mortality [25]. A Cochrane review of 31 trials across multiple specialities provides a good evidence that transfusion threshold of 7–8 g/dL with allogenic PRBCs is adequate for most patients [26]. Therefore, it would be prudent to adopt a restrictive approach to transfusion in patients undergoing CRS and HIPEC, so as to reduce the incidence of MBT.

Intraoperative blood losses can be minimized by improved surgical techniques and maintaining a prothrombotic state intra-operatively. Surgically, losses can be minimized by effective sealing of vessels using energy devices and double ligation, packing and compression of the operative field with dry gauzes after excision and by application of hemostatic materials. A balanced pro-thrombotic state can be achieved intraoperatively by appropriate transfusion of fibrinogen, prothrombin and calcium during peritonectomy. Sargant et al. [27] described a protocol to maintain a higher average fibrinogen levels intraoperatively and postoperatively. As per the protocol, Tranexemic acid is administered at the beginning of surgery and repeated at 4 h into the surgery. Throughout the surgery, the goal is to maintain the patient's fibrinogen level at 2 g/dL.

Alleviation of anemia preoperatively can significantly reduce requirement of peri-operative transfusion. In a Greek study, patients of gastro-intestinal tract cancer-induced anemia were randomised in a double-blind fashion to receive preoperative iron and recombinant erythropoietin (rEPO) or else placebo and iron. The patients who received rEPO received significantly fewer transfusions intraoperatively and postoperatively. Also, these patients experienced lower post-operative morbidity and improved 1-year survival [28].

39.4.5 Analgesia Modalities and Advantages

Pain after CRS and HIPEC is caused both due to inflammation caused by surgical injuries and chemotherapy agents which result in stimulation of peripheral as well as central nociceptors.

The optimal analgesic regimen for a major surgery should provide good pain relief, facilitate early mobilisation, early return of gut function and to prevent respiratory complications [29]. There are no randomised trials providing evidence for superior analgesic regimen in CRS & HIPEC. Multimodal analgesia (regional analgesia and local anesthesia), in order to reduce doses of parenteral opioids, remains the cornerstone of analgesia management.

Thoracic epidural anesthesia (TEA) containing short acting opiates and local anesthetics should be administered for at least 72 h after surgery [30]. TEA aids in recovery of gut function, improves the stability of anastomosis by aiding early recovery of gut function and reduces pulmonary complications [31–33]. Epidural block should be administered before incision and should include segments T5 to T11 [34]. An improved survival was noted when TEA was used for a minimum of 48 h postoperatively, among colorectal cancer and ovarian cancer patients undergoing HIPEC, upon retrospective analysis.

Combination of short-acting opioids and local anesthetics is considered the best for TEA, as this combination reduces the risk of hypotension and motor block due to sympathetic blockade [35]. In comparison to conventional continuous epidural infusion, patient controlled epidural analgesia is gaining popularity [36]. TEA should be removed 48–72 h postoperatively. Breakthrough pain, hypotension and neurological side effects of TEA should be treated as per local policy [34].

As HIPEC can potentially affect hemostasis and cause thrombocytopenia, administration of TEA is potentially unsafe. Korakiantis et al., in a prospective study, demonstrated that TEA is a safe option in patients undergoing CRS & HIPEC [37]. In a retrospective study evaluating 4277 patients who underwent CRS & HIPEC, none of the patient had postoperative epidural hematoma [38].

Transversus abdominal plane (TAP) block was found to be non-inferior to TEA in a study evaluating the postoperative analgesic effects of the two modalities in open colorectal surgery. TAP block produces analgesic effects on anterior abdominal wall skin, muscle and parietal peritoneum by acting on lower thoracic nerves (T7 to T12) and the anterior branch of first lumbar nerve (L1). Requirement of parenteral opioids can be effectively reduced by TAP block [39].

Paracetamol is a vital part of multimodal analgesia. NSAIDs can be given but careful consideration should be made in patients with renal dysfunction. Use of alternative analgesic drugs such as lidocaine, ketamine or gabapentin are presently not recommended, awaiting further studies.

39.4.6 Extubation Planning

Among patients undergoing CRS & HIPEC, the rate of extubation varies from 62 to 100%, depending upon institutional policy [40–42]. Most patients undergoing CRS & HIPEC can be extubated after surgery. A few patients, who are clinically unstable, require ionotropic support, had diaphragmatic resection or multiple comorbidities, remain intubated and are shifted to ICU for postoperative ventilation.

Criteria for extubation in CRS & HIPEC patients have not been defined and differ with institutional practices and anesthesiologist's comfort and experience. In a retrospective study by Balakrishnan et al. [42], higher PCI, longer duration of surgery, higher delta temperature, increased estimated blood loss, high intraoperative fluid requirement, lower mean arterial pressure and higher blood product requirement were associated with prolonged post-operative ventilation (>24 h) and longer ICU stay.

The advantages of early extubation include early ambulation and shorter duration of sedation, resulting in earlier return of bowel function and shorter duration of hospitalisation. Opioid requirement in perioperative period is reduced upon use of TEA and local anesthetic infusion, thereby facilitating early extubation.

ERAS guidelines for perioperative care in CRS & HIPEC recommend early extubation to be performed routinely in absence of contra-indications [43].

39.4.7 Thromboprophylaxis

Stasis, hypercoagulability and endothelial injury are the classic risk factors associated with venous thromboembolism (VTE) and are usually present in patients after CRS & HIPEC. Western data suggest that without thromboprophylaxis, 30–50% of patients of peritoneal malignancy undergoing surgery may experience VTE [44]. It is the most common cause of death in perioperative period [45].

Risk factors for VTE include disease burden, blood transfusion and extent of surgery, PCI, blood loss, operative time, length of hospital and ICU stay and lack of administration of anticoagulant on discharge [46]. Standard guidelines for thromboprophylaxis among patients undergoing major cancer surgery can be extrapolated to patients undergoing CRS & HIPEC.

It is observed that 2/3rd of cases of VTE occur in patients 'after' discharge. Extended thromboprophylaxis reduce the 60 day VTE rate from 10 to 5% and post discharge VTE rate from 8 to 2%. ERAS guidelines for CRS & HIPEC strongly recommend use of peri-operative mechanical and pharmacological thromboprophylaxis and also recommend extended pharmacological thromboprophylaxis [30].

39.4.8 Immediate Postoperative Complications

Review of literature reports 18–52% major morbidity in patients undergoing CRS & HIPEC during the post-operative period [47]. Majority of complications are related to surgical procedures and can be handled as per standard guidelines. In this section, we will be focussing on immediate systemic complications caused by HIPEC.

Risk of postoperative renal dysfunction is significant and multifactorial. Nephrotoxicity is the main dose-limiting side effect of cisplatin, especially at doses greater than 240 mg [48]. Sodium thiosulfate can be used to reduce the risk of renal failure [49]. Mitomycin C (MMC) can also less commonly lead to nephrotoxicity. Goal directed fluid resuscitation and optimising oxygen delivery by hemodynamic monitoring is perhaps the most suitable method to prevent and/or treat nephrotoxicity [50]. Use of other nephrotoxic agents in these patients should be avoided. Tissue inhibitor of metalloproteinases-2 (TIMP-2) and insulin-like growth factor binding protein 7 (IGFBP 7) have been approved by USFDA as biomarkers for risk stratification of acute kidney injury (AKI) in critically ill patients and can be extrapolated for use among patients undergoing HIPEC [51].

Respiratory complications are important source of morbidity after CRS & HIPEC and should therefore be prevented by prophylactic usage of non-invasive ventilation (NIV) or HFNC and routine implementation of thoracic epidural analgesia.

Septic shock and multisystem organ failure is the leading cause of mortality in patients undergoing CRS & HIPEC and causative factors include extensive nature of procedure, immunosuppression due to previous chemotherapy, surgical complications as well as extensive peritoneal inflammation and inflammatory response.

Hematological toxicity is a recognised complication of HIPEC and has been reported in up to 10–28% of patients in postoperative period [52]. It appears to be primarily related to the type of chemotherapy agent used for HIPEC. Using a dose of MMC 35 mg/m^2 over 90 min of HIPEC can result in postoperative neutropenia/leukopenia in as many as 27% of patients. Routine prophylactic granulocyte colony-stimulating factor (G-CSF) does not alter neutropenia rates but may be used to avoid or prevent profound aplasia when white cell counts are decreasing [53].

Major surgical complications are anastomotic leaks (0–9%), intraabdominal abscesses (0–37%), intestinal perforation/peritonitis (0–10%), fistulas (0–23%) and prolonged ileus (0–86%). Intra abdominal bleeding, bile leaks, pancreatitis, major wound infections, acalculous cholecystitis, mesenteric ischemia, mechanical intestinal obstruction are other surgical complications that can be encountered after CRS and HIPEC

39.5 Conclusion

Peri-operative management and critical care are extremely important determinants of outcomes following CRS and HIPEC. Dedicated multi-disciplinary teams including Anesthesiologists, and critical care experts play a significant role in the management of these patients. Protocol based management approach and establishment of standard operating procedures is critical for optimal outcomes. Important domains need to be focussed include fluid, blood and protein losses, increased intra-abdominal pressure, systemic hypo-/hyperthermia and increased metabolic rate in patients undergoing HIPEC. TAE and NIV are recommended to ensure adequate pain relief and early post-operative extubation. Postoperatively, volume status optimization, early nutrition support, sufficient anti-coagulation and point of care coagulation management are essential. Systemic toxicities need to be identified early and optimally managed.

References

1. Dedrick RL, Myers CE, Bungay PM, DeVita VT Jr. Pharmacokinetic rationale for peritoneal drug administration in the treatment of ovarian cancer. Cancer Treat Rep. 1978;62(1):1–11. PMID 626987 [Internet] [cited 3 Apr 2021]. Available from: https://pubmed.ncbi.nlm.nih.gov/626987
2. Valle SJ, Alzahrani NA, Liauw W, Sugarbaker PH, Bhatt A, Morris DL. Hyperthermic intraperitoneal chemotherapy (HIPEC) methodology, drugs and bidirectional chemotherapy. Indian J Surg Oncol. 2016;7:152–9.
3. Chua TC, Yan TD, Saxena A, Morris DL. Should the treatment of peritoneal carcinomatosis by cytoreductive surgery and hyperthermic intraperitoneal chemotherapy still be regarded as a highly morbid procedure?: a systematic review of morbidity and mortality. Ann Surg. 2009;249:900.
4. Piccioni F, Casiraghi C, Fumagalli L, Kusamura S, Baratti D, Deraco M, et al. Epidural analgesia for cytoreductive surgery with peritonectomy and heated intraperitoneal chemotherapy. Int J Surg. 2015;16(Pt A):99–106.
5. Solanki SL, Mukherjee S, Agarwal V, Thota RS, Balakrishnan K, Shah SB, Desai N, Garg R, Ambulkar RP, Bhorkar NM, Patro V, Sinukumar S, Venketeswaran MV, Joshi MP, Chikkalingegowda RH, Gottumukkala V, Owusu-Agyemang P, Saklani AP, Mehta SS, Seshadri RA, Bell JC, Bhatnagar S, Divatia JV. Society of Onco-Anaesthesia and Perioperative Care consensus guidelines for perioperative management of patients for cytoreductive surgery and hyperthermic intraperitoneal chemotherapy (CRS-HIPEC). Indian J Anaesth. 2019;63(12):972–87. https://doi.org/10.4103/ija.IJA_765_19. Epub 11 Dec 2019. PMID: 31879421
6. Baratti D, Kusamura S, Laterza B, Balestra MR, Deraco M. Early and long-term postoperative management following cytoreductive surgery and hyperthermic intraperitoneal chemotherapy. World J Gastrointest Oncol. 2010;2:36–43.
7. Padmakumar AV. Intensive care management of patient after cytoreductive surgery and HIPEC—a concise review. Indian J Surg Oncol. 2016;7:244–8.
8. Polderman KH, Varon J, Marik PE. Fluid management decisions should not be guided by fixed central venous pressure targets. Am J Emerg Med. 2015;33:1311.
9. Hakeam HA, Breakiet M, Azzam A, Nadeem A, Amin T. The incidence of cisplatin nephrotoxicity post hyperthermic intraperitoneal chemotherapy (HIPEC) and cytoreductive surgery. Ren Fail. 2014;36:1486–91.
10. Cata JP, Zavala AM, Van Meter A, Williams UU, Soliz J, Hernandez M, Owusu-Agyemang P. Identification of risk factors associated with postoperative acute kidney injury after cytoreductive surgery with hyperthermic intraperitoneal chemotherapy: a retrospective study. Int J Hyperthermia. 2018;34:538–44.
11. Eng OS, Dumitra S, O'Leary M, Raoof M, Wakabayashi M, Dellinger TH, et al. Association of fluid administration with morbidity in cytoreductive surgery with hyperthermic intraperitoneal chemotherapy. JAMA Surg. 2017;152:1156–60.
12. Raspé C, Flöther L, Schneider R, Bucher M, Piso P. Best practice for perioperative management of patients with cytoreductive surgery and HIPEC. Eur J Surg Oncol. 2017;43:1013–27.
13. Reynolds L, Beckmann J, Kurz A. Perioperative complications of hypothermia. Best Pract Res Clin Anaesthesiol. 2008;22:645–57.
14. Bell JC, Rylah BG, Chambers RW, Peet H, Mohamed F, Moran BJ. Perioperative management of patients undergoing cytoreductive surgery combined with heated intraperitoneal chemotherapy for peritoneal surface malignancy: a multi-institutional experience. Ann Surg Oncol. 2012;19:4244–51.
15. Stens J, Hering JP, van der Hoeven CWP, Boom A, Traast HS, Garmers LE, et al. The added value of cardiac index and pulse pressure variation monitoring to mean arterial pressure-guided volume therapy in moderate-risk abdominal surgery (COGUIDE): a pragmatic multicentre randomised controlled trial. Anaesthesia. 2017;72:1078–87.

16. Esquivel J, Angulo F, Bland RK, Stephens AD, Sugarbaker PH. Hemodynamic and cardiac function parameters during heated intraoperative intraperitoneal chemotherapy using the open 'coliseum technique'. Ann Surg Oncol. 2000;7:296–300.
17. Colantonio L, Claroni C, Fabrizi L, Marcelli ME, Sofra M, Giannarelli D, et al. A randomized trial of goal directed vs. standard fluid therapy in cytoreductive surgery with hyperthermic intraperitoneal chemotherapy. J Gastrointest Surg. 2015;19:722–9.
18. Hendrix RJ, Damle A, Williams C, Harris A, Spanakis S, Lambert DH, Lambert LA. Restrictive intraoperative fluid therapy is associated with decreased morbidity and length of stay following hyperthermic intraperitoneal chemoperfusion. Ann Surg Oncol. 2019;26(2): 490–6.
19. Said ET, Sztain JF, Abramson WB, Meineke MN, Furnish TJ, Schmidt UH, et al. A dedicated acute pain service is associated with reduced postoperative opioid requirements in patients undergoing cytoreductive surgery with hyperthermic intraperitoneal chemotherapy. Anesth Analg. 2018;127:1044.
20. Saxena A, Yan TD, Chua TC, et al. Risk factors for massive blood transfusion in cytoreductive surgery: a multivariate analysis of 243 procedures. Ann Surg Oncol. 2009;16:2195–203. https://doi.org/10.1245/s10434-009-0484-7.
21. Acheson AG, Brookes MJ, Spahn DR. Effects of allogeneic red blood cell transfusions on clinical outcomes in patients undergoing colorectal cancer surgery: a systematic review and meta-analysis. Ann Surg. 2012;256:235–44. https://doi.org/10.1097/SLA.0b013e31825b35d5.
22. Amato A, Pescatori M. Perioperative blood transfusions for the recurrence of colorectal cancer. Cochrane Database Syst Rev. 2006;CD005033. https://doi.org/10.1002/14651858.CD005033.pub2.
23. Nizri E, Kusamura S, Fallabrino G, et al. Dose-dependent effect of red blood cells transfusion on perioperative and long-term outcomes in peritoneal surface malignancies treated with cytoreduction and HIPEC. Ann Surg Oncol. 2018;25:3264–70. https://doi.org/10.1245/s10434-018-6630-3.
24. Saxena A, Valle SJ, Liauw W, Morris DL. Allogenic blood transfusion is an independent predictor of poorer peri-operative outcomes and reduced long-term survival after cytoreductive surgery and hyperthermic intraperitoneal chemotherapy: a review of 936 cases. J Gastrointest Surg. 2017;21:1318–27. https://doi.org/10.1007/s11605-017-3444-8.
25. Chen Q-H, Wang H-L, Liu L, et al. Effects of restrictive red blood cell transfusion on the prognoses of adult patients undergoing cardiac surgery: a meta-analysis of randomized controlled trials. Critical Care. 2018;22:142. https://doi.org/10.1186/s13054-018-2062-5.
26. Carson JL, Stanworth SJ, Roubinian N, et al. Transfusion thresholds and other strategies for guiding allogeneic red blood cell transfusion. Cochrane Database Syst Rev. 2016;10(10):CD002042.
27. Sargant N, Roy A, Simpson S, et al. A protocol for management of blood loss in surgical treatment of peritoneal malignancy by cytoreductive surgery and hyperthermic intraperitoneal chemotherapy. Transfus Med. 2016;26:118–22. https://doi.org/10.1111/tme.12301.
28. Kosmadakis N, Messaris E, Maris A, et al. Perioperative erythropoietin administration in patients with gastrointestinal tract cancer: prospective randomized double-blind study. Ann Surg. 2003;237:417–21. https://doi.org/10.1097/01.SLA.0000055275.38740.56.
29. Veenhof AAFA, Vlug MS, van der Pas MHGM, et al. Surgical stress response and postoperative immune function after laparoscopy or open surgery with fast track or standard perioperative care: a randomized trial. Ann Surg. 2012;255:216–21. https://doi.org/10.1097/SLA.0b013e31824336e2.
30. Hübner M, Kusamura S, Villeneuve L, et al. Guidelines for perioperative care in CytoReductive Surgery (CRS) with or without Hyperthermic IntraPEritoneal Chemotherapy (HIPEC): Enhanced Recovery After Surgery (ERAS®) Society recommendations—Part II: Postoperative management and special considerations. Eur J Surg Oncol. 2020;46:2311–23. https://doi.org/10.1016/j.ejso.2020.08.006.
31. Michelet P, D'Journo X-B, Roch A, et al. Perioperative risk factors for anastomotic leakage after esophagectomy. Chest. 2005;128:3461–6. https://doi.org/10.1378/chest.128.5.3461.

32. Pöpping DM, Elia N, Marret E, et al. Protective effects of epidural analgesia on pulmonary complications after abdominal and thoracic surgery: a meta-analysis. Arch Surg. 2008;143:990–9. Discussion 1000. https://doi.org/10.1001/archsurg.143.10.990.
33. Cook TM, Counsell D, Wildsmith JAW. Major complications of central neuraxial block: report on the Third National Audit Project of the Royal College of Anaesthetists. Br J Anaesth. 2009;102:179–90. https://doi.org/10.1093/bja/aen360.
34. Owusu-Agyemang P, Soliz J, Hayes-Jordan A, et al. Safety of epidural analgesia in the perioperative care of patients undergoing cytoreductive surgery with hyperthermic intraperitoneal chemotherapy. Ann Surg Oncol. 2014;21:1487–93. https://doi.org/10.1245/s10434-013-3221-1.
35. Feldheiser A, Aziz O, Baldini G, et al. Enhanced Recovery After Surgery (ERAS) for gastrointestinal surgery, part 2: consensus statement for anaesthesia practice. Acta Anaesthesiol Scand. 2016;60:289–334. https://doi.org/10.1111/aas.12651.
36. Osseis M, Weyrech J, Gayat E, et al. Epidural analgesia combined with a comprehensive physiotherapy program after Cytoreductive Surgery and HIPEC is associated with enhanced postoperative recovery and reduces intensive care unit stay: a retrospective study of 124 patients. Eur J Surg Oncol. 2016;42:1938–43. https://doi.org/10.1016/j.ejso.2016.06.390.
37. Korakianitis O, Daskalou T, Alevizos L, et al. Lack of significant intraoperative coagulopathy in patients undergoing cytoreductive surgery and hyperthermic intraperitoneal chemotherapy (HIPEC) indicates that epidural anaesthesia is a safe option. Int J Hyperthermia. 2015;31:857–62.
38. Wang X, Li T. Postoperative pain pathophysiology and treatment strategies after CRS + HIPEC for peritoneal cancer. World J Surg Oncol. 2020;18:62. https://doi.org/10.1186/s12957-020-01842-7.
39. Jakobsson J, Wickerts L, Forsberg S, Ledin G. Transversus abdominal plane (TAP) block for postoperative pain management: a review. F1000Res. 2015;4 https://doi.org/10.12688/f1000research.7015.1.
40. Cooksley TJ, Haji-Michael P. Post-operative critical care management of patients undergoing cytoreductive surgery and heated intraperitoneal chemotherapy (HIPEC). World J Surg Oncol. 2011;9:169. https://doi.org/10.1186/1477-7819-9-169.
41. Thong SY, Chia CS, Ng O, et al. A review of 111 anaesthetic patients undergoing cytoreductive surgery and hyperthermic intraperitoneal chemotherapy. Singapore Med J. 2017;58:488–96. https://doi.org/10.11622/smedj.2016078.
42. Balakrishnan KP, Survesan S. Anaesthetic management and perioperative outcomes of cytoreductive surgery with hyperthermic intraperitoneal chemotherapy: a retrospective analysis. Indian J Anaesth. 2018;62:188–96. https://doi.org/10.4103/ija.IJA_39_18.
43. Hübner M, Kusamura S, Villeneuve L, et al. Guidelines for perioperative care in CytoReductive Surgery (CRS) with or without Hyperthermic IntraPEritoneal Chemotherapy (HIPEC): Enhanced Recovery After Surgery (ERAS®) Society recommendations—Part I: Preoperative and intraoperative management. Eur J Surg Oncol. 2020;46:2292–310. https://doi.org/10.1016/j.ejso.2020.07.041.
44. Sleightholm R, Watley D, Wahlmeier S, et al. The efficacy of dextran-40 as a venous thromboembolism prophylaxis strategy in cytoreductive surgery and hyperthermic intraperitoneal chemotherapy. Am Surg. 2017;83:134–40.
45. Agnelli G, Bolis G, Capussotti L, et al. A clinical outcome-based prospective study on venous thromboembolism after cancer surgery: the @RISTOS project. Ann Surg. 2006;243:89–95. https://doi.org/10.1097/01.sla.0000193959.44677.48.
46. Rottenstreich A, Kalish Y, Kleinstern G, et al. Factors associated with thromboembolic events following cytoreductive surgery and hyperthermic intraperitoneal chemotherapy. J Surg Oncol. 2017;116:914–20. https://doi.org/10.1002/jso.24746.
47. Baratti D, Kusamura S, Pietrantonio F, et al. Progress in treatments for colorectal cancer peritoneal metastases during the years 2010–2015. A systematic review. Crit Rev Oncol Hematol. 2016;100:209–22.
48. Kusamura S, Baratti D, Younan R, et al. Impact of cytoreductive surgery and hyperthermic intraperitoneal chemotherapy on systemic toxicity. Ann Surg Oncol. 2007;14:2550–8.

49. Van Driel WJ, Koole SN, Sikorska K, et al. Hyperthermic intraperitoneal chemotherapy in ovarian cancer. N Engl J Med. 2018;378:230–40.
50. Raspé C, Flöther L, Schneider R, et al. Best practice for perioperative management of patients with cytoreductive surgery and HIPEC. Eur J Surg Oncol. 2017;43:1013–27. https://doi.org/10.1016/j.ejso.2016.09.008.
51. Kashani K, Al-Khafaji A, Ardiles T, et al. Discovery and validation of cell cycle arrest biomarkers in human acute kidney injury. Crit Care. 2013;17:R25. https://doi.org/10.1186/cc12503.
52. Yan TD, Deraco M, Baratti D, et al. Cytoreductive surgery and hyperthermic intraperitoneal chemotherapy for malignant peritoneal mesothelioma: multi-institutional experience. J Clin Oncol. 2009;27:6237–42. https://doi.org/10.1200/JCO.2009.23.9640.
53. Feferman Y, Bhagwandin S, Kim J, et al. Conflicting data on the incidence of leukopenia and neutropenia after heated intraperitoneal chemotherapy with mitomycin C. Ann Surg Oncol. 2017;24:3831–6.

40 Communication with Patient and Family in ICU

Vikas Kumar

40.1 Communication in Intensive Care Unit

Communication is a mutual exchange of information between two or more individuals—a basic requirement of life and vital in truly commenting with the patient and their family members. The intensive care unit (ICU) environment can be very overwhelming, introducing high levels of stress, anxiety, and depression and effective communication improves decision-making and contributes to patient and family satisfaction as well as their psychological well-being [1–3].

This can also ease the transition from curative to palliative care and reduce the use of futile therapies. Even though communication between healthcare providers, patients, and families has been identified as critically important, it is also the least accomplished factor in the quality of care in intensive care units because of lack of education and training. Inadequate communication is one of the important reasons for treatment conflicts. It is recommended that proactive communication should be implemented to prevent intractable treatment conflicts [4].

> *The single biggest problem with communication is the illusion that it has taken place.*
> *George Bernard Shaw.*

Some of the problems in intensive care unit communications are unfamiliar surroundings from alarms, the severity of illness, altered mental status from sedatives or illness, and barriers of verbal communication because of the endotracheal tube. The communication between family members and clinicians is often time confusing because of various communication techniques, physician workload, and

V. Kumar (✉)
Department of Anesthesiology & Critical Care Medicine, Medical College of Georgia at Augusta University, Augusta, GA, USA
e-mail: vikkumar@augusta.edu

V. Kumar et al. (eds.), *Onco-critical Care*,
https://doi.org/10.1007/978-981-16-9929-0_40

multi-disciplinary team managing the patients [5]. Transparent communication improves patient understanding and supports autonomy, informed decision-making, and relationship development [6, 7]. Proactive transparency appears promising to increase understanding and collaboration. More than 50% of family members do not understand a diagnosis, prognosis, or treatment. The clinician-family communication can be improved with standard scheduled family-centered rounds, interdisciplinary family meetings, daily updates, and electronic patient portals. This has been shown to improve patient-family satisfaction scores in intensive care units. It is important to understand the barriers and facilitate family participation in intensive care unit rounds. The day may sound like a daily routine for the ICU team but not for patients or family members. Empathetic communication is often lacking because of barriers like time constraints, chaotic environment, managing own emotions, and patient's negative affect and empathetic communication benefits both patients and physicians. Physicians with higher empathy scores have lower burnout, a higher sense of well-being.

Telemedicine options may facilitate family participation for families who live far away or have time constraints [8]. There are multiple apps and online resources available as well to achieve communication goals and decrease barriers like language. Family members can also participate virtually during daily rounds and get updates.

The American Thoracic Society, Society of Critical Care Medicine, and European Society of Critical Care Medicine recommended practices for improving communication and support in the intensive care unit. This includes conducting regular, interprofessional family meetings in a dedicated meeting space. It is important to establish consensus among treating clinicians before the meeting. The physicians should use family-centered communication strategies and foster shared decision-making. While communicating to the family members or surrogates, provide information in small chunks, acknowledge and address emotion and support religious/spiritual needs and concerns.

40.2 Realistic Hope

The communication of distressing news with patients can be very stressful to physicians, patients, and family members. There is a delicate balance between fostering realistic hope and unethically creating unrealistic expectations. A study by Hegarty et al. [9] showed the majority of patients preferred a realistic and individualized approach with detailed information when discussing prognosis. Research is lacking in determining how patients define hope and how healthcare professionals communicate hope to patients. Hope is a core need and tool for dealing with cancer illness and promotes cancer patient's adaptability to their illness [10].

40.3 The Psychological Aspect of Cancer Diagnosis

A cancer diagnosis can cause stress, anxiety, and depression (SAD) in patients, families, and caregivers. It is vital to provide psycho-educational and psychosocial support and psychotherapy for cancer patients and their families. Depressive feelings and disappointment were reported by 90% of patients while 85% of them reported fear, hopelessness, and emptiness in a study by Klikovac et al. [11]. Many people experience shock, anxiety, denial, and depression as stages of adjustment. This is followed by withdrawal, anger, acknowledgment, acceptance, and adjustment. The prevalence of psychological symptoms in family caregivers of critically ill patients in ICU vary widely and includes depression, anxiety, post-traumatic stress disorder [12] and it is directly proportional to ICU length of stay.

The cancer diagnosis leads to a potential for an unpredictable course [13] and a complex set of issues, including dealing with physical symptoms from the disease and treatment. The six feared "D"—discomfort, dependency, disfigurement, disability, disruption, disengagement, and death mentioned by Holland et al., [14]. The complexity and variability of psychological issues associated with cancer have created the demand for highly skilled practitioners who are trained to provide multilevel assessment and intervention throughout the illness continuum. Cancer has more than a physical impact, there are psychological, social, spiritual, informational, physical, emotional, and practical consequences as well.

The survivors from cancer have fear and uncertainty, changes in family roles, changes in employment, and increased risk for additional cancers [15]. Encouraging patients and caregivers to discuss personal cancer-related concerns may improve their ability to cope with the illness together [16].

40.4 Medical Ethics

Ethics are a cornerstone to the proper and professional practice of medicine. We often face ethical and decision-making challenges in intensive care units. Conflicts happen with the right to refuse or the right to demand treatment. An unconscious patient who has no close relatives or friends, no power of attorney, the clinical team cannot make decisions. For example, an elderly woman in ICU after cardiac arrest, confirmed hypoxic brain injury, no advance directive, and lack of surrogate brings ethical challenges with decision-making regarding continuation or discontinuation of care. An unrepresented patient lacks decision-making capacity, has no advance directive or surrogate decision-maker.

An increasing number of patients are dying in intensive care units and up to 90% of ICU deaths occur after the decision to withdraw life support and of those up to 95% of patients are not capable of making decisions [17, 18]. Ethical dilemmas have increased significantly since the early 1990s mainly because of the development of advanced medical technologies and therapies. Medical ethics guide decision-making and provide a moral compass to use in not so straightforward situations.

The 6 basic principles of medical ethics include autonomy, beneficence, nonmaleficence, veracity, distributive justice, and proportionality.

Autonomy is a patient's right to make decisions for themselves according to their morals and beliefs. Patient education and informed consent are important elements of autonomy. There are exceptions to autonomy and challenges when a patient is legally deemed unable to make rational decisions for themselves such as dementia (Incompetence) or clinically due to delirium, psychosis, lack of consciousness (Incapacity). The criteria for adequate decision-making include the ability to comprehend information relevant to the decision, the ability to compare alternatives of the decision with personal values and goals, and the ability to communicate in a consistent and meaningful manner. If there is any doubt regarding capacity, formal psychiatric consultation should be obtained to evaluate decision-making capacity. If the patient is incapacitated, respect for the patient's autonomy can be preserved through the use of surrogate decision-makers. This can be done in advance formally by creating an advanced directive or durable power of attorney. Paternalism is making decisions for the patient without seeking their input.

Beneficence is a value in which providers take actions or recommend courses in the patient's best interest. When patient autonomy is compromised, beneficence needs to be the guiding ethics. Beneficence promotes patients' best interest by understanding patient perspective, addressing misunderstanding and concern, and letting the patient decide.

Nonmaleficence is closely related to beneficence. It is abstaining from any action that may bring harm to the patient. "*Do no harm*". Beneficence is what you do and nonmaleficence is what you don't do.

Nonmaleficence forbids physicians from providing ineffective therapies.

Veracity (truth-telling) is honesty and revealing all pertinent details of a patient's medical conditions to them, as well as risks and benefits of a procedure, and their prognosis. It is never OK to lie to or deceive a patient, for any reason.

Distributive justice is the proper allocation of resources in a manner that is fair and justified. It is not necessarily equal allocation of resources.

Proportionality is a principle that ensures a medical treatment or plan is commensurate with the illness and with the goals of treatment. This is to ensure that benefits are maximized (beneficence) and risks are minimized (nonmaleficence).

Physicians have no obligation to provide treatments that offer no benefit and are potentially inappropriate (futile) and providing care to such patients is a major source of burnout among healthcare providers in intensive care units. There should be a case review by an interdisciplinary institutional committee and clinicians should obtain a second medical opinion to verify the prognosis and the judgment that the requested treatment is inappropriate (Society of Critical Care Medicine guideline). The ethics committee consultation should be sought to provide guidance in ethical dilemmas. In a study by Schneiderman et al. [19], there was no difference in mortality but the reduction in hospital, ICU, and ventilator days concluded that ethics consultation is helpful.

In intensive care units, predictive scoring systems like Acute Physiology and Chronic Health Evaluation (APACHE) III predict the probability of survival for populations and should be used cautiously to guide the prognosis of critically ill patients.

40.5 Advance Care Planning

Advance care planning is making decisions about the healthcare a patient would want to receive when facing a medical crisis based on personal values and preferences. This includes completing advance directives for types of treatments and assigning a decision-maker when a patient is unable to speak because of critical conditions. Sharing personal values with loved ones helps prevent an emotional burden on family members when they are asked to make tough decisions regarding the care of their loved ones. Advance care planning allows the person to have more choice and improve the quality of the end-of-life care. Everyone regardless of age or health should consider advance care planning. Some of the triggers for initiation include when the patients' medical condition changes, deterioration of cognitive function, and poor prognostication [20]. Advance care planning plays an essential role in maintaining autonomy when people are no longer able to communicate wishes directly and support treatment decisions in healthcare delivery during legal and ethical dilemmas.

Although advance care planning is a novel concept to meaningful advance directives, it is still not widely practiced. It requires facilitated discussions with patients or their proxies and medical professionals. This is necessary but often not an easy conversation.

40.6 Surrogate Decision Making

An increasing number of deaths in intensive care units occur after decisions to withdraw life support and more than 90% of those patients are not capable of autonomous choice [17, 18]. Surrogate decision-maker, also known as health care proxy, is an advocate for incompetent adults. Ideally, patients will have created a durable power of attorney for health care. In case of no legal document, the current spouse can serve as a surrogate. Clinicians may want to include surrogates in advance care planning before decision-making and identify and address surrogate stressors during decision-making. Studies have estimated that surrogates make approximately 75% of decisions for hospitalized patients with a life-threatening illness.

Surrogate decision-making has two standards—substituted judgment standard and best interests standard. Substituted judgment standard is based on what the patient would have decided if they had been able to and the best interest standard is when we don't have any idea of what the patient would have wished. Advance directives like the durable power of attorney or living will guide decision-making with substituted judgment standards and patients can decide what medical interventions. The best interest standard is vague and causes inconsistency in the treatment of medically identical patients.

When surrogates have unilateral decision capacity, it can cause strong emotional challenges to forgoing life-prolonging treatment for a loved one which is most of the time an emotional decision. Physicians should not have unilateral decision-making capacity as well because of significant practice variability among them.

In the case of no designated surrogate, the typical rank order is spouse, adult child, parent, adult sibling, grandparent, adult grandchild, and adult close friend. End-of-life decision-making should not be done solely by the medical team even if this is in the best interest standard.

Patients lack decision-making capacity from critical illness or medications in intensive care units, but may still possess the capacity to designate a surrogate. Decision-making capacity is lost in many cognitive illnesses, but patients can still understand and express a preference regarding choosing a surrogate and they may still understand the role of a surrogate in their care. Patients who won't be able to make medical decisions should not be prevented from selecting a surrogate [21].

References

1. Lilly CM, De Meo DL, Sonna LA, Haley KJ, Massaro AF, Wallace RF, et al. An intensive communication intervention for the critically ill. Am J Med. 2000;109(6):469–75.
2. Ong LM, de Haes JC, Hoos AM, Lammes FB. Doctor-patient communication: a review of the literature. Soc Sci Med. 1995;40(7):903–18.
3. Stewart MA. Effective physician-patient communication and health outcomes: a review. CMAJ. 1995;152(9):1423–33.
4. Bosslet GT, Pope TM, Rubenfeld GD, Lo B, Truog RD, Rushton CH, et al. An official ATS/AACN/ACCP/ESICM/SCCM policy statement: responding to requests for potentially inappropriate treatments in intensive care units. Am J Respir Crit Care Med. 2015;191(11):1318–30.
5. Odeniyi F, Nathanson PG, Schall TE, Walter JK. Communication challenges of oncologists and intensivists caring for Pediatric oncology patients: a qualitative study. J Pain Symptom Manag. 2017;54(6):909–15.
6. Carmel S, Singer Y, Yosef-Sela N, Bachner YG. Open communication between caregivers' and terminally ill cancer patients about illness and death: the role of gender—a correlational study. Eur J Oncol Nurs. 2020;49:101828.
7. Robins L, Witteborn S, Miner L, Mauksch L, Edwards K, Brock D. Identifying transparency in physician communication. Patient Educ Couns. 2011;83(1):73–9.
8. Stelson EA, Carr BG, Golden KE, Martin N, Richmond TS, Delgado MK, et al. Perceptions of family participation in intensive care unit rounds and telemedicine: a qualitative assessment. Am J Crit Care. 2016;25(5):440–7.
9. Hagerty RG, Butow PN, Ellis PM, Lobb EA, Pendlebury SC, Leighl N, et al. Communicating with realism and hope: incurable cancer patients' views on the disclosure of prognosis. J Clin Oncol. 2005;23(6):1278–88.
10. Bovero A, Opezzo M, Botto R, Gottardo F, Torta R. Hope in end-of-life cancer patients: a cross-sectional analysis. Palliat Support Care. 2021:1–7.

11. Klikovac T, Djurdjevic A. Psychological aspects of the cancer patients' education: thoughts, feelings, behavior and body reactions of patients faced with diagnosis of cancer. J BUON. 2010;15(1):153–6.
12. Johnson CC, Suchyta MR, Darowski ES, Collar EM, Kiehl AL, Van J, et al. Psychological sequelae in family caregivers of critically III intensive care unit patients. A systematic review. Ann Am Thorac Soc. 2019;16(7):894–909.
13. Dankert A, Duran G, Engst-Hastreiter U, Keller M, Waadt S, Henrich G, et al. Fear of progression in patients with cancer, diabetes mellitus and chronic arthritis. Rehabilitation (Stuttg). 2003;42(3):155–63.
14. Holland JC. Improving the human side of cancer care: psycho-oncology's contribution. Cancer J. 2001;7(6):4.
15. Ganz PA. Late effects of cancer and its treatment. Semin Oncol Nurs. 2001;17(4):241–8.
16. Tiete J, Delvaux N, Lienard A, Razavi D. Efficacy of a dyadic intervention to improve communication between patients with cancer and their caregivers: a randomized pilot trial. Patient Educ Couns. 2020;
17. White DB, Curtis JR. Establishing an evidence base for physician-family communication and shared decision making in the intensive care unit. Crit Care Med. 2006;34(9):2500–1.
18. White DB, Curtis JR, Lo B, Luce JM. Decisions to limit life-sustaining treatment for critically ill patients who lack both decision-making capacity and surrogate decision-makers. Crit Care Med. 2006;34(8):2053–9.
19. Schneiderman LJ, Gilmer T, Teetzel HD, Dugan DO, Blustein J, Cranford R, et al. Effect of ethics consultations on nonbeneficial life-sustaining treatments in the intensive care setting: a randomized controlled trial. JAMA. 2003;290(9):1166–72.
20. Bovero A, Opezzo M, Botto R, Gottardo F, Torta R. Hope in end-of-life cancer patients: a cross-sectional analysis. Palliat Support Care. 2021:1–7.
21. Navin M, Wasserman JA, Stahl D, Tomlinson T. The capacity to designate a surrogate is distinct from decisional capacity: normative and empirical considerations. J Med Ethics. 2021;

Palliative Care in Intensive Care Unit

41

Swati Bhan, Rudranil Nandi, Saurabh Vig, and Seema Mishra

41.1 Introduction

The Intensive Care Unit (ICU) in a hospital serves and cares for critically ill, debilitated, and most sick patients. Thus, these units witness a high rate of mortality of around 20 percent of all admissions [1]. Of all the patients admitted in a medical or surgical ICU, not all have a good prognosis or disease amenable to cure. Some patients are terminally sick and nearing the end of life. An approach that differs from the standard curative intent for an ICU patient is required for these patients for optimal utilization of ICU and hospital resources. Palliative care with a focus on the end of life care and symptom control to improve quality of life in terminal sickness and alleviate the suffering of patients and care-giver is the ideal approach for such patients. Thus, ICUs are critically important locations for providing effective, high-quality end-of-life and palliative care [2].

Despite developments in the field of palliative care and critical care medicine, the role of palliative care in the ICU setting is still not recognized and there is no consensus on the basics of palliative care practice in the ICU.

Palliative care is not an alternative to critical care but both specialties go hand in hand as a part of comprehensive care from the time of admission to ICU of patients who are at the end-stage of a chronic illness or suffer from advanced malignancy beyond curative treatment. Therefore, from the time of admission to ICU, patients

S. Bhan · S. Vig
Onco-Anaesthesia and Palliative Medicine, NCI Jhajjar, AIIMS, New Delhi, India

R. Nandi
Tata Medical Center, Kolkata, West Bengal, India

S. Mishra (✉)
Department of Onco-Anesthesia and Palliative Medicine, Dr. B.R.A. Institute Rotary Cancer Hospital, All India Institute of Medical Sciences, New Delhi, India

V. Kumar et al. (eds.), *Onco-critical Care*,
https://doi.org/10.1007/978-981-16-9929-0_41

with an incurable disease and at the end stages of life should be identified and integrated with palliative care [3]. The aim of integrated palliative care in the ICU is to encourage the development of better quality, cost-effective, patient and family-centric care to improve the quality of care and aid in optimum utilization of ICU infrastructure.

41.2 Components of Palliative Care in ICU [4]

Palliative care in the ICU comprises of these basic components—[1] decision making which revolves around preferences of the patient and the caregiver [2] proper communication to establish continuity of care [3] emotional and practical support to patient and caregivers [4] symptom management and comfort care [5] emotional and organizational support for the clinicians and other workforce of ICU.

Worldwide, three models are described for the integration and implementation of palliative care and ICU. These are—1. Integrative model, 2. Consultative model and 3. Mixed model.

The salient features of each of these models are summarized below.

41.2.1 Integrative Model

- This model aims to integrate the basic essence of palliative care and supportive management into the working curriculum and daily practices of the ICU.
- The basic need in this approach is the training of the critical care specialists in the basics of palliative care and symptom management to empower them to provide end-of-life care and palliative care to their patients.
- A separate palliative care ward/area in the ICU is not required as palliative care is integrated into day to day functioning of the ICU.
- Suitable for a '*closed system*' of ICU care.

41.2.2 Consultative Model

- This model states that palliative care for ICU patients and their families should be dealt with by personnel specialized in palliative medicine to effectively tackle difficult situations like decision making at the end of life, and withdrawal of organ support systems, etc.
- Two approaches of working are described—(a) consult-based approach—palliative care specialists are consulted by the intensivists from time to time to impart palliative care in selected patients. (b) daily presence of a palliative care physician in the ICU rounds—this method would aid in early identification of palliative care concerns and their management.

- This latter approach would also make interdisciplinary coordination easier as the palliative care physician would be present in daily ICU rounds and their viewpoint would be acknowledged and implemented by the critical care physicians at the earliest and will lead to reduced length of ICU stay in a terminal patient, better end of life care in ICU, avoidance of unnecessary ventilation and aggressive management in a select group of terminal patients and thus lead to better utilization of ICU resources.
- The majority of situations requiring palliative care consultation can be summarized as [1] Prolonged ICU stay of more than 10 days [2]. Multisystem organ failure (3 or more systems involved) [3] Intracerebral hemorrhage with patient dependent on mechanical ventilation [4]. Stage 4 malignancy [5] Post cardiac arrest status

41.2.3 Mixed Model

- This model incorporates features of both the above-described models and is largely agreed upon as the most appropriate and acceptable model to deliver palliative care in the ICU.
- model imparts a basic training of palliative care to the intensivists to handle day to needs like symptom management etc. in terminally ill patients in the ICU. Difficult scenarios like the initiation of end-of-life care, advanced life directives, etc. can be handled by palliative care specialists on a consultation basis.
- This approach would increase the palliative care skills of the intensivist and also bring down routine palliative care needs (like pain management, breathlessness, etc.) being referred to a palliative care specialist, thus bringing down costs.
- This is the most effective model to deliver palliative care in ICU as the primary physician manages straightforward palliative care needs and refers a palliative care specialist for more complex or refractory problems.
- This "mixed model" closely resembles the referral to a specialist approach practiced for complex problems related to infectious disease, cardiology, nephrology, and other specialties in the care of critically ill patients.

41.3 Role of Palliative Physician in ICU [5]

A palliative care physician or an intensivist trained in palliative care has multiple roles in the ICU which can be summarized in the following headings.

(a) Communication and Surrogate decision making
(b) Basic symptom management in terminal stage patients.
(c) End-of-life care/terminal sedation.
(d) Palliative/supportive care in non-malignant diseases.
(e) Psychological support to intensivists

41.3.1 Communication and Surrogate Decision Making

A terminally ill patient in the ICU will not be in a mental state to make its own decisions in the majority of ICU admissions. Caregivers and the immediate family are the surrogate decision-makers for the patient. A properly structured communication with the caregivers is thus essential to explain the patient's prognosis, and further care plan in a crisp clear manner with minimum communication gaps so that the caregivers can take decisions keeping the best interest of the patient in mind.

Intensive care physicians are usually well versed in prognosticating and communicating with families of patients with curable conditions or having a short duration of expected stay in the ICU. In the subset of patients having chronic debilitating conditions at the end stage of life and admitted to the ICU, the primary physician—oncologist or the intensivist may find it difficult to realistically communicate with the family of the patient regarding the disease stage and the expected life duration of the patient. In these conditions, palliative care physicians may be the best people to facilitate communication between the patient's family and the intensive care team. Daily family meetings may or orchestrated and coordinated by the palliative care team between the ICU core team and the main decision-makers of the patient's family.

The onus of identification of the main decision-maker in the patient's family, maintenance of continuity of this family member in daily family meetings and guiding the patient's family in difficult decisions like the decision to not escalate treatment, palliative end of life sedation, do not into intubate and resuscitate, etc. lies with the palliative care specialist.

This integration of the palliative approach into terminal patients counseling will lead to minimal communication gaps between the patient's family and the treating team thus leading to an easier transition into comfort care and terminal symptom management from an aggressive curative approach in a terminally ill patient in the ICU.

41.3.2 Basic Symptom Management in Terminal Stage Patients

A palliative care physician with basic knowledge about the safe use of opioids and pathophysiology of various debilitating symptoms like pain, nausea, vomiting, etc. in the end stages of malignant and chronic nonmalignant diseases is the best person for symptomatic management of such patients in the ICU. Basic concepts of symptom management in terminally ill patients are—medications should be started at their lowest doses and gradually titrated up to get the desired effect, patients not tolerating oral route may be managed with sublingual, subcutaneous, or rectal preparations of drugs.

Common distressing symptoms seen in terminally ill patients and their management are summarized in Table 41.1.

Table 41.1 Common symptoms and their management in a terminally sick patient [6]

S.No	Distressing Symptom	Etiopathogenesis	Management
1	Pain	Most common symptom at end of life [6]. The concept of 'total pain' must be adhered to for proper management [7].	Opioids are the drugs of choice for management. Initial titration of the required dose for analgesia is usually done through the intravenous route. Long-acting or extended-release preparations are usually avoided in the initial management.
2	Dyspnea [8]	Often seen with end-stage pulmonary and cardiac diseases. Can also be seen in malignancies and cerebrovascular disease. Clinical manifestations may include tachypnea, restlessness, and grunting.	Opioids are the drug of choice for managing dyspnea at end of life. Started at low doses and on a need basis. In appropriate doses, they do not suppress the respiratory drive but act by reducing the air hunger of the patient.
3	Delirium and agitation [9]	*Reversible causes*—uncontrolled pain, electrolyte imbalance, drug adverse effects, urinary retention, constipation, etc. *Irreversible/disease-related causes*—dementia, cerebrovascular disorders, etc.	The first step—look for and treat reversible causes. Drug therapy in severe/refractory cases. Antipsychotics (haloperidol) drug of choice. Benzodiazepines—can aggravate symptoms, can be used to alleviate anxiety.
4	Nausea and vomiting	Causes—most commonly due to malignant bowel obstruction, pelvic and genitourinary obstruction.	Drug therapy—antidopaminergic (haloperidol, risperidone, prochlorperazine, metoclopramide) are among the first choice. Corticosteroids and octreotide can be used in the medical management of mechanical bowel obstruction [10].
5	Constipation.	Poor oral intake, dehydration at end of life, and adverse effects of drugs (e.g. Opioids) are the most common causes.	Preventive measures—adequate hydration and combination of stimulant laxative with stool softener and polyethylene glycol [11]. Stronger laxatives, suppositories, or enemas may be used in refractory cases.
6	Oropharyngeal secretions.	Inability to clear oral secretions at the terminal stages leads to accumulation of these and leads to a bothersome gurgling noise with respiration called as 'death rattle'.	Anticholinergic medications to dry up these secretions—glycopyrrolate, atropine or scopolamine transdermal patches may be used [12].

41.3.3 End of Life Care/Terminal Sedation

A trained palliative care physician is the most suitable person to identify terminally ill patients in the ICU, initiate and coordinate the multispecialty interaction in declaring the futility of further aggressive management and reaching a consensus to initiate end-of-life care in such patients.

Terminal sedation with drugs like opioids, symptom management like a death rattle, maintaining hydration and managing nutrition, etc. at the end of life are best dealt with by the palliative care team thus giving a dignified death to the patient.

The real meaning of good and dignified death is perhaps best understood by the palliative care team as unlike the intensivists they have more time in hand to have multiple meaningful conversations showing empathy with the caregivers and giving real bereavement care and counseling to the family after the patient's death, thus minimizing distress of the family [13].

41.3.4 Palliative Care in Nonmalignant Diseases

Chronically ill patients staring at the end of life are not specific to malignancies alone. Other specialties dealing with chronically sick patients and their related issues are summarized in Table 41.2.

Table 41.2 Nonmalignant conditions in ICU requiring palliative care support

S.no	Specialty	Diseases	Palliative care issues
1	Neurology and neurosurgery [14]	• Stroke patients with ventilator dependence. • Head injury Post craniotomy dependent on a ventilator • Guillain Barre syndrome • Other demyelinating disorders and myopathies.	• Decision on continuing ventilatory support • Home-based ventilation—preparation and planning
2	Pulmonology [15]	• Interstitial lung diseases with severe restrictive pattern and dependent on a ventilator • COPD on ventilator	• Palliative extubation or home-based ventilation/oxygenation—preparation and planning. • Opioids in management of dyspnea
3	Cardiology [16]	– Heart failure not responding to medications in terminal stages	– Dyspnea management – Diuresis for edema management
4	Nephrology [17]	– Dialysis-dependent chronic kidney condition in the acute decompensated state.	– Planning for continuation or termination of dialysis
5	Others.	– HIV patients in end stages of life [18].	– Management of opportunistic infections.

41.3.5 Psychological Support to Intensivists

the palliative care team also plays an important role to recognize burnout in intensivists and provide them with psychological support as the palliative care team is well versed in dealing with terminal patients near death and facilitating a dignified death in these patients. This close contact with a dying patient with no cure is an emotionally and psychologically taxing experience for intensivists not used to dealing with such patients.

41.4 Barriers to Integration of Palliative Care in ICU [19, 20]

The environment in a conventional ICU setup is full of challenges that impair the proper amalgamation of palliative care services in the conventional care algorithms which are established in the ICU. These barriers or hindrances to the incorporation of palliative care in the ICU may be described under 3 main headings

1. Deficiencies at the level of doctors/treating physicians.
2. Deficiencies at the level of patients and caregivers.
3. Policy-based deficiencies.

41.4.1 Deficiencies at the Level of Doctors/Treating Physicians

The knowledge regarding palliative care and symptom management in a terminally sick patient is sparse among the medical fraternity. The medical curriculum and teaching across various specialties are yet to accept and inculcate the role of palliative medicine in their respective fields. Thus, the lack of basic knowledge among doctors trained in various fields about the role of palliative medicine in their respective fields.

This problem intensifies further in the ICU where the percentage of sick and terminally ill patients is more which require high-quality palliative care but are denied the same due to lack of physician awareness.

Also, communication with the caregivers, giving a realistic hope with clearly explained disease stage and the expected future course is an essential skill imparted in the palliative care curriculum. Sadly, the intensivists and the primary caregivers may not be well versed in effective communication with the caregivers of a terminally sick patient. This problem may be further intensified in a cancer patient where the oncologist being the primary care provider since the start of anticancer therapy may be overzealous and unrealistically aggressive at the terminal stage of illness. This may increase the communication gap between the caregivers and the clinicians and give rise to false and unrealistic hope and thus prolonging the patient's misery and leading to an undignified end to life.

A palliative physician stationed in the ICU or a timely consultation with the palliative care team essentially prevents this sad chain of events.

41.4.2 Deficiencies at the Level of Patients and Caregivers

There are various shortcomings on the part of the family and caregivers of a terminally sick patient in the ICU. Patients especially in the Indian setup where health resources are minimal present late for treatment in the advanced stages of malignancy and have unrealistic hope of cure thus pressurizing physicians to continue aggressive therapy in a terminal patient and widening the communication gap. Also, the caregivers do not have basic knowledge about the rights of a terminally ill patient like advanced care directives and the role of a palliative care physician in aiding surrogate decision-making.

Due to this basic lack of awareness caregivers are unable to actively seek the help of palliative care even if it is available in multidisciplinary care centers.

41.4.3 Policy-Based Deficiencies

Numerous hurdles to the practice of palliative medicine exist on the higher organizational and policy-based levels. The scope of palliative medicine is not clearly defined and its acceptance as a supportive branch helping inpatient management is poor.

The acceptance of the positive and constructive role of palliative medicine aiding inpatient care is poor among intensivists, oncologists, and other specialists specially in branches like nephrology, neurology which have a large burden of terminally sick patients needing symptom management, counseling, and other supportive measures to ease the pain and enhance the quality of life.

A comprehensive change in the medical curriculum is the need of the hour to impart training in palliative care to every specialty which will help in recognition of the need and its integration in respective specialties of this under-utilized branch.

41.5 Directions for Future Research

The palliative care team is an indispensable part of the multidisciplinary management team of the ICU. This nascent concept in its budding stages will gain widespread acceptance only if it is supported by data showing positive outcomes for patients in the ICU and the hospital when palliative care is integrated with ICU.

Theoretically, integration and amalgamation of palliative care with ICU will have multiple benefits like avoidance of prolonged life support and ventilation in a terminally sick patient, better symptom management at the end of life, lesser ICU death in terminally sick patients, and acceptance of end-of-life care. These will minimize the costs of maintaining ICU infrastructure, better utilization of existing scarce ICU resources for deserving patients with a reversible pathology, and better caregiver satisfaction.

Studies should be targeted to generate data in these areas like reduction in duration of ICU stay in terminally sick patients after initiation of palliative care services in ICU, utilization of end of life and advanced care directives, generation of caregiver satisfaction scores, etc.

Palliative care in ICU may aid in generating benchmark data in the field of health economics and ICU resource utilization for deserving patients as ICU beds are a scarce and costly to maintain commodity for the health care setups across the globe.

41.6 Summary

Palliative care as a specialty has a definitive place in managing terminally ill critically sick patients admitted in the ICU. However, in the present-day scenario, the acceptance of this branch as a part of the multispecialty team in the ICU is next to none. Concrete efforts are needed to bring about administrative and personal level changes to integrate this branch into the critical care curriculum.

Institutes and hospitals may start working on their level to set up protocols in their ICUs for integration of palliative care. Hospitals functioning as exclusive cancer centers should lead the way in this aspect as the maximum need for palliative care is in the cancer patients in the ICU. We should not wait for a large administrative push for palliative care integration in critical care but start working on our hospital and workplace level.

Changes even if microscopic and on the ground level will serve as a push for larger administrative and policy-based changes in the future.

References

1. Angus DC, Barnato AE, Linde-Zwirble WT, Weissfeld LA, Watson RS, Rickert T, et al. Use of intensive care at the end of life in the United States: an epidemiologic study*. Crit Care Med [Internet]. 2004;32(3). Available from: https://journals.lww.com/ccmjournal/Fulltext/2004/03000/Use_of_intensive_care_at_the_end_of_life_in_the.3.aspx
2. Aslakson RA, Curtis JR, Nelson JE. The changing role of palliative care in the ICU. Crit Care Med [Internet]. 2014;42(11) Available from: https://journals.lww.com/ccmjournal/Fulltext/2014/11000/The_Changing_Role_of_Palliative_Care_in_the_ICU.13.aspx
3. Kelley AS, Morrison RS. Palliative care for the seriously ill. N Engl J Med. 2015;373(8):747–55.
4. Nelson JE, Bassett R, Boss RD, Brasel KJ, Campbell ML, Cortez TB, et al. Models for structuring a clinical initiative to enhance palliative care in the intensive care unit: a report from the IPAL-ICU Project (Improving Palliative Care in the ICU). Crit Care Med. 2010;38(9):1765–72.
5. Truog RD, Campbell ML, Curtis JR, Haas CE, Luce JM, Rubenfeld GD, et al. Recommendations for end-of-life care in the intensive care unit: a consensus statement by the American College of Critical Care Medicine. Crit Care Med [Internet]. 2008;36(3) Available from: https://journals.lww.com/ccmjournal/Fulltext/2008/03000/Recommendations_for_end_of_life_care_in_the.41.aspx
6. Wilkie DJ, Ezenwa MO. Pain and symptom management in palliative care and at end of life. Nurs Outlook. 2012;60(6):357–64.
7. Ong C-K, Forbes D. Embracing Cicely Saunders's concept of total pain. BMJ. 2005;331(7516):576.
8. Mahler DA. Opioids for refractory dyspnea. Expert Rev Respir Med. 2013;7(2):123–35.
9. Hosker CMG, Bennett MI. Delirium and agitation at the end of life. BMJ. 2016 Jun 9;353:i3085.

10. Ferguson HJM, Ferguson CI, Speakman J, Ismail T. Management of intestinal obstruction in advanced malignancy. Ann Med Surg. 2012. 2015;4(3):264–70.
11. Sizar O, Genova R, Gupta M. Opioid induced constipation. In: StatPearls [Internet]. Treasure Island (FL): StatPearls Publishing; 2021 [cited 2021 Jun 14]. Available from: http://www.ncbi.nlm.nih.gov/books/NBK493184/
12. Twomey S, Dowling M. Management of death rattle at end of life. Br J Nurs. 2013;22(2):81–5.
13. Rietjens JAC, van Delden JJM, van der Heide A, Vrakking AM, Onwuteaka-Philipsen BD, van der Maas PJ, et al. Terminal sedation and euthanasia: a comparison of clinical practices. Arch Intern Med. 2006;166(7):749–53.
14. Mosenthal AC, Weissman DE, Curtis JR, Hays RM, Lustbader DR, Mulkerin C, et al. Integrating palliative care in the surgical and trauma intensive care unit: a report from the Improving Palliative Care in the Intensive Care Unit (IPAL-ICU) Project Advisory Board and the Center to Advance Palliative Care*. Crit Care Med [Internet]. 2012;40(4) Available from: https://journals.lww.com/ccmjournal/Fulltext/2012/04000/Integrating_palliative_care_in_the_surgical_and.21.aspx
15. Narsavage GL, Chen Y-J, Korn B, Elk R. The potential of palliative care for patients with respiratory diseases. Breathe. 2017;13(4):278.
16. Sobański P, Brzezińska Rajszys G, Grodzicki T, Jakubów P, Jankowski P, Kurzyna M, et al. Palliative care for people living with cardiac disease. Kardiologia Pol Pol Heart J. 2020;78(4):364–73.
17. Brown EA, Chambers EJ, Eggeling C. Palliative care in nephrology. Nephrol Dial Transplant. 2008;23(3):789–91.
18. Merlins JS, Tucker RO, Saag MS, Selwyn PA. The role of palliative care in the current HIV treatment era in developed countries. Top Antivir Med. 2013;21(1):20–6.
19. White DB, Luce JM. Palliative care in the intensive care unit: barriers, advances, and unmet needs. Crit Care Clin. 2004;20(3):329–43.
20. Singer PA, Martin DK, Kelner M. Quality end-of-life carepatients' perspectives. JAMA. 1999;281(2):163–8.

Ethical Issues at End of Life Care in the ICU

42

Brajesh Kumar Ratre and Sushma Bhatnagar

42.1 Introduction

Dying was a 'natural' process before the modernization of medicine and advancement in medical technologies. Now with the help of modern medicine and newer medical technologies the life expectancy of population has increased and with the help of newer medical gadgets one can prolong the dying process. Along with ageing of population this will also increases the number of patient with chronic condition with little or no chance of survival. Intensive care unit plays a major role in this. The central purpose of intensive care unit is to provide short term, life saving services to patients with acute illness or severe injury but in modern intensive care unit the number of patients with chronic condition is increasing, although the newer technologies and medicine do not cure the patient but it prolongs the life of patients by providing secondary support [1, 2].

A significant number of patients with chronic illness i.e. cancer, chronic lung disease, congestive heart failure, nervous system disorder, AIDS require multiple hospitalization and many of these patients are shifted to intensive care units at the time of death. At the end of life secondary support intervention will not reduce the suffering rather it will increase the burden of prolonged process of dying. Patient's family member, friends and caregivers may also experience multiple problems. In addition, many of patients do not have any medical insurance so the health expenses are borne by patient or by their family members. At the end of life shifting the patient to intensive care unit with aggressive medical interventions will further drain the resources of family members [3]. Rising cost of treatment during chronic illness will force the patient to leave the hospital against medical advice without even getting supportive treatment for their symptoms [4].

B. K. Ratre (✉) · S. Bhatnagar
Oncoanaesthesia & Palliative Medicine AIIMS Delhi, New Delhi, India

V. Kumar et al. (eds.), *Onco-critical Care*,
https://doi.org/10.1007/978-981-16-9929-0_42

End of life care in an important topic for discussion in modern medical practice. When patient is diagnose with terminal illness (cancer, chronic renal failure, COPD, ILD), patient along with their family members experiences a high level of stress that can be presented in form of anger, depression and other psychosomatic problems (Kubler-Ross five stage of grief) [5]. Family members are foremost caregiver for terminally ill patient. They may feel hopelessness, helplessness, guilt and even anger when they understand the graveness of the disease and not able to relieve the patient from suffering.

From ethical prospective patient is the best person for decision making about the treatment limitation or withholding the life prolonging supportive treatment. But at the end of life patient may lost the ability to take such decision, at that time family members, primary caregivers or treating physician will have to take the decision for the patient [6, 7]. Family member who is called for decision making is already under great fear, sadness and stressed out and if they are not aware of patient's decision at the end of life they may confused for taking further decision. Sometime family members may have different opinion for care planning and many a time relative ask treating physician to give most appropriate treatment to the patient. In such scenario, oncologist or intensive care physician will be in difficult situation [8].

There are multiple levels at which different ethical issues may be precipitate during treatment of critically ill cancer patient. There may be lack of understanding or therapeutic misconception and also lack of decision making capacity at patient level. At family members level, they may be in guilt or in burden regarding therapeutic decisions for their loved one. There may be lack of communication between oncologist and the care provider of patient and many a time oncologist are in moral distress that may leads to ethical issues. Without proper communication request of some intervention, excessive end of life care counselling, avoiding analgesics, withholding or withdrawing life sustaining therapies may triggers ethical issues [9].

For any cancer patient who is at the end of life, there are two major concerns one is the cost of hospital stay that will be bear by patient and family member who are already being drained due to the prolong illness and multiple sessions of treatment, and the second is the comfort of patient at the end of life. Aggressive medical intervention at the end of life will not only increase the suffering of patient but also increases the cost. There are evidences that support that the physician in intensive care units are incompatible in providing end of life care support after decision taken by family members to withheld life support interventions [10–12]. End of life care in Intensive care unit is an area for intensive care physician, which requires same high level of knowledge and comprehension as other area of critical care practice [13]. It is important for ICU physician to recognize the process of dying and efficient to start advance care planning in form of palliation and providing comfort care. He/she must have effective communication about the advance directive with primary care team and with the family member. Physician should understand the spiritual and religious concern of family member.

42.2 Recognizing the Dying Patient

It is very important for critical care physician to recognize the terminally ill patient who is dying. Oncologist who provide care from the beginning of diagnosis often overestimate patient's survival [14]. So this may be a challenge for transition of patient from definitive care to supportive or palliative care [15]. Accurate prognostication by oncologist at advance stage of disease has a good influence on patient's and family's decision regarding end of life care and preparation for the same. Oncologist can use different prognostication tools and performance status scales for prognostication [16]. In a dying audit done by royal college of physician about 45% patients were actually recognize that they are dying [17]. A majority of patient does not want to die in intensive care unit rather they wish to die in home in presence of their loved one. Finally, it depends upon clinician to recognize the dying patient and how they communicate for the preparation of end of life.

42.3 Ethical Principals

There are four universally accepted principal for bioethics, they are (1) Autonomy, (2) Beneficence, (3) Nonmaleficence, and (4) Justice [18].

Autonomy: Everyone has the right to take self-decision, about their level of care. Respecting patient's autonomy is well established ethical principal in medicine [8]. This is also applicable for life prolonging interventions. Oncologist's approach should be patient centered and they must inform the trajectory of disease and all available treatment modalities for the disease and their future consequences so that it is possible for patient to decide the treatment of advance malignancy. Many patients are not able to take their decision about further care planning they may depend upon their treating oncologist and family member to help to take the decision and at the terminal stage patients is not in the stage to take decision regarding end of life care.

Advance directive is derived from patient's autonomy which empower oncologist to respect the autonomy of their patient who is not able to take decision for end of life care planning due to any reason [8]. Advance directive or advance bill is permitted in united states of America which is a lawful document prepared during full mental status of patient regarding patient's preference during advance stage of disease and about end of life decision. In intensive care setting when patient is not in the state to take decision then decision will be taken by family member or close family friend, this is called surrogate decision making.

Beneficence: It is oncologist or intensive care physician's moral obligation to provide best care to patient and family member at the end of life [19]. When patient is not able to express their wish or not in a state of decision making specially in intensive care setting and at the end of life then the decision should be made by the treating oncologist, intensive care physician after detailed discussion with family members to alleviate patients suffering and to provide the treatment that will give maximum benefit to patient [6–8, 19]. There may be conflict in decision between oncologist, intensive care physician and family member, even in between the family members, this conflict can be solved by a family meeting with involving treating oncologist and intensive care physician.

Nonmaleficence: It is ethical obligation of physician to not to harm the patient during treatment [20, 21]. This should be more strictly practice than beneficence. Nonmaleficence support few moral responsibilities of physician i.e. not to harm, do not kill, do not cause suffering to patient, not to do offence, patient should not be deprived of good and conform. Nonmaleficence should be practice in a way to make a balance between all available intervention and to choose the best one so that the benefits after that intervention should more than the harm. This is particularly more important at the end of life where decision making is difficult i.e. intervention for pain management (difficult pain), withholding or to continue life prolonging interventions, providing artificial nutrition or hydration [22]. Similarly like beneficence there is also conflict for nonmaleficence between the oncologist and intensive care physician to decide the best intervention for a critically ill patient for providing the intervention with maximum benefits and minimum harm.

Justice: Justice is fourth fundamental ethical principal in bioethics and it is most difficult to implement specially at the end of life. Distributive justice is type of justice that implies appropriate, fare and equitable health care services to the patient [23]. Distribution justice is focus on individual patient and care should be given in terms of equal share, according to need of patient, merit, contribution and efforts [20]. There is also a concept of social justice, which implies justice to society specially in a society with limited medical resources [24]. Inappropriate treatment may waste the resources for any appropriate candidate, similarly life prolonging or sustaining intervention in ICU may engage the resources which may be beneficial for some other individuals. It is very difficult to choose the appropriate intervention at the end of life i.e. withholding or withdrawing ventilator support, withdrawal some life sustaining drug etc.

42.4 Role on Oncologist and Intensive Care Physician

Oncologist play an important role in resolving ethical issues at the end of life by providing detail information and expected trajectory of the patient during early medical treatment of patient [25]. They must discuss the all available possible treatment for the disease along with their benefits, limitation and side effect if any and respect patients autonomy to choose the treatment modality. Early integration of palliative medicine physician will improve the understanding about the disease, its futility and alleviate the suffering of patient and family member [26]. During further advancement of disease oncologist's approach should be patient centered and advance care planning and/or end of life care decision must be discuss in advance with patient and their relatives so that they can prepare for end of life decision [25].

At the end of life communication between the oncologist, intensive care physician and nurses are very crucial [27]. There may be conflict between the opinions about the end of life intervention between the medical team. A respectful communication between the team members with detail discussion about the patient status and exchange of their ideas can be a great help for the patient and family member. While communicating with family member all team members should be in same platform and all aspect of available intervention should be discussion to alleviate the maximum suffering of patient [28].

At the end of life if patient or family member insist for intensive care treatment and advance medical intervention and if it is futile according to oncologist or intensive care physician's evaluation it should be well explain to patient or family member. Before withholding or withdrawing any treatment or giving instruction for do not resuscitate, intensive care physician must respect the belief and value of patient and their family members. Intensive care physician must explain the drawback of futile treatment and unrealistic expectations with the advance medical intervention i.e. ventilation, artificial nutrition etc. there must be a mutual understanding between the patient or family member with intensive care physician about the withholding or withdrawing life sustaining modalities [29]. Along with saving patient's life it is intensive care physician's additional responsibility to judicious use of resources and also judge between the expenditure and benefits of advance medical interventions as advancement and innovation in health care technology i.e. mechanical ventilation, artificial nutrition, ECMO may prolong the life but also increase the suffering of patient and increase the emotional stress of family members [30, 31].

42.5 Conclusion

Malignancy is a broad disease that encompasses a wide range of disease involvement and varieties of treatment modalities. When presented in advance stage or after recurrence patient develop critical illness that may require intensive care services. Intensive care services should not be limited to resuscitation or prolonging the life it should also address the end of life issues of patient and to provide a comfort care to the patient. The goal of end of life care is to relieves the suffering of patient and their family members with respective patients desire about the end of life. Intensive care physician may face many ethical problems while dealing a terminal advance cancer patient, they mostly face uncertainty about when to shift patient from curative to palliative treatment and when to start end of life discussion with patient and family member. Good effective communication between family member, oncologist, intensive care nurse and physician will improve end of life decision making. Open communication in form of family meeting and active participation of all health care providers who are involve in patient care i.e. oncologist, intensive care physician, palliative medicine physician, intensive care nurse, ancillary staff may avoid many ethical issues at the end of life. Intensive care physician can play an important role in promoting communication, education of other ancillary health staff related to end of life discussion.

References

1. Karnik S, Kanekar A. Ethical issues surrounding end of life care: a narrative review. Healthcare. 2016;4(2):24.
2. Thorns A. Ethical and legal issues in end-of-life care. Clin Med. 2010;10(3):282–5.
3. Jayaram R, Ramakrishnan N. Cost of intensive care in India. Indian J Crit Care Med. 2008;12:55–61.
4. Mani RK. Limitation of life support in the ICU. Indian J Crit Care Med. 2003;7:112–7.
5. Newman L. Elisabeth Kübler-Ross. BMJ. 2004;329(7466):627.
6. Crane MK, Witting M, Doukas DJ. Respecting end-of-lifetreatment preferences. Am Fam Physician. 2005;72:1263–8.
7. Cavalieri TA. Ethical issues at the end of life. J Am Osteopath Assoc. 2001;101(10):616–22.
8. OrnekBuken N. Clinical ethical decision making process and determining factors at the end of life. Turkiye Klin J Med Ethics Law Hist-Special Top. 2016;2(3):24–33.
9. Riches JC, Voigt LP. Palliative, ethics, and end-of-life care issues in the cancer patient. Crit Care Clin. 2021 Jan;37(1):105–15.
10. A controlled trial to improve care for seriously ill hospitalized patients: The study to understand prognoses and preferences for outcomes and risks of treatments (SUPPORT). SUPPORT Principal Investigators. JAMA. 1995;274:1591–1598.
11. Hall RI, Rocker GM, Murray D. Simple changes can improve conduct of end-of-life care in the intensive care unit. Can J Anaesth. 2004;51:631–6.
12. Wood KA, Marik PE. ICU care at the end of life. Chest. 2004;126:1403–6.
13. Truog RD, Campbell ML, Curtis JR, Haas CE, Luce JM, Rubenfeld GD, et al. Recommendations for end-of-life care in the intensive care unit: a consensus statement by the American College [corrected] of Critical Care Medicine. Crit Care Med. 2008;36:953–63.
14. Glare P, Virik K, Jones M, Hudson M, Eychmuller S, Simes J, et al. A systematic review of physicians' survival predictions in terminally ill cancer patients. BMJ. 2003;327:195–8.
15. Munday D, Petrova M, Dale J. Exploring preferences for place of death with terminally ill patients: qualitative study of experiences of general practitioners and community nurses in England. BMJ. 2009;339:b2391.
16. Boyd K, Murray SA. Recognising and managing key transitions in end of life care. BMJ. 2010;341:c4863.
17. National care of the dying audit-hospitals (NCDAH) In Royal College of Physicians: Summary report. 2007.
18. Page K. The four principles: can they be measured and do they predict ethical decision making? BMC Med Ethics. 2012;13:10.
19. McDaniel SH, Campbell TL, Hepworth J, et al. Looking death in the eye: facilitating end-of-life care and the grieving process. In: Mc Daniel SH, Campbell TL, Hepworth J, et al., editors. Family oriented primary care. 2nd ed. New York: Springer; 2005. p. 261–84.
20. Varkey B. Principles of clinical ethics and their application to practice. Med Princ Pract. 2021;30(1):17–28.
21. Beauchamp TL, Childress JF. Principles of biomedical ethics. New York (NY): Oxford University Press; 2009. p. 162–4.
22. Mularski RA, Puntillo K, Varkey B, Erstad BL, Grap MJ, Gilbert HC, et al. Pain management within the palliative and end-of-life care experience in the ICU. Chest. 2009 May;135(5):1360–9.
23. Fleishacker S. A short history of distributive justice. Cambridge (MA): Harvard University Press; 2005.
24. Gavrin JR. Ethical considerations at the end of life in the intensive care unit. Crit Care Med. 2007 Feb;35(2 Suppl):S85–94.
25. Committee on Improving the Quality of Cancer Care: Addressing the Challenges of an Aging Population; Board on Health Care Services; Institute of Medicine; Levit L, Balogh E, Nass S, et al., editors. Delivering high-quality cancer care: charting a new course for a system in

crisis. Washington (DC): National Academies Press (US); 2013 Dec 27. 3, Patient-Centered Communication and Shared Decision Making.

26. Kain DA, Eisenhauer EA. Early integration of palliative care into standard oncology care: evidence and overcoming barriers to implementation. Curr Oncol. 2016;23(6):374–7.
27. Baggs JG, Schmitt MH, Mushlin AI, Mitchell PH, Eldredge DH, Oakes D, et al. Association between nurse-physician collaboration and patient outcomes in three intensive care units. Crit Care Med. 1999;27:1991–8.
28. Jacobowski NL, Girard TD, Mulder JA, Ely EW. Communication in critical care: family rounds in the intensive care unit. Am J Crit Care. 2010;19:421–30.
29. Winzelberg G, Hanson L, Tulsky J. Beyond autonomy: diversifying end-of-life decision-making approaches to serve patients and families. J Am Geriatr Soc. 2005;53:1046–50.
30. Thorns A. Ethical and legal issues in end-of-life care. Clin Med. 2010;10:282–5.
31. Baily M. Futility, autonomy, and cost in end-of-life care. J Law Med Ethics. 2011;39:172–82.

Clinical Research in Onco-Critical Care 43

P. V. Sai Saran, Mohd Saif Khan, and Mohan Gurjar

43.1 Introduction

Advancements in immunopharmacology, targeted chemotherapy, cancer surgery, and precision radiotherapy have increased the cure rates and survival in malignancies [1]. According to a recent estimate from American Association for Cancer Research (AACR), the number of alive Americans with a history of cancer is expected to increase by 76.5% in the span of 11 years, from 2019 to 2030 [1]. As life expectancy prolongs in cancer patients, utilization of life supports in intensive care units (ICU) will be stepped up. However, there is always a dearth of intensive care beds in mixed medical-surgical ICU, due to constant admissions with non-oncological diagnoses. Therefore, health administrators, health policymakers and physicians (oncologists, onco-surgeons, general physicians, and hospitalists) would be concerned to know the outcome (length of stay, mortality), quality of life post-discharge and cost of admitting the cancer patients to ICU. Cancer is a multisystem chronic disease that is often kept in remission with a variety of treatment options such as radiation, chemotherapy, and surgery. In cancer patients, critical illness transpires either due to the disease itself (progression of cancer, treatments-related); or unrelated to cancer (acute illness, exacerbations of other chronic illnesses, trauma etc.) [2].

P. V. Sai Saran
Department of Critical Care Medicine, King George Medical University, Lucknow, Uttar Pradesh, India

M. Saif Khan
Department of Critical Care Medicine, Trauma Centre and Central Emergency, Rajendra Institute of Medical Sciences, Ranchi, Jharkhand, India

M. Gurjar (✉)
Department of Critical Care Medicine, Sanjay Gandhi Post Graduate Institute of Medical Sciences (SGPGIMS), Lucknow, Uttar Pradesh, India

V. Kumar et al. (eds.), *Onco-critical Care*,
https://doi.org/10.1007/978-981-16-9929-0_43

There has been a vast expansion of health care services provided to oncology patients in the last 50 years. With the expansion of a growing number of dedicated, state of the art oncology setups across the world, we have witnessed the parallel enthusiasm in providing cutting edge critical care services to oncology patients. This has led to the birth of a new subspecialty of medicine/critical care called "Onco-critical care". However, there will be a difference in critical care provided at a multispecialty facility compared to that at a dedicated and specialized oncology ICU in terms of regular multidisciplinary rounds, cancer-specific protocols, palliative care services, and daily meeting between intensivists and oncologists [3]. Faced with new challenges, meeting the growing demands of an array of critical care services among oncology patients, in such dedicated oncologic facilities are evolving with invasion of evidence-based medicine and best practices. High quality research in this young subspecialty is much desirable as the problems and issues of critically ill oncology patients are unique and require entirely different approach. Onco-critical care has broad room for extensive research to resolve dilemmas and controversies related to various critical care aspects such as determination of optimal patient population in which full code 'ICU trial' can be given, development of unique early warning scores to recognize sick cancer patients in the ward, triage rules to rationalize the admissions to ICU, the timing of the use and duration of life-sustaining therapies (e.g.; mechanical ventilation, renal replacement therapy), development of cancer-specific severity of illness scoring systems and formulation of cancer-specific guidelines and care bundles [4, 5].

In this chapter, the authors made an attempt to categorize the various evidence gaps in onco-critical care available for exploration and enumerated the requirement of addition of new knowledge by a young generation of critical care specialists, oncologists, medical scientists, and researchers, mentioned as various domains in Table 43.1.

Table 43.1 Research domains with various knowledge-gaps in onco-critical care

Research domain	Possible research questions specific to onco-critical care
ICU organization	• Development of dedicated ICUs with positive and negative pressure isolation cubicles along with their evidence in infection control practices
ICU admission and prognostication	• Development of specific screening scoring systems or early warning scores and severity scores in onco-critical care
Acute respiratory failure	• Modified definition for ARDS • Which patients for NIV and HFNC and how long? • Role of diagnostic strategies • Role of recruitment manoeuvres, inhaled nitric oxide and prone position • Role of adjunctive therapy • Role of extracorporeal therapies
Onco-emergencies	• New definition applicable to febrile neutropenia • Role of colony stimulating factors (CSF) in critically ill patients • Rasburicase over allopurinol in the prevention of TLS

Table 43.1 (continued)

Research domain	Possible research questions specific to onco-critical care
Transfusion triggers	• Indications and thresholds for various blood product transfusions (leuko-reduced and irradiated blood products), specific to malignancies
Acute kidney injury	• Development of AKI prediction models incorporating various biomarker
Nutritional aspects	• Development of screening tools to identify cancer patients who are malnourished
Infection Control & Sepsis	• Diagnostic methods for various bacterial, fungal and viral infections with rapid turnaround time and higher diagnostic performance are needed
Post ICU discharge life	• Study assessing QOL in cancer survivors post ICU discharge, evaluating the impact of the ICU support on long-term and disease-free survival
End of Life Care & Palliative Care	• Studies assessing qualitative outcomes like quality of dying are much awaited

43.2 Research Domains in Onco-Critical Care

43.2.1 Organizational Aspects

The ICU structure and organizational factors such as the use of protocols, care bundles, and staffing design have potential roles in patient outcomes [6, 7]. Unfortunately, a limited number of studies have explored this aspect for critically ill cancer patients [8, 9]. It is yet to be determined whether specialized onco-ICUs outperform general ICUs [10]. A Brazilian, multicentric, retrospective observational study (ORCHESTRA), found that the presence of clinical pharmacists, ICU protocols, and regular meetings between oncologists and intensivists were associated with better clinical outcomes [3]. However, due to the presence of confounders (being nation-specific, having less number of patients with hematological malignancies, inability to audit the ICU protocol implementation and many studies being retrospective in nature), there exists a grey zone area where researchers should study the impact of various ICU organizational aspects on cancer patient outcomes such as staffing pattern, presence of infectious disease specialist, nutritionist, multidisciplinary grand rounds, closed versus open ICU concept, bedside renal replacement therapy and bedside CT scan facility. Single isolation cubicles (positive pressure (post bone marrow transplant receipts) and negative pressure (respiratory infectious diseases), with waste disposal systems and hand wash facilities bedside along with a highly efficient heating ventilation and air conditioning system (HVAC system) is needful in critically ill oncological patients, as they are immunocompromised [11, 12]. Studies examining the efficacy of such organizational aspects are lacking.

43.2.2 Triage for ICU Admission

About 20% of patients admitted to ICU are reported to have underlying cancer [13]. Repeated discussions and conflicts between the ICU team and the oncologists occur for the admission of critically ill cancer patients, even in dedicated oncology centers, thereby resulting in a cascade of delayed ICU admission, higher severity of illness at presentation, and poor outcomes. This fiery issue can only be resolved by designing oncocritical-care-specific screening scoring systems that may significantly contribute to faster and comprehensive care upon admission to ICU. Nevertheless, in patients with an uncertain prognosis (grey zone), an '*ICU trial*' is said to be decisive, which encompasses *'full code'* management in the first few days [4]. Further research is required to determine the optimal duration of the ICU trial period, although, limited data suggest that less severe illness or malignant neoplasms seem to benefit from the longer duration of 'ICU trial' [14]. Besides, there are various other ICU admission policies like '*exceptional ICU admission*' and '*heroic ICU admission*'. In former admission policy, a newly available potential therapy is tested in a patient with severe limitation of performance status due to malignancy, whereas in later ICU admission is granted until the conflict between intensivist and hemato-oncologist or between patient and physician about actual prognosis is resolved [4, 5]. Other ICU admission categories which have never been formally evaluated in cancer patients are, *'prophylactic'*, '*early'*, *'palliative'* and '*terminal'* categories [15]. Unfortunately, ICU admission criteria are fundamentally based upon '*expert opinion*' which is highly subjective and biased, as sufficient scientific evidence is lacking. Very few conditions benefit hugely from urgent ICU admissions such as tumor lysis syndrome, macrophage activation syndrome, superior vena cava obstruction, and leukostasis. A randomized controlled trial (RCT) designed to admit patients with cancer at the early stages of malignancy (before or within a few days of cancer chemotherapy), can give evidence for such admissions [16]. Incorporation of physical changes that can alert the physician for ICU referral may be a necessity. The criteria for ICU referral and admission decisions require close and fortnight collaboration between oncology and ICU teams.

Early warning scores (EWS) to activate the rapid response teams (RRT), such as Modified Early Warning Score (MEWS), National Early warning score (NEWS), VitalPAC Early Warning score (ViEWS), which exist in other domains of critical care, require validation in onco-critical care [17]. These scores, unfortunately, have demonstrated poor performance with low discriminatory power in identifying oncological patients at risk of deterioration [18]. Thus, constant scrutiny is required to develop a cancer-specific EWS.

43.2.3 Severity of Illness Scores in Onco-Critical Care

Even though specific scoring system like ICU Cancer Mortality Model (CMM), was developed, along with the existing scoring systems available, for instance, the Acute

Physiology and Chronic Health Evaluation (APACHE), Simplified Acute Physiology Score (SAPS), Mortality Prediction Models (MPM), no specific severity-of-illness scoring systems were able to reliably predict the outcome of critically ill cancer patients [19]. Of various scoring systems used in the ICU, very few incorporate malignancy in details (like APACHE III incorporates "malignancy as hematological-disseminated" as a severity item for score calculation) [20]. Thus, a scoring system, incorporating cancer-specific prognostic variables such as performance status, presence of graft versus host disease (GVHD), is highly desirable which will potentially assist the intensivist deciding critical treatment pathways thoughtfully. Further examples of cancer-specific prognostic factors to be considered for development of such a scoring system are bedridden status, life expectancy less than 6 months, newly diagnosed malignancy unresponsive to chemo-radiotherapy [21]. Such a scoring system would definitely help to recognize patients who are unlikely to benefit from ICU admission, in order to conserve costly ICU resources. Additional multi-centre cohort studies evaluating the ASSESS criteria, needs to be done [22]. This includes

- triage criteria for ICU **A**dmission by oncologists/hematologists and ICU physicians;
- code **S**tatus implemented at ICU admission (full code, ICU trial, or early treatment limitation);
- ICU **S**upport; and patient's **E**volution;
- short- and long-term **S**urvival;
- appropriate description of ICU **S**urvivors.

43.2.4 Acute Respiratory Failure

Acute respiratory failure (ARF) is the most common cause of ICU admission among cancer patients [23]. Various aspects of this entity remained unexplored, which are as follows:

43.2.4.1 Definition and Treatment of Acute Respiratory Distress Syndrome (ARDS)

Causes of ARDS in cancer patients are uniquely described as pulmonary metastases (lymphangitic carcinomatosis), drug-induced lung injury (DILI), active GVHD, radiation toxicity, in addition to traditional aetiologies such as infection, trauma, transfusion, sepsis, or surgery. Therefore, the definition of ARDS in cancer needs modification as the prognosis varies with the type of malignancy associated with or chemo-radiotherapy. ARDS management strategies for such patients may be unique and different from those in the general population and studies focussing on such treatment modifications are needed [24].

43.2.4.2 Role of Alternatives to Invasive Mechanical Ventilation in Cancer Patients

Use of invasive mechanical ventilation is linked to higher mortality in immunocompromised patients including those having malignancy [25]. Earlier, it was believed that non-invasive ventilation (NIV) is associated with more benefits or at least no harm to patients with immunodeficiency [26]. Later, the evidence was conflicting especially in ARDS, with no benefits and a few studies demonstrated higher mortality [27]. High degree of clarity is needed in identifying patients who may benefit from NIV application, and also in determining the duration of NIV trial. The other alternative to invasive mechanical ventilation is heated high flow oxygen therapy (HFNC) which requires further explorative studies after the two RCTs revealing conflicting results, comparing it with standard oxygen therapy and NIV [27, 28].

43.2.4.3 Role of Diagnostic Strategies

Prevalence, aetiology and prognostic implications of pneumonia in immunocompromised cancer patients are entirely different from general critically ill population. Infectious or non-infectious pathologies masquerading pneumonia may be simultaneously present and hence, requirement of various diagnostic interventions is highly desirable such as early bronchoscopy guided sampling or broncho alveolar lavage (BAL), thoracic ultrasound, trans-bronchial or open lung biopsy, along with early CT imaging [29]. Regrettably, not every patient can be subjected to such diagnostic interventions, therefore, future research should highlight who may benefit from such interventions after ICU admission [4]; for instance, BAL is indicated in evaluating the cause of non-resolving pneumonia caused by Invasive Pulmonary Aspergillosis (IPA) and Pneumocystis jirovecii pneumonia (PJP) [30].

43.2.4.4 Role of Recruitment Manoeuvres, Inhaled Nitric Oxide and Prone Position

No prospective randomised controlled trial has yet assessed the efficacy and safety of these interventions in critically ill cancer patients with severe ARDS. Data from observational and retrospective studies reveal that prone positioning may improve mortality in cancer patients [4, 5].

43.2.4.5 Corticosteroids in Pneumonia

Available evidence for role of coticosteroids in ARDS caused by PJP, diffuse alveolar hemorrhage, acute interstitial pneumonia or DILI are weak, and hence, require further exploration. Nevertheless, utility of steroids needs to be always balanced against the risk of infections [31].

43.2.4.6 Extra Corporeal Membrane Oxygenation (ECMO)

In case of severe ARDS requiring mechanical ventilation, the mortality can be as high as 60–100% [32]. Utility of ECMO in hematologic malignancies was reported with poor results, a well-designed prospective randomised controlled trial is needed to explain the outcome in cancer patients [33].

43.2.5 Oncological Emergencies

In order to promote the research in oncological emergencies, Comprehensive Oncologic Emergencies Research Network (CONCERN)—an open scientific forum for oncology and emergency medicine was created [34]. We have reviewed few sub-domains related to research in oncological emergencies:

43.2.5.1 Febrile Neutropenia

This condition is well documented in immunocompromised cancer patients, which is defined as a single oral temperature of >38.3 °C or a temperature of >38.0 °C sustained for more than 1 h. In critically ill patients, this definition needs a modification to include core body temperature, as oral temperature is not reliable in critically ill patients [35]. Granulocyte Monocyte Colony Stimulating Factor (GM CSF), is indicated in severe febrile neutropenia when the absolute neutrophil count (ANC) is less than <500 cells/microL or ANC that is expected to decrease to <500 cells/microL over the next 48 hours associated with critical illness or high risk (expected to persist for more than 7 days). With the advances in the diagnosis of sepsis, the role of colony stimulating factors becomes questionable. Again, evidence assessing the clinical value of Colony Stimulating Factor (CSF), is lacking in critically ill neutropenic patients [36]. Studies to determine the optimal route of administration of such molecular therapies in critically ill patients with multi-organ dysfunction syndrome (MODS) and shock, where subcutaneous absorption is questionable, are awaited. Further studies are required comparing G-CSF versus GM-CSF as the data is contradictory. Moreover, the duration of therapy requires resilient evidence. Deterioration of respiratory status during the recovery from neutropenia, treated with G-CSF is a concern which needs to be specifically elucidated by further studies [37].

43.2.5.2 Tumor Lysis Syndrome (TLS)

The superiority of rasburicase over allopurinol in the prevention of TLS is still unclear, whether it reduces the intensity of clinical TLS, acute kidney injury or mortality, with very limited data in paediatric as well as adult population [32, 37, 38].

43.2.6 Acute Kidney Injury (AKI) and Renal Replacement Therapy (RRT)

Malignancies (such as multiple myeloma), related complications (TLS, infections, compression and obstruction from a tumour, thrombotic microangiopathy, radio-contrast nephropathy, nephrotoxic chemotherapeutics) and major cancer surgeries, enormously predispose cancer patients to a uniquely recognized entity of acute kidney injury, labelled as "*Malignancy Related Acute Kidney Injury (MR-AKI)*" [39]. Critically ill cancer patients were reported to have a 54% risk of developing AKI

[34]. Utility of biomarkers in the early detection of MR-AKI has to be investigated in prospectively designed research. Furthermore, an AKI prediction model is desirable by incorporating various biomarkers in critically ill cancer patients in order to detect and treat AKI timely [40].

43.2.7 Transfusion Medicine

Baseline prevalence of anaemia, thrombocytopenia and neutropenia due to myelosuppression is high in cancer patients, which gets amplified during critical illness [41]. As transfusion of the blood and blood component increases the risk of transfusion associated lung injury (TRALI), transfusion associated circulatory overload (TACO) apart from various infectious complications, a definite transfusion threshold needs to be established for these patients. Apart from this blood transfusion can increase the risk of cancer progression. The age of packed red blood cells (PRBC) plays a major role in determining above risks [42]. Therefore, fresh PRBC transfusion is indicated in order to prevent such progression, however, further studies delineating the underlying mechanisms through which storage of blood products can impact the rate of complications needs to be conducted in future [42]. Leukoreduced PRBC have decreased rates of transfusion related immune modulation (TRIM) by decreased HLA sensitization of recipients, apart from reduced incidence of febrile-non hemolytic reactions. Their preference in cancer patients cannot be quoted as a standard of care, until further studies with high level of evidence appear in upcoming years [42, 43]. Again, evidence is weak regarding recommendations to transfuse irradiated blood products to reduce the risk of TA-GVHD (Transfusion associated GVHD) in recipients of bone marrow transplantations, and further explorative work needs to be done in this area.

Whether restrictive transfusion (Haemoglobin cut-off at 7 g/dL) strategy is appropriate in patients with advanced cancer needs further research. No structured study has established unsafe INR (international normalized ratio) triggering transfusion of fresh frozen plasma before invasive procedures. Studies to clarify indications and thresholds for various blood product transfusions (leukoreduced and irradiated blood products), specific to malignancies in situations explained as above, are much needed and awaited. Leukoreduced and irradiated platelets can also decrease the alloimmunization and platelet transfusion refractoriness, but their prescription in specific clinical contexts needs to be addressed [42].

43.2.8 Nutritional Aspects

The prevalence of malnutrition in cancer patients admitted to ICU is exceedingly high (86%) [44]. Cancer as well as critical illness is systemic hyper inflammatory state which creates a high energy and protein demand leading to high risk of malnutrition. The Nutrition Risk Score 2002 (NRS-2002) and NUTRIC score (Nutrition

Risk in the Critically Ill) are valid screening tools that take into account of severity of illness [45]. However, in hospitalized cancer patients, Patient-Generated Subjective Global Assessment (PG-SGA) has been accepted as a malnutrition assessment tool [46]. NUTRIC score may not be applicable as IL-6 is usually high due to cancer induced inflammation. Other conditions which impair the assessment of nutritional status in cancer patients are fluid retention, tumour burden, excessive vomiting, anorexia, fatigue and depression, and organ toxicities. Composite of weight loss, serum CRP, albumin, urea, creatinine and alkaline phosphatase, in junction with various assessment tools such as PG-SGA, and Glasgow Prognostic Score (GPS) may be useful in grading malnutrition, and link that with mortality [47]. Therefore, we require development of new scoring systems for onco-critically ill patients, which needs further research in this field.

43.2.9 Infection Control and Diagnosis

Incidence of infections in cancer patients is high due to various factors (neutropenia, functional deficits in humoral and cellular immunity and complement kinetics) [48]. Many factors such as invasive catheters, drains and tubes, organ support devices, contribute to the escalating incidence of polymicrobial infections in such patients. Multicentric studies with prospectively collected data to delineate those factors that predispose cancer patients to sepsis, along with their risk stratification are required to be conducted. Diagnostic techniques for various bacterial, fungal and viral infections with rapid turnaround time with higher diagnostic performance are to be subjected to further research. Additionally, sampling methodology needs revamp in development of cost-effective and non-invasive techniques. Interventional trials converging on evaluation of the sensitivity and specificity of such rapid diagnostic methods, specifically applicable in cancer patients are desirable. Biomarkers as well as molecular techniques, with high negative predictive value, are needed, in order to reduce the burden of polypharmacy, undue treatment toxicity and extra costs [49]. Furthermore, research addressing the safety and efficacy of antibiotic de-escalation in cancer patients with neutropenia is also desirable.

43.2.10 Post ICU Discharge Life

Limited literature is available regarding quality of life post ICU discharge, post ICU-burden, prevalence of post-traumatic stress disorder (PTSD) and post-intensive care syndrome (PICS) [50, 51]. The prevalence of various symptoms and signs like pain, disturbed sleep, anxiety, depression and activities based physical limitations due to contractures or development of critical illness neuromyopathy (CINM) at 6-months or 1-year post ICU discharge need to be assessed. Another interesting focus of future research could be to evaluate the impact of the ICU support on long-term and disease-free survival among cancer patients [5, 15].

43.2.11 Prognostication of Survival in Patients with Cancer

Survival time point, like '28-day', which is commonly used in research related to the general ICU population cannot hold true in these patients. More pragmatic data like hospital discharge, post ICU survival time along with quality of life. There are well established prognostic scores such as "the palliative prognostic score' and 'Glasgow Prognostic Score', but their performance and validity in ICU patients are questionable. "*Onco score*", was designed to predict post ICU discharge outcome of solid organ cancers at 120-day, needs to be evaluated through prospective studies, for other types of malignancies as well. Such scores can help the intensivists is to identify which patients with cancers would benefit from ICU care [52]. Future research in identifying and validating novel prognostic factors, and linking prognostication to clinical decision making will be greatly appreciated.

43.2.12 End of Life Care (EOLC) and Palliative Care

A cancer patient is admitted to ICU with curative intent in mind, however, at times, the critical illness does not respond to even best treatments available in ICU and at such crossroads of oncology and acute illness, opportunities of providing the "best end of life care" emerge [53]. The pathway to providing the end of life care in ICU patients is full of challenges and uncertainties. It is wrong to state that ICU is not the place for palliative care and should be restricted to cancer patients with full code. Studies assessing the quality of collaborative decision making from the perspective of physicians, nurses and families along with qualitative outcomes like quality of death are much awaited. Further, the biological basis of non-pain symptoms (vomiting, fatigue, delirium, breathlessness, and thirst), a critically ill palliative patient need further exploration in future clinical research. Various aspects of palliative care in ICU such as assessment and treatment of patient symptoms, psychosocial support for patients and families are the targets of future research [54].

43.3 Conclusion

Onco-critical care being a new sub-speciality has broad room for extensive research to resolve dilemmas and controversies in critically ill oncological patients related to various aspects such as development of dedicated ICUs, early screening tools to recognise patients at risk of deterioration in wards, cancer-specific severity scoring systems needful for prognostication and deciding the level of care in ICU, alternatives to invasive mechanical ventilation, transfusion thresholds and type of blood products needed, development of malnutrition screening tools, quality of life post ICU discharge, formulation of cancer-specific guidelines and care bundles.

References

1. Arnold M, Rutherford MJ, Bardot A, et al. Progress in cancer survival, mortality, and incidence in seven high-income countries 1995–2014 (ICBP SURVMARK-2): a population-based study. Lancet Oncol. 2019;20:1493–1505. http://www.ncbi.nlm.nih.gov/pubmed/31521509.
2. Soares M, Caruso P, Silva E, et al. Characteristics and outcomes of patients with cancer requiring admission to intensive care units: a prospective multicenter study. Crit Care Med. 2010;38:9–15. http://www.ncbi.nlm.nih.gov/pubmed/19829101.
3. Soares M, Bozza FA, Azevedo LCP, et al. Effects of organizational characteristics on outcomes and resource use in patients with cancer admitted to intensive care units. J Clin Oncol. 2016;34:3315–3324. http://www.ncbi.nlm.nih.gov/pubmed/27432921.
4. Azoulay E, Soares M, Darmon M, et al. Intensive care of the cancer patient: recent achievements and remaining challenges. Ann Intensive Care. 2011;1:5. http://www.ncbi.nlm.nih.gov/pubmed/21906331.
5. Azoulay E, Schellongowski P, Darmon M, et al. The intensive care medicine research agenda on critically ill oncology and hematology patients. Intensive Care Med. 2017;43:1366–1382. http://link.springer.com/10.1007/s00134-017-4884-z.
6. Sakr Y, Moreira CL, Rhodes A, et al. The impact of hospital and ICU organizational factors on outcome in critically ill patients: results from the extended prevalence of infection in intensive care study. Crit Care Med. 2015;43:519–526. http://www.ncbi.nlm.nih.gov/pubmed/25479111.
7. Checkley W, Martin GS, Brown SM, et al. Structure, process, and annual ICU mortality across 69 centers: United States critical illness and injury trials group critical illness outcomes study. Crit Care Med. 2014;42:344–356. http://www.ncbi.nlm.nih.gov/pubmed/24145833.
8. Hawari FI, Al Najjar TI, Zaru L, et al. The effect of implementing high-intensity intensive care unit staffing model on outcome of critically ill oncology patients*. Crit Care Med. 2009;37:1967–1971. http://journals.lww.com/00003246-200906000-00021.
9. Zuber B, Tran T-C, Aegerter P, et al. Impact of case volume on survival of septic shock in patients with malignancies. Crit Care Med. 2012;40:55–62. http://www.ncbi.nlm.nih.gov/pubmed/21926606.
10. Koch A, Checkley W. Do hospitals need oncological critical care units? J Thorac Dis. 2017;9:E304–E309. http://jtd.amegroups.com/article/view/12495/10677.
11. Saran S, Gurjar M, Azim A, et al. Structural risk factors for hospital-acquired infections in intensive care unit. HERD Heal Environ Res Des J. 2020;193758672097882. http://journals.sagepub.com/doi/10.1177/1937586720978825.
12. Saran S, Gurjar M, Baronia A, et al. Heating, ventilation and air conditioning (HVAC) in intensive care unit. Crit Care. 2020;24:194. https://ccforum.biomedcentral.com/articles/10.1186/s13054-020-02907-5.
13. Soares M, Bozza FA, Angus DC, et al. Organizational characteristics, outcomes, and resource use in 78 Brazilian intensive care units: the ORCHESTRA study. Intensive Care Med. 2015;41:2149–2160. http://www.ncbi.nlm.nih.gov/pubmed/26499477.
14. Shrime MG, Ferket BS, Scott DJ, et al. Time-limited trials of intensive care for critically ill patients with cancer: how long is long enough? JAMA Oncol. 2016;2:76–83. http://www.ncbi.nlm.nih.gov/pubmed/26469222.
15. Azoulay E, Soares M, Darmon M, et al. Intensive care of the cancer patient: recent achievements and remaining challenges. Ann Intensive Care. 2011;1:5. https://annalsofintensivecare.springeropen.com/articles/10.1186/2110-5820-1-5.
16. Hourmant Y, Kouatchet A, López R, et al. Impact of early ICU admission for critically ill cancer patients: post-hoc analysis of a prospective multicenter multinational dataset. J Crit Care. 2020;62:6–11. http://www.ncbi.nlm.nih.gov/pubmed/33227593.
17. Gerry S, Bonnici T, Birks J, et al. Early warning scores for detecting deterioration in adult hospital patients: systematic review and critical appraisal of methodology. BMJ. 2020;m1501. https://www.bmj.com/lookup/doi/10.1136/bmj.m1501.

18. Cooksley T, Kitlowski E, Haji-Michael P. Effectiveness of modified early warning score in predicting outcomes in oncology patients. QJM. 2012;105:1083–1088. http://www.ncbi.nlm.nih.gov/pubmed/22855285.
19. Soares M, Fontes F, Dantas J, et al. Performance of six severity-of-illness scores in cancer patients requiring admission to the intensive care unit: a prospective observational study. Crit Care. 2004;8:R194–203. http://www.ncbi.nlm.nih.gov/pubmed/15312218.
20. Bouch DC, Thompson JP. Severity scoring systems in the critically ill. Contin Educ Anaesth Crit Care Pain. 2008;8:181–185. https://linkinghub.elsevier.com/retrieve/pii/S1743181617304663.
21. Azoulay E, Pène F, Darmon M, et al. Managing critically ill hematology patients: time to think differently. Blood Rev. 2015;29:359–367. http://www.ncbi.nlm.nih.gov/pubmed/25998991.
22. Soares M, Azoulay É. Critical care management of lung cancer patients to prolong life without prolonging dying. Intensive Care Med. 2009;35:2012–2014. http://link.springer.com/10.1007/s00134-009-1633-y.
23. Pastores SM, Voigt LP. Acute respiratory failure in the patient with cancer: diagnostic and management strategies. Crit Care Clin. 2010;26:21–40. http://www.ncbi.nlm.nih.gov/pubmed/19944274.
24. Young AY, Shannon VR. Acute respiratory distress syndrome in cancer patients. oncol crit care. Cham: Springer; 2020. p. 557–582. http://link.springer.com/10.1007/978-3-319-74588-6_48.
25. Wang T, Zhang L, Luo K, et al. Noninvasive versus invasive mechanical ventilation for immunocompromised patients with acute respiratory failure: a systematic review and meta-analysis. BMC Pulm Med. 2016;16:129. http://www.ncbi.nlm.nih.gov/pubmed/27567894.
26. Wang T, Zhang L, Luo K, et al. Noninvasive versus invasive mechanical ventilation for immunocompromised patients with acute respiratory failure: a systematic review and meta-analysis. BMC Pulm Med. 2016;16:129. http://bmcpulmmed.biomedcentral.com/articles/10.1186/s12890-016-0289-y.
27. Lemiale V, Mokart D, Resche-Rigon M, et al. Effect of noninvasive ventilation vs oxygen therapy on mortality among immunocompromised patients with acute respiratory failure: a randomized clinical trial. JAMA. 2015;314:1711–1719. http://www.ncbi.nlm.nih.gov/pubmed/26444879.
28. Frat J-P, Coudroy R, Marjanovic N, et al. High-flow nasal oxygen therapy and noninvasive ventilation in the management of acute hypoxemic respiratory failure. Ann Transl Med. 2017;5:297–297. http://atm.amegroups.com/article/view/15608/15789.
29. Williams D, Yungbluth M, Adams G, et al. The role of fiberoptic bronchoscopy in the evaluation of immunocompromised hosts with diffuse pulmonary infiltrates. Am Rev Respir Dis. 1985;131:880–885. http://www.ncbi.nlm.nih.gov/pubmed/4003940.
30. Svensson T, Lundström KL, Höglund M, et al. Utility of bronchoalveolar lavage in diagnosing respiratory tract infections in patients with hematological malignancies: are invasive diagnostics still needed? Ups J Med Sci. 2017;122:56–60. https://ujms.net/index.php/ujms/article/view/6258.
31. Kim S, Oh I-J, Park S-Y, et al. Corticosteroid therapy against treatment-related pulmonary toxicities in patients with lung cancer. J Thorac Dis. 2014;6:1209–1217. http://www.ncbi.nlm.nih.gov/pubmed/25276362.
32. Soeteman M, Potratz J, Nielsen JSA, et al. Research priorities in pediatric onco-critical care: an international Delphi consensus study. Intensive Care Med. 2019;45:1681–1683. http://link.springer.com/10.1007/s00134-019-05706-x.
33. Kang HS, Rhee CK, Lee HY, et al. Clinical outcomes of extracorporeal membrane oxygenation support in patients with hematologic malignancies. Korean J Intern Med. 2015;30:478–488. http://www.ncbi.nlm.nih.gov/pubmed/26161014.
34. NCID of CC& PS. Comprehensive oncologic emergencies research network (CONCERN). https://epi.grants.cancer.gov/concern/.
35. Chacko B, Peter J. Temperature monitoring in the intensive care unit. Indian J Respir Care. 2018;7:28. http://www.ijrconline.org/text.asp?2018/7/1/28/224399.
36. Darmon M, Azoulay E, Alberti C, et al. Impact of neutropenia duration on short-term mortality in neutropenic critically ill cancer patients. Intensive Care Med. 2002;28:1775–1780. http://www.ncbi.nlm.nih.gov/pubmed/12447522.

37. Azoulay E, Attalah H, Harf A, et al. Granulocyte colony-stimulating factor or neutrophil-induced pulmonary toxicity: myth or reality? Chest. 2001;120:1695–1701. https://linkinghub.elsevier.com/retrieve/pii/S0012369215363819.
38. Bose P, Dinnel J, Moore B, et al. Rasburicase in the management of tumor lysis: an evidence-based review of its place in therapy. Core Evid. 2015;23. http://www.dovepress.com/rasburicase-in-the-management-of-tumor-lysis-an-evidence-based-review%2D%2Dpeer-reviewed-article-CE.
39. Rosner MH, Perazella MA. Acute kidney injury in the patient with cancer. Kidney Res. Clin. Pract. The Korean Society of Nephrology; 2019 [cited 2021 Feb 3]. p. 295–308. /pmc/articles/PMC6727896/?report=abstract.
40. Park N, Kang E, Park M, et al. Predicting acute kidney injury in cancer patients using heterogeneous and irregular data. In Burdmann EA, editor. PLoS One. 2018;13:e0199839. https://dx.plos.org/10.1371/journal.pone.0199839.
41. Epstein RS, Aapro MS, Basu Roy UK, et al. Patient burden and real-world management of chemotherapy-induced myelosuppression: results from an online survey of patients with solid tumors. Adv Ther. 2020;37:3606–3618. /pmc/articles/PMC7340862/?report=abstract.
42. Atzil S, Arad M, Glasner A, et al. Blood transfusion promotes cancer progression: a critical role for aged erythrocytes. Anesthesiology. 2008;109:989–997. http://www.ncbi.nlm.nih.gov/pubmed/19034095.
43. Watkins T, Surowiecka MK, McCullough J. Transfusion indications for patients with cancer. Cancer Control. 2015;22:38–46. http://www.ncbi.nlm.nih.gov/pubmed/25504277.
44. Goswami L, Chakravarty C, Hazarika B. Prevalence of malnutrition in a tertiary care hospital in India. Indian J Crit Care Med. 2013;17:170–173. https://www.ijccm.org/doi/10.4103/0972-5229.117058.
45. Canales C, Elsayes A, Yeh DD, et al. Nutrition risk in critically ill versus the nutritional risk screening 2002: are they comparable for assessing risk of malnutrition in critically ill patients? J Parenter Enter Nutr. 2019;43:81–87. https://pubmed.ncbi.nlm.nih.gov/29846011/.
46. Jager-Wittenaar H, Ottery FD. Assessing nutritional status in cancer: role of the patient-generated subjective global assessment. Curr Opin Clin Nutr Metab Care. 2017;20:322–329. http://www.ncbi.nlm.nih.gov/pubmed/28562490.
47. Fruchtenicht AVG, Poziomyck AK, Kabke GB, et al. Nutritional risk assessment in critically ill cancer patients: systematic review. Rev Bras Ter Intensiva. 2015; http://www.gnresearch.org/doi/10.5935/0103-507X.20150032.
48. Zembower TR. Epidemiology of infections in cancer patients. Cancer Treat Res. 2014;161:43–89. /pmc/articles/PMC7120867/?report=abstract.
49. Brzeźniakiewicz-Janus K, Lancé MD, Tukiendorf A, et al. Clinical profiles of selected biomarkers identifying infection and cancer patients: a Gorzów hospital example. Dis Markers. 2019;
50. Gayat E, Cariou A, Deye N, et al. Determinants of long-term outcome in ICU survivors: results from the FROG-ICU study. Crit Care. 2018;22:8. https://ccforum.biomedcentral.com/articles/10.1186/s13054-017-1922-8.
51. Ryu JH, Kredentser MS, Bienvenu OJ, et al. Post-traumatic stress disorder in survivors of critical illness. Compr guid to post-traumatic stress disord. Cham: Springer; 2016. p. 263–280. http://link.springer.com/10.1007/978-3-319-08359-9_81.
52. Oeyen SG, Benoit DD, Annemans L, et al. Long-term outcomes and quality of life in critically ill patients with hematological or solid malignancies: a single center study. Intensive Care Med. 2013;39:889–898. http://www.ncbi.nlm.nih.gov/pubmed/23248039.
53. Dalal S, Bruera E. End-of-life care matters: palliative cancer care results in better care and lower costs. Oncologist. 2017;22:361–368. https://onlinelibrary.wiley.com/doi/abs/10.1634/theoncologist.2016-0277.
54. Metaxa V, Anagnostou D, Vlachos S, et al. Palliative care interventions in intensive care unit patients—a systematic review protocol. Syst Rev. 2019;8:148. https://systematicreviewsjournal.biomedcentral.com/articles/10.1186/s13643-019-1064-y.

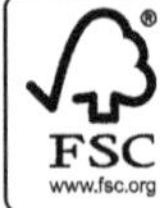

MIX
Papier aus verantwortungsvollen Quellen
Paper from responsible sources
FSC® C105338

If you have any concerns about our products,
you can contact us on
ProductSafety@springernature.com

In case Publisher is established outside the EU,
the EU authorized representative is:
Springer Nature Customer Service Center GmbH
Europaplatz 3, 69115 Heidelberg, Germany

Printed by Libri Plureos GmbH
in Hamburg, Germany